Pathology of the Ear

This volume is published as part of a long-standing cooperative program between Harvard University Press and the Commonwealth Fund, a philanthropic foundation, to encourage the publication of significant scholarly books in medicine and health.

Pathology of the Ear

Harold F. Schuknecht, M.D.

 A Commonwealth Fund Book   Harvard University Press, Cambridge, Massachusetts

1974

75-61048

Preface

It is my firm conviction that a knowledge of pathophysiology forms the basis for intelligent and successful prevention and management of disease. The source of such knowledge derives principally from laboratory research performed by individuals who are trained in scientific methodology. Recent years have brought from many laboratories a burgeoning mass of information on the embryology, anatomy, physiology, biochemistry, and pathology of the auditory and vestibular systems. I have taken the privilege of compiling what I think are the most significant facts from these basic sciences and interpreted them in the light of my clinical experiences. It is my hope that this book will be useful to both researchers and clinicians who concern themselves with the function of these sensory systems.

I first viewed this book as an accumulation of case reports with selected photomicrographs in a loose leaf format, to which could be added new and interesting cases as they became available. It soon became apparent to me however that this type of presentation would limit the opportunity for personal interpretation and integration of the material. The result therefore is a textbook, in which the material is organized into twelve chapters. For orientation, there are chapters on histological methods, anatomy, and pathophysiology. Following are nine chapters on otological diseases classified on the basis of pathogenesis, in so far as that is possible. In some instances, of course, the causes for diseases are only presumed and require confirmation. The final chapter is entitled, Disease of Unknown or Multiple Cause and includes those disorders which do not fall clearly into a specific category.

Frequently I have taken author's license to derive an interpretation on pathogenesis based on the correlation of morphological changes with clinical manifestations. These discussions are clearly couched in terminology which will inform the reader as to what is factual and what is hypothetical. Considering the significance of pathology as a determinant or mode of therapy, it seemed reasonable that some comments on treatment would be pertinent to the objectives of this book. In general, these statements are based on pathological and clinical evidence which will withstand harsh scientific scrutiny. Hopefully, the contents of this book will provide the basis for a more logical therapeutic armamentarium than is now advocated for some otologic disorders. Certainly many medical regimens now in common use cannot be supported by the available pathological or clinical data. In many instances, this will mean discarding popular but unproven therapies which not only instill false hope but strain the economics of medical care.

The writing of a medical textbook will always remain an imperfect art by reason of the mass of knowledge extant which seems to be accumulating in logarithmic proportions. The bibliography consists of references considered to be either original or classical works on a subject. It is impossible to give bibliographical note to all who have contributed to our knowledge of ear disease, for there are many. For blatant omissions, I ask your indulgence.

I view this work as my *opus magnum*. The probability of publishing revised editions will be determined in large part by whether our temporal bone laboratory will continue to receive financial support. This work would not have been possible without substantial grants from the National Institutes of Health of the Public Health Service, the Deafness Research Foundation, the Research Fund of the American Otological Society, and private funds from the University of Chicago, Henry Ford Hospital, Harvard Medical School, and the Massachusetts Eye and Ear Infirmary.

A great many individuals have contributed in one way or another to the culmination of this work. For demonstrating to me the importance of teaching and research in medicine as a means of improving man's existence, for instilling in me some capability for judgment of evidence, and for teaching me basic truths regarding clinical otology and research, I am especially indebted to John Lindsay, William D. Neff, Henry Perlman, Joseph Hind, Heinrich Kobrak, Hallowell Davis, Robert Kimura, Richard Gacek and Nelson Kiang. Alfred Weiss gave valuable advice on clinical neuro-otology. Above all, it was the exciting concepts and infectious enthusiasm of John Lindsay which stimulated me to pursue pathology of the ear as a principal research interest. Throughout the years many Research Fellows and Residents at the Henry Ford Hospital and the Massachusetts Eye and Ear Infirmary have assisted in the acquisition and study of both animal and human ear preparations for which I am very grateful. Their work has led to many publications, most of which are listed in the bibliography of this book. Among those to be mentioned are Stanley Oleksiuk, George Singleton, Michael Paparella, T. Manford McGee, Jaime Benitez, Bernard Colman, Albert Hohman, Makoto Igarashi, Alaa El Seifi, Eugene Myers, Shiro Fujita, Herbert Silverstein, Roger Lindeman, George Miller, Isamu Sando, Heinrich H. Spoendlin, Werner Chasin, Yasuya Nomura, Collingwood Karmody, Ronald McNeill, Arthur Kos, Charles Gross, Tetsuo Ishii, Joel Bernstein, Alan Kerr, Warren Griffin, Garfield Davies, Roger Kaufman, Herbert Fields, Yoshihiko Murakami, Abdel Allam, Harold Holden, Earl Singleton, Edward Applebaum, Keatjin Lee, Pierre Naufal, Charles Cummings, Manuel Mock, Andrew Baxter, Ralph Ruby, Bjorn Etholm, Haruo Saito, Luiz DeMoura, Pierre Montandon, Daiji Ishii, John Wright, Kozo Watanuki, Aziz Belal, Didier Péron, Terence Stewart, Sun Yuen, Jorge Otte, and Francisco Antoli-Candela, Jr.

I greatly appreciate the assistance of Elaine Joseph, Elaine Meade, Julie Barrett, Sandra Fitch, Carol Ota, Sandra Feibelkorn and Lorraine Marchand Kidder in organizing and maintaining the temporal bone collection and in typing and editing the manuscript.

Certainly much of the success of the histological preparations must be attributed to the care and experience given this aspect of the work by Clarinda Northrop, Richard Begin, Michael Lyon, and Diane DeLeo Jones. The enormous task of preparing serial sections of over 800 human temporal bones and an equal number of animal specimens fell to them and to their assistants.

Almost all of the photomicrographs were made by Arthur Bowden. In photomicrography of this difficult material, he has no peer. None of the photographs in this book have been touched-up, cropped, or altered in any way. Edward Gadowski, Roger Lancaster and James Schuknecht prepared the photographs for most of the charts, drawings, and other material. The art work was done by David Tilden and Norman Archambault. To all of them, I am grateful.

Those at the Harvard Press who have performed the laborious task of designing and editing are David Ford and Kathleen Ahern.

The financial support of the Commonwealth Fund is greatly appreciated for this has made it possible to produce this book at a cost which will make it available to all who have a serious interest in the behavior of the ear in health and disease.

Finally, thanks to my wife, Anne, for her editorial assistance and for her patience with my preoccupation for the temporal bone.

HFS

Contents

Chapter 5   Infections 215

Pathology of the Ear

1 Histological Method

The current method of preparation of the temporal bone for light microscopy is fundamentally the same as that which has been employed for a
century and consists of treating the tissues by fixation, decalcification, sectioning, staining, and mounting. The refinements in technique which have
evolved may be credited to better microtomes, purer chemicals, alterations in
the application of method, and improved manual skills in the handling
of tissues.

A number of temporal bone collections were in existence in Europe at the
turn of the century; however, because of political events and economic
reasons most of the involved laboratories have since become inactive, and the
collections of specimens lay dormant or have disappeared. A temporal bone
laboratory which is to endure must have continuing institutional support and
energetic direction. In America, federal and private funding has provided
support for many new temporal bone laboratories, most of which are located
in institutions with training programs in Otology. Unfortunately the study
of temporal bone pathology is generally considered to be a research activity
rather than an institutional function, budgeted in conjunction with the
clinical and morbid pathology laboratories which serve the institution.

The accumulation of knowledge of temporal bone pathology has been difficult because (1) the acquisition of specimens is generally only possible when
a complete autopsy, including brain examination, has been granted; (2) time
delays in acquiring the specimens after death often result in severe autolysis
of the membranous labyrinth; (3) histological techniques for preparing the
temporal bone are costly and laborious; and (4) detailed clinical history,
otologic examination, and functional test data are frequently unavailable.

Light microscopy is now being supplemented by other methods which hold
great promise for resolving some of the mysteries which have escaped solution to date. Phase microscopy and the technique of surface preparations
(Engström et al., 1966; Johnsson and Hawkins, 1967a, 1967b; Bredberg,
1968; Lindeman, 1969) provide a new dimension for the acquisition of pathological data. The conventional transmission electron microscope, with its
great resolving power, has been used for some years to elucidate the ultrastructural anatomy of the mammalian ear (Engström, 1951; Engström and

Wersäll, 1953, 1958; Iurato, 1961; Iurato and dePetris, 1967; Smith, 1956, 1957; Hilding, 1965; Kimura, 1966, Duvall et al., 1966; Spoendlin, 1964, 1966). Kimura et al. (1964) first used the electron microscope to study the human temporal bone. The scanning electron microscope, which has been in wide use in metallurgical research, is now being applied to the study of ear anatomy (Lim, 1969; Lim and Lane, 1969a, 1969b; Bredberg et al., 1970; Lindeman and Ades, 1971; Engström et al., 1972). This instrument, which creates an image by secondary electrons emitted from the excited surface of the specimen, has a depth of field about 500 times that of the light microscope, with magnification between 20 and 20,000 and a resolving power of 100 A. Other methods which have come into common use to supplement light microscopy are histochemical techniques and the biochemical analysis of inner ear fluids and tissues. Some of these methods, particularly electron microscopy and chemical analysis, are hampered by the need to acquire specimens soon after death.

A. REMOVAL OF THE TEMPORAL BONE

In most hospitals permission for the removal of the temporal bones is considered to be implied in a complete autopsy permit; however, the policy to be followed must conform to the local laws and practices. Delays in acquiring specimens are often unavoidable because of the need to acquire properly endorsed autopsy permits and because of the work schedules of the pathologists. In many hospitals bodies are placed in cold storage and postmortem examinations are performed at a scheduled time each day; thus the time lapse between death and autopsy may be prolonged. Fortunately, refrigeration greatly retards postmortem autolysis so that useful specimens may be acquired as long as 24 hours after death.

A portion of the temporal bone adequate for routine histological study can be acquired at autopsy without disfigurement of the head after the brain has been removed (Schuknecht, 1968). When removing the brain, the VIIth and VIIIth cranial nerve trunks should be severed with a sharp knife rather than avulsed from the internal auditory canal (Fig. 1.1).

The *block technique* of removal consists of making four linear bone cuts with either the mallet and osteotome or the electrically operated bone saw (Fig. 1.2). The temporal bone is then grasped with a large bone-grasping forceps, and any remaining bony connections are loosened by a gentle rocking motion, thereby freeing the specimen sufficient to permit cutting of the remaining muscular, ligamentous, and fibrous attachments with a knife, scis-

Fig. 1.1: As the brain is being removed, the temporal lobe and cerebellum should be elevated and the surface of the petrous bone inspected for gross pathological changes. The trunks of the VIIth and VIIIth cranial nerves should then be cut at the level of the internal auditory meatus.

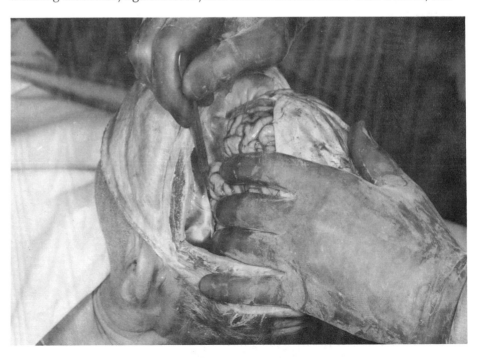

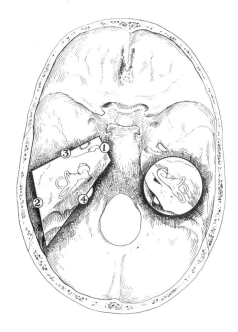

Fig. 1.2: This drawing shows the areas to be removed in the block method and the bone plug method of temporal bone removal.

Block method: Cut 1 is made perpendicular to the long axis of the petrous pyramid at its apex. By making this cut more anteriorly, the eustachian tube can be included in the specimen. *Cut 2* is made in the lateral aspect of the middle cranial fossa, parallel to the squamous portion of the temporal bone. The cut passes through the cartilaginous portion of the external auditory canal and traverses the mastoid cells; thus most of the squamous part of the temporal bone and part of the mastoid cortex is left in continuity with the base of the skull to preserve the lateral contour of the head. *Cut 3* joins *Cuts 1* and *2* and is made in the floor of the middle cranial fossa approximately 1 inch anterior to and parallel to the petrous ridge. *Cut 4* is a horizontal undermining cut made from the posterior cranial fossa in an anterior direction severing the bone from its inferior attachments.

Bone plug method: The bone plug cutter (1½ inches in diameter for adult heads) is centered on the arcuate eminence and directed perpendicular to the floor of the middle cranial fossa.

sors, or sharp osteotome. The internal carotid artery is ligated with a black silk suture. Care must be used to avoid crushing a highly pneumatized and fragile temporal bone.

The *bone plug method* of removal is performed with the oscillating (Stryker) bone plug saw. A 1.5-inch diameter saw, adjusted to a depth of 1.5 inches is used for the adult skull and a 1-inch diameter saw adjusted to a depth of 1 inch for smaller skulls. The saw should be centered precisely over the arcuate eminence (Fig. 1.3) and directed perpendicular to the floor of the middle cranial fossa (Fig. 1.4). The head should be steadied by an assistant because movement leads to damage of the saw blade. The cut is complete when a loss of resistance is felt, indicating penetration of the base of the skull. After removal of the saw, the bone plug is grasped with forceps (Fig. 1.5) and rotated and retracted sufficiently to permit visualization of the internal carotid artery which is attached to its inferior surface. The artery is grasped with a curved hemostat and ligated, and all remaining attachments are severed with a knife, scissors, or osteotome. When properly executed the cut should pass through the cartilaginous rather than the bony part of the external auditory canal (Fig. 1.6).

Following either method of removal, the stump of the cartilaginous part of the external auditory canal should be closed with black silk on a sharp curved suture needle.

These methods of removal provide specimens of adequate size for pathological study (Fig. 1.7). When properly performed the external configuration of the head is not disturbed and embalming procedures are not impaired (Fig. 1.8).

B. PREPARATION OF THE TEMPORAL BONE

Excess soft tissue and bone are trimmed from the specimen, using scissors, rongeur, and bone-cutting forceps.

Fixation is begun immediately by placing the temporal bones separately in 500 cc glass jars (with screw-on lids) containing about 300 cc of Heidenhain-Susa fixative solution. This solution is prepared at the time of use by mixing 240 cc of the stock solution with 60 cc of formaldehyde solution (HCHO—37%). Stock fixative solution is composed of: 45 gm $HgCl_2$; 5 gm NaCl; 800 cc distilled water; 20 gm trichloroacetic acid; and 40 cc glacial acetic acid. The jar with fixative and specimen is stored at 38°F for 48 hours. The solution need not be removed; however, the jar should be shaken once or twice a day to improve penetration of the fixative. Shorter fixation periods may result in incomplete fixation of the specimen while prolonged periods may result in the deposition of mercury salts in the tissue. There is no need to de-gas the distilled water used in preparing the stock solution or the stock solution itself.

The *decalcification* process is started by removing the specimens from the Heidenhain-Susa fixative solution, washing them in tap water, and placing them in 300 cc of 5 percent trichloroacetic acid solution in 500 cc glass jars. The trichloroacetic acid solution is renewed three times per week for six weeks. This procedure, as well as all subsequent procedures, is performed at room temperature. At weekly intervals a single-edged razor blade or similar instrument is used to trim away unwanted tissue. If there is cerumen or epithelial debris in the external auditory canal, it should be removed. When the bone becomes soft the superior semicircular canal is opened by cutting away tissue with a razor blade. If desired, the end-point for decalcification may be determined by either x-ray filming or by a chemical test. The chemical test is performed by mixing 2 cc of solution from the specimen with 1 cc of 5 percent ammonium oxalate and 1 cc of 5 percent ammonium hydroxide. The formation of a white precipitate indicates incomplete decalcification. The specimens may remain in the trichloroacetic acid solution for a few days beyond complete decalcification without harm to the tissue.

Fig. 1.3: The bone plug cutter should be centered on the arcuate eminence which is indicated by the point of the scissors.

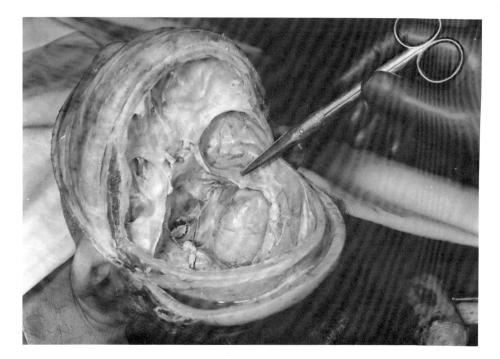

Fig. 1.4: A 1.5 inch diameter bone plug cutter set for a depth of 1.5 inches is directed perpendicular to the floor of the middle cranial cavity.

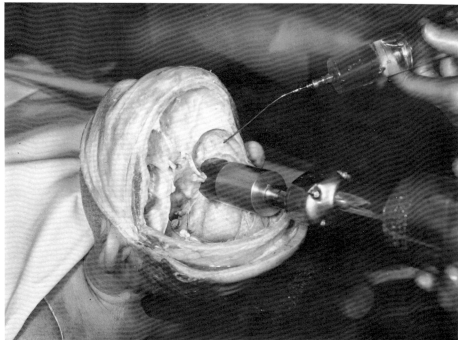

Fig. 1.5: The bone plug is engaged with a large bone grasping forceps and forcefully rotated and retracted until the soft tissues attached to its inferior surface are brought into view.

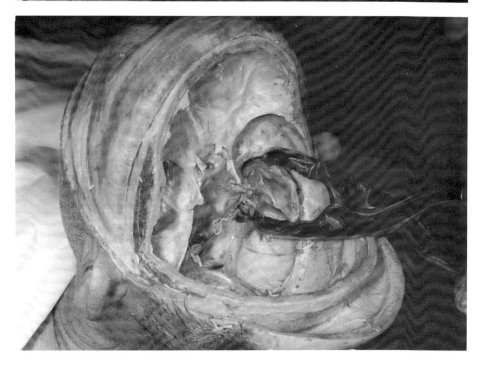

Fig. 1.6: Specimens removed by the 1.5 inch bone plug cutter. Note on the lateral view (left specimen) that the cut extends through the cartilaginous canal.

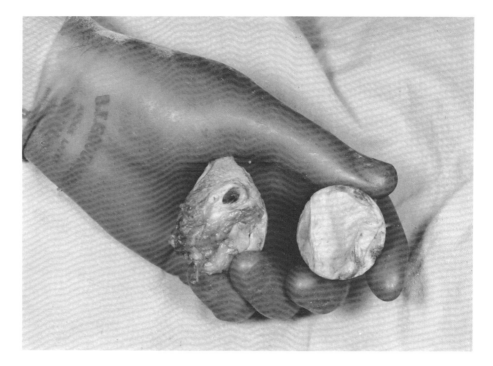

Fig. 1.7: This photomicrograph of a horizontal section of the temporal bone at the mid-modiolar level shows the structure encompassed by the 1.5 inch bone plug cutter. The cartilaginous part of the external auditory canal has been trimmed away in preparation for mounting on the 1 x 3 inch glass slide.

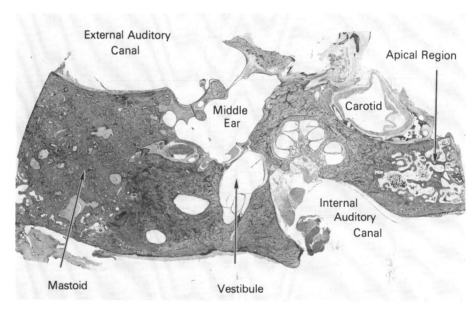

Fig. 1.8: Photograph showing appearance of the base of the skull following removal of the temporal bone specimens by the bone plug method. The internal carotid arteries have been ligated and the cartilaginous external auditory canals have been closed with sutures.

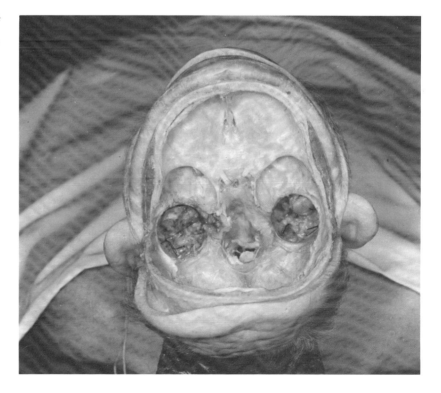

5   Histological Method

Neutralization is performed by removing the specimens from the trichloro-acetic, washing them in running tap water for 24 hours, and placing them in 300 cc of 5 percent sodium sulfate solution for 8 to 24 hours.

If large numbers of specimens are being processed, the work schedules are facilitated by coordinating the various steps. For example, all specimens may be washed on a Monday, and the neutralization procedure may begin on Tuesday morning. On Tuesday evening, at the close of the work day, the specimens may be placed in distilled water overnight prior to the dehydration procedure which may begin on Wednesday morning.

Dehydration is accomplished over a period of ten days during which the specimens are placed in a series of alcohols of increasing concentration in amounts of 300 cc in 500 cc jars according to the following schedule:

(1) 50 percent alcohol, 24 hours (Wednesday morning)
(2) 70 percent alcohol, 24 hours (Thursday morning)
(3) 80 percent alcohol, 3 days (Friday morning to Monday morning)
(4) 95 percent alcohol, 24 hours (Monday morning)
(5) 95 percent alcohol, 24 hours (Tuesday morning)
(6) 100 percent alcohol, 24 hours (Wednesday morning)
(7) 100 percent alcohol, 24 hours (Thursday morning)
(8) Ether-alcohol (1:1), 8 hours (Friday morning)
(9) Ether-alcohol (1:1), 3 days (Friday evening to Monday morning)

Embedding is accomplished during a twelve-week period by placing the specimens in sequence in 300 cc quantities of celloidin preparation according to the following schedule:

(1) 1.5 percent celloidin–1 week
(2) 3 percent celloidin–3 weeks
(3) 6 percent celloidin–4 weeks
(4) 12 percent celloidin–4 weeks

The celloidin solutions are prepared by placing the appropriate amounts of celloidin[1] in a solution of equal amounts of absolute alcohol and ether and agitating on a mechanical shaker until completely dissolved. The specimens are placed in the 12 percent celloidin solutions with the superior surfaces of the petrous bones facing the bottoms of the jars. The ether and alcohol are permitted to evaporate very slowly so as to prevent air bubbles forming in the celloidin. To accomplish this, the lids of the jars should be loosened to permit slow evaporation. The speed of evaporation is determined in part by the temperature of the room. Evaporation should be controlled so that the surface of the celloidin becomes tacky in about two weeks and moderately firm in three weeks. Then to expedite further hardening, chloroform is poured into the jars to form a layer about one-half inch in thickness, after which the jars are tightly capped. Approximately the upper third of the celloidin will be hardened in 24 hours at which time it should be partly trimmed away with a sharp knife to permit better penetration of the chloroform. A layer of chloroform is again placed on the specimens. Part of the surrounding hardened celloidin is trimmed away each day until the specimens are finally embedded in properly hardened celloidin. The celloidin blocks are hardened to the stage where blunt pressure with the finger will not produce an obvious indentation, but where pressure from a fingernail will produce a mark. A sharp knife is used to cut the celloidin blocks from the jar. Excess celloidin is trimmed away to create rectangular blocks measuring about 1½ x 1½ x 2 inches.

When *"blocking"* the specimens (mounting on the cutting blocks) they are oriented to achieve the desired plane of sectioning. For horizontal sections, the celloidin on the inferior surfaces of the temporal bones is cut away so that the modioli of the cochleae will be in a horizontal plane when they are placed on the cutting blocks. The principal anatomical landmarks are the

---

1. Parlodion (Mallinckrodt) is recommended as the celloidin preparation.

internal and external auditory canals and the arcuate eminences. The inferior surfaces of the blocks are softened in an ether-alcohol solution, pressed on a mounting block layered with 12 percent celloidin, and hardened in chloroform. If the specimens are to be stored for longer than a few days they may be placed in 80 percent alcohol solution.

To acquire the desired plane of *sectioning* it may be necessary to make minor adjustments in the position of the specimen during the first stages of cutting to achieve the proper plane. For horizontal sections the proper plane will have been achieved when the ampulla of the superior semicircular canal is reached simultaneously with the superior surface of the malleus and incus. Four representative planes through the labyrinth and their matching photomicrographs are seen in Figs. 1.9 through 1.13.

The microtome knife may require sharpening several times during the cutting of one temporal bone. Usually the sections are cut at a thickness of 20 micra, resulting in about 400 sections from each temporal bone. All sections are placed on numbered pieces of onionskin paper, and every tenth section is removed for preparation of the tracer series of slides. The sections are stored in 80 percent alcohol solution.

The tracer series of sections are floated off the onionskin papers into tap water, and the papers are saved for later reference in numbering the slides. No attempt is made to maintain sequential order.

The sections are *stained* with hematoxylin and eosin by the following method:

(1) Place tissue in Lugol's solution for 10 to 15 minutes.

(2) Place tissues in 5 percent sodium thiosulfate solution until sections lose orange color (about 1 to 2 minutes).

(3) Dip tissues in tap water to remove sodium thiosulfate.

(4) Place tissues in Harris' hematoxylin for 40 to 60 minutes. Harris' hematoxylin stain may be prepared in the following way: (a) dissolve 5 gm of hematoxylin in 50 cc of 100 percent alcohol; (b) dissolve 100 gm aluminum ammonium sulfate in 1000 cc of distilled water by heating; (c) mix the hematoxylin and aluminum ammonium sulfate solutions and bring to a boil; (d) remove from heat and slowly add 2.5 gm of red mercuric oxide; (e) return to heat and bring to the boiling point and remove immediately; (f) filter the hematoxylin solution before each use.

(5) Dip the tissues into a series of dishes of tap water to remove excess hematoxylin.

(6) Decolorize the tissues by passing them singly through a series of four baths, agitating slightly to hasten the process, in the following order: (a) place 0.3 percent solution of hydrochloric acid in 70 percent alcohol until the celloidin is clear and the tissue has acquired the desired shade of purple; (b) rinse in a dish of tap water; (c) place in ammonia solution for several minutes until the tissue turns blue. The ammonia solution is prepared by introducing 5 drops of full strength ammonium hydroxide into each 100 ml of distilled water; (d) dip into several changes of tap water.

(7) Dip the tissue into eosin solution and agitate until the section is well stained. Stock solution of Eosin-Y contains 12 gm of eosin-Y, 100 cc of 95 percent ethyl alcohol, and 900 cc of distilled water. Just before use, the solution is diluted in the proportion of two parts of stock solution to one part of distilled water, with two drops of glacial acetic acid being added to each dish containing dye solution.

(8) Place tissue through three changes of 80 percent alcohol solution until it has the desired stain contrast.

(9) Dip tissue in two changes of 95 percent alcohol.

(10) Place the tissue in a solution containing equal amounts of chloroform and 100 percent alcohol, slide it onto a piece of onionskin paper, and trim with scissors to the desired final size.

With the tissue section still on the paper, place in full strength Terpineol[2] ($C_{10}H_{18}O$; mol wt 154.24) and leave in this solution for at least 40 minutes. Longer periods of exposure to Terpineol will not damage the tissue.

The tissues are *mounted* on the glass slides in a uniform position for the purpose of facilitating subsequent microscopic examination.

The glass slides (3 x 1 inch) and cover slips (24 x 40 mm) are dipped in 80 percent alcohol and wiped with 20-12 mesh cotton gauze until all dust, lint, or other particles are removed. The tissue sections are separated from the papers with a small pick, removed from the Terpineol with a brush and placed on glass slides. Some technicians prefer to float the sections onto the glass slides from the Terpineol. A heavy grade of blotting paper is firmly pressed

Fig. 1.9: Horizontal planes of sectioning for the left ear. The specimen is oriented on the microtome to ensure that the plane of cutting will be parallel to the axis of the modiolus. See Figs. 1.10 to 1.13.

2. This agent is available from Fisher Scientific Co., Fairlawn, New Jersey.

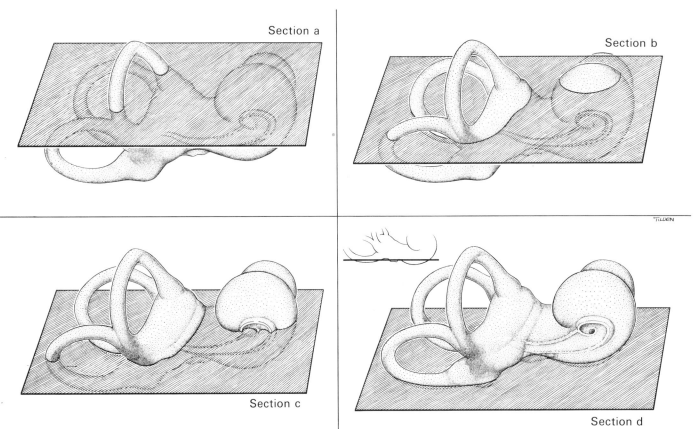

Section a

Section b

Section c

Section d

Fig. 1.10: Section corresponding to level a. of Fig. 1.9

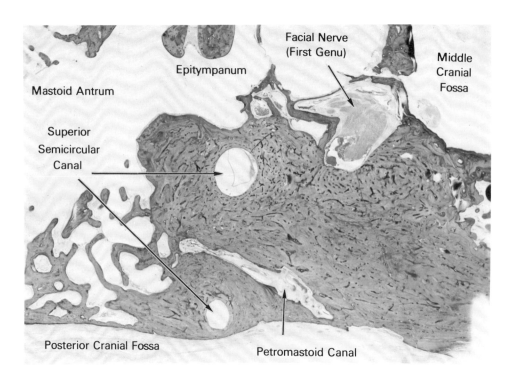

Epitympanum

Facial Nerve
(First Genu)

Middle
Cranial
Fossa

Mastoid Antrum

Superior
Semicircular
Canal

Posterior Cranial Fossa

Petromastoid Canal

Fig. 1.11: Section corresponding to level b. of Fig. 1.9

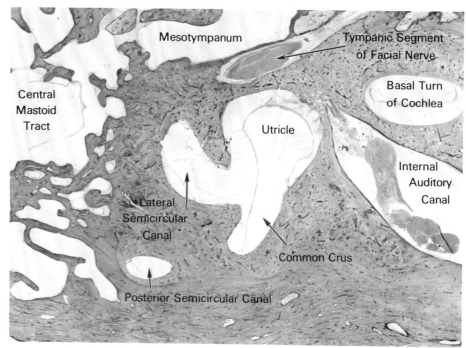

Fig. 1.12: Section corresponding to level c. of Fig. 1.9

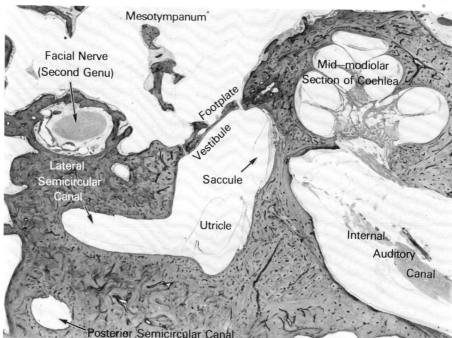

Fig. 1.13: Section corresponding to level d. of Fig. 1.9

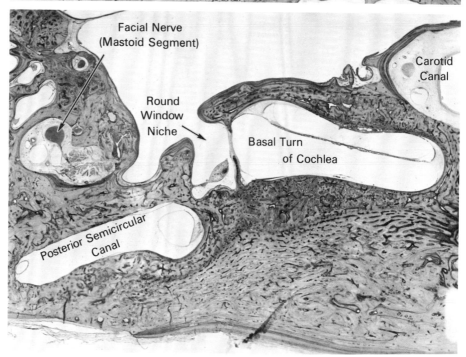

on the tissue to remove the Terpineol. Permount[3] is placed on the section with a dropper, the cover slip is pressed on the tissue, and the excess is removed with a xylene-soaked cotton sponge.

Lead weights are used to compress the cover slips onto the slides and they are permitted to dry for one week (Fig. 1.14). Excess Permount is then removed with xylene-soaked cotton sponges, and they are placed in anatomical sequence and labeled with India ink. The name and section number are written on each slide with India ink or other suitable inscribing method. When ink is used it should be covered with a transparent fingernail polish. The tracer set of slides may be deposited in a cardboard tray[4] which accommodates 48 slides. It has a white background to facilitate anatomical identification of sections during microscopic study (Fig. 1.15).

3. Permount mounting medium is available from Fisher Scientific Co., Fairlawn, New Jersey.

4. Slide trays of this type are available from the Commercial Bindery Corp., 6620 Lonyo St., Dearborn, Michigan.

Fig. 1.14: The tissue sections are carefully oriented on 1 x 3 inch glass slides, they are covered with Permount and 24 x 40 mm glass cover slips. Wooden blocks of appropriate size and lead weights are placed on the cover slips and they are permitted to dry for one week.

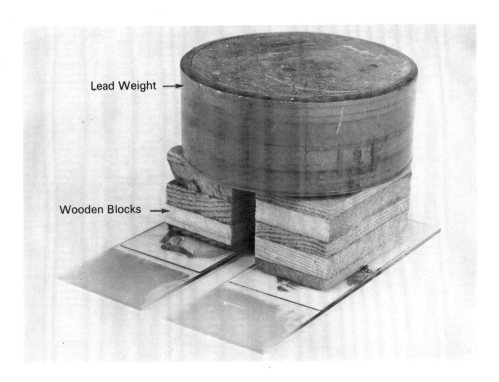

Fig. 1.15: This cardboard tray will accommodate up to 48 sections. The tissues are displayed on a white background, and all are fully in view for rapid identification and removal.

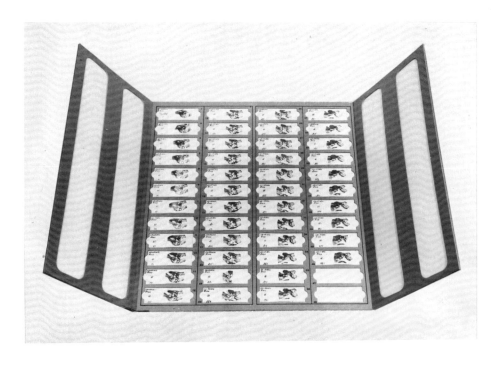

C. ARTIFACTS

Artifacts are changes introduced during the removal and preparation of tissue, and may be classified as primary and secondary (Fernández, 1958a).

Primary artifacts are those changes which are expected to result from tissue preparation and produce the so-called "normal" histological appearance. During fixation the proteins are precipitated in a coarse, sponge-like network (Baker, 1955), and the resulting spaces become filled with mounting medium. The cell walls remain intact, and the nuclei usually retain their normal positions. Intracellular organelles, such as mitochondria, usually are not visible. Fixation results in about 10 percent shrinkage of most tissues, although the tectorial membrane, the otolithic membranes, and the cupulae shrink as much as 50 percent. The tectorial membrane usually becomes detached from the organ of Corti and is retracted toward the limbus. Fixatives produce their own peculiar artifacts; for example, Wittmaack's fluid (Wittmaack and Laurowitsch, 1912) characteristically induces detachment of the inner sulcus cells (Fernández, 1958a).

Secondary artifacts are those tissue changes resulting from removal and preparation which are not "normal" for the technique used and may or may not be avoidable. Secondary artifacts caused by removal of the specimen consist of fractures of bone, tearing of soft tissue (such as the skin of the external auditory canal), and the introduction of fluid, blood, and bone dust into the pneumatized spaces. Inadequate decalcification of bone leads to tearing, and over-decalcification leads to feathery fragmentation during cutting. The formation of gas bubbles in the specimen can be attributed to faulty histologic technique and results in gross distortions of the inner ear structures. A dull microtome knife creates tears and scratches in the tissue and sometimes results in alternate thick and thin sections. Rough handling of the tissue sections during staining and mounting can create tears and wrinkles.

D. POSTMORTEM AUTOLYSIS

When a cell dies and is not preserved by fixation its contents become acid, proteins break down into amino acids which diffuse out of the cells, the cytoplasm becomes homogeneous, the nucleus shrinks and the cell swells (Fernández, 1956,1958b). Unless fixation occurs to interrupt the process these changes continue until the cell has disintegrated. Important determinants of the magnitude of autolytic change are temperature and time lapse between death and fixation. The best tissue preservation is achieved by the technique of intravital perfusion (Fig. 1.16) which obviously is not applicable to the human. Rutledge (1969) has performed arterial perfusion on full-term, stillborn human fetuses immediately after delivery and has achieved excellent histological preservation (Fig. 1.17). Because the temporal bones cannot be removed until the time of autopsy, time lapses of three to four hours are usual and twelve to twenty hours are common.

The cochlear neurons begin to swell soon after death. The nuclei become pyknotic and are surrounded by a clear zone. Finally, the cell walls and nerve fibers disintegrate, and only the pyknotic nuclei are clearly identifiable. Fortunately, the pyknotic nuclei remain intact for many hours, and under conditions of refrigeration, a fairly accurate estimation of cochlear neuron population can be made after prolonged postmortem delays (Fig. 1.18). Autolytic change is less severe for the vestibular ganglion cells presumably because these cells are located in the internal auditory canal where they are more accessible to fixative solutions.

The organ of Corti, as a whole, may appear shrunken (Fig. 1.19) or swollen. The factors which determine these reactions have never been clearly determined. Early changes consist of swelling and homogenization of cytoplasm, detachment of hair cells from Deiters' cells, space formation among the ex-

Fig. 1.16: This photomicrograph of the organ of Corti of a cat shows the excellent preservation of histological detail that can be achieved by intravital perfusion. In this method fixative solution is perfused through the vascular system with the animal under deep general anesthesia.

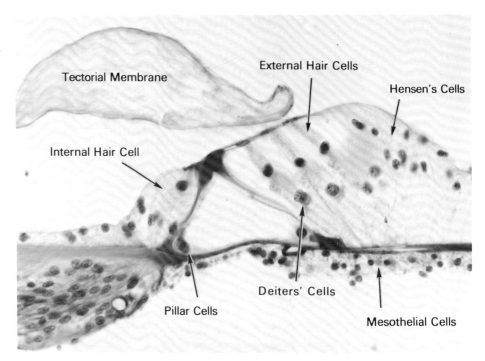

Fig. 1.17: Cochlear duct of a full-term stillborn human fetus subjected to intra-arterial perfusion immediately after birth. Preservation of tissues is excellent and approaches that of intravital perfusion (Courtesy of Rutledge)

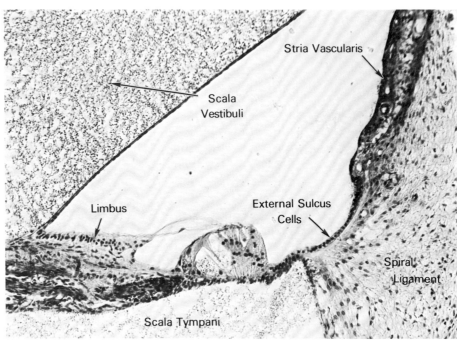

Fig. 1.18: This photomicrograph shows the cochlear neurons of a cat. After this animal was killed its body was permitted to lie at room temperature (70°F) for 24 hours, following which the temporal bones were removed from the skull and immersed in 10 percent formalin solution and prepared in the usual way. The cell bodies are greatly swollen, and the nuclei are pyknotic; however, the neurons can be clearly identified.

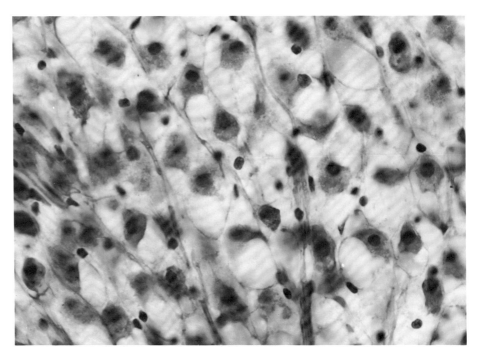

Fig. 1.19: This view shows the organ of Corti of a cat in which the temporal bone was treated by immersion in 10 percent formalin three hours after death. The cells are shrunken, and the cytoarchitecture is greatly disturbed. There is a fine granular precipitate in the scala tympani. In spite of these changes all cytological elements of the organ of Corti can be identified.

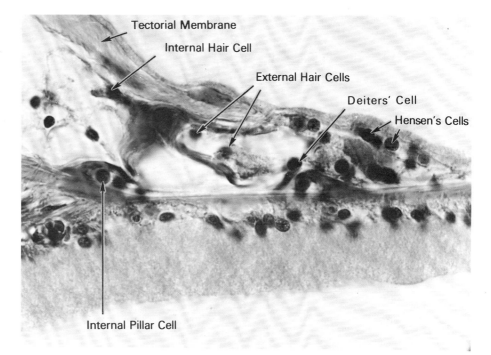

Fig. 1.20: The organ of Corti in this photomicrograph shows the autolytic change occurring after a 12-hour postmortem delay. The cytoplasmic masses are greatly enlarged and homogenized, and the cell walls are beginning to disintegrate with discharge of contents into the fluid spaces. In spite of these changes the cell types are still recognizable.

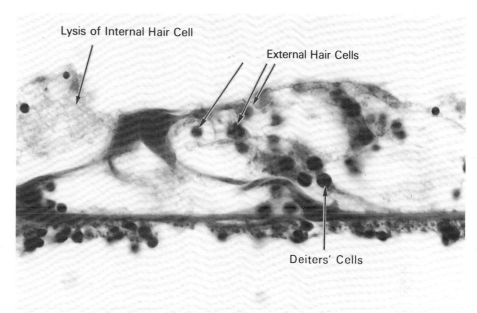

Fig. 1.21: There is total lysis of the organ of Corti of the cat after 24 hours at room temperature without fixation. All that remains of the organ of Corti is a few free-floating degenerating cells and fragments of the tectorial membrane. Some cells of the tympanic lamella remain attached to the basilar membrane.

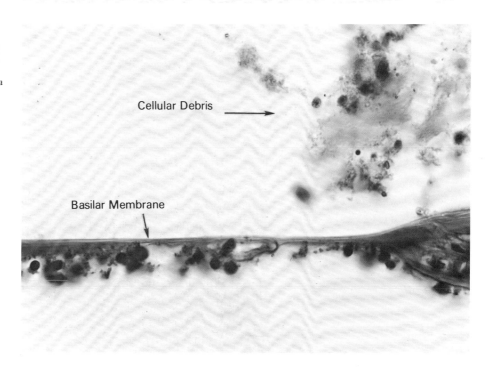

13   Histological Method

ternal and internal sulcus cells, and formation of precipitate in the fluid spaces adjacent to the cells. Later there is detachment of the internal and external sulcus cells. The outer hair cells assume a spherical shape with a centrally located nucleus (Fig. 1.20). Although the walls of the cells become progressively less distinct, the nuclei maintain their relative locations so that cell types can often be identified even when autolysis is severe. The supporting structures, such as the pillars and reticular plate, maintain a normal position until autolysis is far advanced, after which they also disintegrate (Fig. 1.21). The spiral ligament, tectorial membrane, limbus, and basilar membrane persist even after total disintegration of the organ of Corti. The mesothelial cells, which lie on the scala tympani side of the basilar membrane, and Reissner's membrane show progressive cellular swelling and nuclear pyknosis, but are very durable and usually remain intact longer than the cells within the cochlear duct. The position of Reissner's membrane usually does not change as a function of time after death.

The changes in the stria vascularis closely parallel those seen in the cells of the organ of Corti. A common early change is the extrusion of globules on the surface of the stria (Fig. 1.22) followed by a layer of precipitate (Fig. 1.23). As the cells begin to disintegrate, the entire stria detaches from the spiral ligament and becomes separated from it by a zone which contains a fine precipitate (Fig. 1.24).

The pattern of autolytic change in the vestibular sense organs parallels that of the organ of Corti. As swelling of the cells occurs, the sensory epithelium increases in thickness until cellular disintegration occurs. The otolithic membranes and cupulae gradually become detached, and the intervening spaces accumulate a fine precipitate. The otoconial layer can usually be identified until autolysis is far advanced, but eventually the otolithic membranes disintegrate and the otoconia disperse into the endolymph (Figs. 1.25, 1.26, 1.27).

One of the enigmas in the preparation of animal and human temporal bones is "compression artifact" (Fig. 1.28). The term is misleading as there is no evidence that this artifact is actually caused by pressure on the tissues; however, the term is descriptive of the appearance of the tissues. Wittmaack and Laurowitsch (1912), Wittmaack (1956) and Mygind et al. (1945) believe that this condition is an intravital phenomenon, although each gave a different explanation for its etiology. Wittmaack and Laurowitsch termed it "hypotonic degeneration" and believed that a decrease in endolymphatic pressure and an increase in perilymphatic pressure accounted for the change,

Fig. 1.22: Mild postmortem changes in the stria vascularis (cat) after 1½ hours of exposure to room temperature without fixation. There are globular extrusions on the surface and nuclear pyknosis; however, all three cell types can be clearly identified.

Fig. 1.23: There is severe postmortem autolysis of the stria vascularis (cat) after 12 hours of exposure to room temperature without fixation. There is swelling of the cytoplasmic masses of all cells, lysis of some of the marginal cells, and formation of a precipitate in the adjacent fluid.

Fig. 1.24: There are severe lytic changes in the stria vascularis (cat) after 24 hours of exposure to room temperature without fixation. The strial tissue has separated from the spiral ligament. Many cells have disappeared, and others are disintegrating.

1.22

1.23

1.24

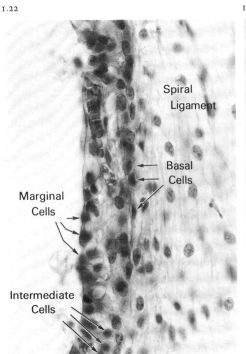

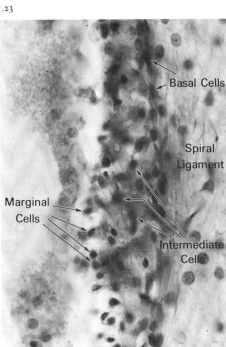

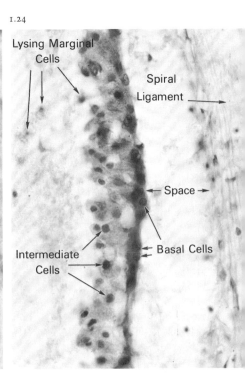

Fig. 1.25: Saccular maculae of the cat. The animal was killed, and 10 percent formalin was injected immediately into the right auditory bulla. After exposure to room temperature for 1½ hours, both temporal bones were removed and immersed in 10 percent formalin solution. The sensory and supporting cells, otolithic membrane, and otoconial layer are clearly visible in both ears but the degenerative change and swelling are greater in the left ear.

Fig. 1.26: Saccular maculae of the cat. The animal was killed, and 10 percent formalin was injected immediately into the right auditory bulla. After exposure to room temperature for 12 hours, both temporal bones were removed and immersed in 10 percent formalin solution. Postmortem autolytic change is much greater in the left ear. Sensory and supporting cells can be clearly differentiated in the right ear. In the left ear the cell walls have disintegrated, and although the nuclei have intermingled to some extent, it is probable that those nuclei located near the surface are from sensory cells.

Fig. 1.27: Saccular maculae of the cat. The animal was killed, and 10 percent formalin was injected immediately into the right auditory bulla. After exposure to room temperature for 24 hours, both temporal bones were removed and immersed in 10 percent formalin solution. The macula of the right ear still shows good cellular preservation; however, the macula of the left ear shows severe cellular disintegration and identification of cell types is difficult.

Fig. 1.28: This photomicrograph shows typical compression artifact of the structures of the cochlear duct in a 72-year-old man. The temporal bones were removed nine hours after death and immersed in Heidenhain-Susa solution. There is shrinkage and agglutination of the soft tissues (organ of Corti, stria vascularis, limbus, tectorial membrane) and decrease in the volume of endolymph so that Reissner's membrane comes to lie on the organ of Corti. The same general changes can be seen in the vestibular labyrinth.

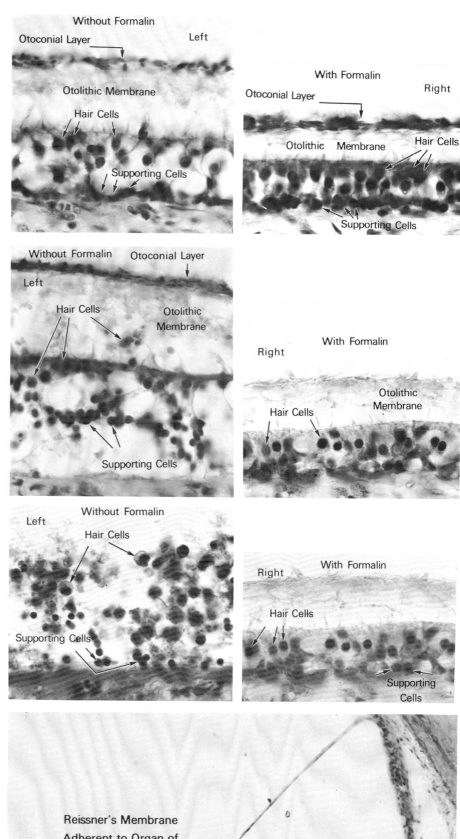

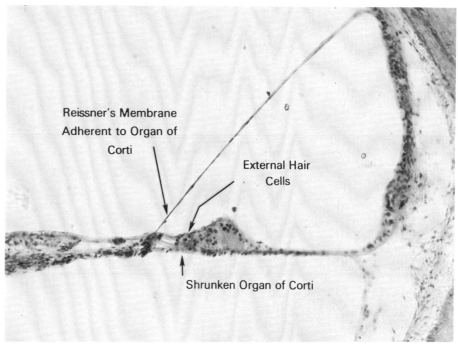

whereas Mygind termed it "endolymphatic compression" and believed it to be due to some caprice of terminal neural activity with filtration dominating over secretion. Fernández (1958a) believes that compression artifact is caused by methods of histological preparation and that it may be an uncontrollable reaction between the reagents and tissues.

Compression artifact may occur in specimens intravitally perfused as well as those treated by immersion fixation and does not appear to be related to time lapse after death. It is characterized by collapse and agglutination of the soft tissues. The cytoplasmic mass is decreased, the nuclei become pyknotic, and the cell outlines become indistinct. The pillars and the reticular lamina collapse so that the tunnel of Corti and Nuel's spaces disappear. The tectorial membrane is flattened into a thin lamina, which often lies in contact with the internal sulcus cells and the organ of Corti. The stria vascularis and vestibular sense organs show similar changes. Reissner's membrane is displaced toward the basilar membrane and often is adherent to the shrunken organ of Corti.

Formalin injection (10 or 20 percent) into the middle ear immediately after death was shown by Fernández (1958) to reduce postmortem change. A similar study was performed by Schuknecht (unpublished data) on humans and animals which consistently demonstrated better preservation in the injected ear than the control ear (See Figs. 1.25, 1.26, 1.27, 1.29, 1.30, 1.31, 1.32 and 1.33). Presumably the fixative solution diffuses into the inner ear through the round window membrane. The method seems to be more effective in guinea pigs and cats than in humans, possibly because the specimens are smaller and the round window membranes are comparatively larger in animals.

Opening the superior semicircular canal at the arcuate eminence prior to immersion also appears to accelerate fixation. Removal of the stapes accomplishes the same effect but is not recommended because the method causes artifacts in the middle ear and vestibule.

Total body refrigeration aids in arresting the temperature sensitive enzymatic reactions which destroy tissue. Fernández (1958) showed that for equal time lapses after death, refrigerated human specimens showed less postmortem autolysis than nonrefrigerated animal specimens.

The following rating of tissue preservation is patterned after that suggested by Fernández (1958):

(1) *Excellent:* These specimens demonstrate the normal microscopic cytology and cytoarchitecture anticipated from successful intravital perfusion.

(2) *Good:* The histological appearance is that anticipated from fixation by immersion soon after death. There may be precipitates in the fluid spaces and some distortion of cells by swelling or shrinking; however, the cell membranes and nuclei, as well as the general cytoarchitecture, are well preserved.

(3) *Fair:* The histological appearance is that anticipated after delayed fixation by immersion. In this stage postmortem autolysis is more advanced with cells showing indistinct outlines, beginning separation and generally disturbed cytoarchitecture; however, the nuclei have maintained their spatial relationships adequately to identify cell types.

(4) *Poor:* This is the stage of severe autolytic change. Disintegration is so severe that evaluation of hair cell and neuronal populations is not possible. Only remnants of the sense organs, stria vascularis and other structures are seen. The tectorial membrane, limbus, basilar membrane, spiral ligament, supporting structures of the maculae, Reissner's membrane, and walls of the membranous labyrinth are still structurally intact but show cellular disintegration. Specimens in this stage of degeneration are mainly useful for the study of bony anatomy and pathology.

Fig. 1.29: This cat was killed and 10 percent formalin was injected immediately into the right auditory bulla. After the body was exposed to room temperature for four hours, both temporal bones were removed and immersed in 10 percent formalin solution. There is greater cytoplasmic swelling of the soft tissues of the uninjected ear (below).

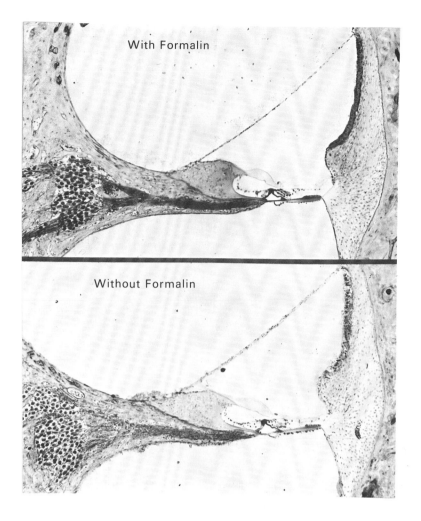

Fig. 1.30: This cat was killed, and 10 percent formalin was injected immediately into the right auditory bulla. After the body was exposed to room temperature for 12 hours, both temporal bones were removed and immersed in 10 percent formalin solution. In the left ear the nuclei of Deiters' cells and the hair cells are present but they are difficult to identify because of the disturbance of cyto-architecture.

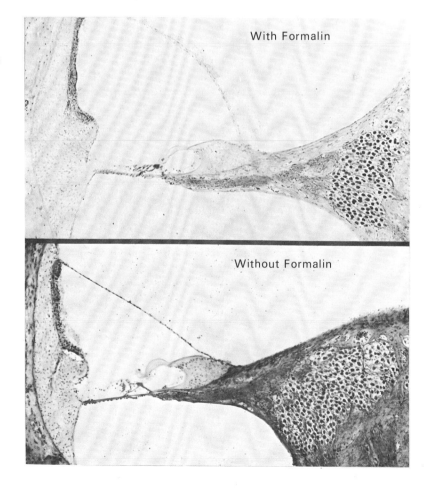

Fig. 1.31: This cat was killed, and 10 percent formalin was injected immediately into the right auditory bulla. After the body was exposed to room temperature for 18 hours, both temporal bones were removed and immersed in 10 percent formalin solution. The tissues of the injected ear (above) are still well preserved. In the uninjected ear (below) the cells of the organ of Corti show severe lysis, and only nuclear fragments remain. The cochlear neurons are swollen but the cell walls and nuclei are intact.

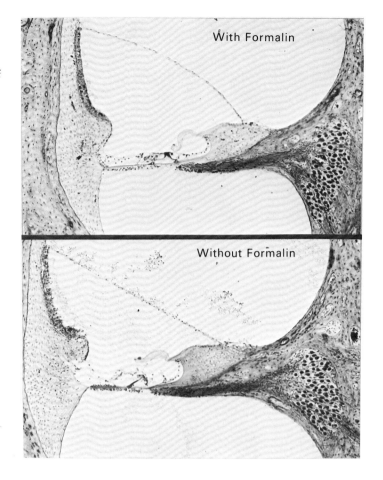

Fig. 1.32: This cat was killed, and 10 percent formalin was injected immediately into the right auditory bulla. After the body was exposed to room temperature for 24 hours, both temporal bones were removed and immersed in 10 percent formalin solution. The injected ear (above) still shows good preservation. The uninjected ear (below) shows total lysis of the organ of Corti, separation of the stria vascularis from the underlying spiral ligament, separation of the tectorial membrane from the limbus, and beginning disintegration of Reissner's membrane. The cochlear neurons are greatly swollen, and the nuclei are pyknotic; however, individual cells can still be identified clearly.

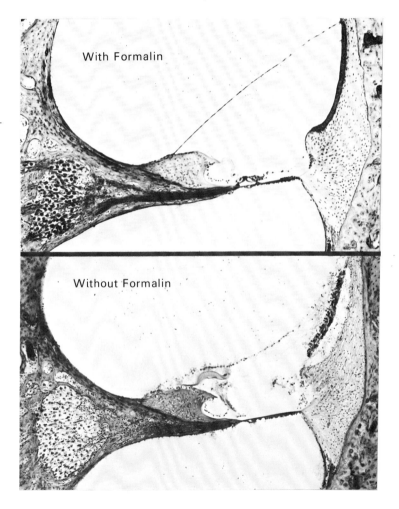

Fig. 1.33: Twenty percent formalin was injected through the right tympanic membrane into the middle ear 25 minutes after the death of this 47-year-old man. The body lay at room temperature for five hours before autopsy was performed, and both temporal bones were removed and immersed in Helly's fixative solution. The injected ear (above) shows excellent preservation, while the uninjected ear (below) shows severe autolysis and compression artifact.

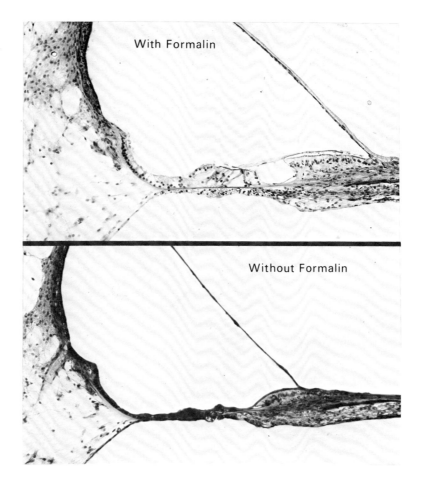

References

Baker, J., 1955: Cytological technique. Methuen, London.

Bredberg, G., 1968: Cellular pattern and nerve supply of the human organ of Corti. Acta oto-laryng. Suppl. 236.

Bredberg, G., Lindeman, H., Ades, H., and West, R., 1970: Scanning electron microscopy of the organ of Corti. Science 170:861.

Duvall, A., III, Flock, Å., and Wersäll, J., 1966: The ultrastructure of the sensory hairs and associated organelles of the cochlear inner hair cell, with reference to directional sensitivity. J. Cell Biol. 29:497.

Engström, H., 1951: Microscopic anatomy of the inner ear. Acta oto-laryng. 40:5.

Engström, H., Ades, H., and Andersson, A., 1966: Structural pattern of the organ of Corti. William and Wilkins, Baltimore, Md.

Engström, H., and Wersäll, J., 1953: Structure of the organ of Corti, I. Outer hair cells. Acta oto-laryng. 43:1.

Engström, H., and Wersall, J., 1958: Structure and innervation of the inner ear sensory epithelia. Int. Cytol. 7:535.

Engström, H., Bergstrom, B., and Ades, H., 1972: Macula utriculi and macula sacculi in the squirrel monkey, in Inner Ear Studies. Acta oto-laryng. Suppl. 301.

Fernández, C., 1956: Postmortem changes in the vestibular and cochlear receptors. Air University, School of Aviation Medicine, USAF, Randolph AFB, Texas, no. 56–118.

Fernández, C., 1958a: Postmortem changes and artifacts in human temporal bones. Laryngoscope 68:1586.

Fernández, C., 1958b: Postmortem changes in the vestibular and cochlear receptors (guinea pig). Arch. Otolaryng. 68:460.

Hilding, D., 1965: Cochlear chromaffin cells. Laryngoscope 75:1.

Iurato, S., 1961: The neurological work of Alfonso Corti. Proc. Int. Symp. Hist. Neurol., Varenna—30.

Iurato, S., and dePetris, S., 1967: Methods. Chap. 2, in Submicroscopic Structure of the Inner Ear, ed. S. Iurato, Pergamon Press, Oxford.

Johnsson, L-G., and Hawkins, J., Jr., 1967a: A direct approach to cochlear anatomy and pathology in man. Arch. Otolaryng. 85:599.

Johnsson, L-G., and Hawkins, J., Jr., 1967b: Otolithic membranes of the saccule and utricle in man. Science 157:1454.

Kimura, R., 1966: Hairs of the cochlear sensory cells and their attachment to the tectorial membrane. Acta oto-laryng. 61:55.

Kimura, R., Schuknecht, H., and Sando, I., 1964: Fine morphology of the sensory cells in the organ of Corti of man. Acta oto-laryng. 58:390.

Lim, D., 1969: Three dimensional observation of the inner ear with the scanning electron microscope. Acta oto-laryng. Suppl. 255.

Lim, D., and Lane, W., 1969a: Cochlear sensory epithelium: a scanning electron microscopic observation. Ann. Otol. Rhinol. Laryng. 78:827.

Lim, D., and Lane, W., 1969b: Vestibular sensory epithelia: a scanning electron microscopic observation. Arch. Otolaryng. 90:283.

Lindeman, H., 1969: Studies on the morphology of the sensory regions of the vestibular apparatus. Adv. Anat. Embry. Cell Biol., Springer-Verlag, Berlin, Heidelberg, New York.

Lindeman, H., and Ades, H., 1971: The sensory hairs and tectorial membrane in the development of the cat's organ of Corti. Acta oto-laryng. 72:229.

Mygind, S., Andersen, H., and Arnvig, J., 1945: Experimental histological studies on the labyrinth: V. Comparison between the results of fixation with Wittmaack's fluid and with "susa". Acta oto-laryng. 33:273.

Rutledge, L., 1969: Histologic study of the perfused human temporal bone. Laryngoscope 79:2104.

Schuknecht, H., 1968: Temporal bone removal at autopsy: preparation and uses. Arch. Otolaryng. 87:129.

Smith, C., 1956: Microscopic structure of the utricle. Ann. Otol. Rhinol. Laryng. 65:450.

Smith, C., 1957: Structure of the stria vascularis and the spiral prominence. Ann. Otol. Rhinol. Laryng. 66:521.

Spoendlin, H., 1964: Organization of the sensory hairs in the gravity receptors in utricle and saccule of the squirrel monkey. Z. Zellforsch. 62:701.

Spoendlin, H., 1966: The organization of the cochlear receptor. Adv. Oto-Rhino-Laryng. S. Karger, Basel.

Wittmaack, K., 1956: Die Ortho-und Pathobiologie des Labyrinthes. Georg Thieme Verlag, Stuttgart.

Wittmaack, K., and Laurowitsch, Z., 1912: Über artifizielle postmortale und aganale Beeinflussung der histologischen Befunde im membranösen Labyrinthe, Z. Ohrenheilk. 65:157.

2 Anatomy

The primary concern of this book is with pathology so that no attempt will be made to present a detailed account of the embryology and anatomy of the ear. A review of current knowledge in this area, however, will help orient the reader and provide terminology as a basis for the descriptions of pathology which follow.

In its phylogenetically simplest form, the otocyst retains its original connection with the parent ectoderm. Thus in the shark, the primitive auditory pit becomes a vesicle containing fluid in continuity with the environmental water. In man this ectodermal continuity is lost early in the embryo and is followed by a series of developmental changes in which the branchial arch system is remodeled into the external and middle ear. The otocyst develops into the membranous labyrinth and retains its aqueous system in the form of endolymph. In this sequestered state the labyrinth can serve as an equilibratory apparatus but is not suited to perform as an auditory organ. Auditory function requires a sound-transmitting mechanism to bring the environmental air into contact with the sense organ. The development of the eustachian tube and tympanic cavity from the first branchial pouch and the ossicles from the first and second branchial arches achieved this end (Anson et al., 1967) (Figs. 2.1, 2.2).

The membranous labyrinth begins as ectodermal thickenings (otic placodes) on each side of the rhombencephalon. The primitive otocyst is formed by invagination of the otic placode which becomes the inner layer of the walls in the membranous labyrinth. This layer is enveloped in a sheath of mesenchymal tissue and then, through infolding of the walls of the otocyst, develops into three primary parts: (1) the endolymphatic duct and sac, (2) the utricle and semicircular canals, and (3) the saccule and the cochlear duct. Thus the walls of the membranous labyrinth are constituted of two layers—an inner layer of ectodermal origin and an outer layer of mesodermal origin, separated by a basement membrane. The inner layer, which originally consists chiefly of polygonal squamous cells, differentiates in certain areas into the sense organs. The membranous labyrinth is enclosed within a bony labyrinth and in most areas is separated from the bony walls by a space containing perilymph. Among those making original observations on the anatomy of

Fig. 2.1: In the shark the auditory pit becomes a vesicle which contains fluid in continuity with environmental water. In man, this ectodermal continuity is lost as the otocyst develops into the membranous labyrinth. The endolymphatic system derives from the otocyst, the tympanic cavity from the first branchial pouch, the external auditory canal from the first branchial groove, the ossicles from the first and second branchial arches, and the perilymphatic space and otic capsule from surrounding mesenchyme. (After Anson et al., 1967)

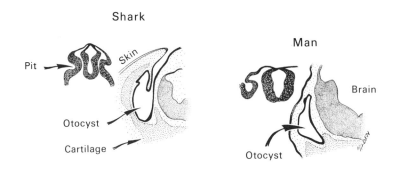

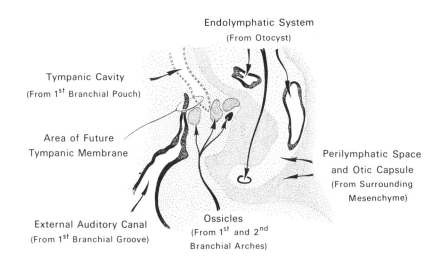

Fig. 2.2: Transverse section through the skull showing the structures of the ear in a human fetus (crown-rump length, 165 mm, about 7 months). The auricle and external auditory canal are well developed. The eustachian tube and anterior mesotympanum show cavitation. The ossicles are embedded in mesenchyme and show foci of ossification. The otic capsule has well-defined endosteal, endochondral, and periosteal bone layers.

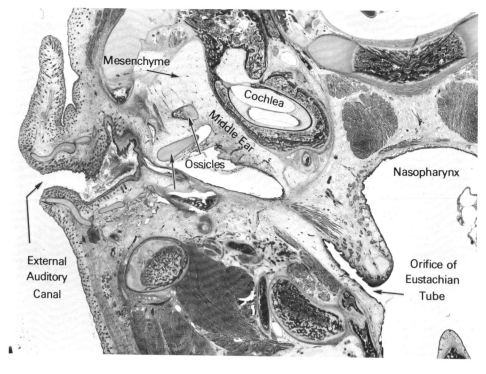

Fig. 2.3: Diagrammatic sketch of the histological components of the tympanic membrane (squirrel monkey). (Courtesy of Lim, 1968)

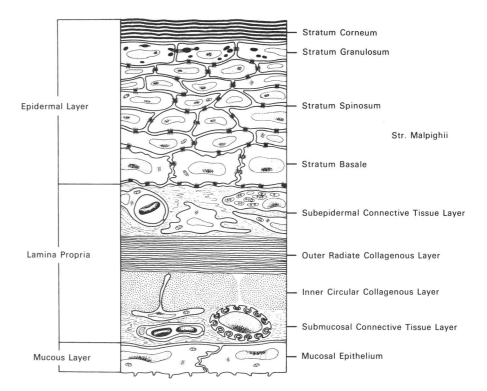

the membranous labyrinth are Scarpa (1800), Steifensand (1835), and Retzius (1881, 1884). A detailed account of the embryology of the ear appears in a book by Bast and Anson (1949) and in a movie film by the American Academy of Ophthalmology and Otolaryngology, edited by Altmann.

A. THE MIDDLE EAR

1. THE TYMPANIC MEMBRANE

The tympanic membrane is irregularly round and slightly conical in shape. It varies somewhat in thickness and elasticity, being thicker in the center and periphery than in the intermediate area. Wever and Lawrence (1954) found the vertical diameter of the tympanic membrane as measured along the axis of the manubrium to range from 8.5 to 10 mm and the horizontal diameter to range from 8 to 9 mm. The average weight of the tympanic membrane was found to be 14 mg. Békésy and Rosenblith (1951) determined the total area of the tympanic membrane to be 85 sq mm and the physiologically effective area to be 55 sq mm. The elasticity of the tympanic membrane is stated to be 4.9 x 10^{-8} dynes per sq cm (Kirikae, 1969) which is close to that of rubber.

The three layers of the pars tensa (epidermis, lamina propria, mucosa), as well as the inner circular and outer radiate lamina, have been known to exist for a century (Politzer, 1869; Gerlach, 1869). In electron microscopic studies, Lim (1968, 1970) elucidated the ultrastructural details of the pars tensa (Fig. 2.3). The epidermal layer consists of the four strata characteristic of skin (corneum, granulosum, spinosum, and basale). The stratum granulosum contains keratin granules in association with fine cytoplasmic microfilaments attached to desmosomes. The lamina propria is composed of a varying mixture of collagen fibers and fine fibrils of unknown nature. The outer radiate stratum contains more fine fibrils, and the inner circular stratum contains more collagen fibers. Elastic fibers are rare in the pars tensa (Lim, 1970). There is a layer of connective tissue on each side of the lamina propria. The mucous layer consists of a single stratum of simple squamous cells having numerous microvilli on their free cell surfaces.

The pars flaccida first described by Shrapnell (1832) consists of epidermis, lamina propria and mucous layers. The epidermis is composed of five to ten layers of desquamating epithelial cells. Its lamina propria consists of abun-

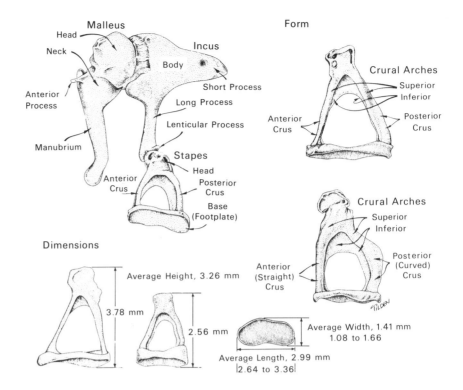

Fig. 2.4: Sketches showing the articulated ossicles and the form and dimension of the stapes. (After Anson and Donaldson, 1967)

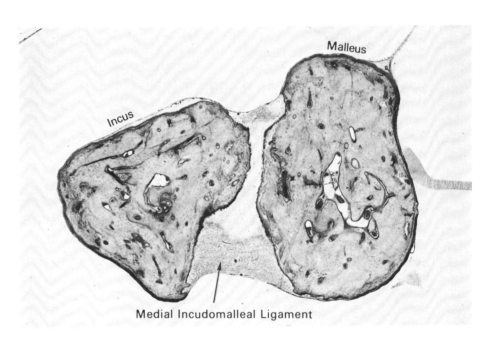

Fig. 2.5: Photomicrograph showing the medial incudomalleal ligament.

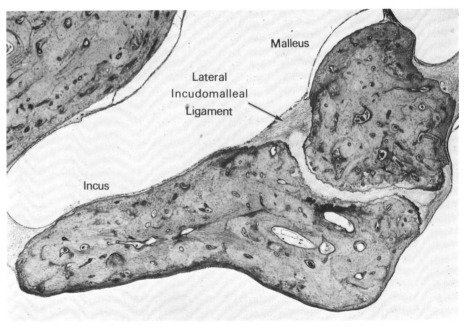

Fig. 2.6: Photomicrograph showing the lateral incudomalleal ligament.

dant irregularly arranged collagen and elastic fibers, large numbers of capillaries, and myelinated and unmyelinated nerve fibers. The mucous layer of the pars flaccida is formed mainly by simple squamous cells. The pars flaccida, contrary to popular conception, is thicker than the pars tensa (Lim, 1970).

2. THE OSSICLES AND MUSCLES

The ossicles (malleus, incus, and stapes) are arranged to form a lever mechanism by which sound energy is transmitted from the tympanic membrane to the inner ear fluids. The malleus has a head, neck, lateral process, anterior process, and manubrium; the incus has a body, short process, long process, and lenticular process, and the stapes consists of the head, anterior crus, posterior crus, and footplate (Fig. 2.4).

The incus and malleus are bound together at their articular surfaces to form a diarthrodial joint known as the incudomalleal articulation. In the adult this joint has incomplete cartilaginous surfaces. The capsule is thickened on both its medial and lateral aspects to form the incudomalleal ligaments (Figs. 2.5, 2.6). The lenticular process of the incus articulates with the head of the stapes in another diarthrodial joint termed the incudostapedial articulation. The articular surfaces are cartilaginous at an early age but consist partly of bone in adult life. The footplate of the stapes articulates with the walls of the oval window in a syndesmotic joint known as the stapediovestibular articulation. This articulation is held together by the annular ligament. In some adult specimens a space lined by connective tissue cells forms in the anterior part of the annular ligament (Bolz and Lim, 1972), but it is not clear whether this space should be considered a modified synovial joint, a bursa, or a degenerative change caused by use and aging. The position of the ossicles is maintained by the superior, anterior, and lateral malleal ligaments, the posterior incudal ligament, the annular ligament of the oval window, the tensor tympani muscle, and the stapedius muscle (Wolff and Belluci, 1956).

Various investigators have given somewhat different values for the weights of the ossicles, the average being about 23 mg for the malleus, 27 mg for the incus, and 2.5 mg for the stapes. The size and weight of the ossicles of Japanese individuals as measured by Kojo (1954) were found to be consistently less than those of investigators who measured Caucasian populations.

Two muscles, the tensor tympani muscle and the stapedius muscle, modify the action of the ossicles. The tensor tympani muscle is penniform (feather-shaped) and is about 2 cm in length. Most of the muscle lies within a bony channel (semicanal) parallel with the eustachian tube. It arises from the bony wall of the semicanal, the adjacent part of the greater wing of the sphenoid, and from the cartilage of the eustachian tube. The muscle fibers converge onto a central fibrous core, which proceeds posteriorly to form the tendon of the tensor tympani muscle. The peripheral fibers of the tendon are firmly attached to the concave surface of the cochleariform (spoon-shaped) process. Here the tendon turns laterally to attach to the medial and anterior surface of the neck and superior part of the manubrium of the malleus (Fig. 2.7). Contraction of the muscle draws the manubrium medially and thus tenses the tympanic membrane (Fig. 2.7).

The stapedius muscle lies in the posterior wall of the tympanic cavity in a bony sulcus adjacent to the facial canal. The muscle fibers arise from the walls of the sulcus and converge into a round tendon which passes anteriorly to emerge from the pyramidal eminence. The tendon attaches to the stapes in the region of the capitulum and upper part of the posterior surface of the posterior crus and occasionally to the capsule of the incudostapedial joint (Figs. 2.8 and 2.9).

Fig. 2.7: Photomicrograph illustrating the tensor tympani muscle and tendon.

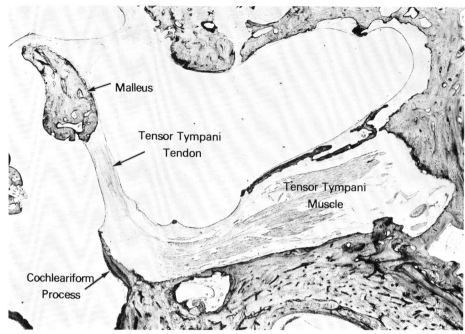

Fig. 2.8: Photomicrograph of the posterior mesotympanum showing the stapedius muscle and the attachment of its tendon to the head.

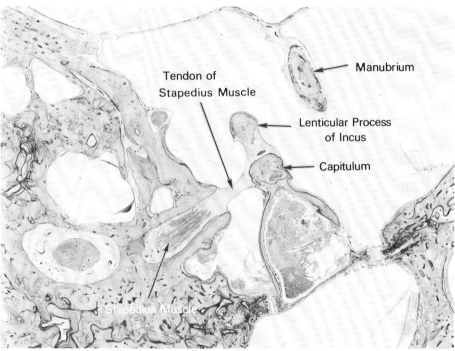

Fig. 2.9: Photomicrograph illustrating attachment of the stapedius tendon to the posterior crus of the stapes.

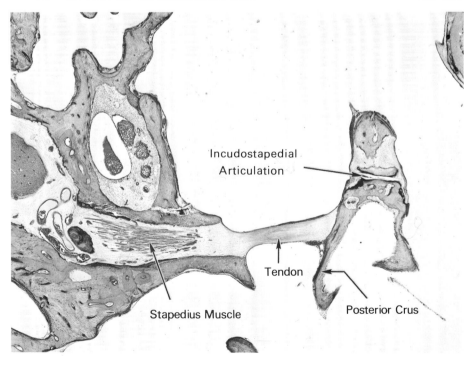

The tympanic cavity is a flat cleft with vertical and anteroposterior diameters of about 15 mm and a transverse diameter varying from 2 to 6 mm. The roof is formed by the tegmental wall (tegmen tympani), which is a thin plate of bone separating the tympanic cavity from the middle cranial fossa. The floor is formed by the jugular bulb upon which are located a number of irregular pneumatized cells. The posterior aspect of the floor consists of the stylomastoid prominence. The posterior wall of the tympanic cavity is more narrow inferiorly and is marked by a number of anatomical features, including the pyramidal eminence, iter chordae posterius, facial recess, and tympanic sinus (Proctor, 1969). The anterior boundary is marked by three important structures: the tensor tympani muscle, the wall of the carotid canal, and the eustachian tube orifice. The medial wall presents various features, including the promontory (basal turn of the cochlea), the oval and round windows, the fallopian canal, and the cochleariform process with its tensor tympani tendon. The lateral boundary of the tympanic cavity is formed by the tympanic membrane, tympanic annulus, and scutum.

The superior recess of the tympanic membrane, commonly called Prussak's space (Prussak, 1867), has been described in detail by Proctor (1968) (Fig. 2.10). The space is limited laterally by the pars flaccida which is attached superiorly along the edge of the notch of Rivinus. The superior and anterior walls are formed by the lateral malleal ligament which radiates from its site of origin on the neck of the malleus and from the anterior and posterior malleal folds. Posteriorly, Prussak's space opens into the epitympanum. The inferior margin of the posterior malleal fold extends from the pretympanic spine to the manubrium and lies in close lateral relationship to the chorda tympani nerve (Fig. 2.11).

The medial wall of the posterior mesotympanum is divided into three main depressions by a bridge of bone superiorly, the ponticulus, and a ridge of bone inferiorly, the subiculum (Platzer, 1961). These depressions are the round window niche inferior to the subiculum, the tympanic sinus between the subiculum and ponticulus, and the oval window niche superior to the ponticulus (Donaldson et al., 1968) (Fig. 2.12). The tympanic sinus lies between the bony labyrinth medially and the pyramidal eminence laterally. It is limited superiorly by the ponticulus and horizontal semicircular canal, posteriorly by the posterior semicircular canal, and inferiorly by the subiculum, styloid eminence, and jugular wall (Saito et al., 1971). The tympanic sinus is of surgical significance in that it may contain diseased tissue and is not directly visible by the usual surgical approaches to this area (Cheatle, 1907; Ballance, 1919; Dworacek, 1960).

The space, which is limited medially by the styloid complex and facial canal and laterally by the bony tympanic annulus, is termed the facial recess (Fig. 2.13).

The mucosal folds of the middle ear occur in rather constant anatomical positions which can be explained by the embryological development of the middle ear (Proctor, 1964). Between the third and seventh month of fetal life, the gelatinous tissues of the middle ear are slowly absorbed, and simultaneously the tympanic cavity develops by the ingrowth of four endothelial-lined pouches from the eustachian tube. The anterior sac extends superiorly, anterior to the tensor tendon, to form the anterior pouch of von Troeltsch. The medial sac forms much of the epitympanic space, including Prussak's space, and extends posteriorly to pneumatize that portion of the mastoid air cell system which derives from the petrous part of the temporal bone. The superior sac extends posteriorly between the manubrium and long process of the incus to the region of the pyramidal eminence, and eventually pneumatizes that portion of the mastoid which is derived from the squamous part of the temporal bone. The posterior sac extends along the hypotympanum to form the round and oval window niches and the sinuses of the posterior mesotympanum. Mucosal folds are formed where these endothelial-lined pouches con-

Fig. 2.10: Sketch showing the superior, anterior, and inferior walls of Prussak's space. The lateral wall (not shown) consists of Shrapnell's membrane which extends from the anterior and posterior tympanic striae to the margins of the notch of Rivinus. (After Proctor, 1968)

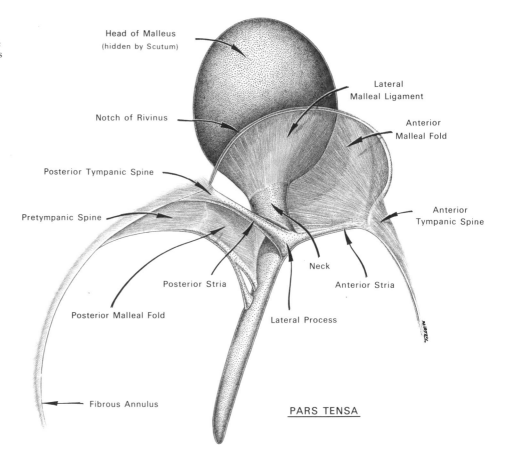

Head of Malleus
(hidden by Scutum)

Lateral
Malleal Ligament

Notch of Rivinus

Anterior
Malleal Fold

Posterior Tympanic Spine

Pretympanic Spine

Anterior
Tympanic Spine

Posterior Stria

Neck

Anterior Stria

Posterior Malleal Fold

Lateral Process

Fibrous Annulus

PARS TENSA

Fig. 2.11: Photomicrograph showing the relationship of the pretympanic spine to the tympanic membrane, chorda tympani nerve, and thickened inferior margin of the posterior malleal fold. See also Fig. 2.10.

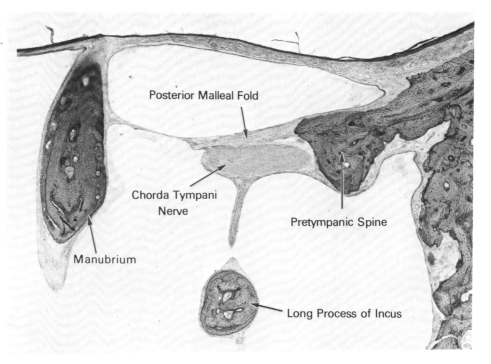

Posterior Malleal Fold

Chorda Tympani
Nerve

Pretympanic Spine

Manubrium

Long Process of Incus

28 Anatomy

Fig. 2.12: This sketch illustrates the anatomical relationships of the tympanic sinus. It is limited superiorly by the ponticulus and inferiorly by the subiculum and may extend several millimeters posterior to the pyramidal eminence. (After Donaldson et al., 1968)

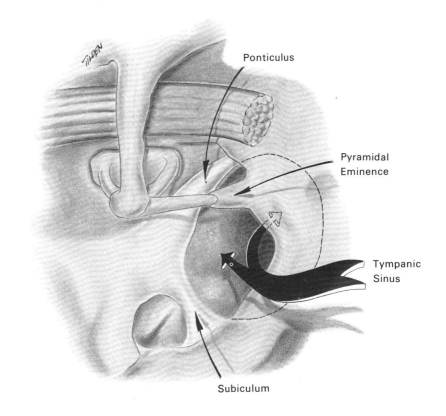

Fig. 2.13: Photomicrograph showing the anatomical relationships of facial recess, sinus tympani, and round window niche.

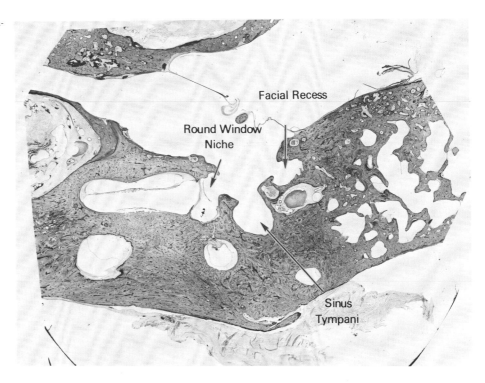

tact each other. They envelop remnants of mesoderm containing the ossicles, tendons of the tympanic muscles, chorda tympani nerve, and blood vessels. They influence in some degree the location and extension of disease processes such as secondary keratoma (cholesteatoma).

In an electron microscopic study, Hentzer (1970) found five types of cells in the mucosa of the human middle ear, mastoid and eustachian tube. These cell types are: (1) the nonciliated cell without secretory granules, (2) the nonciliated cell with secretory granules (including the goblet cell), (3) the ciliated cell, (4) the intermediate cell, and (5) the basal cell. The mastoid cavity has predominantly simple squamous or cuboidal epithelium, although ciliated cells can be found in some specimens. The posterior part of the mesotympanum and the epitympanum have taller epithelium, which is often ciliated. The promontory has secretory and nonsecretory columnar cells, occasional ciliated cells, and rarely goblet cells and glands (Kaneko et al., 1971; Shimada and Lim, 1972). In the eustachian tube the epithelium is of the pseudostratified ciliated columnar type with scattered goblet cells and glands (Tos, 1971). Hentzer concluded that the middle ear mucosa is a modified respiratory mucosa and that the nonciliated cell is the principal secretory cell of the middle ear. In its most active secretory phase the nonciliated cell has the cytological characteristics of a goblet cell.

4. THE VASCULAR SYSTEM

a. Arterial system

In a detailed study Nager and Nager (1953) traced the arteries supplying the middle ear and mastoid from serial sections of human temporal bones. Their findings are in general agreement with those of Nabeya (1923) and others (Hyrtl, 1835; Bast and Anson, 1949).

The anterior tympanic artery. The anterior tympanic artery is a branch of the mandibular division of the internal maxillary artery. While in the petrotympanic (glaserian) fissure, it gives rise to three major branches which enter the ear via the tympanosquamosal and other small fissures (Fig. 2.14). The superior branch supplies the bone and mucosa of the anterior and lateral walls of the epitympanum, and an anastomotic branch is sent to the superior tympanic artery through the posterior squamosal suture. The posterior branch supplies the bone and mucosa of the lateral wall of the epitympanum. A small descending tributary anastomoses with a vessel from the mastoid to supply the mucous membrane of the medial aspect of the tympanic membrane. The ossicular branch divides into separate branches which provide the main blood supply for the malleus and incus. The malleal artery reaches the malleus in the mucosa of the lateral malleal ligament and sends its main vessel into a nutrient foramen at the anterolateral aspect of the neck of the malleus. The incudal artery enters a mucosal fold in the lateral epitympanic wall to reach the lateral aspect of the body of the incus where it sends a branch into a nutrient foramen at the anterolateral aspect of the body.

The tubal artery. The tubal artery is a branch of the accessory meningeal artery and enters the middle ear in the wall of the eustachian tube to supply the tympanic part of the tube and the bone and mucosa of the protympanum. Its terminal branches anastomose with branches of the caroticotympanic arteries (Fig. 2.15).

The caroticotympanic arteries. The caroticotympanic arteries are usually two in number and arise as separate branches of the internal carotid artery. They enter the middle ear through separate bony channels in the partition between the carotid canal and cochlea and course posteriorly in the mucosa of the promontory to anastomose with branches of the inferior tympanic and tubal arteries, all of which supply the anterior part of the middle ear.

The superficial petrosal artery. The superficial petrosal artery arises from the middle meningeal artery and enters the facial hiatus adjacent to the greater superficial petrosal nerve, sends an anastomotic branch to the superior tym-

Fig. 2.14: Sketch showing the branches and distribution of the anterior tympanic artery. (After Nager and Nager, 1953)

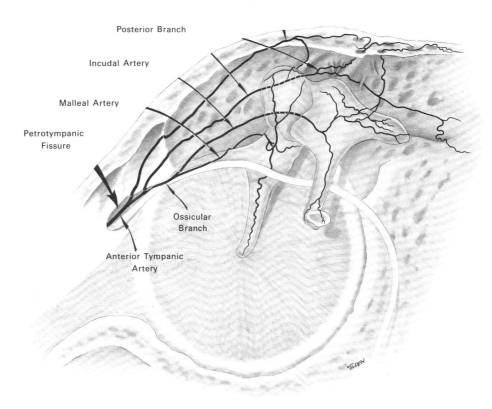

Superior Branch

Posterior Branch

Incudal Artery

Malleal Artery

Petrotympanic Fissure

Ossicular Branch

Anterior Tympanic Artery

Fig. 2.15: This sketch shows the usual arterial supply of the middle ear and mastoid exclusive of the anterior tympanic and deep auricular arteries. (After Nager and Nager, 1953)

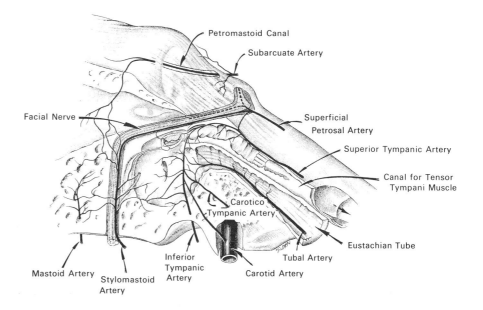

Petromastoid Canal

Subarcuate Artery

Facial Nerve

Superficial Petrosal Artery

Superior Tympanic Artery

Canal for Tensor Tympani Muscle

Carotico-Tympanic Artery

Eustachian Tube

Mastoid Artery

Stylomastoid Artery

Inferior Tympanic Artery

Carotid Artery

Tubal Artery

31   Anatomy

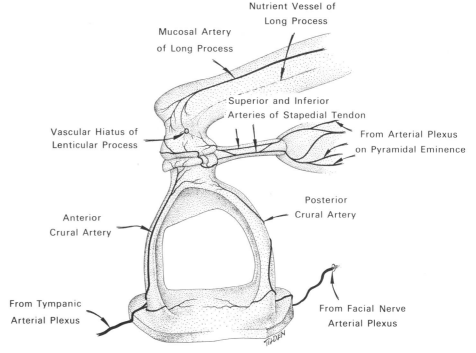

Nutrient Vessel of
Long Process

Mucosal Artery
of Long Process

Superior and Inferior
Arteries of Stapedial Tendon

Vascular Hiatus of
Lenticular Process

From Arterial Plexus
on Pyramidal Eminence

Posterior
Crural Artery

Anterior
Crural Artery

From Tympanic
Arterial Plexus

From Facial Nerve
Arterial Plexus

panic artery, and divides into main branches. One of these main branches enters the geniculate ganglion and divides into two vessels which pass within the facial nerve, one coursing in the direction of the internal auditory canal and the other toward the periphery. The other main branch bypasses the geniculate ganglion and continues as a descending branch in the space between the trunk of the facial nerve and the bony wall of the fallopian canal to anastomose with the stylomastoid artery in the upper third of the vertical part of the canal.

The vascular supply to the incudostapedial joint area has attracted the attention of anatomists and otologic surgeons because of occasional resorption of the long process of the incus in association with chronic infection and following prosthetic replacement of the stapes. The blood supply derives in part from the superior and inferior arteries of the stapedial tendon and from the posterior crural artery, all of which originate from the arterial plexus within the fallopian canal, which in turn is supplied by the superficial petrosal artery and the stylomastoid artery. The anterior crural artery arises from the tympanic arterial plexus (Alberti, 1963; Anson et al., 1962) (Fig. 2.16).

The superior tympanic artery. The superior tympanic artery arises from the middle meningeal artery and enters the middle ear adjacent to the lesser superficial petrosal nerve through the superior tympanic canaliculus. It supplies the tensor tympani muscle, the medial half of the roof, and the medial wall of the epitympanic space, and then accompanies the lesser superficial petrosal nerve and the nerve of Jacobson to anastomose with the inferior tympanic artery at the level of the oval window. The anastomotic plexus formed by the superior and inferior tympanic arteries gives rise to the anterior stapedial artery, which in turn gives origin to the anterior crural artery.

The inferior tympanic artery. The inferior tympanic artery is a branch of the ascending pharyngeal artery and enters the anterior part of the middle ear with the nerve of Jacobson through the inferior tympanic canaliculus. It ascends over the promontory in a bony groove (occasionally a canal) and anastomoses with branches of the caroticotympanic and superior tympanic arteries. It supplies the mucosa and bone of the adjacent hypotympanum and promontory.

The deep auricular artery. The deep auricular artery arises from the mandibular branch of the internal maxillary artery and enters the temporal bone at the inferior aspect of the osseous portion of the external auditory canal. It divides into two branches which contribute to the peripheral vascular ring of the tympanic membrane. The posterior branch, after ascending in the posterior wall of the bony canal, descends between the skin and radiate fibers of the tympanic membrane close to the manubrium, to supply a large part of the tympanic membrane. The anterior branch supplies a lesser part of the inferior and anterior part of the tympanic membrane.

The stylomastoid artery. The stylomastoid artery is a branch of the posterior auricular artery and enters the fallopian canal through the stylomastoid foramen, coursing upward in the canal between the nerve trunk and bony walls to terminate by anastomosing with the superficial petrosal artery. The vessel supplies the facial nerve as well as the bone and mucosa of the adjacent mastoid region and otic capsule and gives a branch to the stapedius muscle. It gives off the posterior tympanic branch which enters the middle ear via the iter chordae posterius to supply the postero-inferior part of the tympanic cavity.

The subarcuate artery. The subarcuate artery, which occasionally consists of more than one branch, most commonly arises from the labyrinthine artery, but may come from the anterior inferior cerebellar artery and enters the petromastoid canal. Near its origin it gives vessels to the dura mater of the posterior and middle cranial fossi and usually a branch to the petrous apex. Terminal vessels supply the adjacent area of the otic capsule and the anteromedial part of the mastoid (Mazzoni, 1969a).

The mastoid artery. The mastoid artery arises from the occipital artery and with numerous ramifications supplies the posterior part of the mastoid bone.

b. Venous system

The veins which drain the middle ear and mastoid are more variable than the arteries but, in general, follow the arterial distribution. They drain principally into the lateral sinus, jugular bulb, superior and inferior petrosal sinuses, the pterygoid plexus of veins, and the middle meningeal veins.

c. The major vessels

The major blood vessels anatomically related to the temporal bone and consequently of great importance to the otologic surgeon are the carotid artery, jugular bulb, and sigmoid sinus.

The carotid artery is located in the petrous apex region of the temporal bone and may be encountered in temporal bone resections for neoplasm as well as in other operative procedures at the petrous apex. Injury or obstruction of this vessel carries a high incidence of morbidity and mortality as this vessel provides the main blood supply to the cerebral hemisphere.

The middle meningeal artery or an accessory meningeal artery may occasionally be found in temporal bone sections. When present it is located in the petrous apex region lateral to the facial hiatus (Fig. 2.17).

Fig. 2.17: As shown in this photomicrograph, the middle meningeal artery may occasionally be seen in a bony canal lateral to the facial hiatus.

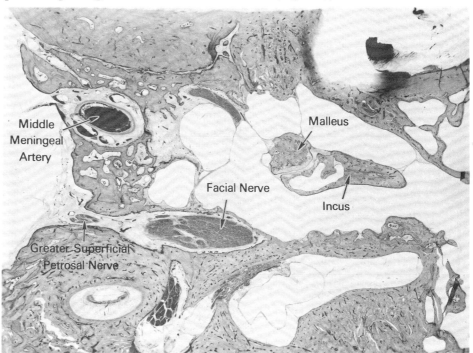

The cranial venous sinuses are the collecting veins from the brain, temporal bone, and orbit. These sinuses are located within split layers of the dura mater, principally in the areas where the tentorium cerebelli, falx cerebelli, and falx cerebri are attached to the skull. The lateral sinuses are the largest and are responsible for delivering most of the venous blood from the head to the neck. These sinuses begin at the occipital protuberance and pass anteriorly in the posterior walls of the mastoids to reach the jugular bulbs. The S-shaped segment of the lateral sinus which lies in the sigmoid sulcus of the mastoid part of the temporal bone is known as the sigmoid sinus (Fig. 2.18). The mastoid emissary vein carries blood from the scalp and penetrates the posterior part of the mastoid cortex to enter the lateral sinus in its sigmoid portion. The jugular bulb is located in the floor of the hypotympanum and marks the beginning of the internal jugular vein.

The superior petrosal sinus lies in the attachment of the tentorium cerebelli to the petrous ridge and drains into the lateral sinus. The inferior petro-

Fig. 2.18: The sigmoid sinus is that curved part of the lateral venous sinus which occupies the sigmoid sulcus. Often it protrudes prominently into the posterior part of the mastoid air cell system as shown in this photomicrograph.

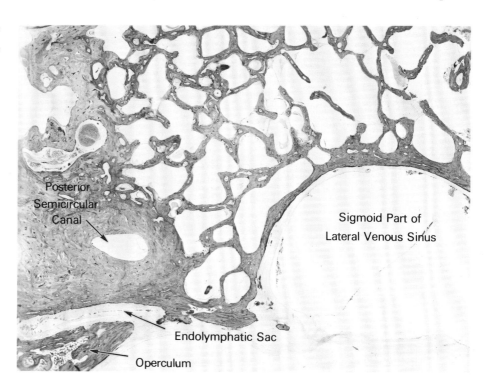

Fig. 2.19: This view shows the jugular bulb extending into the hypotympanic space. In this ear the wall of the jugular vein abuts the tympanic annulus.

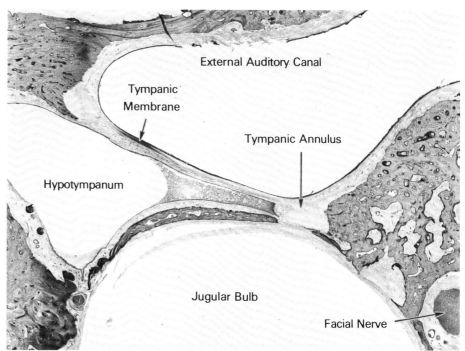

Fig. 2.20: This sketch shows most of the sensory nerves of the middle ear. GSPN is the greater superficial petrosal nerve, and LSPN is the lesser superficial petrosal nerve. OW indicates the oval window and RW the round window. (Courtesy of Montandon, unpublished).

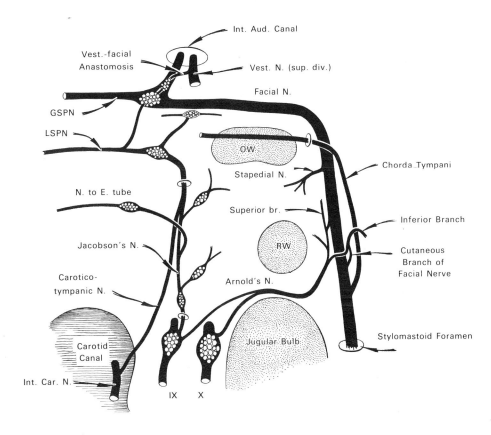

sal sinus passes along the postero-inferior border of the temporal bone in the petrosal sulcus and drains into the jugular bulb. Both carry blood from the cavernous sinus and from adjacent parts of the temporal bone.

5. THE SENSORY NERVES

The nervus intermedius constitutes the sensory root of the facial nerve. It contains sensory taste fibers, secretory fibers, and cutaneous sensory fibers (Van Buskirk, 1945; Foley, 1948; Rhoton et al., 1968; Sunderland and Cossar, 1953). In the internal auditory canal it is joined by a small bundle of fibers from the superior division of the vestibular nerve, which is termed the vestibulo-facial anastomosis (Fig. 2.20). Orzalesi and Pellegrini (1933) observed that part of the intermediate nerve emerges from the brain stem with the vestibular root and then, via this anastomosis, rejoins the main bundle of intermediate nerve fibers in the facial nerve trunk. The neurons for the vestibulo-facial anastomosis are located in a medial extension of the geniculate ganglion. Gacek (1961a) demonstrated in the cat that this anastomotic bundle also contains efferent fibers, the terminations of which are not known.

Those fibers of the nervus intermedius which pass anteriorly from the geniculate ganglion form the greater superficial petrosal nerve. It exits through the facial hiatus, traverses the superior surface of the petrous apex, and enters the foramen lacerum. Here it joins the deep petrosal nerve to form the Vidian nerve which traverses the Vidian canal to reach the sphenopalatine ganglion. Its sensory (taste) fibers have their cell bodies in the geniculate ganglion and, after passing through the sphenopalatine ganglion, are distributed to the soft palate and glossopalatine arches. Its preganglionic secretory fibers have their cell bodies in the superior salivatory nucleus and end in the sphenopalatine ganglion. The postganglionic fibers carry secretory impulses to the lacrimal gland and seromucinous glands in the nasal cavity.

Those fibers of the nervus intermedius which pass posteriorly from the geniculate ganglion form a bundle within the facial nerve trunk and exit as the chorda tympani nerve. This sensory bundle occupies about 10 percent of the cross-sectional area of the facial nerve trunk (Saito et al., 1970) (Fig. 2.21).

Although the chorda tympani nerve may arise almost anywhere along the course of the facial nerve trunk, Kullman et al. (1971) found the average location to be 5.3 mm proximal to the stylomastoid foramen. In two of their specimens the nerve arose outside the temporal bone, and in both instances the nerve had its own separate bony canal parallel to the fallopian canal leading back to the iter chordae posterius. As it passes anteriorly in the tympanic cavity it lies lateral to the long process of the incus and medial to the superior part of the manubrium. Near the petrotympanic fissure it enters the canal of Huguier at the iter chordae anterius. The sensory (taste) fibers of this branch

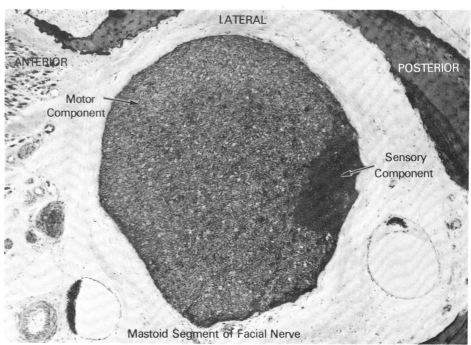

Fig. 2.21: Photomicrograph of the mastoid segment of the facial nerve showing the sensory bundle. The bundle lies in the posterolateral part of the nerve trunk and occupies about 10 percent of the total cross-sectional area of the nerve. (Saito et al., 1970)

have their cell bodies in the geniculate ganglion and are distributed to the anterior two-thirds of the tongue. The preganglionic secretory fibers of the chorda tympani have their cell bodies in the superior salivatory nucleus and end in the submaxillary ganglion. The postganglionic fibers carry secretory impulses to the submandibular and sublingual salivary glands and to the minor salivary glands in the oral cavity.

The tympanic nerve (Jacobson's nerve) arises from the inferior ganglion of the IXth nerve, enters the tympanic cavity through the inferior tympanic canaliculus and ascends in a groove or canal on the medial wall of the middle ear. It provides the main sensory fibers to the mucosa of the mesotympanum and eustachian tube. Along the course of the tympanic nerve there are numerous groups of ganglion cells sometimes referred to as the tympanic ganglia. This nerve is joined by the caroticotympanic nerve which arises from the sympathetic plexus of the internal carotid artery. Both nerves pass superiorly and then join near the superior tympanic canaliculus at the level of the cochleariform process to form the lesser superficial petrosal nerve. The lesser superficial petrosal nerve passes superiorly for a short distance, where it lies medial to the cochleariform process and then turns anteriorly to travel either within the canal but do not appear to join the facial nerve. The tympanic nerve provides preganglionic parotid secretory fibers to the otic ganglion. cells. The most posterior group of ganglion cells provides a twig which enters the fallopian canal and divides into bundles which pass centrally and distally within the canal but do not appear to join the facial nerve. The tympanic nerve provides preganglionic parotid secretory fibers to the otic ganglion.

The auricular branch of the vagus nerve (Arnold's nerve) is formed by a large main branch from the superior ganglion (nodosa) of the Xth nerve and a small branch from the inferior ganglion of the IXth nerve (Arnold, 1831). It passes posteriorly over the dome of the jugular bulb and proceeds within a small bony channel to the fallopian canal where it divides into superior and inferior branches. The superior branch gives off twigs which appear to end in the facial nerve sheath. The inferior branch is joined by a twig from the facial nerve and continues in a bony channel to provide cutaneous sensation to a region of the posterior surface of the external auditory canal (Foley and Dubois, 1943). Hunt (1915) proposed that these fibers were responsible for the cutaneous eruption in the ear canal so commonly seen in herpes zoster oticus.

B. THE EUSTACHIAN TUBE

The primary function of the eustachian tube is to provide ventilation for the pneumatized spaces of the temporal bone. In the adult, the tube varies in length from 31 to 38 mm (1¼″ to 1½″) with the cartilaginous portion constituting two-thirds and the osseous portion one-third of its total length (Graves and Edwards, 1944). The cartilage is shaped like a shepherd's crook with a larger medial and smaller lateral laminae, producing a groove which opens inferiorly and laterally. A dense fibrous membrane, the salpingopharyngeal fascia, is attached to the free edge of the hook-like lateral lamina of the cartilage and to the inferior free edge of the medial lamina. The cartilage is mostly of hyaline structure with an elastic component which is richest along the line of junction of the medial and lateral laminae (Aschan, 1954). The mucous membrane consists of pseudo-stratified ciliated columnar epithelium on a tunica propria of varying thickness. The tunica propria has three layers: (1) a basement membrane immediately beneath the epithelium, (2) a layer of lymphoid tissue of varying thickness, depending upon the age of the individual, and (3) a layer of compound tubulo-alveolar glands (Figs. 2.22, 2.23).

Fig. 2.22: The tunica propria of the eustachian tube consists of a basement membrane immediately beneath the epithelium and a layer of compound tubulo-alveolar glands. A layer of lymphoid tissue is often present, presumably in amounts determined by the response of the reticuloendothelial system to local inflammation. The fossa of Rosenmueller is located immediately posterior to the tubal orifice.

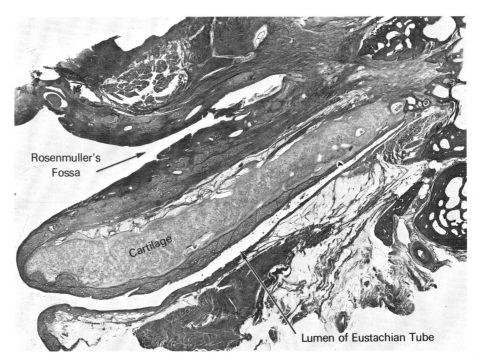

Fig. 2.23: The mucous membrane of the eustachian tube consists of pseudostratified ciliated columnar epithelium on a tunica propria of varying thickness.

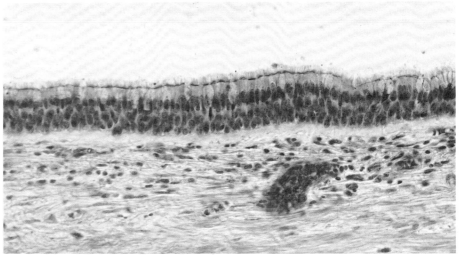

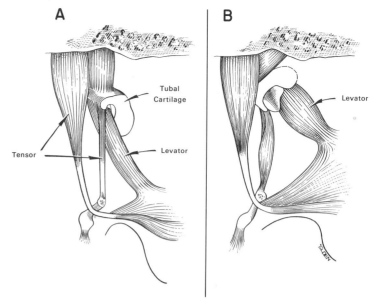

Lymphatic tissue located in the lateral pharyngeal walls surrounding the eustachian tube was first described by Rüdinger (1870) and by Gerlach (1875) and has been referred to as "Gerlach's tubal tonsil." More recent studies (Aschan, 1954, Farrior, 1943) have failed to reveal a discrete lymphatic structure in this region which could be considered to be analogous to the palatine tonsils. Aschan points out that the collections of lymphocytes found in the submucosal layers of the eustachian tube and surrounding areas represent a cellular proliferation from the reticulo-endothelial system in response to inflammation and is approximately termed lymphoid tissue. Most studies showing lymphoid tissue in the submucosa of the eustachian tube (Fowler, 1944, 1945, 1946) involve specimens from patients suffering from inflammatory disease of the pharynx or ear. Eggston and Wolff (1947) and Aschan (1954) have found no evidence on histological studies to indicate that lymphatic tissue of the nasopharynx ever extends as far as the pharyngeal orifice of the eustachian tube or invades it.

The osseous portion of the tube opens obliquely in an anterolateral direction at its junction with the tubal cartilage. This region marks the isthmus, or narrowest region of the tube, and is bounded posteromedially and inferiorly by bone, and anterolaterally and superiorly by cartilage. The tympanic ostium of the tube is located in the anterior wall of the tympanic cavity about 4 mm above the most inferior part of the floor of the cavity. The ostium is triangular in shape and measures 3 to 5 mm in diameter. The lumen gradually narrows to the isthmus where it is 2 to 3 mm in vertical dimension and 1 to 1½ mm in width. The epithelium of the osseous portion is a low columnar ciliated type with numerous goblet cells. The tunica propria consists of a basement membrane and loose connective tissue.

An exhaustive description of the relationships of the eustachian tube to the palatal muscles and other adjacent structures can be found in a manuscript by Proctor (1967) (Fig. 2.24). Normally, in the resting position the eustachian tube is closed by the passive spring effect of the cartilage and by the pressure of surrounding tissues (Zöllner, 1942; Guild, 1955). During deglutition, three muscles—the tensor veli palati, the levator veli palati, and the salpingopharyngeus—cause the tube to open. The tensor veli palati, the most important muscle involved in tubal opening, takes origin from the spine of the sphenoid bone, the scaphoid fossa, the lateral lamina of the tubal cartilage, and the salpingopharyngeal fascia (Graves and Edwards, 1944). Its flat belly projects antero-inferiorly to form a tendon which hooks around the hamulus of the medial pterygoid plate and passes medially to insert into the soft palate (Holborrow, 1962; Rich, 1920). The muscle is supplied by the mandibular division of the trigeminal nerve. Some of the muscle bundles of the tensor veli palati extend superiorly to become contiguous with the tensor tympani muscle (Lupin, 1969). The levator veli palati muscle takes origin from the inferior surface of the petrous bone and from the inferior border of the medial lamina of the tubal cartilage and passes inferior and parallel to the cartilage to end in the soft palate where the muscle bundles interdigitate with those of the opposite side. The salpingopharyngeus muscle takes origin from the most medial and inferior aspect of the medial lamina of the tubal cartilage and passes inferiorly to blend with the palatopharyngeus muscle.

C. THE FACIAL NERVE

The facial nerve arises from the second branchial arch along with the facial musculature (Jepsen, 1965). Its fibers provide the following functions: (1) efferent fibers, which have an orderly arrangement in the facial nerve trunk (May, 1973), to the striated musculature of the face and neck, to the stylohyoid, to the posterior belly of the digastric, and to the stapedius muscles; (2) efferent preganglionic fibers of secretory function for the lacrimal glands and seromucinous glands of the nasal cavity via the greater superficial petrosal nerve and for the submaxillary and sublingual glands via the chorda tympani nerve; (3) afferent fibers conveying taste impulses from the anterior two-thirds of the tongue via the chorda tympani nerve and from the palate and tonsilar fossae via the greater superficial petrosal nerve; and (4) afferent fibers carrying proprioceptive sensation from the facial muscles and cutaneous sensation from the external auditory canal and adjacent conchal region.

Three nuclei supply the facial nerve: (1) the motor nucleus, which is located in the caudal part of the pons with its superior part receiving bilateral innervation from the motor cortex and supplying the frontal and orbicularis oculi muscles, and its inferior part receiving unilateral uncrossed cortical innervation; (2) the superior salivatory nucleus, which is located dorsal to the motor nucleus and conveys parasympathetic secretory impulses to the lacrimal glands, seromucinous glands of the nasal cavity, and submaxillary and sublingual glands; (3) the nucleus of the solitary tract, which lies in the medulla oblongata and receives taste, proprioceptive, and cutaneous sensory fibers from the facial nerve.

The facial nerve arises at the inferior border of the pons. As it proceeds toward the internal auditory canal, it lies in a groove on the superior surface of the cochlear nerve. This intracranial segment is 23 to 24 mm in length. The internal auditory canal segment is 7 to 8 mm in length and lies in a superior relationship to the cochlear nerve, passing above the transverse crest to enter the area nervi facialis. The labyrinthine segment, which is 3 to 4 mm in length, begins at the area nervi facialis and passes forward and laterally at nearly right angles to the petrous pyramid, just superior to the cochlea and vestibule, to reach the geniculate ganglion. At the geniculate ganglion the nerve makes a sharp posterior angulation. This first genu marks the beginning of the tympanic segment, which is 12 to 13 mm in length and passes posteriorly and laterally, parallel to the longitudinal axis of the petrous bone, on the medial wall of the tympanic cavity superior to the oval window and inferior to the lateral semicircular canal. At the sinus tympani the nerve bends inferiorly. This second genu marks the beginning of the mastoid segment, which is 15 to 20 mm in length and passes vertically downward in the posterior wall of the tympanic cavity and anterior wall of the mastoid to reach the stylomastoid foramen where it exits from the skull.

The primary branches of the facial nerve are (1) the greater superficial petrosal, which arises from the geniculate ganglion and ends in the sphenopalatine ganglion in the pterygopalatine fossa; (2) the nerve to the stapedius muscle which leaves the mastoid segment in the region of the pyramidal eminence to supply this muscle; and (3) the chorda tympani, which leaves the facial nerve about 5 mm above the stylomastoid foramen and ends in the lingual nerve in the parapharyngeal space.

The facial nerve may pursue anomalous courses through the petrous bone (Basek, 1962); Duncan et al., 1967; Shambaugh, 1967; Wright et al., 1967). The main nerve trunk may take a devious course, the most common being anterior and inferior to the oval window. A deviant course anterior to both windows is extremely rare (Dickinson et al., 1968; Fowler, 1961). It may divide into two or more branches at any position along its course, and these branches may proceed in juxtaposition or become widely divergent.

Jepsen (1965) presented the following scheme for the topographic diagnosis of lesions along the facial nerve: (1) *infrachordal*—this lesion is located inferior to the chorda tympani branch and does not alter taste, lacrimation, or the stapedial reflex; (2) *infrastapedial*—this lesion is located between the chorda tympani branch and the nerve to the stapedius muscle and affects taste but has no affect on lacrimation or the stapedial reflex; (3) *suprastapedial*—such a lesion is located between the nerve to the stapedius muscle and the geniculate ganglion and affects taste and the stapedial reflex but has no affect on lacrimation; (4) *suprageniculate*—this lesion is located between the geniculate ganglion and motor nucleus and affects taste, lacrimation, and the stapedial reflex. Methods for the testing of taste, lacrimation, and stapedial reflexes, as well as motor and cutaneous functions, are clearly described in several publications (Kettel, 1959, Meihlke, 1960, Copenhagen Symposium, 1965; Symposium of Otoneurology Group, 1970).

Gabriele Falloppio (cited by Politzer, 1907) first described the facial canal as an "aquaeductus" because it reminded him of a water pipe; however, he did not allude to any gaps in its walls. In an earlier textbook, Politzer (1894) wrote of "congenital gaps in the facial canal" and observed that "part of the canal which traverses the tympanic cavity sometimes presents dihiscences of varying sizes." Baxter (1971) found dehiscences in 294 (55 percent) of 535 temporal bones studied from microscopic sections. Dehiscences were common in the oval window region and occasional in the vertical segment as well as in the region of the genu of the nerve (Fig. 2.25). He found the average width of the dehiscences to be 0.92 mm in the region of the oval window and 0.73 mm in the vertical segment. From histological studies (Kikuchi, 1907; Iida, 1951) and from other observations (Fowler, 1947; Guild, 1949; Hough, 1958; Kaplan, 1960; Beddard and Saunders, 1962) the area of the canal near the oval window has been recognized as the most common site for dehiscence. The total myelinated nerve fiber population (sensory and motor) in the facial nerve trunk distal to the geniculate ganglion ranges from about 12,000 to 20,000 and decreases after the fourth decade of life (Van Buskirk, 1945; Kullman et al., 1971).

D. THE INNER EAR

1. THE BONY LABYRINTH

The bony labyrinth develops from the primitive otic capsule and consists of the vestibule, semicircular canals, and cochlea (Fig. 2.26).

The vestibule measures about 4 mm in diameter and leads anteriorly into the cochlea and posteriorly into the semicircular canals. The wall of the vestibule is marked by the elliptical recess for the utricle and the spherical recess for the saccule. Between these recesses lies the vestibular crest, which divides posteriorly into two limbs between which is located the cochlear recess for the vestibular cecum of the cochlear duct. The cribrose areas consist of groups of small foramina through which the vestibular nerve bundles enter the vestibule. Other openings in the vestibule are the vestibular aqueduct and the oval window.

Each of the three bony semicircular canals makes two-thirds of a circle, lies at right angles to the other two, and measures about 1 mm in diameter. Each is enlarged at one end to form the bony ampulla. The nonampullated ends of the superior and posterior semicircular canals join to form the common crus.

The bony cochlea contains a base lying at the anterolateral aspect of the internal auditory canal and an apex directed anterolaterally and inferiorly.

The axial length of the cochlea is about 5 mm. It is shaped into a spiral canal about 31 to 33 mm in length which winds 2½ turns around the modiolus and ends at the apex in the hook-like hamulus. The osseous lamina spirals about the modiolus, incompletely subdividing the spiral canal into the scala vestibuli and scala tympani which join at the helicotrema.

2. THE MEMBRANOUS LABYRINTH

The membranous labyrinth is enclosed within the bony labyrinth. The outer layer is generally separated from the periosteum of the bony labyrinth by a space containing perilymphatic fluid and is supported in this fluid by a weblike network containing blood vessels (Bast and Anson, 1949). Among the early investigators who made important observations on the membranous

Fig. 2.25: Photomicrograph of the anterior epitympanic area showing a dehiscence in the facial canal near the genu of the facial nerve (Female, age 72).

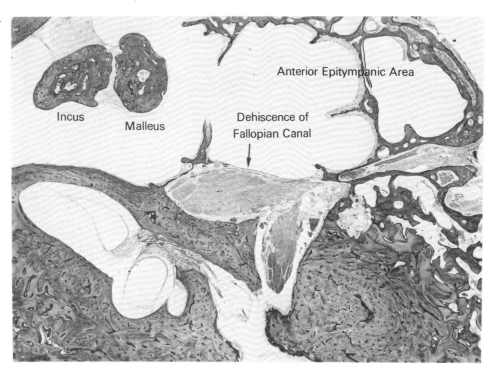

Fig. 2.26: This sketch shows the bony labyrinth. (Drawing after Sobotta, 1957)

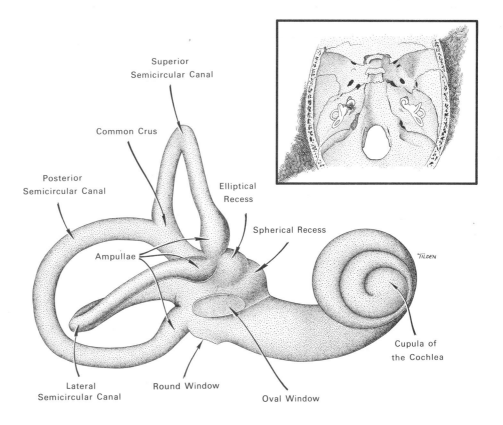

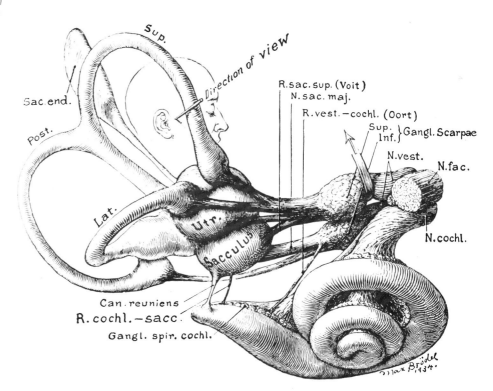

Fig. 2.27: This drawing is by Max Brödel (1946) and shows the membranous labyrinth and its afferent nerve supply.

Fig. 2.28: This photograph shows the human membranous labyrinth stained with Sudan black and dissected from the bony labyrinth. (Courtesy of Gacek).

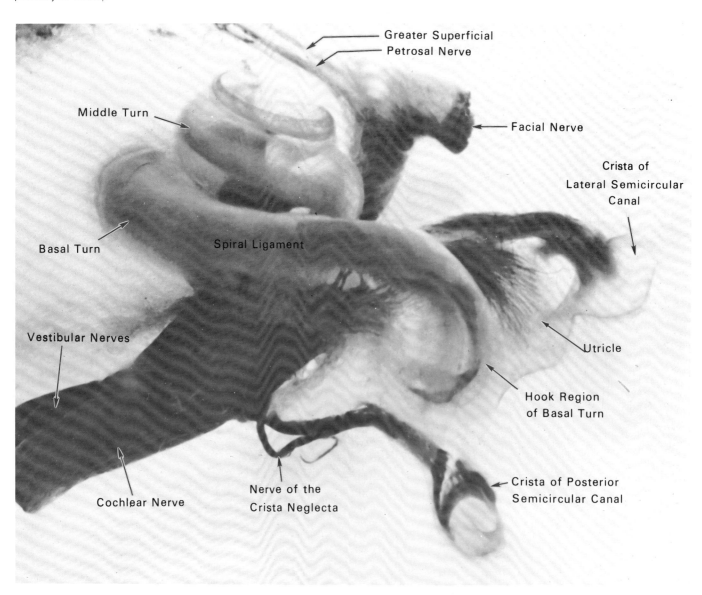

labyrinth are Steifensand (1835), Scarpa (1800), and Retzius (1881, 1884). A drawing of the membranous labyrinth by Brödel appears in Fig. 2.27 and a photograph of a dissected preparation by Gacek in Fig. 2.28.

a. The cochlear duct

The cochlear duct is a spiral membranous canal located between the osseous spiral lamina and external bony wall of the cochlea (Fig. 2.29). With the osseous spiral lamina it completes the subdivision of the bony spiral canal into the scala vestibuli and scala tympani. The basal end of the cochlear duct terminates in the vestibular cecum, from which it communicates with the saccule via the ductus reuniens. The apical end terminates blindly in the cupular cecum. The spiral ligament is located in a sulcus on the external wall of the bony cochlear duct and is lined on its internal surface by the stria vascularis, spiral prominence, and external sulcus cells. It serves for the external attachments of the basilar membrane and Reissner's membrane.

Reissner's membrane is a thin membrane extending obliquely from the vestibular crest of the spiral ligament to the spiral limbus. The spiral limbus is situated on the osseous spiral lamina and has an inner sulcus covered with epithelial cells and a free surface lined with interdental cells to which is attached the tectorial membrane.

The basilar membrane extends from the tympanic lip of the osseous spiral lamina to the basilar crest of the spiral ligament and carries the organ of Corti on the scala media side.

Huschke (1824) was the first to mention the basilar papilla and to consider it as the excitatory structure of the cochlea. Utilizing a technique of microdissection, Corti (1851) provided the first description of the cytoarchitecture of this structure after which it has been termed Corti's organ. Later studies by Boettcher (1869), Retzius (1884), Held (1926), and Kolmer (1927) provided a description of the detailed structure of the organ of Corti as it is currently known by light microscopy.

The principal cytological structures include the pillar cells, Deiters' cells, Hensen's cells, hair cells, and internal and external sulcus cells (Figs. 2.30,

Fig. 2.29: Diagrammatic sketch showing the cytological structures of the cochlear duct. (Courtesy of Davis, 1962)

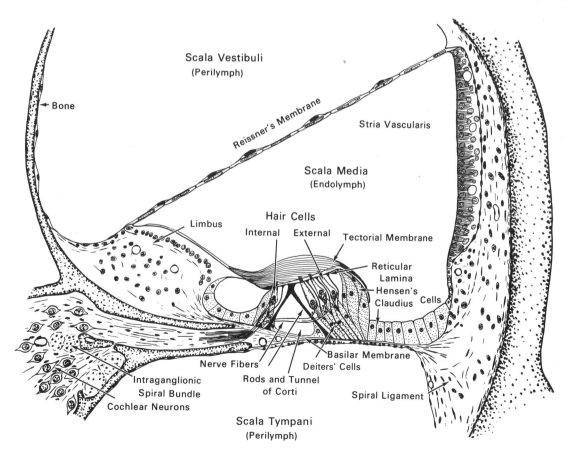

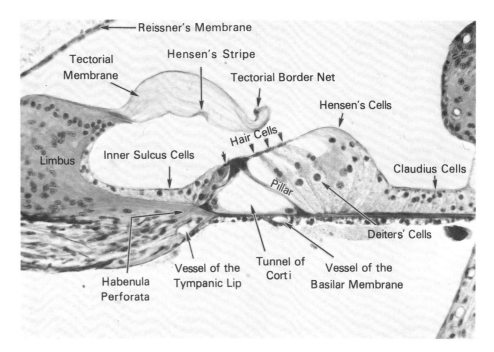

Fig. 2.30: Photomicrograph of the organ of Corti of the cat. Fixation was performed by intravital arterial perfusion with Heidenhain-Susa solution.

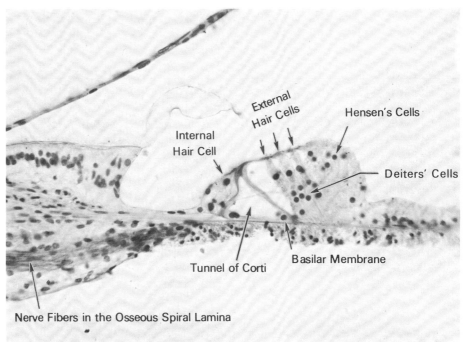

Fig. 2.31: Photomicrograph of the organ of Corti of a 28-year-old human. The temporal bone was removed and placed in 10 percent formalin solution one hour and 15 minutes after death.

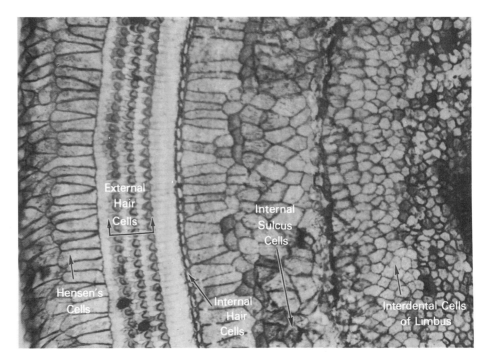

Fig. 2.32: Surface preparation showing the cellular structures on the basilar membrane of the guinea pig. Silver-hematoxylin-eosin stain (Courtesy of Watanuki, 1968)

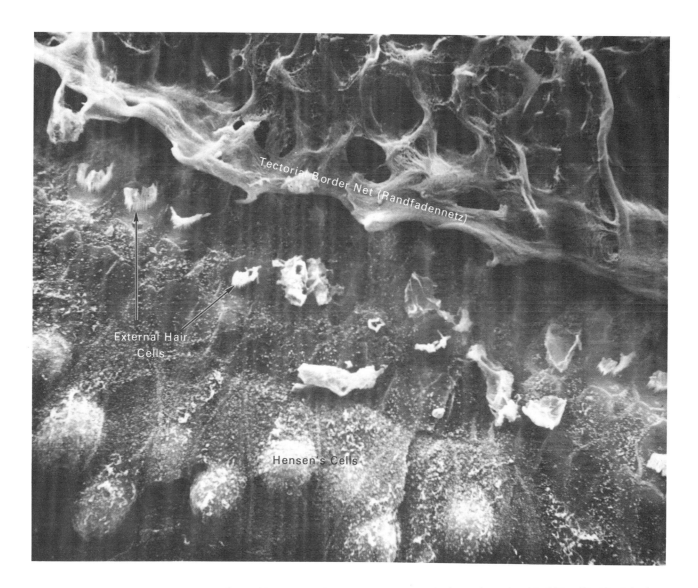

Fig. 2.33: Transmission electron micrograph showing the tectorial border net (Randfadennezt). (Courtesy of Lim)

2.31, 2.32). According to Retzius (1884), the basilar membrane in man is 33½ mm in length and its width is 104 microns at the basal end and 504 microns at the apical end. He found the human cochlea to contain 3,500 internal hair cells and 12,000 external hair cells.

The tectorial membrane is a gelatinous structure extending from the vestibular lip of the limbus over the organ of Corti and ending in the border net (Randfadennetz) which overlies Hensen's cells (Fig. 2.33).

Far greater details have subsequently been elucidated through the use of transmission electron microscopy (Smith, 1957; Engström and Wersäll, 1958a, 1958b; Friedmann, 1959; Wersäll, 1960; Lundquist, 1965; Flock, 1965; Hilding, 1965; Spoendlin, 1966; Kimura, 1966; Iurato 1967; Duvall, 1969) and scanning electron microscopy (Lim, 1969; Bredberg et al., 1970).

The external hair cells in mature form contain no internal supporting structure and maintain their elongated cylindrical shape by support from adjacent cells. The apices of these cells are held by the reticular membrane (Fig. 2.34) and the bases by the shallow cups of Deiters' cells. The hair cells contain only stereocilia, being devoid of kinocilia. These cilia stand perpendicular to the sensory cell surface, and each cilium is anchored by a dense tubular-like rootlet within the cuticular plate. Each external hair cell carries from 46 to 148 stereocilia in a W-shaped pattern (Figs. 2.35, 2.36, 2.37). In cats and guinea pigs the "W" contains about three rows of cilia, whereas in human beings there are six to seven rows (Kimura et al., 1964). These cilia measure about 2 microns in length in the basal turn and about 6 microns in the apical turn. In the external hair cells the mitochondria are concentrated in the subapical area and the infranuclear area (Retzius body). Other cytoplasmic organelles are concentrated along the cell walls, whereas the supranuclear

Fig. 2.34: Surface preparation showing hair cells of the organ of Corti of a 45-year-old man with normal hearing. (Courtesy of Johnsson)

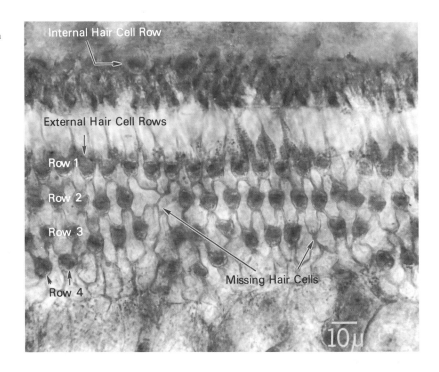

Fig. 2.35: Scanning electron micrograph showing the ciliary tufts of three rows of external hair cells near the apex of the guinea pig cochlea. They are arranged in a W formation with the point of the W facing the spiral ligament. The gradations in height are clearly evident in this view (7,200 x). (Courtesy of Lim)

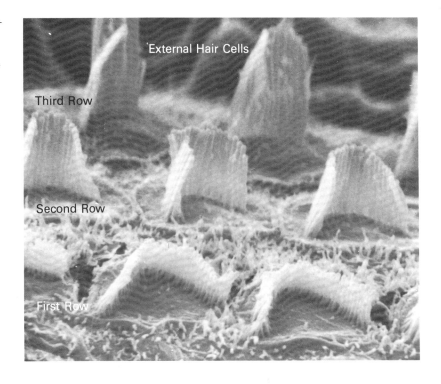

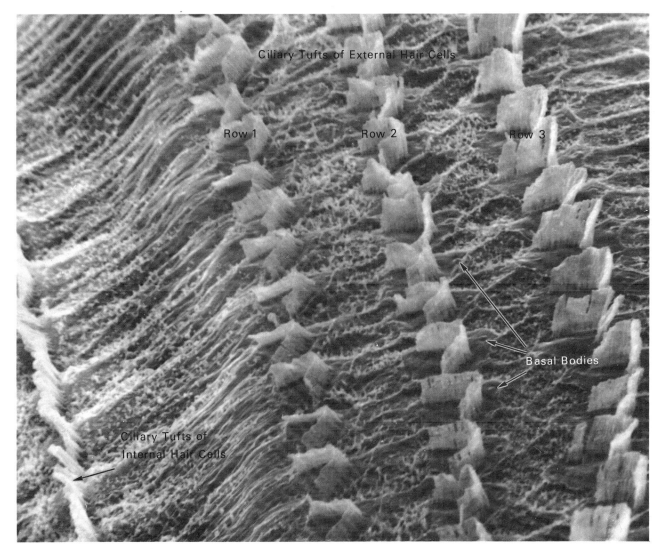

Fig. 2.36: **Scanning** electron micrograph show-ing the ciliary tufts of the three rows of outer **hair** cells of the guinea pig. (Courtesy of **Lim**)

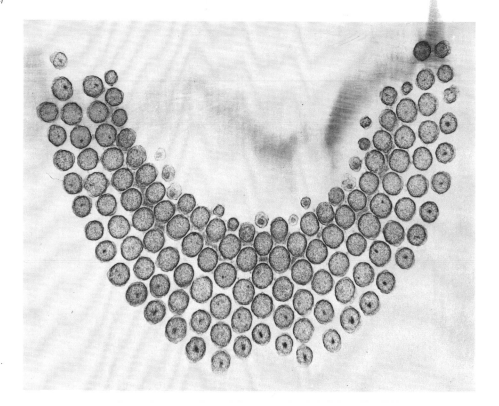

Fig. 2.37: Electron micrograph of cross section of ciliary tuft of human external hair cells. (Courtesy of Kimura and Ota)

Fig. 2.38: This is a conceptual diagram of the external hair cell showing the intracellular organelles and the relationship to the afferent and efferent nerve endings. (Courtesy of Lim and Melnick, 1971)

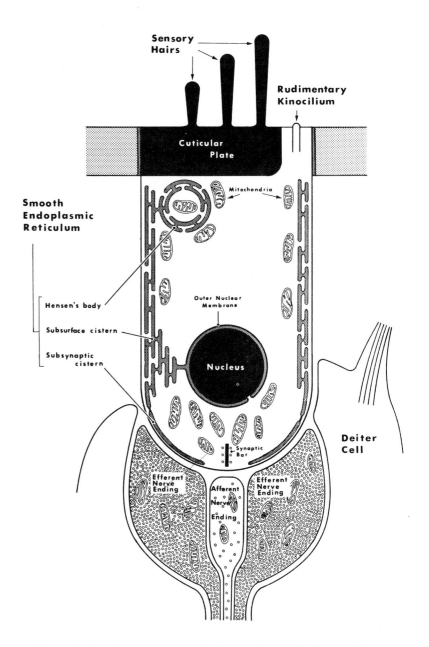

area is relatively free (Figs. 2.38, 2.39). The nuclei of the hair cells are usually rich in chromatin and contain distinct nucleoli.

The internal hair cells have a pear-like shape and, except at the apex, are completely surrounded by internal pillar cells, internal phalangeal cells, and border cells (Fig. 2.40). Their stereocilia number about 120 and are coarser than those of the external hair cells (Fig. 2.41). The mitochondria of the internal hair cells are irregularly distributed; the nucleus is centrally located, and many Golgi structures are seen in the supranuclear zone.

The pillar cells perform a predominantly supportive function. Their cell bodies are very small and sit on the basilar membrane. A great number of supporting filaments constitute the main internal structure of the pillars. These filaments extend to a large, homogeneous basal foot which rests on the basilar membrane. At their opposite ends the pillars widen into massive pillar heads which have a structure comparable to the cuticular plates of the hair cells.

Deiters' cells have very large cell bodies which rest on the basilar membrane and extend to the bases of the external hair cells, where they form cups for the support of the hair cells. The upper portions of the cell bodies have numerous cytoplasmic organelles. They contain bundles of supporting filaments which originate above the basilar membrane, some of which extend to the supporting cup and others through Nuel's space to the apices of the external hair cells where they help to form the reticular membrane (Ades et al., 1972). The reticular membrane is formed by the combined extensions of the pillar cells and Deiters' cells and fills the spaces between the apical portions of the external hair cells. The reticular membrane provides a tight

2.39

Fig. 2.39: Transmission electron micrograph of the external hair cells of the guinea pig (4,300 x). (Courtesy of Kimura and Ota)

Fig. 2.40: Transmission electron micrograph of internal hair cell area. (Courtesy of Kimura and Ota, 1971)

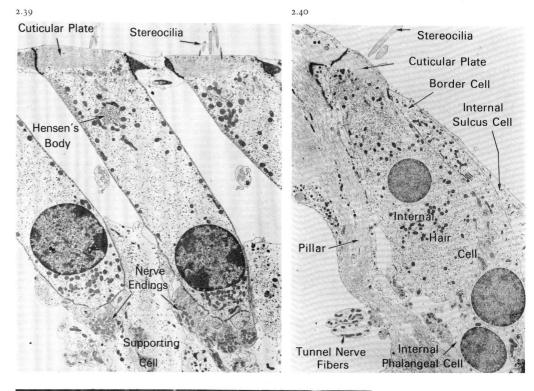

Fig. 2.41: Scanning electron micrograph of the ciliary tuft of an internal hair cell of the guinea pig (15,400 x). (Courtesy of Lim)

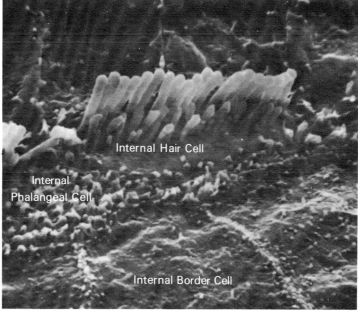

closure between the endolymphatic surface of the organ of Corti and its interior extracellular spaces (Spoendlin, 1966).

Hensen's cells and the inner sulcus cells are the least differentiated of the cell types in the organ of Corti. Hensen's cells are characterized by a lack of cytoplasmic organelles. They consist mainly of the cell membrane, nucleus, and translucent cytoplasm. The cells have a very elongated form in the basilar turn, becoming flatter toward the apical region. Their endolymphatic surfaces contain numerous microvilli (Engström and Wersäll, 1953).

The basilar membrane consists of extracellular material and connective tissue cell layers. It has bundles of fine (50 A) radially oriented fibrils, a rather amorphous ground substance, and, along the vestibular surface, a thick membrane resembling a basement membrane which is separated from the plasma membrane of the cells of the organ of Corti (Iurato, 1967). The basilar membrane is narrower and thicker at the basal end and thinner and wider in the apical region.

The surface of the limbus can be divided into three zones: (1) the zone facing the scala media, (2) the zone facing the inner spiral sulcus, and (3) the zone facing the scala vestibuli. Borghesan (1950) termed the latter zone the vasculo-epithelial zone. Ishiyama et al. (1970) found the vasculo-epithelial

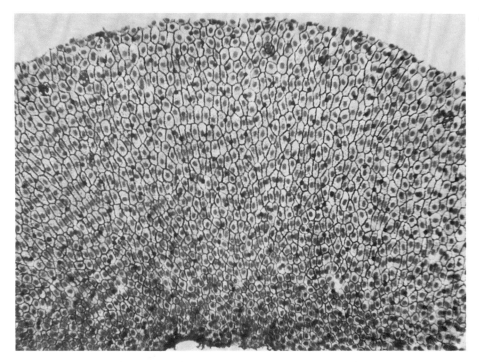

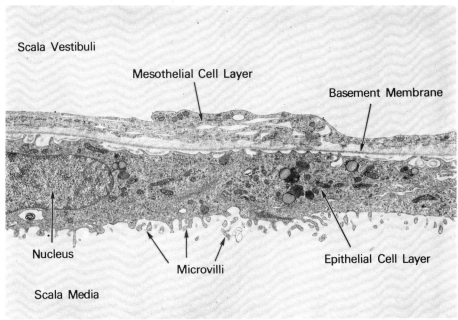

zone to be composed of osmiophilic (dark) and osmiophobic (light) cells. The ultrastructural characteristics of these cells suggests that this zone may be capable of active fluid transport.

The spiral ligament consists of a complicated arrangement of connective tissue cells, intercellular substances, and blood vessels. The connective tissue cells (fibrocytes) are of two types and establish numerous attachments with each other (fascia occludens, fascia adherens, macula adherens) (Takahashi and Kimura, 1970; Takahashi, 1971).

The external sulcus cells form a continuous band throughout the cochlear duct extending from the basilar membrane to the middle of the spiral prominence (Shambaugh, 1908). These cells abut the endolymphatic surface and contain pegs which extend deeply into the spiral ligament and are surrounded by a network of capillaries (Duvall, 1969).

Reissner's membrane is 2 to 3 microns in thickness and consists of a simple squamous epithelium with numerous microvilli on the endolymphatic surface and a layer of connective tissue cells on the perilymphatic surface. The two layers are separated by a distinct basement membrane (Figs. 2.42, 2.43).

The stria vascularis consists of a band of superficial specific tissue, lying on the internal surface of the spiral ligament and extending from the spiral prominence to Reissner's membrane. Light microscopic preparations reveal the stria to be very dense with numerous capillaries passing mainly in the longitudinal direction. Three types of cells may be identified in the stria vascularis proper, these being the marginal (chromophil) cells on the endolymphatic surface, the intermediate (chromophobe) cells, and the basal cells adjacent to the spiral ligament (Smith, 1957). The marginal cells are characterized by a very dark osmiophilic appearance and have nuclei close to the endolymphatic surface with large basal extensions which interdigitate with the intermediate cells. The intermediate cells contain nuclei which lie in the middle part of the stria, and both the nucleus and cytoplasm are much less dense than the marginal cells (Fig. 2.44). They never extend to the endolymphatic surface and frequently contain large amounts of melanin pigment. The basal cells lie on the spiral ligament, and their nuclei and cytoplasm resemble the fibrocytes of the spiral ligament (Kimura and Schuknecht, 1970a, 1970b).

The spiral prominence has a single surface layer of small cuboidal cells which lie between the stria on one side and the outer sulcus cells on the other.

The tectorial membrane consists of three zones (Iurato, 1960; Lim, 1972): (1) the inner limbal zone, which is inserted into the horizontal part of the interdental cells; (2) the middle zone, which is situated on the organ of Corti; and (3) the outer marginal zone, which consists of outer edge of the membrane and corresponds to the border plexus (Löwemberg, 1864) or "randfadennetz" (Held, 1926; Kolmer, 1927; deVries, 1949). Iurato (1960) found the tectorial membrane to be made up of submicroscopic non-anastomosing filaments of indeterminate length embedded in an amorphous substance. These filaments run transversely, following a rather wavy course.

Fig. 2.44: Transmission electron micrograph of the stria vascularis of the squirrel monkey. (Courtesy of Kimura and Ota)

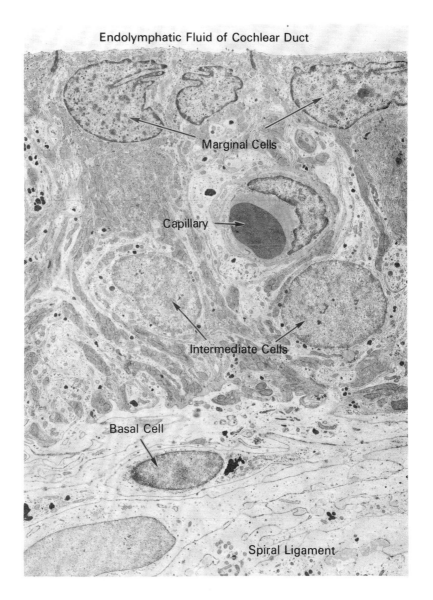

Endolymphatic Fluid of Cochlear Duct

Marginal Cells

Capillary

Intermediate Cells

Basal Cell

Spiral Ligament

Lim (1972) found the tallest rows of the external hair cell stereocilia to be firmly embedded in the Hardesty's membrane, which is part of the marginal zone, and noted that Hensen's stripe is the area where the tectorial membrane is anchored to the internal phalangeal and border cells.

b. The vestibular sense organs

The saccule is a flattened, irregularly shaped sac which lies in the spherical recess on the medial wall of the vestibule (Fig. 2.45). Its membranous wall projects superiorly to reach the wall of the utricle where it has a broad attachment without any communication. The lateral part of the saccular wall, adjacent to the vestibular wall, shows a well-defined thickening termed the "reinforced area" (Perlman, 1940). The macula sacculi is hook-shaped and lies in a predominantly vertical position. The saccule communicates with the sinus of the endolymphatic duct by the saccular duct and with the cochlear duct by the ductus reuniens.

The utricle is an irregular oval-shaped tube lying superior to the saccule in the elliptical recess of the medial wall of the vestibule. The macula of the utricle lies mainly in the horizontal plane and is located in the utricular recess which is the dilated anterior portion of the utricle (Fig. 2.46). The utricular duct leaves the inferior part of the utricle via a cleft-shaped opening and passes close to the utricular wall to enter the sinus of the endolymphatic duct. A thickened part of the utricular wall at this cleft-shaped opening forms the utriculo-endolymphatic valve (Retzius, 1884; Werner, 1940).

The three semicircular canals communicate with the utricle via five openings, one of which is formed by the union of the nonampullated ends of the superior and posterior canals and is termed the common crus. The membranous canals assume an eccentric position in contact with the external surfaces of the bony canals. In man, with the head in the erect position, the lateral canal forms a 30° angle from the horizontal plane. Near the utricular opening each canal is enlarged to form a membranous ampulla, the base of which is attached to bone. A crest-like septum (crista) crosses the base of the ampulla, is made up of sensory epithelium distributed on a mound of connective tissue, blood vessels, and nerve fibers, and covered by the gelatinous

Fig. 2.45: Sketch of the vestibular part of the membranous labyrinth. (After Brödel, 1946)

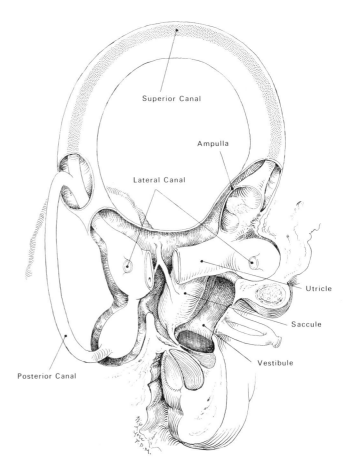

Fig. 2.46: Vertical section through the temporal bone showing the relationship of the utricle and posterior canal ampulla to the oval and round windows.

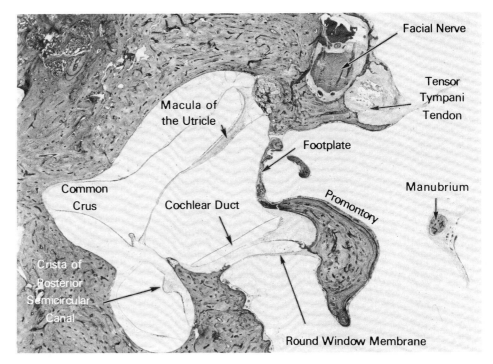

cupula. This cupula extends to the opposing wall of the ampulla (Steinhausen, 1933; Dohlman, 1938). In some species (birds, turtles, some mammals but not man), the sensory epithelium of the posterior and superior canal is divided by a transverse bar of cylindrical cells referred to as the septum cruciatum (Steifensand, 1835; Gacek 1961b; Igarashi and Yoshinobu, 1966). On the ampullary walls at each end of the crista is a zone of cubical or cylindrical cells which form a half-moon-shaped area termed the semilunar planes (Fig. 2.47). A zone of transitional epithelium is located along the sides of the crista beyond which is a zone containing dark cells (Kimura et al., 1963; Mira and dal Negro, 1969). The dark cells are characterized by numerous basal plasma membrane infoldings and are thought to have a secretory function (Kimura, 1969).

The vestibular sensory epithelia are located on the macula sacculi, the macula utriculi, and the ampullae of the three semicircular canals. Retzius (1881; 1884) found a uniformity of structure in the vestibular sense organs of all vertebrates.

The vestibular sense organs, like the organ of Corti, contain two types of hair cells (Wersäll, 1956), presumably of different functional significance (Fig. 2.48). The type I hair cells, which correspond to the internal hair cells of the organ of Corti, are shaped like ancient Greek wine bottles, with round bottoms, thin necks, and wider heads (Fig. 2.49). Each cell is surrounded by a nerve chalice from one of the terminal branches of a thick or medium nerve

Fig. 2.47: Sketch demonstrating the structural organization of the ampulla and crista. (After Mira and dal Negro, 1969)

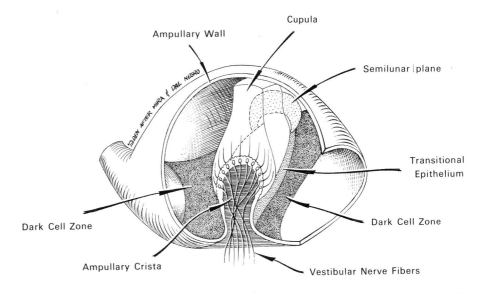

fiber of the vestibular nerve. Occasionally two or three hair cells may be included in the same nerve chalice. The type II hair cells correspond to the external hair cells of the organ of Corti and are shaped like cylinders with a flat upper surface covered by a cuticle. A tuft of cilia protrudes from the free ends of each hair cell.

It was already known early in this century (van der Stricht, 1908; Held, 1909) that in each tuft there was one cilium that was different from the others. This special cilium, known as the kinocilium, emerges from the basal body of the cell. It is unlikely that the kinocilium is actively motile in the fully differentiated hair cell as it does not have an identical structure with

Fig. 2.48: Schematic drawing of the vestibular sensory epithelium. The type I hair cell has a flask-shaped form and is enveloped by a calyciform nerve ending. The type II hair cell is cylindrical in shape and is innervated by numerous small afferent and efferent nerve endings. (Courtesy of Wersäll, 1956)

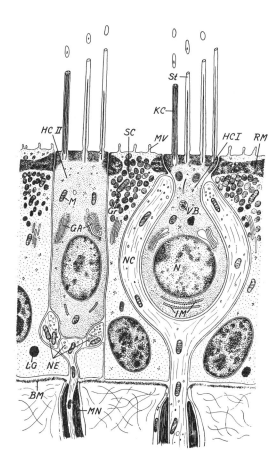

Fig. 2.49: Type I hair cells in the crista of the squirrel monkey. (Courtesy of Kimura)

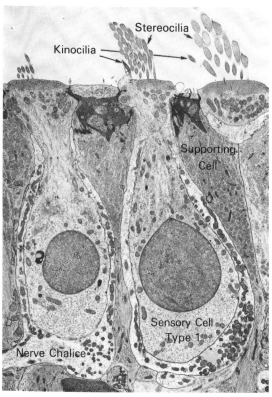

54   Anatomy

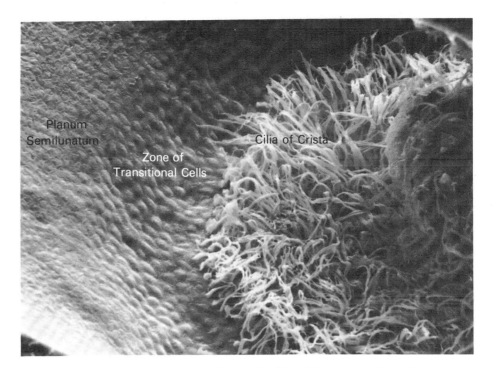

the motile kinocilia of various other epithelia of the human body. It is composed of nine peripheral dense fibers and an intermittent central density
(Hamilton, 1969). The kinocilium is always located at the periphery of the
bundle of stereocilia.

The stereocilia vary in length in the different sense organs, being shortest
in the maculae where they are only a few microns long. Here they are embedded in the gelatinous otolithic membrane. The stereocilia of the cristae measure up to 36 microns in length and protrude into the gelatinous cupula (Lim,
1971) (Fig. 2.50).

Wersäll (1956) and Spoendlin (1965) reported finding a concentration of
type I hair cells on the summit of the cristae. Lindeman (1969a, 1969b), on the
other hand, found the distribution of type I and type II hair cells to be uniform throughout the cristae although 60 percent were type I cells. He also
found the surface areas of the cristae of the guinea pig to measure about 0.360
sq mm with a total number of about 5,500 hair cells.

In the cristae of the lateral semicircular canal the polarization is toward the
utricle, that is, the kinocilium is located on the utricular side of the ciliary
tuft, whereas for the superior and posterior canal cristae, the polarization is
away from the utricle (Figs. 2.51, 2.52). The functional significance of sensory
polarization of the vestibular system is discussed in Chapter 3B, The Vestibular System.

Smith (1956) demonstrated that the sensory epithelium of the maculae has
the same general morphological structure as the cristae. Werner (1933) and
others (Engström et al., 1962; Spoendlin, 1965) have shown that, on a morphological basis, each macula may be divided into two areas by a narrow
curved zone which extends through its middle. This zone has been termed
the striola. Lindeman (1969a, 1969b) found that the striola of the guinea pig
constitutes 13 percent of the macula sacculi and 8 percent of the macula utriculi. He termed that part of the macula on the convex side of the striola as
the "pars externa" and that on the concave side as the "pars interna." He
found the macula sacculi of the guinea pig had an average surface area of
0.495 sq mm and contained about 7,500 hair cells, while the macula utriculi
had a surface area of 0.541 sq mm and contained about 9,000 hair cells.

Engström and Wersäll (1958a, 1958b) and Lindeman (1969a, 1969b) reported a higher concentration of type I hair cells in the striolae and an equal
distribution of type I and type II hair cells elsewhere in the maculae. Each
bundle of sensory hairs protruding from the free surfaces of the hair cells
of the maculae was composed of 50 to 110 stereocilia and 1 kinocilium. In
each bundle of stereocilia those closest to the kinocilium were the longest,

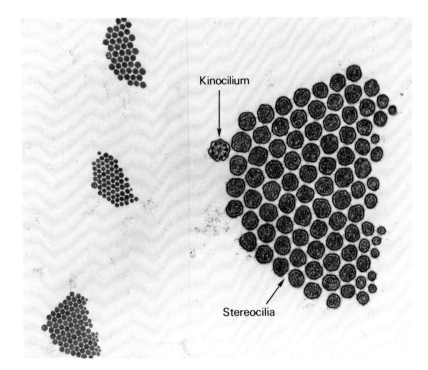

Fig. 2.51: Transmission electron micrograph showing cilia of a crista of the squirrel monkey. Each hair cell contains one kinocilium and about 50 to 100 stereocilia. In the crista of the lateral semicircular canal the kinocilium is located on the utricular side of the hair cell tuft whereas the opposite is true for the superior and posterior canals. (Courtesy of Spoendlin, 1965)

Kinocilium

Stereocilia

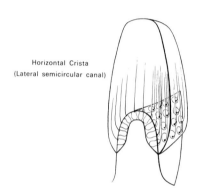

Horizontal Crista
(Lateral semicircular canal)

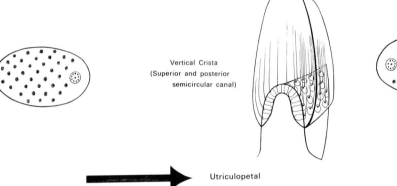

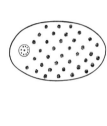

Vertical Crista
(Superior and posterior semicircular canal)

Utriculopetal

Fig. 2.52: Sketch illustrating ciliary polarization of the semicircular canals. (After Spoendlin, 1965)

their lengths becoming progressively shorter as the distance increased from the kinocilium (Fig. 2.53). Each hair cell was morphologically polarized with respect to the location of its kinocilium. In the macula utriculi the hair cells were found to be polarized with the kinocilium facing the striola, whereas in the macula sacculi the kinocilium of each cell faced away from the striola.

The precise morphological and biochemical structure of the otolithic membranes and cupulae is not known. Wersäll (1956) and Iurato (1967) have found these structures to contain filaments arranged in all directions forming a network. Dohlman et al. (1959) and Jensen and Vilstrup (1960) found acid mucopolysaccharides in the maculae and cupulae.

The otoconial layer is thinner in the striola of the utricle and thicker in the striola of the saccule (Figs. 2.54, 2.55). The otoconia are smaller near the surface and, in general, the larger crystals are located near the hair cells. In the guinea pig they vary in size from about 0.5 to 30 microns. In mammals, birds, and sharks, the otoconia are composed of calcium carbonate having a specific gravity of about 2.71 showing the calcite crystalline structure (Lim, 1972) (Figs. 2.56, 2.57). The otoconia of amphibia have the aragonite crystalline structure.

The crista neglecta is a small vestibular endorgan which occurs regularly in lower forms (Gacek, 1961b) and recently has been described in the human (Montandon et al., 1970) (Figs. 2.58, 2.59). A review of serial sections of 500 human temporal bones in the collection at the Massachusetts Eye and Ear Infirmary reveals a distinct crista neglecta in five ears. In the cat, the crista neglecta occurs consistently in the floor of the posterior recess of the utricle, and

Fig. 2.53: Scanning electron micrograph showing a ciliary tuft from the macula of the guinea pig. Note the pipe organ arrangement with fragments of the otolithic membrane attached to the longest cilia (15,400 x). (Courtesy of Lim)

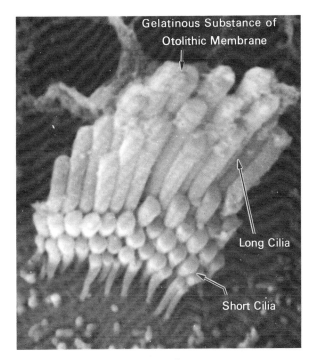

Gelatinous Substance of Otolithic Membrane

Long Cilia

Short Cilia

UTRICLE

Fig. 2.54: Sketch illustrating the morphology of the macula of the utricle and its otolithic membrane. In the region of the striola the otoconial layer is thinner and the crystals are smaller. Type I hair cells and larger nerve fibers dominate in this region. Ciliary polarization is toward the striola. (After Lindeman, 1969a)

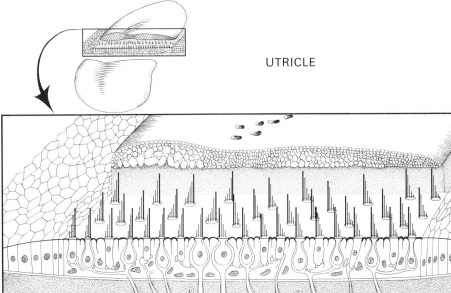

SACCULE

Fig. 2.55: Sketch showing the regional morphology of the macula of the saccule and its otolithic membrane. In the region of the striola the otoconial layer is thicker and the crystals are smaller. There is a predominance of type I hair cells and large nerve fibers in the region of the striola, and the ciliary tufts are polarized away from the striola. (After Lindeman, 1969a)

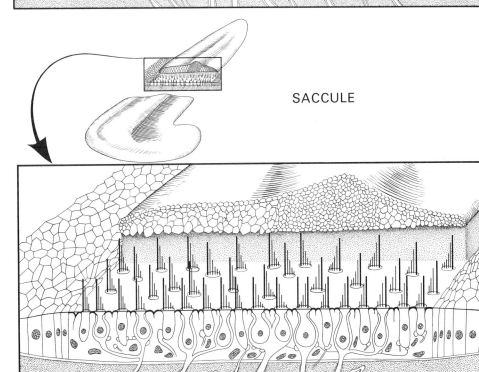

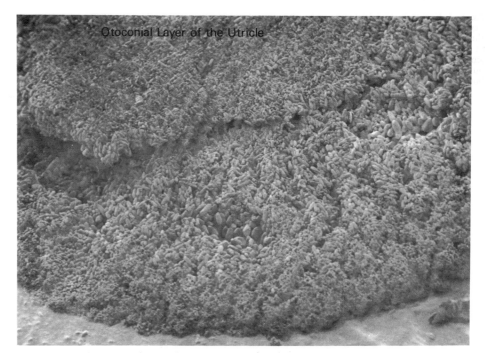

Fig. 2.57: Scanning electron micrograph of human otoconia. Each crystal has an oblong form, and the tips have three surfaces.

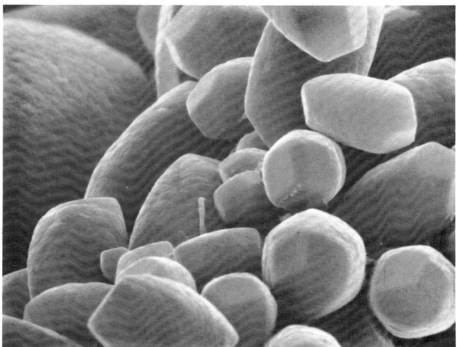

has all the morphological characteristics of a crista ampullaris, including both an afferent and efferent nerve supply and type I and type II hair cells (Montandon et al., 1970). In the human this endorgan does not occur regularly as a separate sense organ but probably is incorporated into the crista of the posterior semicircular canal. This is supported by the fact that there is frequently a small nerve bundle in a separate bony canal running parallel to the nerve to the posterior canal crista which joins the main nerve near the crista. This separate bundle is distinctly shown in Fig. 2.28. In the cat this small nerve bundle consistently innervates the crista neglecta.

c. The endolymphatic duct and sac

The endolymphatic sac lies partly within a bony niche on the posterior surface of the petrous bone and partly within the layers of the dura mater of the posterior cranial fossa (Fig. 2.60). It is connected to the endolymphatic system by the endolymphatic duct which lies in a bony canal known as the vestibular aqueduct and is lined by squamous or cuboidal cells. Lundquist (1965) divides the endolymphatic sac into three parts. The proximal part lies within a bony niche and has epithelial cells which are slightly taller than those of the

Fig. 2.58: Photomicrograph showing the crista neglecta of the cat. It is located in the floor of the posterior recess of the utricle and has all of the morphological characteristics of a crista ampullaris. It is innervated by a separate nerve bundle, and the sensory epithelium contains both type I and type II hair cells.

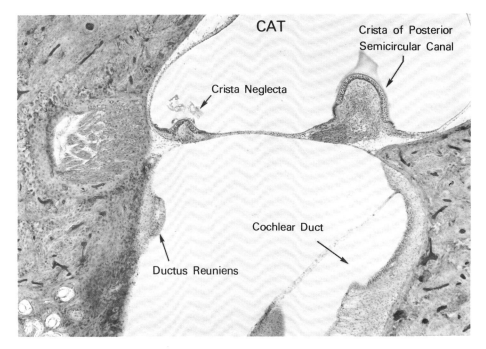

Fig. 2.59: Photomicrograph of the crista neglecta in the human ear. This structure does not occur regularly as a separate sense organ in the human ear but probably is incorporated into the crista of the semicircular canal.

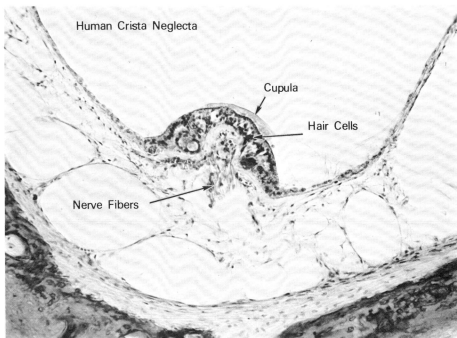

duct. The intermediate part lies partly within the bony niche and partly between layers of the dura mater and has an epithelial lining of tall cylindrical cells irregularly arranged in papillae and crypts. These cells are of two types—the light cells having a rather clear cytoplasm, many pinocytotic vesicles and vacuoles, numerous microvilli and various inclusion bodies, and the dark cells having a dense cytoplasm and somewhat fewer organelles, microvilli, and pinocytotic vesicles (Fig. 2.61). The distal part is located within layers of the dura mater over the transverse venous sinus and has epithelium which is more cuboidal in form and has both light and dark cell types, with the light cells in greater number. The walls of the distal part are normally juxtaposed so that no space exists in this area. The lumen of the endolymphatic sac contains cellular debris, free-floating macrophages exhibiting marked pinocytotic activity, and various blood cells, most of which are leucocytes.

The most highly differentiated part of the sac, the intermediate portion, has pinocytosis as its main activity (Lundquist et al., 1964; Adlington, 1967). In the adult this part of the sac often has villous and polypoid structures protruding into the lumen. The cores of these irregularly shaped structures frequently consist of dense fibrous tissue of sparse cellularity and vascularity (Gussen, 1971).

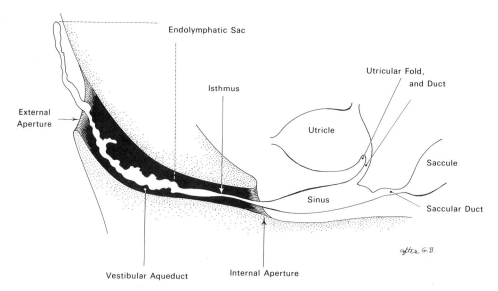

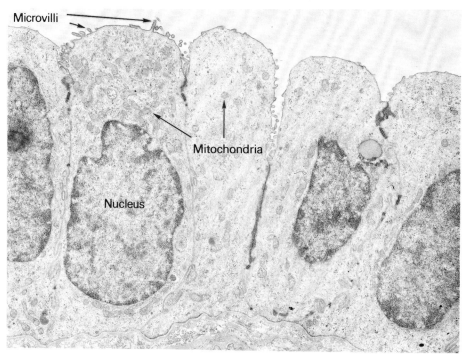

d. The round window membrane

The round window membrane is of particular importance for its role in the transmission of acoustic energy to the inner ear where it performs as a yielding area of the bony labyrinth to permit movement of inner ear fluids in association with movement of the stapedial footplate. Also it is of importance as a site by which toxic substances (bacterial exotoxins, chemical solutions) may enter the inner ear. Finally, recent reports (Goodhill, 1971; Pullen, 1972) indicate that rupture of the round window membrane may result from middle ear pressure changes. The round window membrane measures about 3 mm in its horizontal axis and about 1.5 mm in transverse axis (Kobrak, 1959). The ultrastructure of the round window membrane in guinea pigs has been described by Richardson et al. (1971) and by Kawabata and Paparella (1971).

The membrane consists of three layers. The external layer, which faces the tympanic cavity, has four types of cells: osmiophilic, osmiophobic, dark granulated, and goblet cells. The free surface has numerous microvilli. The cells are of the flat, squamous type and most are nonciliated. The intermediate layer consists of a network of fibrocytes with large intercellular spaces containing collagen and elastic fibers, blood vessels, and both myelinated and unmyelinated nerve fibers. The internal layer, which faces the scala tympani, is composed of a single layer of thin cells having long, thin cytoplasmic extensions and extensive endoplasmic reticulum.

e. The vascular system

The arterial blood supply to the membranous labyrinth originates within the cranial cavity, and while it is principally separate from the vessels that supply the otic capsule and the tympanic cavity, there are some terminal branches which penetrate the endosteal layer (Hansen, 1971). Mazzoni (1969b) in a study of 100 human specimens, consistently found an arterial loop in the region of the internal auditory canal. This arterial loop was the main trunk or a branch of the anterior inferior cerebellar artery in 80 percent of the cases, the accessory anterior cerebellar artery in 17 percent, and a branch of the posterior inferior cerebellar artery in 3 percent. The loop was found inside the internal auditory canal in 40 percent (Fig. 2.62), at the meatus in 27 percent, and in the cerebellopontine angle in 33 percent. In the cat, there are frequent anastomoses between the anterior inferior cerebellar artery, on the one hand, and the posterior superior and accessory cerebellar arteries on the other (Bernstein and Silverstein, 1966).

Fig. 2.62: Photomicrograph showing the anterior inferior cerebellar artery deeply within the internal auditory canal. This artery, or one of its main branches, is found within the internal auditory canal in 40 percent of specimens. (Mazzoni, 1969b)

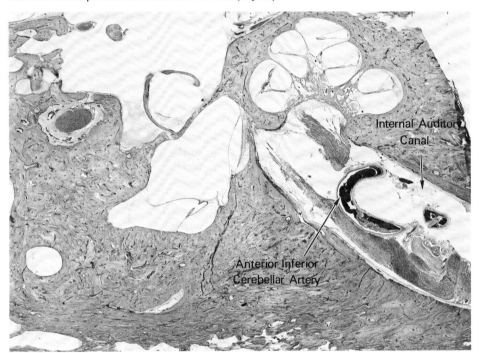

The anterior inferior cerebellar arterial loop gives rise to the labyrinthine artery (also termed internal auditory artery) and also frequently the subarcuate artery before taking a recurrent course to the cerebellum. The labyrinthine artery distributes to the dura and nerves in the internal auditory canal and to adjacent bone around the internal auditory canal and medial aspect of the inner ear before dividing into the common cochlear artery and the anterior vestibular artery (Mazzoni, 1972). The common cochlear artery divides into the main cochlear and vestibulocochlear branches (Fig. 2.63). The vestibulocochlear artery branches into the posterior vestibular artery and the cochlear ramus (Siebenmann, 1894; Shambaugh, 1903, 1905; Asai, 1908a, 1908b; Nabeya, 1923).

The usual distribution of these vessels as outlined by Hawkins (1967) is as follows:

(1) The main cochlear artery supplies three-fourths of the cochlea including the modiolus.

(2) The cochlear ramus supplies the basal one-fourth of the cochlea and adjacent modiolus.

(3) The anterior vestibular artery supplies the macula of the utricle, a small part of the macula of the saccule, the cristae and membranous canals of the superior and lateral semicircular canals, and the superior surfaces of the utricle and saccule.

(4) The posterior vestibular artery supplies the macula of the saccule, the

Fig. 2.63: Diagrammatic sketch showing the arterial system of the mammalian membranous labyrinth. (After Siebenman, Shambaugh, Asai and Nabeya)

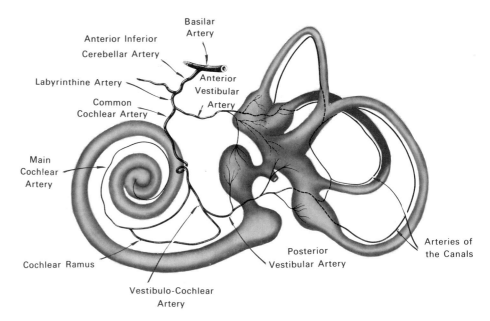

Fig. 2.63: Diagrammatic sketch showing the arterial system of the mammalian membranous labyrinth. (After Siebenman, Shambaugh, Asai and Nabeya)

crista and membranous canal of the posterior semicircular canal, and the inferior surfaces of the utricle and saccule.

The main cochlear artery enters the central canal of the modiolus and gives off several primary and many secondary arteries. The radiating arterioles are tertiary or further ramifications of the main cochlear artery and consist of two sets, one of which supplies the structures of the external wall and the other the structures of the medial wall of the cochlea (Smith, 1951) (Fig. 2.64).

The external radiating arterioles arch over the scala vestibuli within the intracochlear partition and, after providing vessels to the walls of the scala vestibuli, enter the uppermost part of the spiral ligament. These vessels then divide to form the following four groups of capillary networks: (1) spiraling vessels within the spiral ligament in the area where the ligament faces the scala vestibuli and near the vestibular crest (vessels of the scala vestibuli, vessels at Reissner's membrane); (2) the capillary network of the stria vascularis; (3) the vessels in the spiral prominence; and (4) those vessels that are located within the spiral ligament on the scala tympani side of the basilar crest, which serve as collecting venules and are morphologically identical to capillaries.

The capillaries of the stria vascularis pursue a serpentine course in a spiral direction, are extensively connected with each other, and give the appearance of a network having boundaries which are rather straight and parallel (Smith, 1957). Usually each radiating arteriole supplies a branch to the vessel of the

Fig. 2.64: Sketch showing the arterial and venous systems of the cochlea. (After Smith, 1951, 1954)

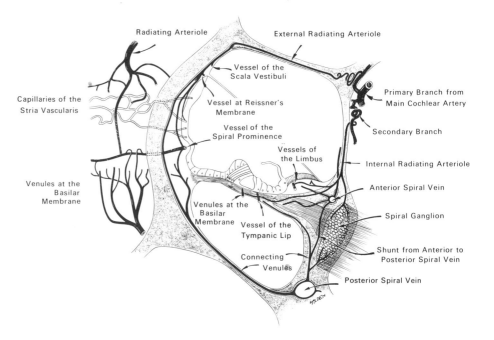

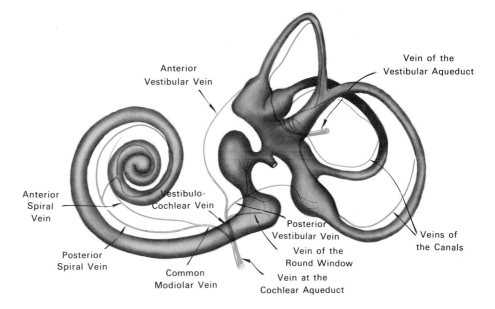

Fig. 2.65: Diagrammatic sketch showing the venous system of mammalian membranous labyrinth. (After Siebenmann, Shambaugh, Asai, and Nabeya)

Anterior Vestibular Vein

Vein of the Vestibular Aqueduct

Anterior Spiral Vein

Vestibulo-Cochlear Vein

Posterior Vestibular Vein

Veins of the Canals

Posterior Spiral Vein

Vein of the Round Window

Common Modiolar Vein

Vein at the Cochlear Aqueduct

spiral prominence. This vessel spirals parallel to the network of the stria vascularis but is not connected with it.

The internal radiating arterioles pass toward the base within the modiolus, giving branches to the spiral ganglion, and enter the vestibular lamina of the osseous spiral lamina to provide the limbus vessels and the marginal vessels (Axelsson, 1968). The marginal vessels form two sets of independent arcades, which function both as arterial and venous channels; one set forms the vessel of the basilar membrane, and the other the vessel of the tympanic lip.

The arterial supply to the macula of the utricle is provided entirely by the anterior vestibular artery. Several arterioles from this vessel descend in bony canals toward the neuroepithelium and form a dense capillary bed located below the hair cell area.

The supply to the macula of the saccule is mainly from the posterior vestibular artery with a minor contribution from the anterior vestibular artery. The arterioles enter the supporting tissue of the macula along with the myelinated nerve fibers and branch into an extensive subepithelial capillary network in the hair cell area.

The semicircular canals are supplied by arterioles which approach the ampullae in coiled bony channels apart from the nerve fibers. Several arterioles pass toward each ampulla and supply the capillary networks of the cristae and domes of the ampullae. Near the midlines of the cristae the arterioles branch to provide capillary networks between the sensory epithelium and nerve fibers. One or two arterioles extend throughout the length of each canal to provide a system of loosely connected capillaries.

The main venous channels of the cochlea are the posterior and anterior spiral veins (Fig. 2.65). The posterior spiral vein drains the spiral ganglion, external wall of the scala media, and the scala tympani. The anterior spiral vein drains the spiral lamina and scala vestibuli. There are several shunts from the anterior to the posterior spiral vein before they join near the basal end of the cochlea to form the common modiolar vein. The common modiolar vein is joined by the vestibulo-cochlear vein to become the vein at the cochlear aqueduct. This main channel then enters a bony canal (canal of Cotugno) near the cochlear aqueduct to empty into the inferior petrosal sinus.

The anterior vestibular vein carries blood from the utricle and the ampullae of the superior and lateral canals (Smith, 1953). The posterior vestibular vein drains the saccule, ampulla of the posterior canal, and the basal end of the cochlea. The confluence of these two vessels is joined by the vein of the round window to become the vestibulo-cochlear vein. The semi-circular canals are drained by vessels which pass toward their utricular ends to form the vein of the vestibular aqueduct which accompanies the endolymphatic duct and drains into the lateral venous sinus. Bast and Anson (1949) also describe an internal auditory vein which drains the apical and middle turns of the cochlea, traverses the internal auditory canal, and enters the inferior petrosal sinus; however, this vessel does not seem to be constant.

E. THE NEURAL PATHWAYS

1. THE AUDITORY PATHWAYS

a. *Afferent auditory pathways*

Light microscopic studies (Lorente de No, 1933a; Rasmussen, 1940; Fernández, 1951) supplemented with recent electron microscopic contributions (Spoendlin, 1956, 1971; Engström, 1958; Smith, 1961), have fairly accurately elicited the neuronal supply of the organ of Corti.

The afferent innervation of the organ of Corti consists of the dendritic terminals of the bipolar cochlear neurons whose cell bodies comprise the cochlear neurons in Rosenthal's canal in the modiolus. The cochlear neuronal population of the cat was found by Howe (1935) to vary from 44,298 to 57,494 and in a single specimen by Schuknecht (1960) to be 38,760. Gacek (1961a) found cat cochlear nerves to contain an average of 51,755 myelinated nerve fibers. Boord and Rasmussen (1958) reported an average of 23,554 myelinated fibers in cochlear nerves of the chinchilla, and Gacek (1961a) counted an average of 24,011 in the guinea pig and 31,400 in the monkey. In a study of 40 human cochlear nerves, Rasmussen (1940) found the number of myelinated cochlear nerve fibers to vary from 22,800 to 40,000 with an average of 31,400.

On the basis of degeneration studies, Spoendlin (1971) has described two types of cochlear afferent neurons. Type I, which constitute 95 percent of the total, have large cell bodies with myelin sheaths and are connected exclusively to internal hair cells. Type II, which constitute the remaining 5 percent of the neurons, do not have myelin sheaths surrounding the cell bodies and provide the entire afferent nerve supply to the external hair cells, with 0.5 percent ending on internal hair cells. Each internal hair cell appears to be innervated by about 20 type I neurons, whereas each type II neuron appears to be connected to about 10 external hair cells.

The afferent dendrites for the internal hair cells have chalice-like endings at the bases of the hair cells. The afferent fibers for the external hair cells have smaller endings at the bases of the hair cells, and assume a spiral course between Deiters' cells to form the three external spiral bundles, each consisting of ten to twenty fibers. The afferent fibers remain near the basilar membrane as they traverse the tunnel of Corti (Fig. 2.66). All of the afferent nerve endings are nonvesiculated.

The classical auditory pathways described originally by Held (1893), Lorente de No (1933b), and Cajal (1909) have been restudied in recent years with techniques which stain degenerating nerve fibers. Most investigators have used either the Marchi method, which stains degenerated myelinated fibers of medium and large size, or the Nauta silver impregnation technique (Nauta and Gygax, 1954; Nauta, 1957), which stains even the smallest unmyelinated degenerated fibers.

The orderly spatial arrangement of the cochlear neurons is maintained in the nerve trunk and continues into the cochlear nuclei (Figs. 2.67 to 2.72). The nerve fibers from the basal turn of the cochlea are located in the peripheral and inferior portions of the nerve trunk, and the apical fibers are in the central region. On entering the brain stem each fiber divides into an anterior and posterior branch. While the shorter anterior branch terminates in the anterior part of the ventral cochlear nucleus, the longer posterior branch divides again, one fiber terminating in the posterior part of the ventral cochlear nucleus and the other in the dorsal cochlear nucleus (Lorente de No, 1937; Rasmussen, 1940; Sando, 1965). Thus the major projection of the affer-

Fig. 2.66: *Above:* Nerve fibers crossing the base of the tunnel of Corti in the 5 mm area of the human cochlea. They pass in a basal direction and are predominantly of the afferent type. *Below:* Nerve fibers crossing the middle of the tunnel of Corti in the 15 mm region of the human cochlea. They pass in an apical direction and are predominantly of the efferent type. (Courtesy of Nomura and Kirikae, 1967)

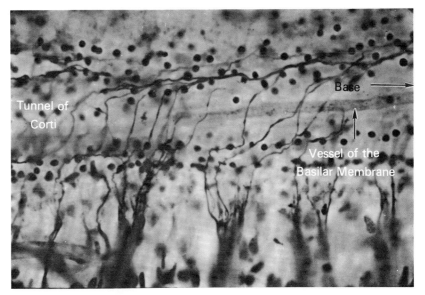

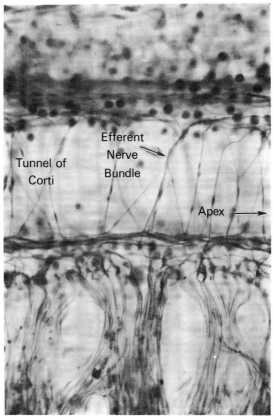

Fig. 2.67: This drawing illustrates the course and termination of the axons of the cochlear neurons which are located at the apex. The fibers are located in the center of the cochlear nerve trunk and upon entering the brain stem divide into anterior and posterior branches. The anterior branch ends in the anterior ventral cochlear nucleus, and the posterior branch divides again to send a branch to the posterior ventral cochlear nucleus and another to the dorsal cochlear nucleus. (After Sando)

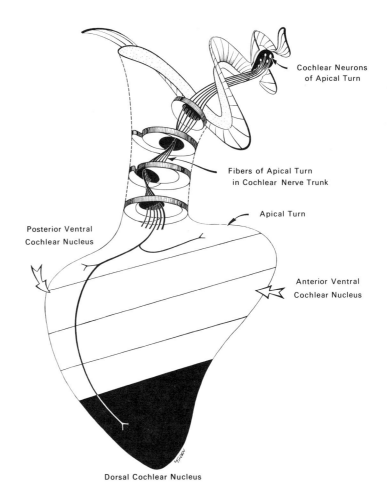

Cochlear Neurons
of Apical Turn

Fibers of Apical Turn
in Cochlear Nerve Trunk

Apical Turn

Posterior Ventral
Cochlear Nucleus

Anterior Ventral
Cochlear Nucleus

Dorsal Cochlear Nucleus

Fig. 2.68: The axons from the cochlear neurons of the middle turn pursue a slightly off-center course within the nerve trunk. Their terminations have a slightly more medial and rostral location in the cochlear nuclei than the apical fibers. (After Sando)

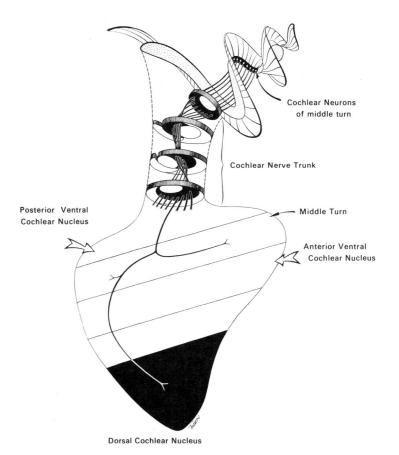

Cochlear Neurons
of middle turn

Cochlear Nerve Trunk

Middle Turn

Posterior Ventral
Cochlear Nucleus

Anterior Ventral
Cochlear Nucleus

Dorsal Cochlear Nucleus

Fig. 2.69: The axons from the cochlear neurons of the superior part of the basal turn assume a peripheral location in the anterior part of the nerve trunk, and their terminations are located in the middle regions of the ventral and dorsal cochlear nuclei. (After Sando)

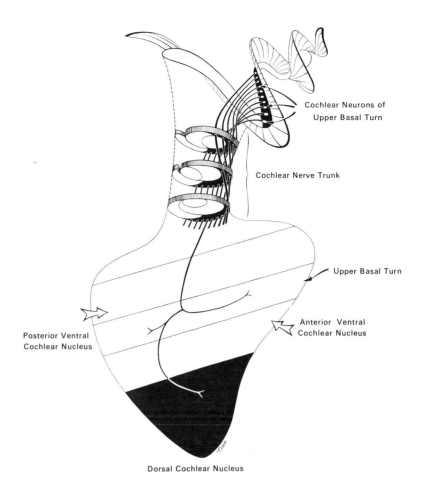

Cochlear Neurons of
Upper Basal Turn

Cochlear Nerve Trunk

Upper Basal Turn

Anterior Ventral
Cochlear Nucleus

Posterior Ventral
Cochlear Nucleus

Dorsal Cochlear Nucleus

Fig. 2.70: The axons which originate from cochlear neurons at the basal end are located at the periphery of the posterior part of the nerve trunk. Their terminations are located in the most medial and rostral areas of the cochlear nuclei. (After Sando)

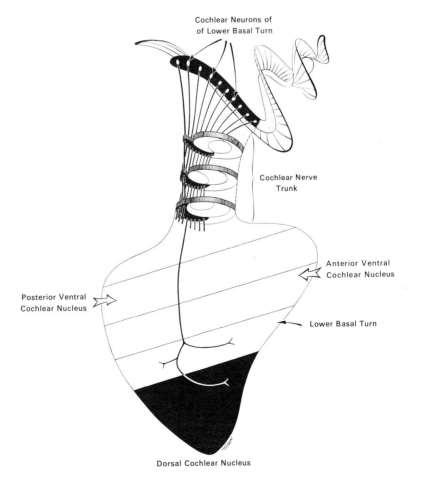

Cochlear Neurons of
of Lower Basal Turn

Cochlear Nerve
Trunk

Anterior Ventral
Cochlear Nucleus

Posterior Ventral
Cochlear Nucleus

Lower Basal Turn

Dorsal Cochlear Nucleus

ent input is to the ventral cochlear nucleus. No primary cochlear neurons bypass or send collaterals beyond the cochlear nuclei.

The dorsal cochlear nucleus contains three layers of cells, the most prominent being a layer of small granular cells while the larger ventral cochlear nucleus has mainly large cells. The cells of the dorsal cochlear nucleus send their axons into the dorsal acoustic stria where they cross the midline and then ascend in the medial division of the contralateral lateral lemniscus (Monakow's area). The lateral lemniscus is divided into medial and lateral portions by the nuclei of this lemniscus. These ascending axons from the dorsal cochlear nucleus finally terminate in the dorsal nucleus of the lateral lemniscus and in the inferior colliculus.

The cell bodies of the ventral cochlear nucleus send axons to the homolateral accessory olive and to the medial dendrites of the cells of the contralateral accessory olive (Rasmussen, 1946). There appears to be an orderly point-to-point spatial projection from the anterior ventral cochlear nucleus

Fig. 2.71: Diagram showing the principal afferent auditory pathways. An orderly spatial arrangement is maintained at all levels. Detailed description in text.

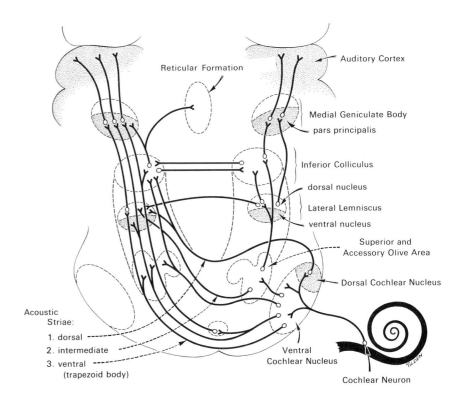

Fig. 2.72: Transmission electron micrograph showing the ultrastructural detail of the cochlear neuron of the squirrel monkey. (Courtesy of Kimura and Ota)

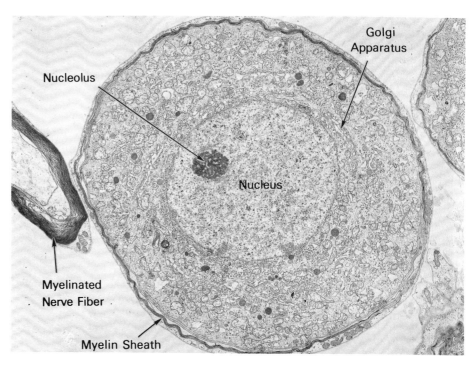

to the superior olivary complex. Some fibers of the intermediate and ventral acoustic stria traverse the superior olivary complex to enter the contralateral lateral lemniscus and the inferior colliculus.

The superior olive is thought to function as both a relay center for the auditory pathway and as a reflex center. The accessory superior olive projects bilaterally in the medial divisions of the lateral lemnisci to terminate primarily in the dorsal nuclei of the lateral lemnisci and inferior colliculi. The lateral superior olive projects homolaterally in the lateral division of the lateral lemniscus to terminate in the dorsal nucleus of the lateral lemniscus with some fibers continuing on to terminate in the inferior colliculus. No superior olivary neurons project beyond the inferior colliculus.

The distant projections from the inferior colliculus are mainly to the medial geniculate body with lesser connections to the superior colliculus and lower centers. No neurons from the cochlear nuclei or superior olive (hindbrain levels) reach the medial geniculate body, for the neurons terminating there originate either in the inferior colliculus or the dorsal and ventral nuclei of the lateral lemniscus. There are crossover connections between the dorsal nuclei of the lateral lemniscus and between the inferior colliculi. Ascending neurons are richly connected with the reticular formation. No ascending neurons bypass the medial geniculate body. The pars principalis of the inferior lobe of the medial geniculate body is composed of many closely packed small cells which project mainly to the primary auditory center. There is an orderly spatial projection of the neurons so that those from the anterior portion of the pars principalis terminate in the rostral portion of the auditory cortex and those from the posterior part terminate in the caudal end of the cortex. There are no commissural neurons at the medial geniculate body level. Each cochlea has nearly equal bilateral neuronal connections to the level of the medial geniculate bodies and thus to the auditory cortices.

The auditory cortex has been studied in terms of its cytoarchitectonic structure and physiological response characteristics (Rose, 1949; Rose and Woolsey, 1949). There is a primary auditory projection region in which high frequencies are represented rostrally and low frequencies caudally. This area receives its essential projection from the rostral portion of the pars principalis of the medial geniculate body. Although anatomical and physiological studies show the neural linkages to be very complex, an orderly spatial arrangement has been demonstrated in the spiral ganglion, nerve trunk, ventral cochlear nucleus, geniculo-cortical projection, and in the primary auditory cortex (Report on Workshop, 1973). Although it has not yet been shown, it is logical to assume this orderly arrangement also exists between the ventral cochlear nucleus and medial geniculate body.

The auditory nerve fiber system, as it ascends from the cochlea to the cortex, projects into centers having progressively larger populations of neurons. Chow (1951) has estimated the cell counts at various levels in the auditory neural system of the monkey, and his figures are as follows:

Cochlear nuclei	8,800
Superior olivary complex	34,000
Nuclei of lateral lemniscus	38,000
Inferior colliculus	392,000
Medial geniculate body (pars principalis)	364,000
Auditory cortex	10,000,000

b. *Efferent auditory pathways*

Recent studies have shown that a rich population of descending or efferent neurons parallel the ascending pathways and link the auditory cortex with the lower auditory centers and the organ of Corti. Rasmussen (1953, 1960, 1964) has described two separate systems of descending neurons which pass through the same areas as the ascending pathways. These two systems of efferent neurons appear to arise in all regions of the auditory cortex and relay in the several nuclei already described for the afferent system, one terminating as the olivo-cochlear bundle on the hair cells of the organ of Corti and the other on neurons in the dorsal cochlear nucleus.

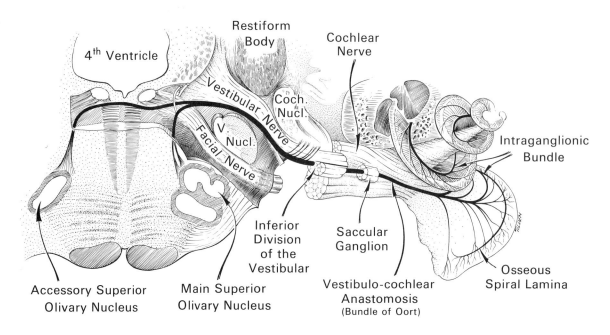

Fig. 2.73: Sketch showing the origin and course of the efferent auditory nerve fibers. Detailed description in text. (After Rasmussen, 1960)

The olivo-cochlear bundle originates in the superior olivary complex. It is composed of about 500 to 600 fibers and has both a homolateral and contralateral origin (Fig. 2.73). Approximately three-fourths of the efferent bundle to one ear originates from small cells located dorsomedial to the contralateral accessory superior olivary nucleus. These fibers ascend in the olivary peduncle, gather into a compact bundle beneath the facial genu, and cross the midline in the floor of the fourth ventricle. Crossing laterally under the homolateral facial genu, the bundle breaks up into several fascicles which interdigitate with the outgoing facial nerve fibers and again merge into a compact bundle which enters the vestibular nerve root. Here it is joined by the homolateral component of the olivo-cochlear bundle which arises from cells dorsal to the main superior olivary nucleus and comprises the remaining one-fourth of the efferent supply to the cochlea. The olivo-cochlear bundle sends collaterals to the ventral cochlear nucleus as it passes beneath it. It travels in the vestibular root to emerge from the brain stem in the inferior division of the vestibular nerve. The bundle leaves this nerve just beyond the saccular ganglion where it becomes the vestibulo-cochlear anastomosis (Oort, 1918). The fibers finally enter the cochlea, where they form the intraganglionic spiral bundles. It is characteristic for the efferent fibers to ramify numerously at every level before terminating. The olivo-cochlear bundle has been demonstrated to exist in species as low on the phylogenetic scale as birds and reptiles and as high as monkey and man, and apparently constitutes an essential part of the neural apparatus in forms that have a cochlea and a superior olive.

Schuknecht and collaborators (Churchill et al., 1956; Schuknecht et al., 1959) first demonstrated the presence of cholinergic fibers in the cochlea and showed that these were the efferent fibers of the olivo-cochlear bundle (Churchill and Schuknecht, 1959) (Figs. 2.74, 2.75). Subsequently, staining methods for acetylcholinesterase have been used extensively to study the course of the efferent fibers. Nomura and Schuknecht (1965) showed that the fibers to the basal end of the cochlea pass singly or in small bundles from the vestibulo-cochlear anastomosis to their terminations in the organ of Corti without forming intraganglionic spiral bundles. The fibers to the remainder of the cochlea enter Rosenthal's canal at various levels to form the intraganglionic bundles from which they pass singly or in small groups into the osseous spiral lamina. Here they again form bundles, taking a spiral course in

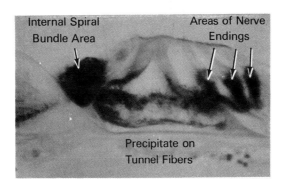

Fig. 2.74: Photomicrograph showing copper sulfide stain on the efferent nerve fibers and endings in the organ of Corti. Acetylcholinesterase stain of Koelle. (Schuknecht et al., 1959)

Internal Spiral
Bundle Area

Areas of Nerve
Endings

Precipitate on
Tunnel Fibers

an apical direction while approaching the rim of the spiral lamina (Fig. 2.76). The efferent fibers branch in the spiral lamina sufficient to provide several fibers in each opening of the habenula perforata (Nomura and Schuknecht, 1965) (Fig. 2.77). Retzius (1927) counted 2,780 openings of the habenula perforata of the cat cochlea. This finding correlates closely with the number of internal hair cells reported by Spoendlin (1966). Taking Rasmussen's figure of 500 to 600 efferent fibers in the internal auditory canal, it appears that there is at least a fivefold increase due to branching.

Efferent fibers enter the internal spiral bundle beneath the internal hair cells and travel for varying distances, mainly in an apical direction. Along this course some provide collaterals which terminate in small vesiculated knobs on either the afferent nerve fibers or their chalice-like endings on the internal hair cells. None of them end on the internal hair cells themselves. Many of the efferent fibers in their spiral course toward the apex, cross the tunnel space in the midtunnel fiber bundle to reach the outer spiral bundles and eventually the external hair cells (Spoendlin and Gacek, 1963; Iurato et al., 1971). Here the fibers contact the external hair cells directly with large vesiculated endings (Iurato, 1962, 1967; Kimura and Wersäll, 1962) (Fig. 2.78). Smith and Sjöstrand (1961) have shown that many efferent endings in the external hair cell area also have contact with the afferent nerve fibers and endings.

Spoendlin (1966) counted a minimum average of three or four efferent nerve endings per external hair cell with the total number estimated to be 40,000. Utilizing histochemical techniques, Ishii and Balogh (1968) studied the efferent nerve density to the external hair cell regions and found decreasing innervation from base to apex, as well as a decreasing innervation from the first to the third row of external hair cells.

Ishii et al. (1967) have also demonstrated acetylcholinesterase-active fibers

Fig. 2.75: Photomicrograph showing near total loss of staining of efferent fibers 14 days following section of both crossed and uncrossed olivo-cochlear bundles. Koelle stain for acetylcholinesterase. A small deposit of copper sulfide remains at the base of the first row of external hair cells. Compare with Fig. 2.74.

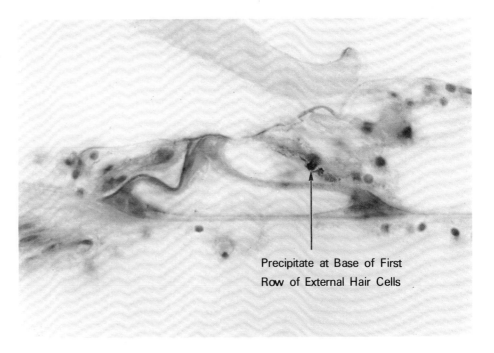

Precipitate at Base of First
Row of External Hair Cells

Fig. 2.76: Efferent fibers in the osseous spiral lamina of the middle turn of the human cochlea. Acetylcholinesterase stain of Koelle. The efferent nerve fiber bundles take a spiral course in the apical direction while approaching the lip of the spiral lamina. (Nomura and Schuknecht, 1965)

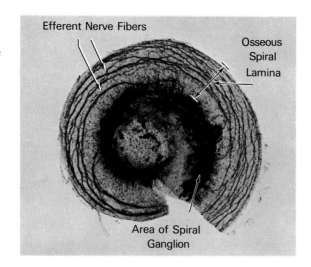

Fig. 2.77: Acetylcholinesterase stain showing efferent nerve fibers at each opening of the habenula perforata in the basal turn of the cat cochlea. (Nomura and Schuknecht, 1965)

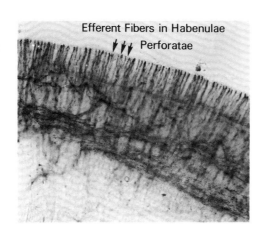

Fig. 2.78: Transmission electron micrograph showing efferent and afferent nerve endings at the base of an external hair cell of the guinea pig. (Courtesy of Kimura)

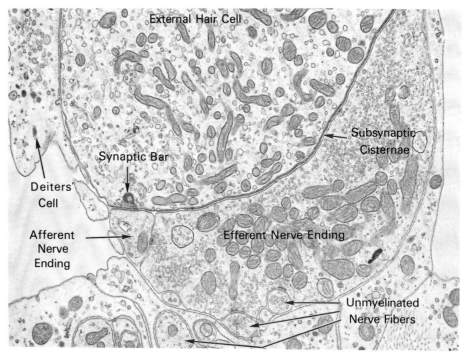

within the cochlear nerve trunk. The origin and termination of these fibers have not been elucidated.

Kimura and Wersäll (1962) found that a midline section of the crossed efferent fibers of the guinea pig resulted in degeneration of a large portion of the vesiculated nerve endings in all turns of the cochlea. The exact distribution of crossed and uncrossed olivo-cochlear nerve bundles is not yet known.

a. Afferent vestibular pathways

The vestibular ganglion consists of bipolar neurons (Fig. 2.79) lying in two linearly arranged cell masses extending in a rostral-caudal direction in the internal auditory canal. It consists of a superior and inferior cell group related to the superior and inferior divisions of the vestibular nerve trunk. The superior division supplies the cristae of the superior and lateral canals, the macula of the utricle, and the anterosuperior part of the macula of the saccule. The inferior division supplies the crista of the posterior canal and the main portion of the macula of the saccule. Medial to the vestibular ganglion the nerve fibers of both divisions merge into a single trunk which enters the brain stem. Boord and Rasmussen (1958) found an average of 7,772 myelinated fibers in the vestibular nerves of eight ears of chinchillas, and Gacek (1961a) found an average of 8,231 vestibular fibers in four guinea pig ears. The average for the monkey was reported by Gacek (1961a) to be 18,271. The average number of vestibular fibers for 37 human ears was reported by Rasmussen (1940) to be 18,500 with a range of 14,200 to 24,000, and by Bergström (cited by Ades et al., 1972) to be 18,000 to 20,000. Naufal and Schuknecht (1972) found the mean total number of Scarpa's ganglion cells in 15 normal human ears to be 18,439.

The early neuroanatomists (Koelliker, 1891; Held, 1892; Cajal, 1909) presented a good general description of the central connections of the vestibular neurons, including the division of these fibers into ascending and descending branches. Lorente de No (1933b), Walberg et al. (1958), Gacek (1969), and Sando et al. (1972) have provided a more complete description of both the peripheral and central projections.

The superior division of the vestibular nerve has large nerve fibers which arise mainly from ganglion cells in the rostral part of the ganglion and small fibers which originate mainly in the caudal portion of the ganglion. The ampullary nerves pass in the rostral part of the nerve trunk. Large fibers become concentrated in the central parts of these nerve branches and are surrounded by the small fibers. This arrangement persists into the cristae, with the large fibers more numerous at the crests and the small fibers more numerous at the slopes of the cristae (Gacek, 1969) (Figs. 2.80, 2.81). The large fibers appear to end predominantly in the large chalice-type endings on type I

Fig. 2.79: Transmission electron micrograph of a neuron of the superior vestibular ganglion of the squirrel monkey.

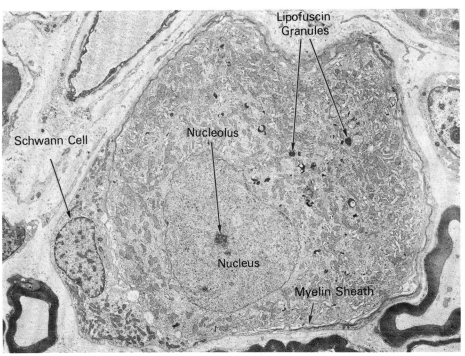

hair cells whereas the small fibers (along with the small efferent fibers) make contact with the type II hair cells. The contention that the type I and II vestibular hair cells have different functional significance is further emphasized by the fact that the large and small afferent fibers have different central terminations. The large fibers terminate on the larger neurons in the central part of the superior vestibular nucleus, while the smaller fibers end on small neurons in the area between the center of the nucleus and the restiform body. These relationships have been established only for the superior and lateral canals but probably are the same for the posterior canal.

Fig. 2.80: Sketch showing the distribution of the afferent nerve supply of the superior division of the vestibular nerve. It innervates the cristae of the superior and lateral canals, the macula of the utricle, and the anterosuperior part of the macula of the saccule. The larger nerve fibers travel mainly to the crest of the cristae while the small fibers are more numerous on the slopes. (Gacek, 1969)

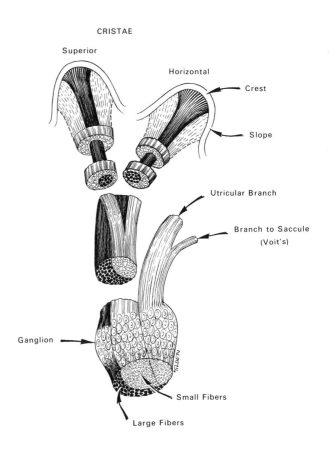

Fig. 2.81: Sudan black stain showing large and small afferent fibers in the superior division of the vestibular nerve. Nauta stain. (Courtesy of Gacek)

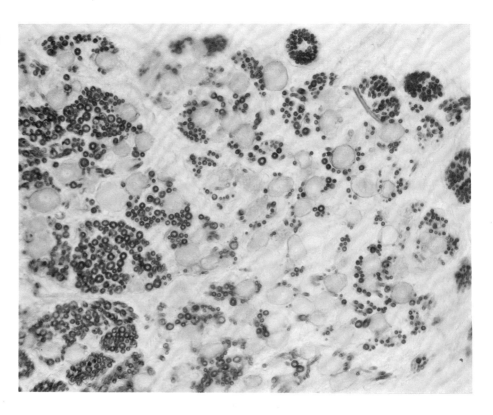

Lindeman's (1969a, 1969b) findings are in general agreement with those of Cajal (1909–1911), Lorente de No (1926, 1931), Poljak (1927), Wersäll (1956), and Gacek (1969) and show that the population of large fibers is greater in the striolae of both maculae where there is a predominance of type I hair cells.

All fibers of the vestibular ganglia, upon entering the brain stem, bifurcate into ascending and descending branches. The ascending branches of the fibers from the superior and lateral canals terminate in the rostral part of the superior vestibular nucleus in a distribution of large and small fibers as already described. After giving off long collaterals in the nucleus, the ascending branches continue on directly to the cerebellum. The incoming fibers from the posterior canal crista bifurcate more medially, and the ascending branches end in a more central and medial region of the superior vestibular nucleus and also probably continue to the cerebellum (Fig. 2.82). The descending branches of fibers from the three cristae give collaterals mainly to the medial vestibular nucleus and to a lesser extent to the lateral and descending vestibular nuclei.

Fibers from all three canals have terminations in the interstitial nucleus of the vestibular root. The connections of this interstitial nucleus are not known, although there is some evidence that, like the lateral vestibular nucleus, it may project to the spinal cord (Brodal and Pompeiano, 1957a). It is associated only with canal function as no fibers from the utricle or saccule terminate in it.

The neurons from the utricular and saccular maculae comprise the caudal part of the vestibular nerve trunk. The ascending rami of the utricular neurons terminate mainly in the rostral part of the medial vestibular nucleus and a small number in the rostroventral part of the lateral vestibular nucleus. The connection to the medial vestibular nucleus presumably mediates compensatory eye movements and that to the lateral nucleus mediates upper spinal cord reflexes. The descending branches of the utricular neurons converge on the medial vestibular nucleus in the same area as the descending branches from the cristae.

The neurons from the saccular macula are smaller in number and are predominantly small in caliber. The main projection of the ascending branches is to the "group y" nucleus. The neural relationships and function of the "y" nucleus are not known but it does not appear to belong to the classical vestibular nuclei (Fuse, 1912; Brodal and Pompeiano, 1957b). The descending branches terminate on a small number of neurons in the lateral and medial vestibular nuclei (Fig. 2.83).

The projections from the vestibular nuclei (second-order vestibular neurons) are fairly well known (Brodal et al., 1962; Carpenter, 1966; Gacek, 1971). These projections extend to the cerebellum, extra-ocular nuclei, and to the spinal cord. The projections to the cerebellum arise only from the medial and descending vestibular nuclei.

The ascending fibers end in the extra-ocular nuclei (IIIrd, IVth, and VIth cranial nerve nuclei). Two sets of fibers travel by way of the medial longitudinal fasciculi to innervate the nuclei of the IIIrd and IVth cranial nerves to supply all muscles innervated by these nuclei exclusive of the inferior rectus (Gacek, 1971). The first set arises from the superior vestibular nucleus and passes in the ipsilateral medial longitudinal fasciculus, and the second arises in the medial vestibular nucleus and passes in the contralateral medial longitudinal fasciculus. Both of these systems also have terminations in the interstitial nucleus of Cajal and the nucleus of Darkshewitsch, which are the most rostral terminals known to exist in the vestibular system (Fig. 2.84).

Two sets of fibers reach the extra-ocular nuclei by routes other than the medial longitudinal fasciculi. The first arises from the lateral vestibular nucleus passing in the "ascending tract of Deiters" to reach the ipsilateral IIIrd nucleus for innervation of the inferior rectus muscle. The second set arises from both the lateral and medial vestibular nuclei and projects directly to the

Fig. 2.82: Schematic drawing showing the central projections of the afferent fibers from the three cristae. Detailed description in text. (After Gacek, 1969)

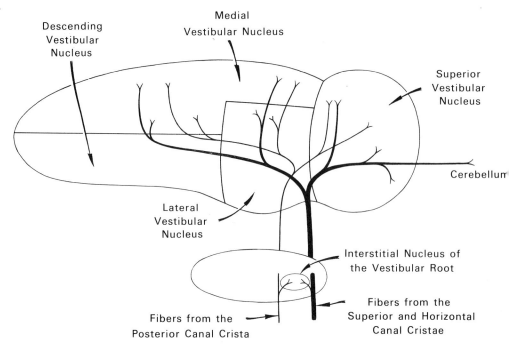

Fig. 2.83: Schematic drawing showing the central projections of the afferent fibers from the maculae. Detailed description in text. (After Gacek, 1969)

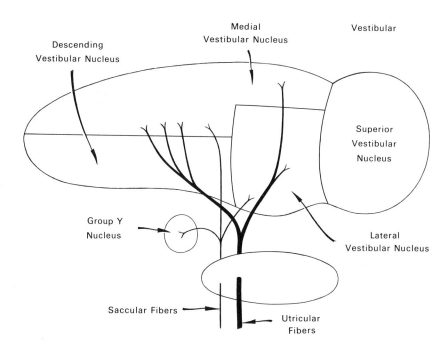

VIth nucleus. The fibers from the lateral vestibular nucleus supply the ipsilateral VIth nucleus, and the fibers from the medial vestibular nucleus provide bilateral supply to the VIth nuclei (Fig. 2.85).

The descending tracts from the vestibular nuclei pass to the anterior horns of the spinal cord and mediate trunk and limb muscle reflexes. From the lateral vestibular nucleus fibers pass in the vestibulo-spinal tract for ipsilateral innervation at all levels of the spinal cord. From the descending and medial vestibular nuclei fibers pass bilaterally via the descending medial longitudinal fasciculi to the cervical and thoracic regions of the spinal cord (Fig. 2.86).

The vestibular area in the cerebral cortex has not been defined by anatomical methods. Electrophysiological studies indicate that the projection area is in the temporal lobe near the auditory cortex (Anderson and Gernandt, 1954).

b. Efferent vestibular pathways

Gacek (1960) studied the pattern and distribution of efferent vestibular fibers obtained after intramedullary transection of the vestibular nerve root. These vestibular efferent fibers accompany the cochlear efferent fibers in the vestibular nerve trunk as far as the saccular ganglion, at which point they

Fig. 2.84: Sketch of projection routes for the ascending fibers of the vestibular nuclei to the nuclei of the extra-ocular muscles. The two sets of fibers reach the nuclei of the IIIrd and IVth cranial nerves by way of the medial longitudinal fasciculi. Detailed description in text. (After Gacek)

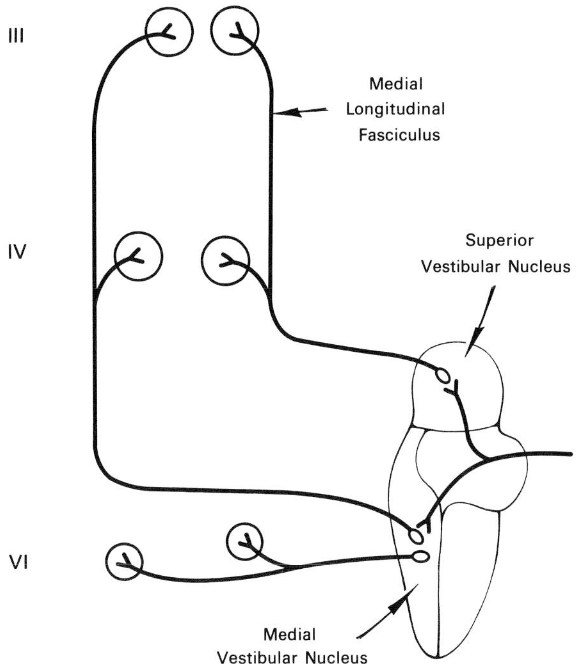

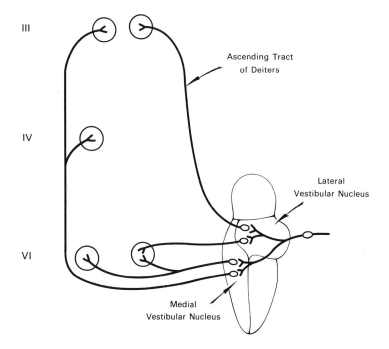

Fig. 2.85: Two sets of fibers reach the extra-ocular nuclei by routes other than the medial longitudinal fasciculi. These are the ascending tracts of Deiters which carry innervation of the ipsilateral inferior rectus and the direct tracts to the VIth nuclei. (After Gacek)

Fig. 2.86: This sketch shows that the descending tracts of the vestibular nuclei end in the anterior horns of the spinal cord. The medial longitudinal fasciculi carry fibers to the cervical and thoracic areas and the vestibulo-spinal tract to all levels of the spinal cord. (After Gacek)

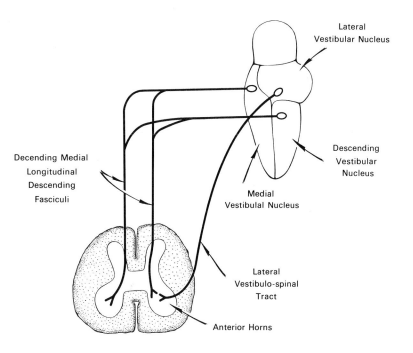

diverge at almost right angles to each other. The bundles of vestibular efferents then disperse as scattered fibers to the rami supplying the maculae and cristae (Gacek et al., 1965; Gacek, 1968). Nomura et al. (1965), utilizing the acetylcholinesterase stain, determined that the fibers richly supply the neuro-epithelium on the slopes of each crista ampullaris as well as the maculae of the utricle and saccule (Fig. 2.87).

The origin of the efferent vestibular system was determined by the use of horseradish peroxidase as a retrograde protein transport tracer after injection into the vestibular of newborn kittens (Gacek and Lyon, 1973). The 200–300 neurons that comprise the efferent supply to one vestibular labyrinth are equally and bilaterally located ventromedial to the ventral portion of the lateral vestibular nucleus (Gacek, 1966).

Fig. 2.87: Surface preparation showing efferent nerve fiber distribution in the macula of the saccule of the guinea pig demonstrated by the acetylcholinesterase stain of Koelle. There is a dual supply of efferent, as well as afferent, fibers via the saccular branch of the inferior division of the vestibular nerve and by a small branch from the superior division of the vestibular nerve. The latter is known as Voit's anastomosis. (Courtesy of Nomura et al., 1965)

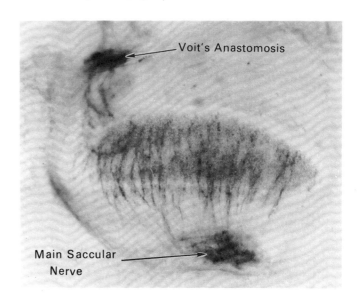

Fig. 2.88: Arrangement of hair cells and nerve endings in the vestibular sense organs (chinchilla). The goblet-shaped type I hair cells are surrounded (except for their hair-bearing ends) by calyciform terminals (C) of afferent function. The type II hair cells are contacted both by vesiculated boutons (VB) of efferent function and nonvesiculated boutons of afferent function. Synaptic bars (SB) are found in the bases of hair cells in relation to nonvesiculated nerve endings. Efferent boutons also end on afferent boutons, on calyciform afferent endings, and on afferent nerve fibers. (After Smith and Rasmussen, 1967)

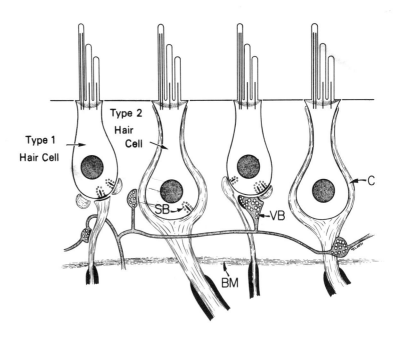

Smith and Rasmussen (1967) studied the maculae and cristae of the chinchilla and found calyciform and bouton-type nerve endings. The calyciform terminals had nonvesiculated neuroplasm and encircled the cell except the hair-bearing end. The boutons were of two types. The first type terminated only on the hair cells, was often associated with an adjacent synaptic bar, and had nonvesiculated neuroplasm. The calyciform and first type boutons are known to have afferent function. The second type, the "vesiculated boutons," contain many small homogeneous vesicles and synapse either by *en passant* endings on hair cells, on other boutons, on calyciform terminals, or on nerve fibers, and are known to be efferent in function (Fig. 2.88).

F. PNEUMATIZATION OF THE TEMPORAL BONE

The extent of pneumatization of the normal human temporal bone varies greatly (Hagens, 1934; Meltzer, 1934; Tremble, 1934; Lindsay, 1940, 1941). The growth pattern is thought to be controlled by heredity, environment, nutrition, bacterial infections, and the adequacy of ventilation as determined by eustachian tube function.

The pneumatized spaces of the temporal bone may be divided into five regions which are further subdivided into areas. A diagrammatic sketch showing most of the regions, areas, and tracts is seen in Fig. 2.89, and the complete classification in Table 2.1 (Allam, 1969).

Table 2.1   Pneumatized Spaces of the Temporal Bone

A. Middle Ear Region
   1. Mesotympanic area
   2. Epitympanic area
   3. Hypotympanic area
   4. Protympanic area
   5. Posterior tympanic area

B. Mastoid Region
   1. Mastoid antrum area
   2. Central mastoid tract
   3. Peripheral mastoid areas
      (a) Tegmental cells
      (b) Sinodural cells
      (c) Sinal cells
      (d) Facial cells
      (e) Tip cells

C. Perilabyrinthine Region
   1. Supralabyrinthine area
   2. Infralabyrinthine area

D. Petrous Apex Region
   1. Peritubal area
   2. Apical area

E. Accessory Region
   1. Zygomatic area
   2. Squamous area
   3. Occipital area
   4. Styloid area

F. Tracts of Pneumatization
   1. Posterosuperior tract
   2. Posteromedial tract
   3. Subarcuate tract
   4. Perilabyrinthine tracts
   5. Peritubal tracts

Fig. 2.89: The mastoid, perilabyrinthine, and petrous apex regions of the petrous bone may be delineated by two vertical planes, one passing through the plane of the superior semicircular canal and the other through the axis of the modiolus. The perilabyrinthine region is further subdivided into the infralabyrinthine and supralabyrinthine areas and the petrous apex region into the peritubal and apical areas.

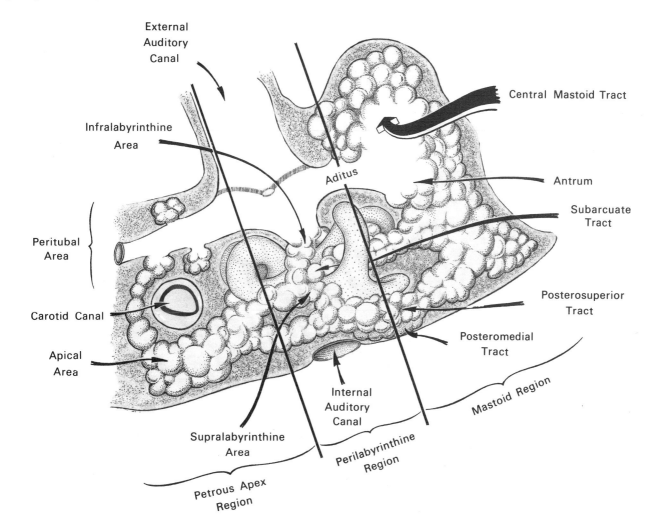

The middle ear region may be divided into five areas:

(a) The mesotympanic area. This space lies medial to the pars tensa.

(b) The epitympanic area. This area lies superior to a horizontal plane passing through the anterior and posterior tympanic striae.

(c) The hypotympanic area. This space lies inferior to a horizontal plane passing through the most inferior level of the tympanic annulus.

(d) The protympanic area. This space lies anterior to a frontal plane passing through the anterior margin of the tympanic annulus.

(e) The posterior tympanic area. This area is located posterior to a frontal plane passing through the posterior margin of the tympanic annulus and includes the sinus tympani and facial recess.

Pneumatization of the ossicles is rare but has been observed in the body of the incus in 3 of 750 temporal bone specimens examined in the collection at the Massachusetts Eye and Ear Infirmary (Fig. 2.90).

Fig. 2.90: Photomicrograph of pneumatization of the body of the incus in a normal adult human temporal bone.

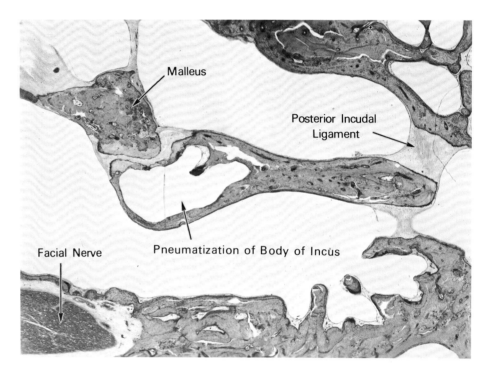

Fig. 2.91: Normal pneumatization in a 41-day-old infant. The external cortical bone of the mastoid is very thin.

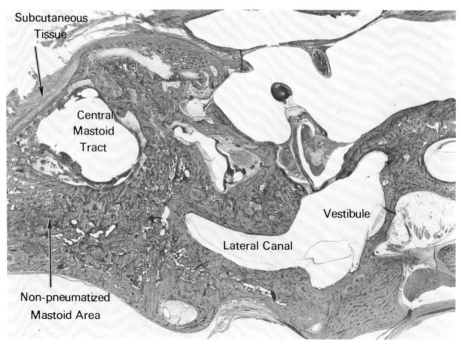

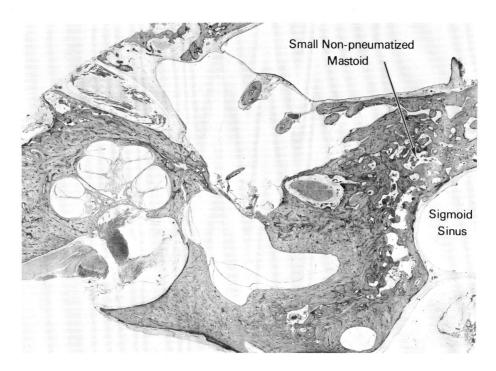

Fig. 2.92: Sclerotic mastoid in an individual with no medical history of ear disease. The sigmoid sinus is located in an anterior and superficial position (male, age 79).

Small Non-pneumatized Mastoid

Sigmoid Sinus

2. THE MASTOID REGION

At birth the mastoid contains a single space consisting of the antrum and adjacent parts of the mastoid. It occupies a superficial position and is surrounded by diploic bone (Fig. 2.91).

In adult life, the normal mastoid may be fully pneumatized, diploic, or sclerotic. In the diploic and sclerotic types, pneumatization is limited mainly to the antra and central mastoid tracts. The diploic type contains abundant soft tissue in the form of bone marrow, whereas the sclerotic type consists predominantly of dense bone (Fig. 2.92). In an examination of 250 human temporal bones, Zuckerkandl (1879) found 36.8 percent to be completely pneumatized, 43.2 percent to be partially pneumatized and partially diploic, and 20 percent to be completely diploic or sclerotic.

The anterolateral portion of the mastoid arises from the squamous part of the temporal bone, and the posteromedial portion, including the mastoid tip, arises from the petrous part of the temporal bone. The delineation of these areas is indicated on the outer surface by the petromastoid fissure, which is usually obliterated in early adult life. In most mastoids the plane of junction of these two parts is marked internally by an incomplete plate of bone, the petrosquamosal septum, also known as Koerner's septum (Moller, 1930). This septum divides the mastoid cells into a superficial squamous group and a deeper petrosal group. The septum may be missing in extensively pneumatized bones. The mastoid region can be divided into the following three areas (Fig. 2.93):

(a) The mastoid antrum. This is a large superior central space which communicates with the middle ear via the aditus. The lateral wall of the antrum is formed by the squamous part of the temporal bone.

(b) The central mastoid tract. This space extends inferiorly from the mastoid antrum. It may consist of a single space of varying size or of a series of cells and may be partly divided by the petrosquamosal septum.

(c) The peripheral mastoid area. This area may be subdivided into five cell groups: (1) the tegmental cells which border the tegmen and thus lie superiorly in the mastoid bone; (2) the sinodural cells which occupy the postero-superior angle of the mastoid bone and are bounded superiorly by the dural plate of bone and

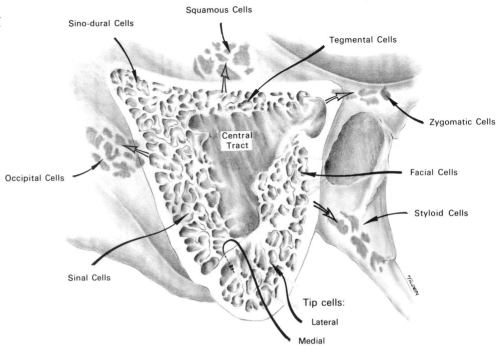

Fig. 2.93: Diagrammatic sketch showing the areas of pneumatization of the mastoid bone. The accessory areas of pneumatization (zygomatic, squamous, occipital, and styloid) are also shown.

postero-inferiorly by the sinus plate of bone; (3) the sinal cells which lie lateral, medial, and posterior to the sigmoid sinus; (4) the facial cells which lie in relation to the mastoid segment of the facial nerve; and (5) the tip cells which occupy the inferior projection of the mastoid bone and are divided by the digastric ridge into medial and lateral groups.

3. THE PERILABYRINTHINE REGION

The perilabyrinthine region is subdivided into: (a) the supralabyrinthine, and (b) the infralabyrinthine areas which lie superior and inferior to the labyrinth respectively (Fig. 2.94).

4. THE PETROUS APEX REGION

The petrous apex region is divided into: (a) the peritubal area, which surrounds the osseous portion of the eustachian tube and lies anterolateral to the carotid canal, and (b) the apical area, which lies posteromedial to the carotid canal (Fig. 2.95). Peritubal pneumatization is common; however, the apical area is rarely pneumatized.

5. THE ACCESSORY REGION

Occasionally, pneumatization extends beyond the middle ear, mastoid, perilabyrinthine and petrous apex regions to involve adjacent portions of the temporal bone and even the adjacent cranial bones, thus forming the accessory cell areas. These are shown in Figure 2.93 and are listed below:

(a) The zygomatic area. This area develops as an anterior extension from either the epitympanic or tegmental cell areas and occupies the root and sometimes the arch of the zygoma.
(b) The squamous area. This space lies in the squamous portion of the temporal bone above the level of the infratemporal line and is a superior extension from the tegmental cells.
(c) The occipital area. This space lies within the occipital bone as a posterior extension from the sinal cells.
(d) The styloid area. This is a rare accessory pneumatization occurring as an extension of the tip cells into the base of the styloid process.

82   Anatomy

6. TRACTS OF PNEUMATIZATION

Pneumatization of the temporal bone is the result of the hollowing-out process in which mesenchyme is resolved to leave spaces. Each space becomes air-containing and is in free communication with all other pneumatized spaces. The tracts of pneumatization are well known to the otologic surgeon for they serve as routes which can be followed to approach diseased areas of the temporal bone (Ziegelmann, 1935; Diamant, 1940; Williams, 1966). These tracts are described below:

(a) The posterosuperior cell tract. This tract passes anteromedially from the superior part of the central mastoid tract. It lies in the angle between the dural plates of bone of the middle and posterior cranial fossae on the one hand, and the superior semicircular canal on the other. The tract usually terminates near the internal auditory canal but may pass superior to the internal auditory canal to reach the supralabyrinthine and apical areas (Fig. 2.96.).

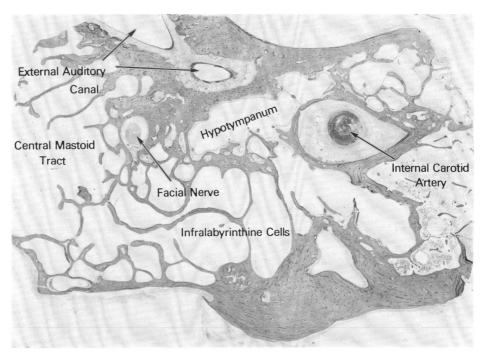

Fig. 2.94: This photomicrograph shows extensive pneumatization of the infralabyrinthine area (male, age 16).

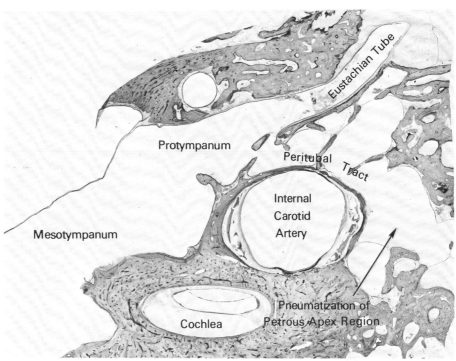

Fig. 2.95: This photomicrograph shows pneumatization of the peritubal and apical areas (female, age 89).

Fig. 2.96: The posterosuperior cell tract extends from the mastoid in an anteromedial direction toward the internal auditory canal along the posteromedial surface of the temporal bone. It lies close to the superior semicircular canal and may extend anteriorly to reach the supralabyrinthine and apical areas (female, age 81).

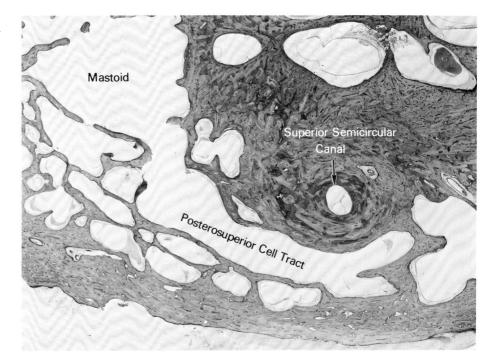

Fig. 2.97: The posteromedial cell tract extends anteromedially from the mastoid along the posteromedial surface of the petrous bone inferior to the posterosuperior cell tract. On one side it is bordered by the endolymphatic duct and sac, and on the other by the bony wall of the posterior cranial fossa. It may extend to the supralabyrinthine and infralabyrinthine areas (male, age 79).

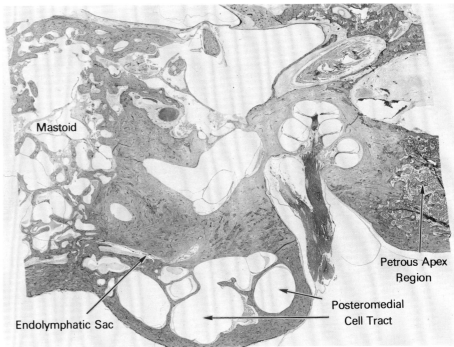

Fig. 2.98: The subarcuate tract extends from the mastoid in an anteromedial direction through the arc of the superior semicircular canal (male, age 44).

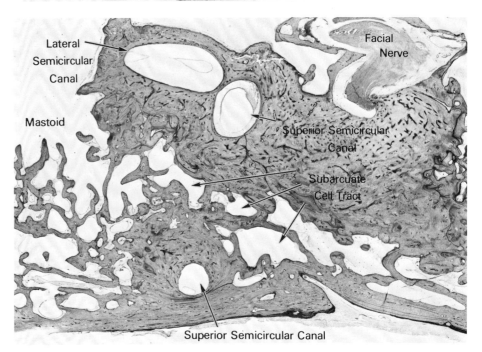

(b) The posteromedial cell tract. This tract extends anteromedially from the central mastoid tract along the posteromedial surface of the petrous bone at a level inferior to the posterosuperior cell tract (Fig. 2.97). On one side it is bordered by the endolymphatic duct and sac, and on the other by the bony wall of the posterior cranial fossa. It frequently leads to the supralabyrinthine and infralabyrinthine areas.

(c) The subarcuate cell tract. This tract extends from the central mastoid tract in an anteromedial direction through the arc of the superior semicircular canal adjacent to the petromastoid canal and may reach the supralabyrinthine area (Fig. 2.98).

(d) The perilabyrinthine tracts. These tracts extend from the epitympanic and hypotympanic areas of the middle ear into the supralabyrinthine and infralabyrinthine areas respectively.

(e) The peritubal tract. This tract arises from the protympanum or eustachian tube and takes a course anterior to the internal carotid artery to reach the apical area (Fig. 2.95).

The apical area of the temporal bone is the most remote and inaccessible area to the surgeon. It may be pneumatized via the peritubal, perilabyrinthine, posterosuperior, posteromedial, and subarcuate cell tracts. Purulent accumulations accompanying infection in the apical area usually can be drained through one of these routes (Jones, 1935; Mayer, 1937).

G. ANATOMY ON SERIAL SECTIONS

The series of photomicrographs in Figs. 2.99 to 2.118 are made from horizontal sections of the right ear of a five-year-old male. The sections were cut at a thickness of 20 microns and every twentieth section photographed for study. The sequence is presented from superior to inferior, and the plane of sectioning is parallel to the axis of the modiolus of the cochlea.

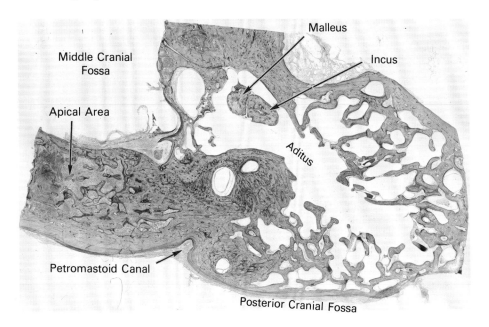

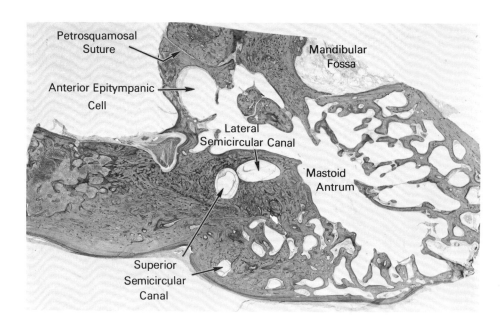

Petrosquamosal Suture

Mandibular Fossa

Anterior Epitympanic Cell

Lateral Semicircular Canal

Mastoid Antrum

Superior Semicircular Canal

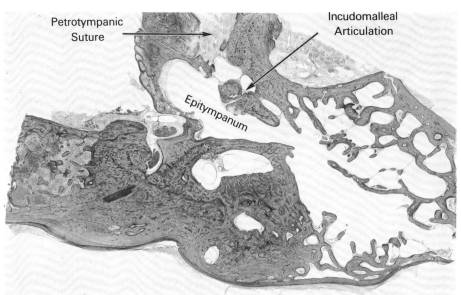

Petrotympanic Suture

Incudomalleal Articulation

Epitympanum

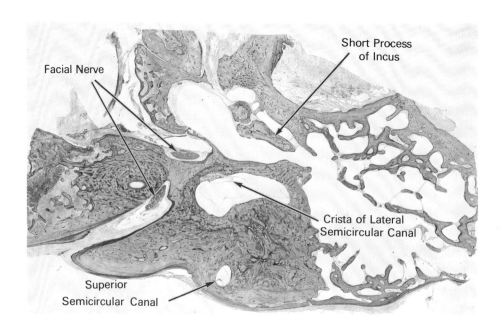

Short Process of Incus

Facial Nerve

Crista of Lateral Semicircular Canal

Superior Semicircular Canal

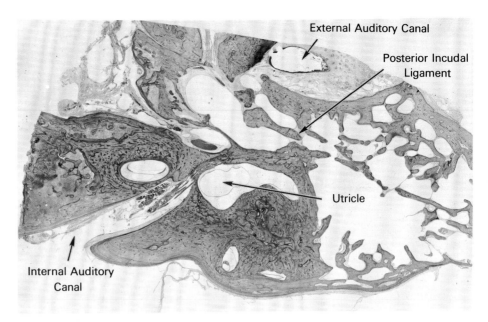

External Auditory Canal

Posterior Incudal Ligament

Utricle

Internal Auditory Canal

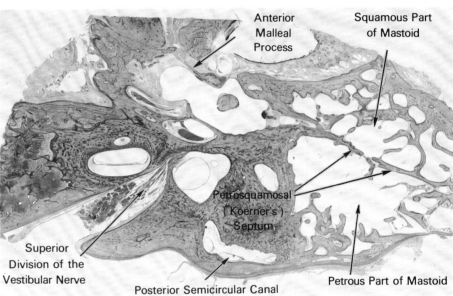

Anterior Malleal Process

Squamous Part of Mastoid

Petrosquamosal (Koerner's) Septum

Superior Division of the Vestibular Nerve

Posterior Semicircular Canal

Petrous Part of Mastoid

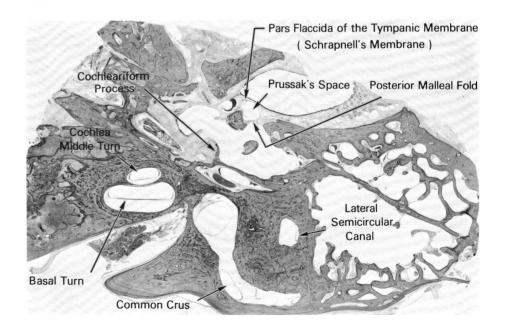

Pars Flaccida of the Tympanic Membrane (Schrapnell's Membrane)

Cochleariform Process

Prussak's Space

Posterior Malleal Fold

Cochlea Middle Turn

Lateral Semicircular Canal

Basal Turn

Common Crus

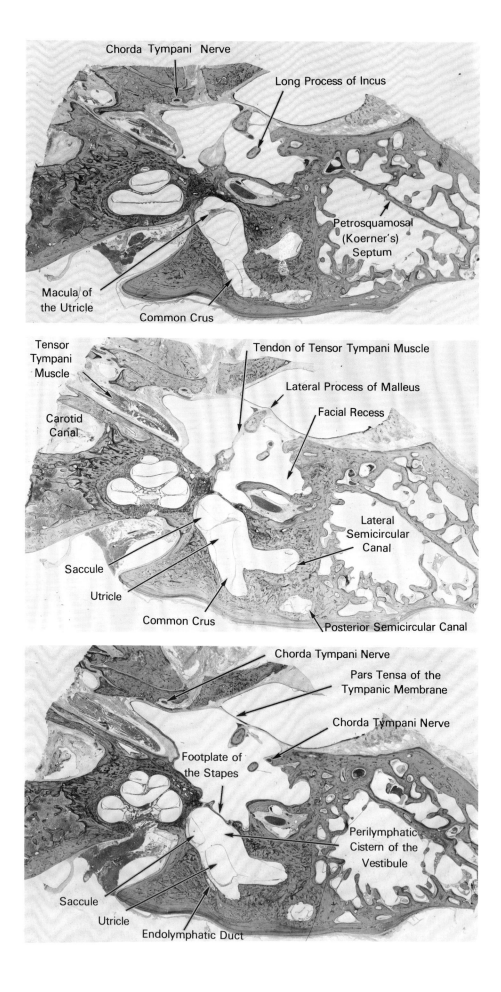

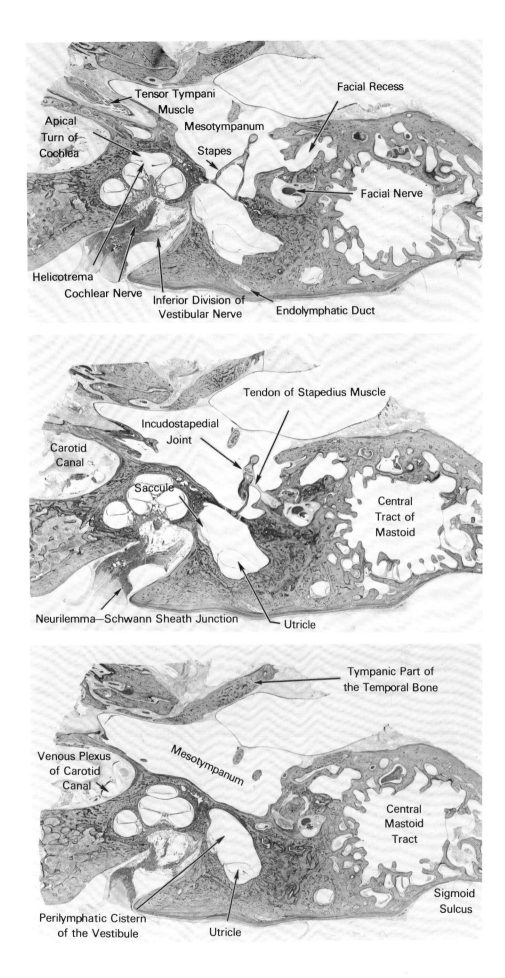

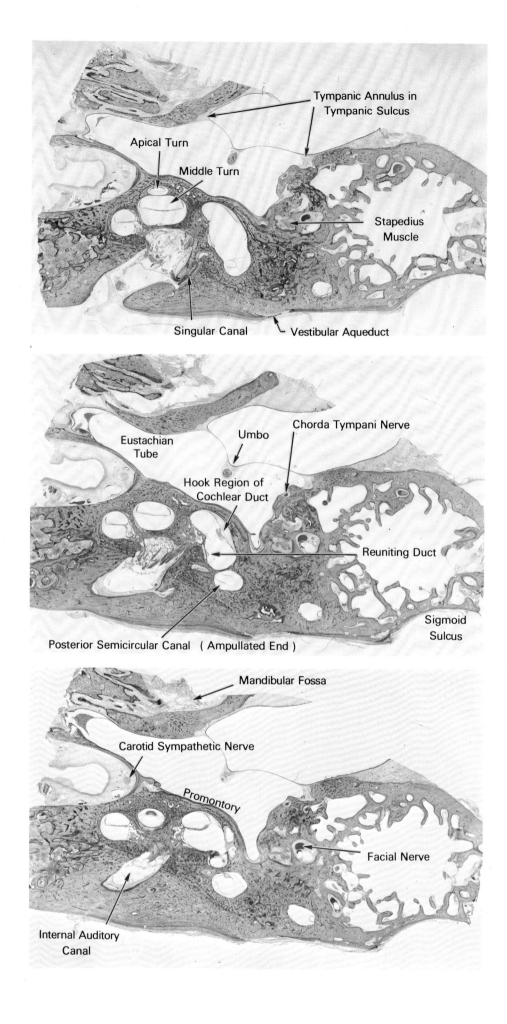

Tympanic Annulus in Tympanic Sulcus

Apical Turn

Middle Turn

Stapedius Muscle

Singular Canal

Vestibular Aqueduct

Eustachian Tube

Umbo

Chorda Tympani Nerve

Hook Region of Cochlear Duct

Reuniting Duct

Posterior Semicircular Canal (Ampullated End)

Sigmoid Sulcus

Mandibular Fossa

Carotid Sympathetic Nerve

Promontory

Facial Nerve

Internal Auditory Canal

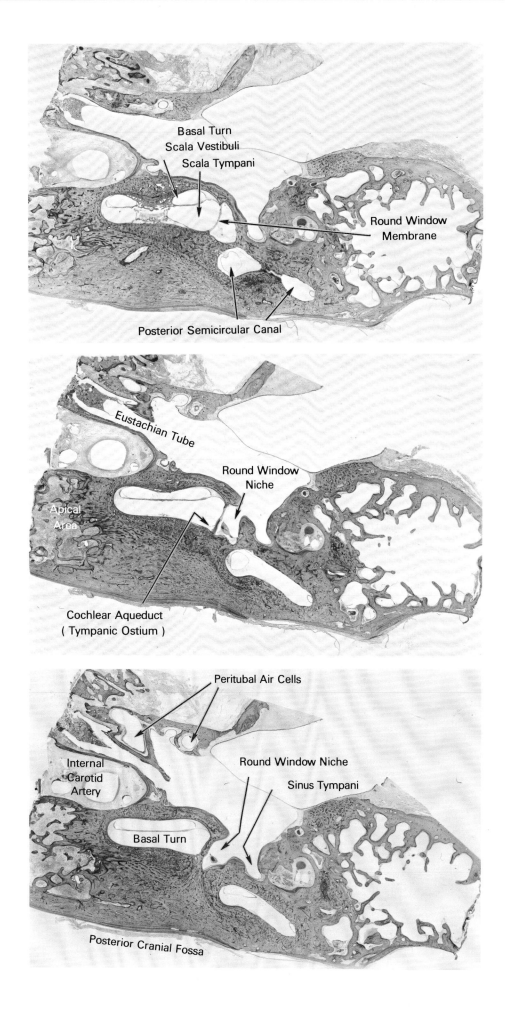

Basal Turn
Scala Vestibuli
Scala Tympani

Round Window
Membrane

Posterior Semicircular Canal

Eustachian Tube

Round Window
Niche

Apical
Area

Cochlear Aqueduct
(Tympanic Ostium)

Peritubal Air Cells

Internal
Carotid
Artery

Round Window Niche

Sinus Tympani

Basal Turn

Posterior Cranial Fossa

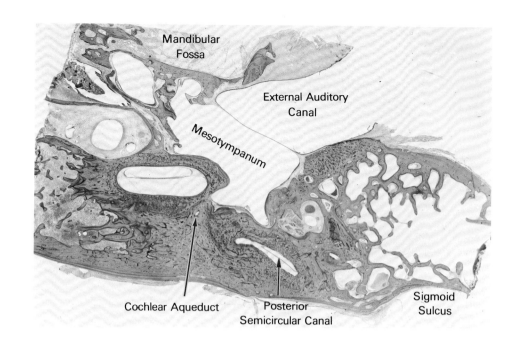

References

Ades, H., Angelborg, C., Bergström, B., Bredberg, G., Engström, H., Stahle, J., and Sugar, J., 1972: Inner ear studies. Acta oto-laryng. Suppl. 301.

Adlington, P., 1967: The ultrastructure and the functions of the saccus endolymphaticus and its decompression in Ménière's disease. J. Laryng. 81:759.

Alberti, P., 1963: The blood supply of the incudostapedial joint and the lenticular process. Laryngoscope 73:605.

Allam, A., 1969: Pneumatization of the temporal bone. Ann. Otol. Rhinol. Laryng. 78:49.

Anderson, S., and Gernandt, B., 1954: Cortical projection of vestibular nerve in cat. Acta oto-laryng. Suppl. 116:10.

Anson, B., and Donaldson, J., 1967: The Surgical Anatomy of the Temporal Bone and Ear. W. B. Saunders, Philadelphia, Pa.

Anson, B., Harper, D., and Hanson, J., 1962: Vascular anatomy of the auditory ossicles and petrous part of the temporal bone in man. Ann. Otol. Rhinol. Laryng. 71:622.

Anson, B., Harper, D., and Winch, T., 1967: The vestibular and cochlear aqueducts: Developmental and adult anatomy of their contents and parietes. IIIrd Symposium on the Role of the Vestibular Organs in Space Exploration. NASA SP-152:125.

Arnold, F., 1831: Der Kopftheil des vegetativen Nervensystems beim Menschen. Karl Groos, Heidelberg and Leipzig.

Asai, K., 1908a: Die Blutgefässe des häutigen Labyrinthes der Ratte. Anat. Hefte 36:711.

Asai, K., 1908b: Die Blutgefässe im häutigen Labyrinthe des Hundes. Anat. Hefte 36:369.

Aschan, G., 1954: The eustachian tube: Histological findings under normal conditions and in otosalpingitis. Acta oto-laryng. 44:295.

Axelsson, A., 1968: The vascular anatomy of the cochlea in the guinea pig and in man. Acta oto-laryng. Suppl. 243.

Ballance, C., 1919: Essays on the Surgery of the Temporal Bone. Macmillan, London.

Basek, M., 1962: Anomalies of the facial nerve in normal temporal bones. Ann. Otol. Rhinol. Laryng. 71:382.

Bast, T., and Anson, B., 1949: The Temporal Bone and the Ear. C. C. Thomas, Springfield, Ill.

Baxter, A., 1971: Dehiscence of the fallopian canal. J. Laryng. 85:587.

Beddard, D., and Saunders, W., 1962: Congenital defects in the fallopian canal. Laryngoscope 72:112.

Békésy, G. von, and Rosenblith, W., 1951: The mechanical properties of the ear. Handbook of Experimental Psychology. Edited by S. Stevens, John Wiley and Sons, New York.

Bernstein, J., and Silverstein, H., 1966: Anterior cerebellar and labyrinthine arteries: A study in the cat. Arch. Otolaryng. 83:422.

Boettcher, A., 1869: Uber Entwicklung und Bau des Gehörlabyrinths nach Untersuchungen an Säugetieran. Nova Acta Academiae cesariae 35:1.

Bolz, E., and Lim, D., 1972: Morphology of the stapediovestibular joint. Acta oto-laryng. 73:10.

Boord, R., and Rasmussen, G., 1958: Analysis of the myelinated fibers of the acoustic nerve of the chinchilla. Anat. Rec. 130:394.

Borghesan, E., 1950: Zona vascola-epithelial della benderella di coniglio considerata probabile sorgente di perilinfa. Atti Clin. Otorinolaring. (University of Palermo) 3:31.

Bredberg, G., Lindeman, H., Ades, H., West, R., and Engström, H., 1970: Scanning electron microscopy of the organ of Corti. Science 170:861.

Brodal, A., and Pompeiano, O., 1957a: The origin of ascending fibres of the medial longitudinal fasciculus from the vestibular nuclei. An experimental study in the cat. Acta morph. neerl. scand. 1:306.

Brodal, A., and Pompeiano, O., 1957b: The vestibular nuclei in the cat. J. Anat. (London) 91:438.

Brodal, A., Pompeiano, O., and Walberg, F., 1962: The vestibular nuclei and their connections, anatomy and functional correlations. The Henderson Trust Lectures, Oliver and Boyd, Edinburgh, Scotland.

Brödel, M., 1946: Three Unpublished Drawings of the Anatomy of the Human Ear. W. B. Saunders, Philadelphia, Pa.

Buskirk, C. van, 1945: The seventh nerve complex. J. comp. Neurol. 82:303.

Cajal, S., 1909: Histologie du système nerveaux de l'homme et des vertébrés. Maloine, Paris, vol. I.

Carpenter, M., 1966: The ascending vestibular system and its relationship to conjugate horizontal eye movements. In The Vestibular System and Its Diseases. Edited by R. Wolfson, University of Pennsylvania Press, Philadelphia, Pa., Chap. III.

Cheatle, A., 1907: Surgical Anatomy of the Temporal Bone. J. and A. Churchill, Ltd., London.

Chow, K., 1951: Numerical estimates of the auditory central nervous system of

rhesus monkey. J. Comp. Neurol. 95:159.

Churchill, J., and Schuknecht, H., 1959: The relationship of acetylcholinesterase in the cochlea to the olivocochlear bundle. Henry Ford Hosp. Med. Bull. 7:202.

Churchill, J., Schuknecht, H., and Doran, R., 1956: Acetylcholinesterase activity in the cochlea. Laryngoscope 66:1.

Corti, A., 1851: Recherches sur l'organe de l'ouie des mammifères. Z. wiss. Zool. 3:109.

Danish Otolaryng. Soc. Symposium, 1965: Management of peripheral facial palsies. Arch. Otolaryng. 81:441.

Davis, H., 1962: Advances in the neurophysiology and neuroanatomy of the cochlea. J. Acoust. Soc. Amer. 34:1377.

Diamant, M., 1940: Otitis and pneumatisation of the mastoid bone, a clinical-statistical analysis. Acta oto-laryng. Suppl. 41.

Dickinson, J., Srisomboon, P., and Kamerer, D., 1968: Congenital anomaly of the facial nerve. Arch. Otolaryng. 88:357.

Dohlman, G., 1938: On the mechanism of transformation into nystagmus on stimulation of the semicircular canals. Acta oto-laryng. 27:425.

Dohlman, G., Ormerod, F., and McLay, K., 1959: The secretory epithelium of the internal ear. Acta oto-laryng. 50:243.

Donaldson, J., Anson, B., Warpeha, R., and Rensink, M., 1968: The perils of the sinus tympani. Trans. Pacific Coast Oto-ophthal. Soc. 49:93.

Durcan, D., Shea, J., and Sleeckx, J., 1967: Bifurcation of the facial nerve. Arch. Otolaryng. 86:619.

Duvall, A., III, 1969: The ultrastructure of the external sulcus in the guinea pig cochlear duct. Laryngoscope 79:1.

Dworacek, H., 1960: Die anatomischen verhältnisse des Mittelohres unter operationsmikroskopischer Betrachtung. Acta oto-laryng. 51:15.

Eggston, A., and Wolff, D., 1947: Histopathology of the Ear, Nose and Throat. Williams and Wilkins, Baltimore, Md.

Engström, H., 1958: On the double innervation of the sensory epithelia of the inner ear. Acta oto-laryng. 49:109.

Engström, H., Ades, H., and Hawkins, J., Jr., 1962: Structure and functions of the sensory hairs of the inner ear. J. Acoust. Soc. Amer. 34:1356.

Engström, H., and Wersäll, J., 1953: Structure of the organ of Corti. I. Outer hair cells. Acta oto-laryng. 43:1.

Engström, H., and Wersäll, J., 1958a: Structure and innervation of the inner ear sensory epithelia. Int. Rev.

Cytol. 7:535.

Engström, H., and Wersäll, J., 1958b: The ultrastructural organization of the organ of Corti and of the vestibular sensory epithelia. Exp. Cell Res. 5:460.

Farrior, J., 1943: Histopathologic considerations in treatment of the eustachian tube. Arch. Otolaryng. 37:609.

Fernández, C., 1951: The innervation of the cochlea (guinea pig). Laryngoscope 61:1152.

Flock, Å., 1965: Electron microscopic and electrophysiological studies on the lateral line canal organ. Acta oto-laryng. Suppl. 199.

Foley, J., 1948: The special visceral efferent zone of the seventh cranial nerve in the canalis facialis. J. Comp. Neurol. 81:169.

Foley, J., and DuBois, F., 1943: An experimental study of the facial nerve. J. Comp. Neurol. 79:79.

Fowler, E., Jr., 1944: Use of radon to prevent otitis media due to hyperplasia of lymphoid tissue and barotrauma (aero-otitis). Arch. Otolaryng. 40:402.

Fowler, E., Jr., 1945: Causes of deafness in flyers. Arch. Otolaryng. 42:21.

Fowler, E., Jr., 1946: Irradiation of the eustachian tube. Arch. Otolaryng. 43:1.

Fowler, E., Jr., 1947: Medicine of the Ear, 1st edition. Thomas Nelson and Sons, New York.

Fowler, E., Jr., 1961: Variations in the temporal bone course of the facial nerve. Laryngoscope 71:937.

Friedmann, I., 1959: Electron microscopic observations on in vitro cultures of the isolated fowl embryo otocyst. J. Biophys. Biochem. Cytol. 5:263.

Fuse, G., 1912: Die innere Abteilung des Kleinhirnstiels (Meynert, IAK) und der Deiterische Kern. Arb. Hirn. Anat. Institut. Zürich 6:28.

Gacek, R., 1960: Efferent component of the vestibular nerve. In Neural Mechanisms of the Auditory and Vestibular Systems. Edited by Rasmussen and W. Windle, Charles C. Thomas, Springfield, Ill., Chap. XX.

Gacek, R., 1961a: The macula neglecta in the feline species. J. Comp. Neurol. 116:317.

Gacek, R., 1961b: The efferent cochlear bundle in man. Arch. Otolaryng. 74:690.

Gacek, R., 1966: The vestibular efferent pathway. In The Vestibular System and Its Diseases. Edited by R. Wolfson, University of Pennsylvania Press, Philadelphia, Pa., p. 99.

Gacek, R., 1968: The innervation of the vestibular labyrinth. Ann. Otol. Rhinol. Laryng. 77:676.

Gacek, R., 1969: The course and central termination of first order neurons supplying vestibular endorgans in the cat. Acta oto-laryng. Suppl. 254.

Gacek, R., 1971: Anatomical demonstration of the vestibulo-ocular projections in the cat. Laryngoscope 81:1559.

Gacek, R., and Lyon, M., 1974: The localization of vestibular efferent neurons in the kitten with horseradish peroxidase. Acta oto-laryng. 77:92.

Gacek, R., Nomura, Y., and Balogh, K., Jr., 1965: Acetylcholinesterase activity in the efferent fibers of the stato-acoustic nerve. Acta oto-laryng. 59:541.

Gerlach, J., 1869: Cited by Politzer, A., The Membrana Tympani in Health and Disease. Trans. A. Mathewson and H. Newton, William Wood and Co. New York, p. 13.

Gerlach, J., 1875: Zur Morphologie der Tuba Eustachii. Mschr. Ohrenheilk. 9:48.

Goodhill, V., 1971: Sudden deafness and round window rupture. Laryngoscope 81:1462.

Graves, G., and Edwards, L., 1944: The eustachian tube: A review of its descriptive, microscopic, topographic and clinical anatomy. Arch. Otolaryng. 39:359.

Guild, S., 1949: Natural absence of part of the bony wall of the facial canal. Laryngoscope 59:668.

Guild, S., 1955: Elastic tissue of the eustachian tube. Ann. Otol. Rhinol. Laryng. 64:537.

Gussen, R., 1971: Tissue changes about the endolymphatic sac. Arch. Otolaryng. 94:406.

Hagens, E., 1934: Anatomy and pathology of the petrous bone: Based on a study of fifty temporal bones. Arch. Otolaryng. 19:556.

Hamilton, D., 1969: The cilium on mammalian vestibular hair cells. Anat. Rec. 164:253.

Hansen, C., 1971: Vascular anatomy of the human temporal bone: I. Anastomoses between the membranous labyrinth and its bony capsule; II. Anastomoses inside the labyrinthine capsule; III. The vascularization of the vestibulo-cochlear nerve. Arch. Ohr. Nas.-Kehlk-Heilk. 200:83.

Hawkins, J., Jr., 1967: Vascular patterns of the membranous labyrinth. IIIrd Symposium on the Role of the Vestibular Organs in Space Exploration. NASA SP-152:241.

Held, H., 1892: Die Endigungsweise der sensiblen Nerven in Gehirn. Arch. Anat. Physiol. (anat./physiol. Abt.) pp. 33–39.

Held, H., 1893: Die centrale Gehörleitung. Arch. Anat. Physiol. (anat./physiol. Abt.) pp. 201.

Held, H., 1909: Untersuchungen über den feineren Bau des Ohrlabyrinthes der Wirbeltiere. II. Zur Entwicklungsgeschichte des Cortischen Organs und der Macula acustica bei Säugetieren und Vögeln. Abh. Sächs. Ges. Wiss. (Leipzig) 31:193.

Held, H., 1926: Die Cochlea der Säuger und der Vögel, ihre entwicklung und ihr Bau. Handbuch der Normalen und Pathologischen Physiologie. Edited by A. Bethe, 11:467, J. Springer, Berlin.

Hentzer, E., 1970: Ultrastructure of the normal mucosa in the human middle ear, mastoid cavities and eustachian tube. Ann. Otol. Rhinol. Laryng. 79:1143.

Hilding, D., 1965: Cochlear chromoffin cells. Laryngoscope 75:1.

Holborow, C., 1962: Deafness associated with cleft palate. J. Laryng. 76:762.

Hough, J., 1958: Malformations and anatomical variations seen in the middle ear during the operation for mobilization of the stapes. Laryngoscope 68:1337.

Howe, H., 1935: The reaction of the cochlear nerve to destruction of its endorgans: A study of deaf albino cats. J. Comp. Neurol. 62:73.

Hunt, H., 1915: The sensory field of the facial nerve: a further contribution to the symptomatology of the geniculate ganglion. Brain 38:418.

Huschke, E., 1824: Über die Hörwerkzeuge. Beitr. Physiol. p. 35.

Hyrtl, J., 1835: Neue Beobachtungen aus dem Gebiete der Menschlichen und Vergleichenden Anatomie, Medizinische , Jahrbücher des Kaiserl.-Königl. Oest. reichischen Staates 19:457.

Igarashi, M., and Yoshinobu, T., 1966: Comparative observations of the eminentia cruciata in birds and mammals. Anat. Rec. 155:269.

Iida, H., 1951: Topographic anatomy of the middle ear. Pract. oto-laryng., Kyoto 44:420.

Ishii, D., and Balogh, K., Jr., 1968: Distribution of efferent nerve endings in the organ of Corti: Their graphic reconstruction in cochleae by localization of acetylcholinesterase activity. Acta oto-laryng. 66:282.

Ishii, T., Murakami, Y., and Balogh, K., Jr., 1967: Acetylcholinesterase activity in the efferent nerve fibers of the human inner ear. Ann. Otol. Rhinol. Laryng. 76:69.

Ishiyama, E., Keels, E., and Weibel, J., 1970: New anatomical aspects of the vasculo-epithelial zone of the spiral limbus in mammals. Acta oto-laryng. 70:319.

Iurato, S., 1960: Submicroscopic structure of the membranous labyrinth. I. The tectorial membrane. Z. Zellforsch. 51:105.

Iurato, S., 1962: Efferent fibers to the sensory cells of Corti's organ. Exp. Cell Res. 27:162.

Iurato, S., 1967: Submicroscopic Structure of the Inner Ear. Pergamon Press, Long Island City, N.Y.

Iurato, S., Luciano, L., Pannese, E., and Reale, E., 1971: Histochemical localization of acetylcholinesterase (AChE) activity in the inner ear. Acta oto-laryng. Suppl. 279.

Jensen, C., and Vilstrup, T., 1960: On the chemistry of human cupulae. Acta oto-laryng. 52:383.

Jepsen, O., 1965: Topognosis (topographic diagnosis) of facial nerve lesions. Arch. Otolaryng. 81:446.

Jones, M., 1935: Pathways of approach to the petrous pyramid. Ann. Otol. Rhinol. Laryng. 44:458.

Kaneko, Y., Hiraide, F., and Paparella, M., 1971: Middle ear epithelium of squirrel monkey. Acta oto-laryng. 72:85.

Kaplan, J., 1960: Congenital dehiscence of the fallopian canal in middle ear surgery. Arch. Otolaryng. 72:197.

Kawabata, I., and Paparella, M., 1971: Fine structure of the round window membrane. Ann. Otol. Rhinol. Laryng. 80:13.

Kettel, K., 1959: Peripheral facial palsy: Pathology and Surgery. Munksgaard, Copenhagen.

Kikuchi, J., 1907: Topographic anatomy of the temporal bone of Japanese. Jap. J. Otolaryng. 13:605.

Kimura, R., 1966: Hairs of the cochlear sensory cells and their attachment to the tectorial membrane. Acta oto-laryng. 61:55.

Kimura, R., 1969: Distribution, structure, and function of dark cells in the vestibular labyrinth. Ann. Otol. Rhinol. Laryng. 78:542.

Kimura, R., Lundquist, P., and Wersäll, J., 1963: Secretory epithelial linings in the ampullae of the guinea pig labyrinth. Acta oto-laryng. 57:517.

Kimura, R., Schuknecht, H., and Sando, I., 1964: Fine morphology of the sensory cells in the organ of Corti of man. Acta oto-laryng. 58:390.

Kimura, R., and Wersäll, J., 1962: Termination of the olivo-cochlear bundle in relation to the outer hair cells of the organ of Corti in guinea pig. Acta oto-laryng. 55:11.

Kimura, R., and Schuknecht, H., 1970a: The ultrastructure of the human stria vascularis, Part I. Acta oto-laryng. 69:415.

Kimura, R., and Schuknecht, H., 1970b: The ultrastructure of the human stria vascularis, Part II. Acta oto-laryng. 70:301.

Kirikae, I., 1969: Physiopathology of the middle ear. Refresher Audio-visual Course (Mexico). University of Tokyo Press, Tokyo, Japan.

Kobrak, H., 1959: The Middle Ear. University of Chicago Press, Chicago, Ill.

Koelliker, A., 1891: Der feinere Bau des verlängerten Markes. Anat. Anz. 6:427.

Kojo, Y., 1954: Morphological studies of the human tympanic membrane. J. Oto-rhinolaryng. Soc. Jap. 57:121.

Kolmer, W., 1927: Gehörorgan. Handbuch der Mikroskopischen Anatomie des Menschen. 3:250. Edited by W. von Mollendorf, Springer, Berlin.

Kullman, G., Dyck, P., and Cody, D., 1971: Anatomy of the mastoid portion of the facial nerve. Arch. Otolaryng. 93:29.

Lim, D., 1968: Tympanic membrane: Electron microscopic observation. Part I: Pars tensa. Acta oto-laryng. 66:181.

Lim, D., 1969: Three dimensional observation of the inner ear with the scanning electron microscope. Acta oto-laryng. Suppl. 255.

Lim, D., 1970: Human tympanic membrane: An ultrastructural observation. Acta oto-laryng. 70:176.

Lim, D., 1971: Vestibular sensory organs: A scanning electron microscopic investigation. Arch. Otolaryng. 94:69.

Lim, D., 1972: Fine morphology of the tectorial membrane: its relationship to the organ of Corti. Arch. Otolaryng. 96:199.

Lim, D., 1973: Formation and fate of the otoconia—scanning and transmission electron microscopy. Ann. Otol. Rhinol. Laryng. 82:23.

Lim, D., and Lane, W., 1969: Three-dimensional observation of the inner ear with the scanning electron microscope. Trans. Amer. Acad. Ophthal. Otolaryng. 73:842.

Lindeman, H., 1969a: Regional differences in structure of the vestibular sensory regions. J. Laryng. 83:1.

Lindeman, H., 1969b: Studies on the morphology of the sensory regions of the vestibular apparatus. Adv. Anat. Embry. Cell Biol. 42:1.

Lindsay, J., 1940: Petrous pyramid of the temporal bone: Pneumatization and roentgenologic appearance. Arch. Otolaryng. 31:231.

Lindsay, J., 1941: Pneumatization of the petrous pyramid. Ann. Otol. Rhinol. Laryng. 50:1109.

Lorente de No, R., 1926: Etudes sur l'anatomie et la physiologie du labyrinthe de l'oreille et du VIIIe nerf. Deuxième partie. Quelques données au sujet de l'anatomie des organes sensoriels du labyrinthe. Trav. Lab. Rech. Biol. Univ. Madr. 24:53.

Lorente de No, R., 1931: Ausgewählte Kapitel aus der vergleichenden Physiologie des Labyrinthes. Die Augenmuskelreflexe beim Kaninchen und ihre Grundlagen. Ergebn. Physiol. 32:73.

Lorente de No, R., 1933a: Studies in hearing: Anatomy of the eighth nerve: III. General plan of structure of the primary cochlear nuclei. Laryngoscope 43:327.

Lorente de No, R., 1933b: Anatomy of the eighth nerve. The central projection of the nerve endings of the internal ear. Laryngoscope 43:1.

Lorente de No, R., 1937: Symposium: I. Anatomy and physiology. b. The sensory endings in the cochlea. Laryngoscope 47:373.

Löwemberg, B., 1864: Beiträge zur Anatomie der Schnecke. 1. Membranen und

Kanäle. Arch. Ohr. Nas.-Kehlk-Heilk. 1:175.

Lundquist, P-G., 1965: The endolymphatic duct and sac in the guinea pig: An electron microscopic and experimental investigation. Acta oto-laryng. Suppl. 201.

Lundquist, P-G., Kimura, R., and Wersäll, J., 1964: Ultrastructural organization of the epithelial lining in the endolymphatic duct and sac in the guinea pig. Acta oto-laryng. 57:65.

Lupin, A., 1969: The relationship of the tensor tympani and tensor palati muscles. Ann. Otol. Rhinol. Laryng. 78:792.

May, M., 1973: Anatomy of the facial nerve (spatial orientation of fibers in the temporal bone). Laryngoscope 83:1311.

Mayer, O., 1937: Die Pyramidenzelleneiterungen. Z. Hals-Nas.-Ohrenheilk. 42:1.

Mazzoni, A., 1969a: The subarcuate artery in man. Laryngoscope 80:69.

Mazzoni, A., 1969b: Internal auditory canal, arterial relations at the porus acusticus. Ann. Otol. Rhinol. Laryng. 78:797.

Mazzoni, A., 1972: Internal auditory artery supply to the petrous bone. Ann. Otol. Rhinol. Laryng. 81:13.

Meltzer, P., 1934: The mastoid cells: Their arrangement in relation to the sigmoid portion of the transverse sinus. Arch. Otolaryng. 19:326.

Miehlke, A., 1960: Die Chirurgie des Nervus Facialis. Urban and Schwartzenberg, Munich and Berlin.

Mira, E., and Negro, F. dal, 1969: Die histochemischen und histoenzymologischen Eigenschaften des Epithels der Ubergangszone der Crista ampullaris. Arch. Ohr. Nas.-Kehlk-Heilk. 193:322.

Møller, J., 1930: Le septum de Körner. Acta oto-laryng. 14:213.

Montandon, P., Gacek, R., and Kimura., R., 1970: Crista neglecta in the cat and human. Ann. Otol. Rhinol. Laryng. 79:105.

Nabeya, D., 1923: A study in the comparative anatomy of the blood-vascular system of the internal ear in Mammalia and in Homo (Japanese). Acta Sch. med. Univ. Kioto 6:1.

Nager, G., and Nager, M., 1953: The arteries of the human middle ear, with particular regard to the blood supply of the auditory ossicles. Ann. Otol. Rhinol. Laryng. 62:923.

Naufal, P., and Schuknecht, H., 1972: Vestibular, facial, and oculomotor neuropathy in diabetes mellitus. Arch. Otolaryng. 96:468.

Nauta, W., 1957: Silver impregnation of degenerating axons. New Research Techniques of Neuroanatomy, p. 17. Edited by W. Windle. Charles C. Thomas, Springfield, Ill.

Nauta, W., and Gygax, P., 1954: Silver impregnation of degenerated axons in the central nervous system. A modified technique. Stain Technology 29:91.

Nomura, Y., Gacek, R., and Balogh, K., Jr., 1965: Efferent innervation of vestibular labyrinth. Arch. Otolaryng. 81:335.

Nomura, Y., and Kirikae, I., 1967: Innervation of the human cochlea. Ann. Otol. Rhinol. Laryng. 76:57.

Nomura, Y., and Schuknecht, H., 1965: The efferent fibers in the cochlea. Ann. Otol. Rhinol. Laryng. 74:289.

Oort, H., 1918: Über die Verästellung des Nervus octavus bei Säugetieren. Anat. Anz. 51:272.

Orzalesi, F., and Pellegrini, E., 1933: Sci rapporti fra i nervi intermedio e vestibolare, e sulla struttura del ganglio del nervo vestibolare nell'uomo. Arch. Ital. Anat. Embriol. 31:105.

Perlman, H., 1940: The saccule: Observations on a differentiated reinforced area of the saccular wall in man. Arch. Otolaryng. 32:678.

Platzer, W., 1961: Zur Anatomie der Eminentia Pyramidalis und des M. stapedius. Mschr. Ohrenheilk. 95:553.

Politzer, A., 1869: The Membrana Tympani in Health and Disease. William Wood and Co., New York.

Politzer, A., 1894: Diseases of the Ear and Adjacent Organs. Bailliere, Tindall and Cox, London.

Politzer, A., 1907: Geschichte der Ohrenheilkunde. F. Enke (Stuttgart) 2:396.

Poljak, S., 1927: Über die doppelte Innervation der Macula sacculi und über das cochleo-vestibulare Bündel bei den Säugetieren. Z. Anat. EntwGesch. 84:144.

Proctor, B., 1964: The development of the middle ear spaces and their surgical significance. J. Laryng. 78:631.

Proctor, B., 1967: Embryology and anatomy of the eustachian tube. Arch. Otolaryng. 86:503.

Proctor, B., 1968: Alexander Prussak. Ann. Otol. Rhinol. Laryng. 77:344.

Proctor, B., 1969: Surgical anatomy of the posterior tympanum. Ann. Otol. Rhinol. Laryng. 78:1026.

Prussak, A., 1867: Studien über die Anatomie des menschlichen Trommelfells. Arch. Ohr. Nas.-Kehlk-Heilk. 3:255.

Pullen, F., 1972: Round window membrane rupture: a cause of sudden deafness. Trans. Amer. Acad. Ophth. Otol. 76:1444.

Rasmussen, A., 1940: Studies of the VIIIth cranial nerve of man. Laryngoscope 50:67.

Rasmussen, G., 1946: The olivary peduncle and other fiber projections of the superior olivary complex. J. Comp. Neurol. 84:141.

Rasmussen, G. L., 1953: Further observations of the efferent cochlear bundle. J. Comp. Neurol. 99:61.

Rasmussen, G., 1960: Efferent fibers of the cochlear nerve and cochlear nucleus. In Neural Mechanisms of the Auditory and Vestibular Systems. Edited by G. Rasmussen and W. Windle. Charles C. Thomas, Springfield, Ill., Chap. 8.

Rasmussen, G., 1964: Anatomic relationships of the ascending and descending auditory systems. In Neurological Aspects of Auditory and Vestibular Disorders. Edited by W. Fields and B. Alford. Charles C. Thomas, Springfield, Ill., Chap. I.

Report on Workshop, 1973: Neuroanatomy of the auditory system. Arch. Otolaryng. 98:397.

Retzius, G., 1881: Das Gehörorgan der Wirbelthiere. I. Das Gehörorgan der Fische und Amphibien. Samson and Wallin, Stockholm.

Retzius, G., 1884: Das Gehörorgan der Wirbelthiere. II. Das Gehörorgan der Reptilien, der Vögel und der Säugethiere. Samson and Wallin, Stockholm.

Retzius, G., 1927: Handbuch der Mikroskopischen Anatomie des Menschen. Cited by W. Kolmer. Dritter Band, p. 319.

Rhoton, A., Jr., Kobayashi, S., and Hollinshead, W., 1968: Nervus intermedius. J. Neurosurg. 29:609.

Rich, A., 1920: A physiological study of the eustachian tube and its related muscles. Johns Hopkins Hosp. Bull. 31:206.

Richardson, T., Ishiyama, E., and Keels, E., 1971: Submicroscopic studies of the round window membrane. Acta oto-laryng. 71:9.

Rose, J., 1949: The cellular structure of the auditory region of the cat. J. Comp. Neurol. 91:409.

Rose, J., and Woolsey, C., 1949: The relations of thalamic connections, cellular structure and evocable electrical activity in the auditory region of the cat. J. Comp. Neurol. 91:441.

Rüdinger, N., 1870: Beiträge zur Vergleichenden Anatomie und Histologie der Ohrtrompete. J. J. Lentner, Munich.

Saito, H., Ruby, R., and Schuknecht, H., 1970: Course of the sensory component of the nervus intermedius in the temporal bone. Ann. Otol. Rhinol. Laryng. 79:960.

Saito, R., Igarashi, M., Alford, B., and Guilford, F., 1971: Anatomical measurement of the sinus tympani. Arch. Otolaryng. 94:418.

Sando, I., 1965: The anatomical interrelationships of the cochlear nerve fibers. Acta oto-laryng. 59:417.

Sando, I., Black, F., and Hemenway, W., 1972: Spatial distribution of vestibular nerve in internal auditory canal. Ann. Otol. Rhinol. Laryng. 81:305.

Scarpa, A., 1800: Anatomische Untersuchungen des Gehörs und Geruchs. Nürnberg.

Schuknecht, H., 1960: Neuroanatomical correlates of auditory sensitivity and pitch discrimination in the cat. In Neural Mechanisms of the Auditory and Vestibular Systems. Edited by G. Rasmussen and W. Windle. Charles C. Thomas, Springfield, Ill. Chap. VI.

Schuknecht, H., Churchill, J., and Doran, R., 1959: The localization of acetylcholinesterase in the cochlea. Arch. Otolaryng. 69:549.

Shambaugh, G., 1903: Blood-vessels in the labyrinth of the ear. The Decennial publication of the Univerity of Chicago. 10:131.

Shambaugh, G., 1905: The distribution of blood vessels in the labyrinth of the ear of the sheep and the calf. Arch. Otolaryng. 34:71.

Shambaugh, G., 1908: On the structure and function of the epithelium in the sulcus spiralis externus. Arch. Otolaryng. 37:538.

Shambaugh, G., Jr., 1967: Facial nerve decompression and repair. Surgery of the Ear. 2nd ed. W. B. Saunders, Philadelphia, Pa. Chap. XXI.

Shimada, T., and Lim., D., 1972: Distribution of ciliated cells in the human middle ear: electron and light microscopic observations. Ann. Otol. Rhinol. Laryng. 81:203.

Shrapnell, H., 1832: On the form and structure of membrana tympani. London Med. Gaz. 10:120.

Siebenmann, F., 1894: Die Blutgefässe im Labyrinthe des menschlichen Ohres. J. Bergmann, Wiesbaden.

Smith, C., 1951: Capillary areas of the cochlea in the guinea pig. Laryngoscope 61:1073.

Smith, C., 1953: The capillaries of the vestibular membranous labyrinth in the guinea pig. Laryngoscope 63:87.

Smith, C., 1954: Capillary areas of the membranous labyrinth. Ann. Otol. Rhinol. Laryng. 63:435.

Smith, C., 1956: Microscopic structure of the utricle. Ann. Otol. Rhinol. Laryng. 65:450.

Smith, C., 1957: Structure of the stria vascularis and the spiral prominence. Ann. Otol. Rhinol. Laryng. 66:521.

Smith, C., 1961: Innervation pattern of the cochlea: The internal hair cell. Ann. Otol. Rhinol. Laryng. 70:504.

Smith, C., and Rasmussen, G., 1967: Nerve endings in the maculae and cristae of the chinchilla vestibule, with a special reference to the efferents. IIIrd Symposium on the Role of the Vestibular Organs in Space Exploration. NASA SP-152:183.

Smith, C., and Sjöstrand, F., 1961: Structure of the nerve endings on the external hair cells of the guinea pig cochlea as studied by serial sections. J. Ultrastruct. Res. 5:523.

Sobotta, J., 1957: Atlas of Descriptive Human Anatomy. Vol. III—Blood vessels—Nervous system—Sense organs—Integument and lymphatics. p. 309. Edited and trans. by E. Uhlenhuth. Hafner Publishing Co., New York.

Spoendlin, H., 1956: Elecktronenmikroskopische Untersuchungen am Cortischen Organ. Pract. oto-rhino-laryng. 18:246.

Spoendlin, H., 1965: Ultrastructural studies of the labyrinth in squirrel monkeys. The Role of the Vestibular Organs in the Exploration of Space. NASA-SP-77:7.

Spoendlin, H., 1966: The organization of the cochlear receptor. Advances in otolaryngology. S. Karger, Basel, vol. 13.

Spoendlin, H., 1971: Degeneration behaviour of the cochlear nerve. Arch. Ohr. Nas-Kehlk-Heilk. 200:275.

Spoendlin, H., and Gacek, R., 1963: Electronmicroscopic study of the efferent and afferent innervation of the organ of Corti in the cat. Ann. Otol. Rhinol. Laryng. 72:660.

Steifensand, K., 1835: Untersuchungen über die Ampullen des Gehörorgans. Arch. Anat. Physiol. wiss. Med. 171:189.

Steinhausen, W., 1933: Über die Funktion der Cupula in den Bogengangsampullen des Labyrinthes. Z. Hals-Nas.-Ohrenheilk. 34:201.

Stricht, N. van der, 1908: L'Histogenèse des parties constituantes du neuroépithélium acoustique des taches et des crêtes acoustiques et de l'organe de Corti. Arch. Biol. 23:541.

Sunderland, S., and Cossar, D., 1953: The structure of the facial nerve. Anat. Rec. 116:147.

Symposium of Neurotology Group, 1970: On surgical considerations in disorders of the facial nerve. Ann. Otol. Rhinol. Laryng. 79:217.

Takahashi, T., 1971: The ultrastructure of the pathologic stria vascularis and spiral prominence in man. Ann. Otol. Rhinol. Laryng. 80:721.

Takahashi, T., and Kimura, R., 1970: The ultrastructure of the spiral ligament in the Rhesus monkey. Acta oto-laryng. 69:46.

Tos, M., 1971: Distribution of mucous glands in the foetal eustachian tube. Arch. Ohr. Nas.-Kehlk-Heilk. 197:295.

Tremble, G., 1934: Pneumatization of the temporal bone. Arch. Otolaryng. 19:172.

Vries, H. de, 1949: Struktur und Lage der Tektorialmembran in der Schnecke, untersucht mit neueren Hilfsmitteln. Acta oto-laryng. 37:334.

Walberg, F., Bowsher, D., and Brodal, A., 1958: The termination of primary vestibular fibers in the vestibular nuclei in the cat. An experimental study with silver methods. J. Comp. Neurol. 110:391.

Watanuki, K., 1968: Some morphological observations of Reissner's membrane. Acta oto-laryng. 66:40.

Werner, C., 1933: Die Differenzierung der Maculae im Labyrinth insbesondere bei Säugetieren. Z. Anat. EntwGesch. 99:696.

Werner, C., 1940: Das Labyrinth. Thieme, Leipzig.

Wersäll, J., 1956: Studies on the structure and innervation of the sensory epithelium of the cristae ampullares in the guinea pig. A light and electron microscopic investigation. Acta oto-laryng. Suppl. 126.

Wersäll, J., 1960: Electron micrographic studies of vestibular hair cell innervation. In Neural Mechanisms of the Auditory and Vestibular Systems. Edited by Rasmussen and W. Windle. Charles C. Thomas, Springfield, Ill. Chap. 18.

Wever, E., and Lawrence, M., 1954: Physiological Acoustics. Princeton University Press, Princeton, N.J.

Williams, H., 1966: Latent or dormant disease in the pneumatic cell tracts of the temporal bone. Trans. Amer. Acad. Ophthal. Otolaryng. 70:545.

Wolff, D., and Bellucci, R., 1956: The human ossicular ligaments. Ann. Otol. Rhinol. Laryng. 65:895.

Wright, J., Jr., Taylor, C., and McKay, D., 1967: Variations in the course of the facial nerve as illustrated by tomography. Laryngoscope 77:717.

Ziegelmann, E., 1935: The cellular character of one hundred temporal bones: Clinical and Surgical significance. Ann. Otol. Rhinol. Laryng. 44:3.

Zöllner, F., 1942: Anatomie, Physiologie und Klinik der Ohrtrompete. Springer Verlag, Berlin.

Zuckerkandl, E., 1879: Zur Anatomie des Warzenfortsatzes. Mschr. Ohrenheilk. 13:49.

3 Pathophysiology

This chapter will deal with some of the well-known physiological mechanisms of the auditory and vestibular systems and probable explanations for deviations in sensory experience resulting from pathological changes in these systems.

A. THE AUDITORY SYSTEM

1. THE MIDDLE EAR

The malleus and incus are united by a firm pseudoarthrodial joint and move as a unit (Kirikae, 1969) except at extremely high intensities (Kobrak, 1959). The movement or slippage which occurs at high intensities may be regarded as a protective mechanism. At low frequencies all three ossicles move in phase; however, at high frequencies (over 3000 Hz), the stapes and incus lag behind the malleus. Studies on the guinea pig have shown that in the range of 30 to 10,000 Hz and up to 130 db SPL (sound pressure level), the motion of the stapes is predominantly piston-like, and its displacement amplitudes are linearly related to sound pressure (Guinan and Peake, 1967).

Calculations by Kirikae (1960) show that the axis of rotation of the ossicles passes through the center of gravity of the combined mass of ossicles and tympanic membrane (Fig. 3.1).

The middle ear functions primarily as a mechanism by which sound energy is transmitted from air to the inner ear fluids. Without a middle ear mechanism about 0.1 percent of the energy in an air wave would be transmitted into the perilymph and about 99.9 percent would be reflected. This ratio of 1000:1 can be expressed in decibels by saying that if a sound wave travels from air directly into perilymph, energy will enter the perilymph with a transmission loss of about 30 db (Kobrak, 1959).

A transmission problem also exists at the boundary between air and the tympanic membrane, for when sound impinges on the membrane a certain percentage of the sound energy is reflected and the remainder is absorbed. There is an abundance of literature on the mechanical impedance of the

Fig. 3.1: The axis of rotation as related to the center of gravity of the tympanic membrane and ossicles (after Kirikae). A line MI is drawn through centers of gravity of the malleus and incus. Point O is located on this line in accordance with the respective masses of the malleus (23 mg) and incus (27 mg) so that MO:IO = 27:23. The mass of the stapes, which is about 2.5 mg, is considered inconsequential; thus point O represents the center of gravity of the ossicles. The mass of the pars tensa is about 14 mg, and its center of gravity is located at the umbo. Point C is located on the line OU in the ratio CU:CO = 50:14, 50 being the combined weight of the malleus and incus and U the weight of the pars tensa. A straight line extending from the center of the posterior incudal ligament through the center of gravity, point C, passes through the lower part of the anterior malleal ligament. Thus if xy represents the axis of rotation of the ossicular system, it is physiologically effective because the center of gravity falls on this axis.

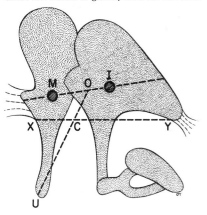

human tympanic membrane beginning with Tröger (1930) and continuing with Metz (1946) and others (Zwislocki, 1957a, 1957b; Møller, 1961).

In recent studies Tonndorf and Khanna (1970) utilizing time-averaged holography determined that the tympanic membrane obeys the mechanism of curved membranes, which implies that part of the transformer action resides in the tympanic membrane. They demonstrated that at low frequencies all parts of the tympanic membrane contribute in equal degrees to the total transformer action of the middle ear. Above 1500 Hz the basic vibratory pattern gradually becomes restricted in size and volume, and above 3000 Hz it breaks up into quasi-independent subpatterns and ceases to contribute to displacement of the manubrium. At these high frequencies the tympanic membrane serves simply as a baffle for the manubrium, which is then driven directly by the incoming sound.

The pars flaccida apparently serves simply to provide freedom of motion for the malleus.

Other mechanisms which are believed to be important for the transfer of sound energy from the air to the inner ear fluid are the lever effect of the ossicular chain and the hydraulic effect of the middle ear. The lever effect is accomplished simply by the fact that the manubrium of the malleus is longer than the long process of the incus in a ratio of 1.3:1, or 2.5 db. The hydraulic effect of the middle ear is achieved by the difference in area of the tympanic membrane and stapes footplate. The effective area of the tympanic membrane is about 55 sq mm and that of the average footplate about 3.2 sq mm, giving a ratio of 17:1, or 25 db. The final transformer ratio of the human tympanic membrane and ossicular chain, therefore, is the product of the lever ratio of 1.3:1 and the hydraulic ratio of 17:1 for a total of 27.5 db (Békésy and Rosenblith, 1951).

The round window is of considerable importance in determining the effectiveness of sound transmission to the inner ear. It has an area of 2 sq mm, is somewhat protected by the overhanging lip of the round window niche, and lies in a horizontal plane at right angles to the oval window. In the normal ear the intact tympanic membrane shields the round window from direct impact of sound. Sound waves reaching the two windows in different phases would tend to enhance sound transmission; however, this effect is minimal in the normal ear because of the great effectiveness of the hydraulic and lever mechanisms. In diseased ears (e.g., perforation of the tympanic membrane), the effect of sound pressure acting on the round window membrane becomes more important. Thus sound vibrations of low frequency reach the head of the stapes and round window at the same phase, whereas higher frequencies may meet these structures at opposite phases. It seems quite clear that to achieve optimum sound transmission to the inner ear, the round window membrane must be free to move against an elastic air cushion and that it must be shielded from the direct impact of sound entering the middle ear.

The measurement of acoustic impedance in the external auditory canal serves some usefulness in the diagnosis of disorders of the tympanic membrane and middle ear. More sound energy is reflected when the tympanic membrane is rigid than when it is yielding. When a vibrating force like sound waves is applied to a vibrating system, the mode of vibration is determined by the friction, mass, and stiffness characteristics of the system. Impedance is a ratio of the force to the velocity of the vibration (Kirikae, 1969).

The factors of friction, mass, stiffness, and frequency interact in accordance with the following equation:

$$\text{Impedance} = \sqrt{\text{friction}^2 + \text{mass} \times \text{frequency} - \frac{\text{stiffness}^2}{\text{frequency}}}$$

The middle ear sound conducting system is a complex vibrating system which comprises the tympanic membrane, ossicles, ligaments, folds of mucous membrane, and tympanic muscles, as well as the air of the external auditory canal, tympanic cavity, and pneumatized spaces of the temporal bone.

Increase of mass improves performance mainly for lower frequencies whereas increase of stiffness enhances resonance mainly for the high frequencies. Increase in friction, on the other hand, has its greatest effect for the mid-frequency area and is less important for both low and high frequencies (Johansen, 1948).

The application of the impedance formula to the problems of sound conduction may aid in the understanding of abnormal threshold curves in conduction deafness; however, it is clearly an oversimplified view and restraint must be used in applying it to clinical otology.

Lesions which occlude the external auditory canal and which are not in contact with the tympanic membrane produce a flat audiometric threshold loss. When there is contact with the tympanic membrane or manubrium, a mass lesion is created with a hearing loss greater for the higher frequencies (Shambaugh, 1967).

Total loss of the pars tensa creates a hearing loss for all frequencies of about 30 db, this being caused by a loss of the hydraulic mechanism and the canceling effect of sound waves striking the round window membrane. For smaller perforations the degree of hearing loss is determined by the size and location of the perforation. Thus a hearing loss will be greater if the perforation is located in the postero-inferior part of the tympanic membrane, permitting ready access of sound waves to the round window. If the perforation is in the far anterior part of the tympanic membrane, the hearing loss is less severe. Interruption of the ossicular chain in the presence of an intact tympanic membrane creates a large conductive hearing loss which may reach a magnitude of 50 to 55 db for some frequencies. In the absence of a tympanic membrane and ossicular chain, direct exposure of the oval window to sound, with the round window protected in an air-containing hypotympanum, causes a loss of about 20 db.

Mass lesions create hearing loss which is greater for high frequencies and may result from edema, serous or hemorrhagic blebs, hyaline plaques in the tympanic membrane, or by serous, mucinous, or purulent fluid in the middle ear. Fluid in the middle ear produces hearing losses of varying degree depending upon the viscosity of the fluid and the ratio of the air to fluid. A middle ear completely filled with fluid exhibits a conductive hearing loss of 30 to 40 db.

Stiffness lesions produce hearing losses which are greater for the low frequencies. Examples of such conditions are stapes fixation due to otosclerosis, fibrous adhesions of the middle ear and negative middle ear pressure (Shambaugh, 1967).

The concept of the decibel has developed because the auditory organ, like all sense organs, operates over a large range of stimulus intensities, making it essential to condense the perceptual range. This has led to the general use of logarithmic scales when recording stimulus-response data.

A commonly accepted method for measuring sound level is the decibel. It does not express an absolute measure of the level of a sound but it is a comparison between the sound being measured and some reference sound.

The Acoustical Society of America has set the reference level at 10^{-16} watts per sq cm, and this value has been generally accepted. A sound in air under standard conditions (temperature $20°C$, 760 mm of mercury barometric pressure) whose power is 10^{-16} watts per sq cm has a pressure of 0.0002 dynes per sq cm and is the usual reference level for sound pressure measurements.

Rating a sound for intensity consists of expressing it in terms of a simple ratio, J/J_0, where J represents the sound level to be rated and J_0 represents the standard reference sound. Because of the tremendous intensity range over which the ear is capable of functioning, such a simple arithmetic ratio would be cumbersome. A logarithmic scale was adopted because intensity changes at low levels of intensity produce greater changes in loudness sensation than the same increments of change at high levels of intensity. Thus we have come to use the logarithm of the ratio to the base 10 in the following formula:

$$\log_{10} \frac{J}{J_0}$$

This unit of one *bel,* named in honor of Alexander Graham Bell, inventor of the telephone, has been found to be a rather large unit; therefore, the decibel has come into standard use. The final formula which is used when the decibel represents power is:

$$\text{decibel} = 10 \times \log_{10} \frac{J}{J_0}$$

When sound pressure is of interest the formula is:

$$\text{decibel} = 20 \log_{10} \frac{P}{P_0}$$

2. THE EUSTACHIAN TUBE

The eustachian tube is opened by the pull of the tensor veli palati muscle on the lateral cartilaginous lamina accompanied by the simultaneous elevation of the medial lamina caused by the bulging contraction of the levator veli palati muscle (see Chapter 2B, The Eustachian Tube). The salpingopharyngeus muscle appears to have little or no effect on tubal opening (Rich, 1920).

In infancy the eustachian tube lies in a horizontal plane so that the lumen is a slit parallel to the base of the skull. In this position the infantile tube opens mainly by the action of the tensor, and action of the levator is minimal (Holborow, 1962b).

A mucous sheath propelled by ciliary activity is located in the anterior part of the middle ear and the eustachian tube (Sade, 1966). Holmgren (1934), Sato (1939), Compere (1958), Rogers et al. (1962) have demonstrated that foreign material introduced into the middle ear is evacuated through the eustachian tube into the nasopharynx within a few minutes.

Normally the ear sucks in air through the eustachian tube during the act of swallowing solely as a consequence of negative pressure prevailing within the middle ear (Ingelstedt, 1964). Failure of the eustachian tube to open during deglutition results in negative pressure in the pneumatized spaces of the temporal bone as a consequence of gases being absorbed into the blood stream.

Interference with opening of the eustachian tube may be due to an inflammatory reaction in the lining membrane such as occurs with viral and bacterial infections and allergic reactions in the upper respiratory tract. Other factors causing narrowing of the lumen are connective tissue hyperplasia or cicatrix associated with chronic inflammatory disorders of the middle ear, hyperplasia of lymphoid tissue, muscle weakness, neoplasms, and developmental anomalies such as those associated with cleft palate (Fig. 3.2).

Flisberg et al. (1963) and Flisberg (1966) demonstrated that during head colds the eustachian tube is more easily locked in the closed position with negative middle ear pressure.

Rundcrantz (1969) studied the ventilatory capacity of the eustachian tube and found that the volume of air passing through the tube during deglutition was reduced to one-third of normal when the patient was placed in the horizontal position. With a head elevation of 20–30° the passage of air was reduced to two-thirds of normal. On the basis of these observations, he suggested that patients with upper respiratory infections utilize pillows at night so that a head position of not less than 20° above the horizontal plane could be maintained.

Silverstein et al. (1966), Baxter (1970), and Westergaard (1970), using a eustachiometer patterned after the design of Miller (1965) and Flisberg (1966), found that most children with seromucinous otitis media are unable to pass air through the eustachian tube during deglutition in the presence of negative middle ear pressure (Fig. 3.3). This observation supports the concept that

Fig. 3.2: Squamous cell carcinoma of the naso-pharynx invading the walls of the osseous part of the eustachian tube. The tube has become obstructed and the pneumatic spaces of the temporal bone contain fluid (female, age 51 years).

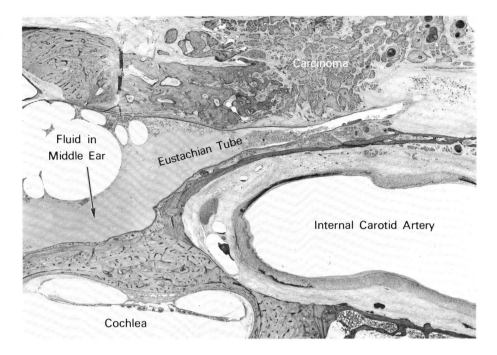

eustachian tube dysfunction is a factor in the etiology of seromucinous otitis media (see Chapter 5B, Seromucinous Otitis Media).

Ingelstedt and Örtegren (1963) and Holmquist (1970) have modified the eustachiometer technique to make it adaptable for ears with intact tympanic membranes. This is accomplished by a device which produces negative pressure in the nasopharynx when the patient swallows. This negative pressure is transmitted to the middle ear and increases the acoustic impedance of the stretched tympanic membrane. When this condition has been accomplished, the patient is directed to swallow. The effectiveness of the eustachian tube in ventilating the middle ear may then be measured as a decrease in acoustic impedance occurring with deglutition.

The capability of the eustachian tube to transmit fluid from the middle ear to the nasopharynx may provide some measure of tubal function. Compere (1958) utilized radio-opaque contrast media, and Rogers et al. (1962) used fluorescein dye; however, further studies are needed to determine whether this method is a useful indicator of the ability of the tube to ventilate the middle ear.

Inadequate ventilative function of the tube in early life is presumed to inhibit pneumatization of the temporal bone (Diamant, 1940) and to lead to the development of chronic middle ear infections (Schuknecht et al., 1966). Holmquist (1970) has found that the size of the mastoid air cell cavity is an important determinant of the success of the myringoplasty. In a test group of 89 ears, myringoplasty was successful in 22 percent of individuals with air

Fig. 3.3: Eustachiometer test equipment (after Miller). Slight negative or positive pressure is introduced into the external auditory canal, and an evaluation is made of the ability of the eustachian tube to reduce the pressures by passing air during the act of deglutition. This test can be used only in the presence of an opening in the tympanic membrane.

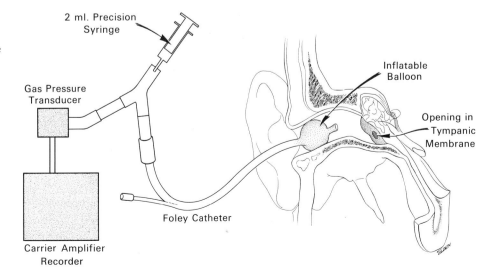

cell systems less than 5 cm, 57 percent of those with air cell systems between 5 and 10 cm, and 71 percent of those with air cell systems greater than 10 cm.

Utilizing the eustachiometer test method, Miller (1965), Flisberg (1966), and Siedentop et al. (1968) found that 50 to 75 percent of patients with chronic otitis media showed a decreased eustachian tube function. Flisberg (1966) and Holmquist (1968) believe that eustachiometer tests are of value in predicting the success of reconstructive surgery for chronic middle ear disease. MacKinnon (1970) found myringoplasty to be successful in 80 percent of individuals with good eustachian tube function and in 29 percent of those with poor eustachian tube function. Miller (1965), Sharp (1970), Ekvall (1970), and Palva and Kärjä (1970), on the other hand, have found that reconstructive procedures are often successful in spite of decreased preoperative eustachian tube function as determined by the eustachiometer technique.

Numerous studies have shown that about one-half of patients with cleft palate show conductive hearing loss (Masters et al., 1960; Holborow, 1962a; Lindsay et al., 1962; Graham, 1963; Bluestone, 1971). It is assumed that the high incidence of middle ear disease in patients with cleft palates is due to eustachian tube dysfunction secondary to the anomalous development of the tensor palati and levator palati muscles. Yules (1970) states that 90 percent of infants with cleft palates develop seromucinous otitis media. Odoi et al. (1971), in an experiment on cats, demonstrated that midline division of the palate resulted in a 50 percent incidence of seromucinous otitis media. Furthermore, pterygoid hamulotomy (which is sometimes performed in cleft palate surgery) caused seromucinous otitis media in 75 percent of the animals. Early and successful closure of congenital cleft palates appears to be associated with decreased hearing loss in later life (Yules, 1970).

The ability to inflate the ear by the Valsalva maneuver or by forced inflation is not a totally adequate method for assessing eustachian tube function. Many ears with chronic inflammatory disease in which air may be forced through the eustachian tube demonstrate poor tubal function on eustachiometer testing. Alternately, the eustachiometer test may be normal in ears in which a successful Valsalva maneuver cannot be accomplished in spite of repeated attempts (MacKinnon, 1970).

Procedures to correct the blocked eustachian tube by bouginage, eustachian tube catheter (Zöllner, 1963), bypass tube to the maxillary sinus (Drettner and Ekvall, 1970) and direct surgical exposure with insertion of a tube (House et al., 1969) have yielded generally disappointing results.

The patulous eustachian tube was first described by Schwartze (1864) and later by Jago (1867). This condition has received some attention in the past (Pitman, 1929; Zöllner, 1963; Shambaugh, 1938; Perlman, 1939); however, only recently has the high incidence of the condition been clearly understood (Flisberg and Ingelstedt, 1970). This is one of the most commonly misdiagnosed conditions in otology.

Patients are frequently treated for a blocked eustachian tube when in fact they have a patent eustachian tube.

The symptoms, which have been clearly described by Flisberg and Ingelstedt (1970), are a feeling of stuffiness in the ear, autophony, tinnitus, and transmission of respiratory noises to the ear. The symptoms are aggravated by exercise, fatigue, and loss of body weight. They are relieved by the edema associated with an upper respiratory infection and the venous congestion occurring in a reclined body position. Sniffing relieves the symptoms momentarily.

Individuals with a patulous tube will exhibit respiratory movements of the tympanic membrane. The condition may occur in asthenic individuals and in those with debilitating disease who have lost weight. The immediate cause is presumed to be loss of adipose tissue in the peritubal region (Lindsay, 1943). In females it may occur during pregnancy and when using oral contraceptive medication (Allen, 1967). Perlman (1939) and Handl (1959) have noted the patulous tube syndrome in patients having had retrogasserian neurectomy for trigeminal neuralgia resulting in atrophy and contracture of the tensor veli palati muscle. Pulec (1967) has been successful in treating the patulous tube by injecting polytetrafluorethylene paste into the tissue adjacent to the eustachian tube. Follow-up studies have shown good results in more than 50 percent of patients treated by this method (Pulec and Simonton, 1964; Pulec and Hahn, 1970). Animal studies have indicated that the injection should be made anterior to the tubal orifice as injections made posterior to the tube resulted in seromucinous otitis media (Reiner and Pulec, 1969).

3. THE MIDDLE EAR MUSCLE REFLEXES

The reflex activity of the stapedius and tensor tympani muscles has been extensively studied in animals and man (Perlman, 1960), and techniques for recording these responses have been found useful in the diagnosis of conductive lesions of the middle ear.

Lüscher (1930) was the first to study the reflex activity of stapedius muscles by inspection through perforated ear drums. The response occurs bilaterally at sound intensities of 70 to 90 db above the threshold of hearing. Several investigators (Metz, 1946; Pichler and Bornschein, 1957; Klockhoff and Anderson, 1959) have observed that the stapedius reflex may also be elicited by tactile stimulation in the external auditory canal. Metz (1951) and others (Okamoto et al., 1954; Møller, 1958) have shown that the acoustic impedance of the middle ear is altered by the stapedius reflex, and furthermore that this alteration does not occur when the ossicles are fixed by disease. Klockhoff and Anderson (1959) studied the stapedius reflex elicited by electrical stimulation with a surface electrode in the external auditory canal. They found that electrical stimuli of 50 pulses per second elicited stapedial contractions for one to three seconds. The responses were transient even with prolonged stimulation. In contrast, reflex activity initiated by acoustic stimulation was found to persist for the duration of the stimulation.

Although numerous investigators have observed contractions of the tensor tympani muscle in response to a sound stimulus (Kato, 1913; Kobrak, 1930; Hallpike and Rawdon-Smith, 1934; Wersäll, 1958), recent studies (Klockhoff, 1961) indicate that this muscle does not respond to acoustic or cutaneous stimuli which are of sufficient magnitude to elicit the stapedius reflex. Klockhoff (1961) demonstrated that stimulation of the orbital region with a jet of air elicited tensor tympani responses. The latency and duration of the responses were shorter and the amplitude generally larger than those observed for the stapedius reflex. He pointed out that the tensor reflex is but one component of the startle reaction and its response to acoustic excitation occurs only if the latter is explosive in character.

It appears that the stapedius reflex is a protective mechanism to limit the movement of the sound transmitting system in the presence of high intensity sound (Sokolovski, 1973). The physiological function of the tensor tympani muscle is less clear; possibly its function is proprioceptive for the purpose of maintaining slight tension in the ossicular system.

4. BONE CONDUCTION

The response of the cochlea to vibrations conducted through the skull is due to the combined effect of several factors. When a vibrator is placed against the head, vibrations travel to the ear as (a) surface waves along the skin and soft tissues, (b) transversal waves by way of the bones of the skull, and (c) pressure waves through the interior of the skull. The first method of transmission is of little importance whereas the other two integrate to either enhance or interfere with each other, depending upon their amplitudes and phase relationships (Tonndorf, 1966). Bone conduction response is brought about by three basic modes: (a) the inertial response of the middle ear ossicles and the inner ear fluids, (b) the distortional response of the cochlear capsule, and (c) irradiation of sound energy into the external auditory canal.

The concept of middle ear ossicular inertia was originally established by Bárány in 1938 on the basis of experiments on human subjects. When the skull undergoes forced vibrations, the ossicles participate in this motion but because of their loose coupling and different resonance properties, they respond in amplitudes and phases which are different from those of the skull. As a consequence, a relative motion is set up between the oval window and the stapes. An inertial effect of the inner ear fluids which interacts strongly with the distortional response of the cochlear capsule was deduced by Wever and Lawrence (1954).

Distortional response of the cochlear capsule was originally considered under the term "inner ear compression." This was first postulated by Reitjö (1914) and clarified by Herzog and Krainz (1926). This concept implies that vibratory energy reaching the cochlea creates alternating compressions and expansions of the cochlear capsule, and because inner ear fluids are incompressible, an alternating fluid displacement occurs in the cochlear windows. Herzog and Krainz pointed out that displacement of the cochlear partition occurred because of two independent mechanisms: (a) during cochlear compression the fluid displacement is preferentially toward the round window because it is more compliant than the oval window (ratio 1:20, according to Kirikae, 1960), and (b) the surface of the contracting walls of the scala vestibuli is larger than that of the scala tympani, the ratio of the two volumes being 5:3 and the areas being 3:2. Consequently, more fluid is displaced into the scala vestibuli, forcing the cochlear partition toward the scala vestibuli.

The radiation of sound energy into the external auditory canal by the vibrating walls of the bony canal results in energy transmission toward the cochlea via the middle ear. Tonndorf (1966) has shown that the open external auditory canal constitutes a high-pass filter, and that its occlusion produces a low-frequency emphasis. The air in the external auditory canal constitutes a load upon the tympanic membrane, and any modifications in the canal such as changes in length or occlusion of the canal will alter the effect. Occlusion of the canal near the tympanic membrane attenuates the bone conduction contribution of the external canal by reducing the radiating wall surface and by loading the tympanic membrane, thus eliminating the occlusion effect. Békésy (1941) showed that irradiation of acoustic energy into the ear canal may be aided by the out-of-phase motion of the mandible; however, this is thought to play only a minor role in the total phenomenon of bone conduction (Allen and Fernández, 1960).

Occlusion of the external auditory canal is known to produce a low-frequency emphasis on bone-conducted signals (Békésy, 1932; Onchi, 1954; Allen and Fernández, 1960; Tonndorf, 1966). A bone-conducted signal applied to the head, particularly when applied to the midline, is perceived with equal intensity by normal ears. The sound image will be shifted toward an ear in which either the intensity is higher or the signal phase is leading.

Based on these concepts of bone conduction, Tonndorf (1966) provided the following explanations for the clinical tests of Bing, Runge, Weber, and Gellé:

In *the test of Bing* (1891), occlusion of the external auditory canal of a normal hearing ear produces lateralization of low-frequency bone-conducted signals to that ear. A failure to lateralize indicates an impairment of middle ear function. Occlusion eliminates the high-pass filter constituted by the external opening of the canal and results in a relative low-frequency emphasis producing an intensity difference between the two ears.

In *the test of Runge* (1923), the ear canal is filled with water producing lateralization of low-frequency bone conduction signals to the involved ear, and failure to lateralize indicates a middle ear conductive lesion. In this situation, mass loading of the tympanic membrane improves low-frequency bone conduction responses due to an increase in the moment of inertia of the ossicular system resulting in intensity differences between the ears.

In *the test of Weber* (1834), bone-conducted signals are lateralized to the side with middle ear pathology. Fluid (serous, mucinous, purulent) in the middle ear results in mass loading of the tympanic membrane (as well as increased friction) which increases the moment of inertia of the ossicular system and leads to intensity differences. With stapedial fixation and ossicular discontinuity there are positive phase shifts in the frequency range below the resonance point of the middle ear for bone conduction; hence phase lead causes lateralization to the involved ear. At frequencies near the resonant point (about 2000 Hz) the response loss is so large that it cannot be overcome by the phase lead phenomenon, and lateralization may occur toward the uninvolved ear.

The test of Gellé (Gellé, 1885), as originally performed, consisted of determining the effect on hearing of increasing air pressure in the external auditory canal. Gellé reported that this maneuver decreased hearing for both air conduction and bone conduction in individuals with normal hearing. In the presence of ossicular fixation or disruption, the phenomenon occurs for air conduction but not for bone conduction and is termed a negative Gellé test (Dankbaar, 1970). Studies by Dishoeck (1937), Aubry and Giraud (1943), and others (Huizing, 1960) have shown that both positive and negative pressure in the middle ear or auditory canal leads to the reduction of auditory acuity and that the effect is more pronounced with low than with high frequencies. Dishoeck (1937) and Perlman (1943) carried the method a step further in the development of the pneumaphone, which measures middle ear pressures. It is based on the principle that when the pressure in the external auditory canal is equal to that in the middle ear the sound-transmitting mechanism functions at its optimum.

5. THE COCHLEA

It is not the purpose of this book to deal in depth with the physical properties, mechanics, and physiology of the cochlea; however, some understanding of these functions is essential for the interpretation of functional disturbances of the different pathologies which are described in the following chapters.

(a) Mechanical properties of the cochlea

Associated with the inward movement of the stapes there is displacement of inner ear fluid toward the round window and outward movement of the round window membrane. This movement of fluid takes place across the cochlear partition and sets into motion a complicated wave form on the basilar membrane which in turn excites the sensory mechanism, resulting in a flow of nerve impulses to the higher centers (Møller, 1972).

Although original studies by Békésy (1936), Fumagalli (1949), and Kobrak (1959) suggested that the human stapes moves by a rocking motion, with the posterior margin being partly fixed and the anterior margin moving in and out of the oval window, it has been demonstrated recently by Guinan and Peake (1967) that within the range of physiological intensities, the movement of the stapes in cats is that of a piston.

The vibratory patterns within the cochlea have been a subject of intense interest for several decades. Helmholtz (1863), who presented the first serious treatise on the subject, assumed that transverse fibers exist in the basilar membrane which act as resonators, each tuned to a different frequency, and that stimulation deflects only a small group of these fibers, with neural excitation taking place only in that localized area. Opponents of this idea postulated the "telephone" theory, which implied that pitch information is presented in the periodicity of neural discharge.

It soon became apparent, however, that the anatomical structure of the cochlea would not support the Helmholtz theory and that the limitations in neural discharge rates in individual fibers would not support the telephone

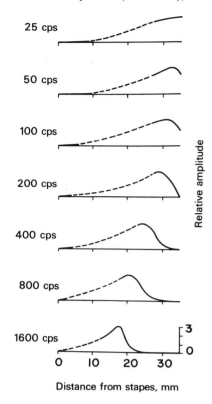

Fig. 3.4: Curves showing patterns of displacement of the cochlear partition of the human ear for seven frequencies. (After Békésy)

25 cps

50 cps

100 cps

200 cps

400 cps

800 cps

1600 cps

Distance from stapes, mm

Relative amplitude

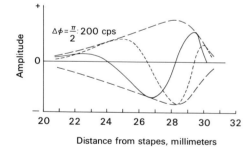

Fig. 3.5: Traveling wave pattern showing movement of the basilar membrane at two instants in time, separated by a phase angle of 90° for the frequency 200 Hz. (After Békésy)

theory. The concept of a volley principle by which a high periodic discharge rate could be represented in a group of nerve fibers, with the different fibers responding to different waves of the tone, provided some relief for the "telephonists"; however, subsequent studies have shown that no such discharge pattern exists for high-frequency stimuli. A nonresonance theory that gained some notice was that of Ewald (1898) and was known as the "sound-pattern" theory. According to this idea, a sinusoidal movement of the stapes sets up a series of standing waves on the basilar membrane which vary in frequency, and the nervous system has the responsibility for resolving the different patterns into tones.

Traveling-wave theories were advanced as far back as 1895 (Hurst, 1895). These theories suggest that a wave of displacement progresses in a systematic way along the cochlear partition and produces a local stimulation in its path. Some theorists proposed that the progression of the wave is a property of the membrane, and others that it is an interaction between fluid and membranes. Because no numerical values had been established relative to the mechanics of the cochlea there were no restrictions on the imagination, and every conceivable theoretical possibility was explored.

Békésy decided that the problem could only be solved by opening the cochlea and observing the action during presentation of a tone. Most of our current knowledge of cochlear mechanics has evolved from his series of experiments which began in 1928.

He measured the movement of the cochlear partition in human and animal cochleae in response to pure tone stimulation (Békésy, 1944). The amplitude of displacement of the cochlear partition was recorded in several regions of the human ear for frequencies in the range from 25 to 1600 Hz. (Fig. 3.4). Observations for higher frequencies were not feasible by the method used. From calculations based on measurements of phase differences and maximum amplitudes of displacement of the basilar membrane, Békésy was able to deduce the form of vibration of the cochlear partition for given frequencies at a given instant in time (Békésy, 1947a). Studies showed that the pattern of movement was indeed that of a traveling wave (Fig. 3.5).

This should not be interpreted to mean that this phenomenon is equal to that of a wave which can be made to travel along a stretched rope. When the sound is introduced through an opening in the apex of the cochlea, the traveling wave on the cochlear partition occurs with exactly the same characteristics. The physical characteristics of the cochlear partition determine the time delay between the stimulus and the response of a particular point on the partition. Actually a large segment of the basal turn responds almost simultaneously, followed by a progressively longer time delay as the displacement moves toward the apex. Observation of these movements gives the impression of a traveling wave.

Iurato (1967) has shown that the basilar membrane is not under tension and is free to yield to fluid movements of physiological magnitude. Although supporting evidence is lacking, it is postulated elsewhere in this book (Chapter 10 J4, Cochlear conductive presbycusis) that stiffening of the basilar membrane as an effect of aging might explain the hearing loss characterized by the descending audiometric pattern. Experimental studies have shown that the basilar membrane of the basal turn of the cochlea can be ruptured by direct mechanical trauma without affecting the threshold of hearing for low tones (Schuknecht and Sutton, 1953). This indicates that local disruptions do not interfere with the progression of traveling waves on the basilar membrane.

The relationship of the tectorial membrane to the hair cells would seem to be an important mechanical feature of inner ear action. The ends of the cilia of the hair cells rest within pockets in the tectorial membrane, and the relationship is sufficiently intimate that when the tectorial membrane is lifted from the organ of Corti, in the course of histological preparations, these cilia may break off and remain attached to this membrane (Fig. 3.6).

The anatomical relationship is such that an upward displacement of the

Fig. 3.6: Electron micrograph demonstrating relationship of cilia of an external hair cell to the tectorial membrane in a rhesus monkey. (Courtesy of Kimura).

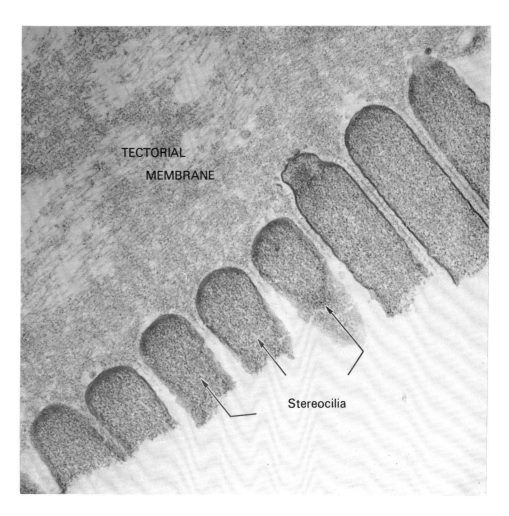

Fig. 3.7: Diagrammatic sketch illustrating how movement of the cochlear partition creates a shearing force between the reticular plate and the tectorial membrane with bending of the cilia of the hair cells (Davis, 1960).

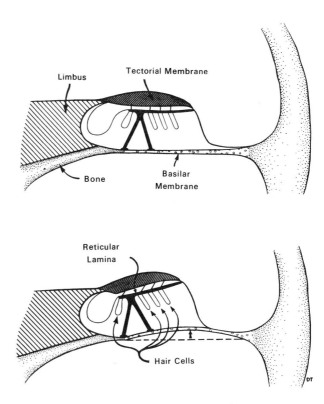

basilar membrane will produce a shearing force between the organ of Corti and the tectorial membrane, resulting in a pushing force on the external hair cell cilia and a pulling force on the internal hair cell cilia (Fig. 3.7). Békésy (1953) demonstrated that the microphonic output from the external hair cells is largest when these cells are stimulated by movement in a radial direction, that is, in a direction from modiolus to stria vascularis. Flock et al. (1962), Wersäll et al. (1965), and Duvall et al. (1966) have shown that the hair cells do not have kinocilia but each has a centriole without a basal foot, which for both internal and external hair cells is located on the side closest to the stria. Avulsion of the tectorial membrane from the organ of Corti has been observed in association with other pathological changes but has not been seen as an isolated phenomenon.

(b) Bioelectric potentials of the cochlea

Since the time that Wever and Bray (1936) first discovered the microphonic response of the cochlea, there has been an intense interest in bioelectric phenomena occurring in the cochlea and their possible relationship to the mechanism of neural excitation and transmission. Because these electrical phenomena are altered by pathological changes in the inner ear, they have been used extensively to assess the functional state of the cochleae of both animal and human subjects. Davis (1960) has postulated that the release of electrical energy from a biological reservoir is controlled by the mechanical bending of the cilia of the hair cells and that the resulting electrical flow in some way excites the nerve fibers.

Four classes of electrical potentials have been identified and associated with particular sources or generators.

The endolymphatic potential is located within the endolymphatic space and within the cells and is about 70 to 90 millivolts positive relative to the perilymph. The investigations of Tasaki and Spyropoulos (1952) indicate that the source of the cochlear endolymphatic DC potential is the stria vascularis.

The cochlear microphonic is an AC response to acoustic stimulation. It appears to be generated at the boundary between the hair cells and the scala media, for it has been found that an electrode, passed through the organ of Corti from the scala tympani, records an abrupt reversal of its electrical sign at this level (Tasaki et al., 1954). The voltage of the response increases with stimulus intensity, in a simple linear relationship up to about 105 db (guinea pig) and then decreases with further increase in intensity.

When differential electrodes are introduced into the cochlea, so that one is located in the scala vestibuli and the other in the scala tympani, it is possible to cancel much of the neural potential and microphonic activity generated from more distant regions of the cochlear partition. Utilizing this method, Tasaki et al. (1952) clearly demonstrated that frequencies differ greatly in the extent of the cochlear partition that they excite, with low frequencies exciting much greater lengths than high frequencies (Fig. 3.8).

The summating potential is a DC response which is usually negative (scala media relative to scala tympani) and is closely related to cochlear microphonics. The summating potential does not have a maximum, as does the cochlear microphonic, but continues to increase with the increasing intensity of the stimulus. Its polarity can be reversed by increasing the hydrostatic pressure in the scala tympani.

The neural action potentials recorded from the cochlea constitute the electrical activity of discharges occurring in the afferent cochlear nerve fibers. These responses represent the synchronized bursts of summed electrical activity occurring in the nerve fibers at the onset of a tone burst. The size of the response is determined by the number of impulses that contribute to it and the degree of synchrony of the impulses.

(c) Ionic gradients and energy sources

The endolymphatic system is lined by epithelial tissue which varies from

Fig. 3.8: Simultaneous oscillograms from turns 1, 2, and 4 of the guinea pig. The amplifications of the three channels were initially adjusted to give approximately equal responses in all three turns at low frequencies. As the frequency was changed, the sound pressure level was adjusted to maintain a constant response (200 microvolts, peak to peak from the basal turn, left column). The findings show that frequencies differ greatly in the length of the partition that they excite, with low frequencies exciting much greater lengths of the cochlear duct than high frequencies (Tasaki et al., 1952).

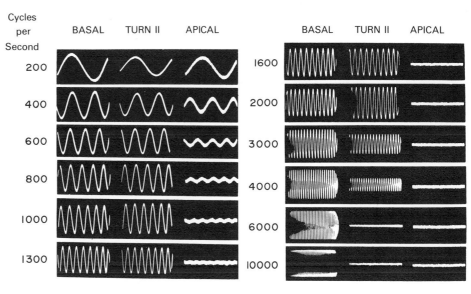

SOUND INTENSITY ADJUSTED FOR CONSTANT RESPONSE IN BASAL TURN

PAIRED ELECTRODES, SCALAE VESTIBULI AND TYMPANI, IN EACH TURN

simple squamous, as in Reissner's membrane, to highly specialized tissue, as in the organ of Corti, cristae, and maculae (Iurato, 1967). The system is sealed from the surrounding areas by tight junctions between the epithelial cells.

Much effort has been expended in attempting to define the permeability of membranes for the various ions, and the sources of energy for an ion pump and the cochlear potentials. Several investigations indicate that K^+ is essential in the scala media to both cochlear microphonic and endolymphatic potential, but that the ionic gradients between endolymph and perilymph can vary independently from endolymphatic potential (Konishi et al., 1966; Bosher and Warren, 1968).

The organ of Corti, the stria vascularis, and Reissner's membrane have been thoroughly searched as places for ion transport (Vosteen, 1970) and the sources of energy for the cochlear potentials. The techniques have consisted of searches for stores of energy in the form of glycogen and glucose, the detection of enzymes that participate in energy-releasing metabolic cycles, and the identification of locations of ATPase as a sign of energy use (Paparella, 1970). Both glycogen and glucose have been found in the organ of Corti of the guinea pig and cat (Matschinsky and Thalmann, 1967; Ishii et al., 1969). Enzymes for glycolysis, the citric acid cycle, and the pentose-P pathway have been found in greater quantities in the organ of Corti and stria vascularis than in Reissner's membrane (Thalmann et al., 1970). Matschinsky and Thalmann (1967) found significant levels of adenoisinetriphosphate and creatine phosphate in both the organ of Corti and stria vascularis. Nakai and Hilding (1967) found histochemical signs of ATPase in the stria vascularis and on the endolymphatic surface of the cells of the organ of Corti. These studies and others indicate a rather high level of activity of respiratory enzymes in the stria vascularis and organ of Corti.

Various methods have been used to block enzyme systems in an attempt to identify how enzyme activity relates to endolymphatic potential, cochlear microphonic, and action potential. The experiments indicate that metabolic energy is essential for cochlear potentials and that the mechanisms underlying the cochlear microphonic and endolymphatic potential differ from those found in nerve action potentials (Kuijpers et al., 1967; Konishi and Kelsey, 1968).

Eldredge and Miller (1971) presented the following model of cochlear metabolic physiology as based on current knowledge: The metabolic energy for endolymphatic potential and the K^+ gradient is supplied in the stria vascularis. Na^+ is actively transported out of the scala media into the blood stream

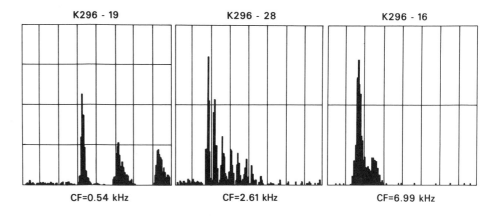

Fig. 3.9: Post-stimulus-time (PST) histograms of responses to clicks for three cochlear nerve fibers of a cat. The characteristic frequencies (CF) of the units were 540 Hz, 2,610 Hz, and 6,990 Hz. The clicks were delivered at a rate of ten per second. The time scale is in milliseconds. For low frequencies the basilar membrane undergoes several oscillations in response to each click and the fiber discharges with each oscillation. The units with high CF have shorter but more variable latencies and are devoid of a periodicity characteristic. (Courtesy of Kiang)

K296 - 19   K296 - 28   K296 - 16

CF=0.54 kHz   CF=2.61 kHz   CF=6.99 kHz

at the stria vascularis. K⁺ and Na⁺ may enter the cochlear duct passively through the walls of the cochlear duct, particularly Reissner's membrane. Cochlear microphonic is produced when the hair cells modulate a direct current at the reticular lamina. Both endolymphatic potential and the intracellular resting potentials of the hair cells are possible sources for this current. Probably a large part of the cochlear microphonic voltage depends upon the endolymphatic potential, and the hair cells primarily modulate this current. Although the energy for the endolymphatic potential and cochlear microphonic is probably provided through the stria vascularis, the metabolic requirements for the organ of Corti appear to be supplied by the capillary loops of the basilar membrane (Lawrence, 1966a).

(d) Activity in single afferent nerve fibers

All cochlear nerve fibers appear to exhibit spontaneous discharges, ranging from a few per minute to more than 100 per second (Kiang, 1965). Each neural unit responds to a certain range of frequencies within which is a frequency of maximum sensitivity termed the characteristic frequency (CF). The latencies for responses to standard clicks are short for all frequencies with a CF above 2000 Hz and systematically longer for lower frequencies, presumably reflecting the characteristics of the traveling wave. When the units respond to noise or frequencies above 5000 Hz, the discharges are irregular and have interval distributions resembling those of spontaneous activity. The discharge rate increases with stimulus intensity to a maximum after which there is no further increase. Some of these properties of single cochlear nerve units are shown in the histograms in Fig. 3.9.

The characteristic frequency (CF) of a unit may be considered to be a reflection of its location longitudinally on the cochlear duct. The location is an important determinant of the pattern of neural response based in part on the nature of the traveling wave. Studies of single unit responses provide no evidence to support the hypothesis of distinct internal and external hair cell innervations. Kiang (1965) found that the sensitivity of the primary units

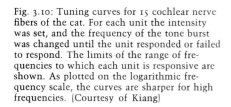

Fig. 3.10: Tuning curves for 15 cochlear nerve fibers of the cat. For each unit the intensity was set, and the frequency of the tone burst was changed until the unit responded or failed to respond. The limits of the range of frequencies to which each unit is responsive are shown. As plotted on the logarithmic frequency scale, the curves are sharper for high frequencies. (Courtesy of Kiang)

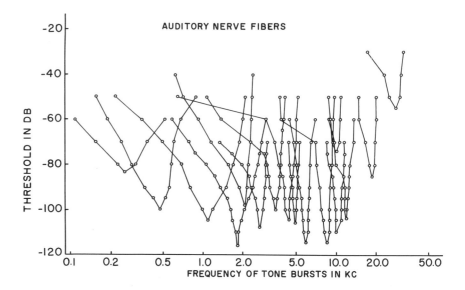

correlated well with the behavioral audiogram. The tuning curves for a family of neural units are shown in Fig. 3.10. It is possible, of course, that more sharpening might occur through inhibitory effects which might become evident if the experiments were performed on the unanesthetized animal. An important part of auditory perception must be involved in neural mechanisms occurring at all levels in the auditory system. Inhibition is an important mechanism occurring in all sensory systems and has been studied in depth by Békésy (1967). The efferent neural pathways, which exist at all levels in the auditory system, may perform some role in the inhibitory phenomenon. The neural processes by which the products of cochlear activity are modified to produce the psychological experience of hearing in all its dimensions are not known.

(e) Frequency localization

Because frequency has a spatial distribution within the cochlea, lesions involving restricted regions of the cochlea are expressed functionally as threshold losses involving part of the auditory spectrum.

Surgically induced lesions in the apical region cause hearing losses for the low frequencies, the magnitude of the threshold loss being proportional to the severity and size of the lesion. This was demonstrated in an experiment on cats in which lesions were created by introducing small needles through bony fistulae in the apical regions of the cochleae (Schuknecht and Neff, 1952). Final hearing tests were made three to six months later, after which the animals were killed and the cochleae prepared for histological study. Pathological changes were plotted on graphic reconstructions to show the severity and spatial limits of the lesions. The hair cells and ganglion cells were judged as being present or missing. The experiment showed that loss of sensory and neural elements in the apical region caused hearing losses for the low frequencies (Figs. 3.11, 3.12).

In another experiment needles were introduced through the round window membrane into the cochlear ducts of the basal ends of the cochleae (Schuknecht and Sutton, 1953). These lesions created severe high-frequency hearing losses which frequently were restricted to a small part of the auditory spectrum (Fig. 3.13).

In chronic experiments, such as the ones described above, the degenerative change spreads somewhat beyond the region of direct trauma. To determine the effects of smaller lesions, an acute experiment was performed in which cortical responses of auditory function were recorded within 15 minutes following injury. This evoked response technique can be used only in acute experiments because of the necessity for exposing the auditory cortex (Hind and Schuknecht, 1954). With this method it is possible to assess the function of cochleae with smaller injuries and thus to demonstrate more accurately the tuning capacity of the cochlea (Sutton and Schuknecht, 1954) (Figs. 3.14, 3.15, 3.16).

Another source of information on frequency localization is available from experiments in which the ear is stimulated with intense pure tone stimuli. In this case the maximum injury is located at or near the points of maximum displacement of the basilar membrane. Wever and Smith's experiment (1944) on guinea pigs is a classic. The location of areas of injury to the organ of Corti for several frequencies is shown in Fig. 3.17.

(f) The anatomical frequency scale

The foregoing studies show that any attempt to correlate cochlear function with cochlear pathology must bring into consideration the location of frequency response within the cochlea. Thus, both researchers and clinicians have found it useful to modify the logarithmic frequency scale to the extent that it expresses the spatial distribution of frequency within the cochlea. This is known as the "anatomical" frequency scale.

Koenig (1949) was the first to use this method. On the basis of limited data,

Fig. 3.11: A lesion was created in the organ of Corti of the apical region of the cochlea by fistulizing the bony labyrinth and introducing a needle into the cochlear duct. The fistula was then covered by a pedicled flap of mucous membrane. Postoperative survival time was three months.

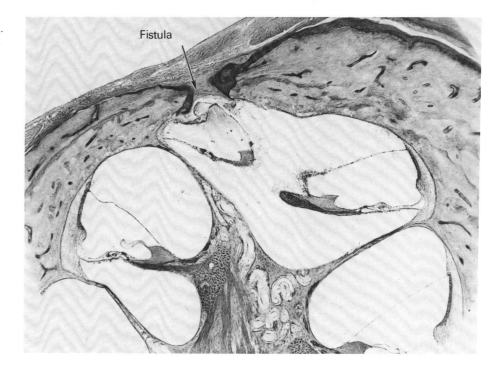

Fig. 3.12: Audiogram and chart of cochlear pathology for a cat with a lesion in the apical region. The injury was created by introducing a needle through a fistula of the bony labyrinth into the apex of the cochlea. The audiogram was made by the conditioned response method and the postoperative survival time was three months. Frequency is plotted on the anatomical frequency scale, and distance along the cochlear duct is shown in millimeters. A total loss of hair cells and partial loss of cochlear neurons in the apical 6 mm have resulted in a 20 to 35 db elevation of threshold for frequencies having their areas of maximum displacement in that region of the cochlea (Schuknecht and Neff, 1952).

Fig. 3.13: Audiogram and chart of cochlear pathology for a cat with a lesion in the basal end of the cochlea. A needle was introduced through the round window into the cochlear duct 2 mm from the basal end. Postoperative survival time was ten weeks. A loss of all of the external hair cells and 30 percent of the internal hair cells in a 6.8 mm region is associated with an abrupt severe hearing loss for frequencies above 8000 Hz (Schuknecht and Sutton, 1953).

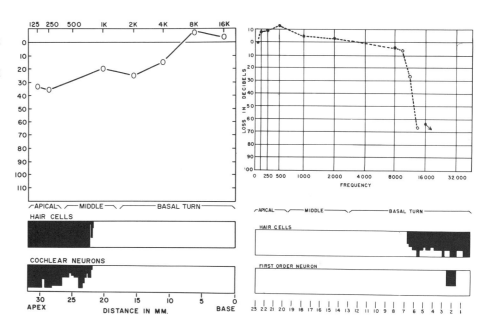

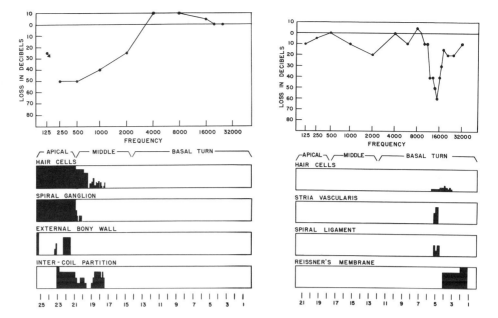

Fig. 3.14: Thresholds of cortical response and charts of cochlear pathology for two cats with needle injuries to the cochleae. A loss of sensory and neural elements in the apical 6 mm of the cochlea (left chart) has caused a severe threshold elevation for the low frequencies. A discrete small lesion in the 5 mm region (right chart) has caused a sharp threshold elevation for a limited range of high frequencies (Sutton and Schuknecht, 1954).

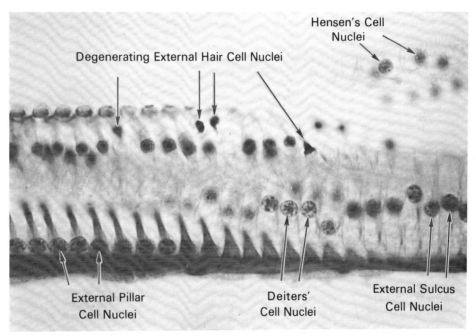

Fig. 3.15: External hair cell injury in the organ of Corti at the margin of a needle injury. The animal was killed by arterial perfusion with Heidenhain-Susa solution 30 minutes after injury. The nuclei of the injured cells are pyknotic and displaced toward the cuticular ends of the cells.

Fig. 3.16: Organ of Corti at the margin of a needle injury showing pyknosis, swelling, fragmentation, and lysis of the nuclei of the external hair cells. The animal was killed by arterial perfusion with Heidenhain-Susa solution 30 minutes after injury.

Fig. 3.17: Location of hair cell injury in guinea pig cochleae following exposure to frequencies of 300, 1,000, 5,000, and 10,000 Hz at high intensities (Wever and Smith, 1944).

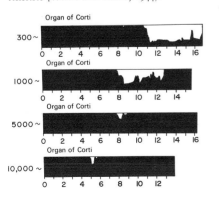

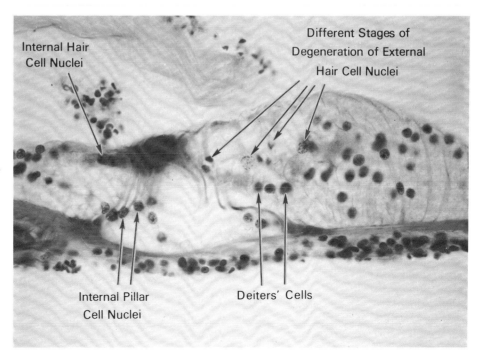

he suggested that a logarithmic scale be employed for frequencies above 900 Hz and a linear scale for frequencies below 900 Hz. Each 100-cycle interval on the linear scale was made equal to the distance between 900 and 1000 on the logarithmic scale. Davis et al. (1949) were the first to make use of Koenig's frequency scale for the presentation of data and bioelectric responses from the guinea pig.

A study of the ears of sixteen cats with abrupt hearing losses, as determined by the conditioned response method, has provided an opportunity to test the validity of the Koenig scale (Schuknecht, 1953a). For most of the ears there were differences in threshold sensitivity greater than 30 db over a frequency range of one octave. In each ear this loss was due to a cochlear lesion of limited size. The margin of the lesion in each instance was characterized by an abrupt transition from normal to abnormal of the sensory and/or neural structures. Correlations were made between the audiograms and cochlear lesions in 20 regions in these 16 ears. For each ear the locations of the margins of the lesions were defined in percentages of the distance from basal to apical ends of the cochlear ducts. Table 3.1 shows, for example, that the ears of five animals had large differences in threshold for 8,000 Hz and 16,000 Hz, which could be correlated with the margins of the cochlear lesions, which were located 6.8, 4.8, 7.7, 6.0, and 8.5 mm from the basal ends of the cochlear ducts. The mean distance was 6.7 mm, or 31 percent of the distance along the cochlear duct as measured from the basal end. Presumably if a sufficient number of correlations could be made, this figure would represent a point on the cochlear duct lying midway between the points of maximum amplitude for 8,000 Hz and 16,000 Hz (Fig. 3.18).

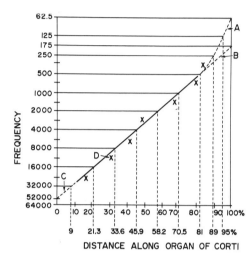

Fig. 3.18: Graph showing method used to determine frequency localization in the cat cochlea. Frequency on the logarithmic scale is plotted against distance along the cochlear duct. The mean locations of the margins of lesions for seven frequency ranges are plotted in accordance with the data appearing in Table 3.1. For example, point D, representing the 8,000 to 16,000 Hz range, is located along a line which extends horizontally from a point midway between 8,000 and 16,000 Hz and 31 percent of the way along the cochlea as measured from the basal end. A visual best-fit line through the seven points shows a nearly linear relationship of log frequency to distance in the range 500 to 32,000 Hz. If one assumes that this linear relationship holds for both ends of the cochlea represented by the broken lines, C and B, then the highest and lowest frequencies still having points of maximum amplitude would be 52,000 and 175 Hz respectively. The upper limit is very close to the highest frequency for which cortical potentials can be recorded from the normal cat ear. The data indicate that the frequencies below 500 Hz are located in the apical 19 percent of the cochlea. Békésy's investigations show the lowest frequency still having a point of maximum displacement in the human cochlea is about 25 to 35 Hz. Thus, because cats appear to have a poorer sensitivity for low frequencies than humans, it seems reasonable to believe that the lowest frequency having a point of maximum displacement is greater than 35 Hz. If this frequency were an octave higher, 62.5 Hz, then the contour line A would indicate the extent of departure from linearity for the frequency-distance function. This does not mean that the cat is incapable of hearing frequencies lower than 62.5 Hz, since lower frequencies would be expected to excite the apical end of the cochlea with the so-called "tail end" of the wave. The low frequency 62.5 is a purely arbitrary end-point subject to correction when more information becomes available.

Horizontal lines have been drawn on the graph from the frequency scale to intersect the contour line and, from these points of intersection, a vertical line intersects the distance scale (abscissa). The lower figures on the abscissa, therefore, show the approximate areas of maximum amplitude for the respective frequencies in terms of the percentage of the distance along the cochlear duct.

Table 3.1   Margin of Cochlear Lesion

Frequency	Cochlea	Total length of cochlea	Location of Margin		
			mm	% of length	mean %
250–500	1	21.6	18.3	84	84
500–1000	2	22.5	16.7	74	78
	3	23.8	20.0	83	
1000–2000	4	21.3	13.7	64	67
	5	22.2	15.5	70	
2000–4000	6	20.0	10.5	52	48
	7	21.3	9.5	44	
	8	21.7	9.5	44	
	9	21.3	11.5	54	
	10	21.5	10.7	50	
4000–8000	11	21.2	5.7	37	44
	12	21.9	10.3	47	
	13	21.4	9.5	44	
	14	22.8	7.0	30	
	15	23.0	6.8	30	
	16	21.5	4.8	22	
8000–16000	17	20.0	7.7	39	31
	18	22.2	6.0	27	
	19	23.1	8.5	37	
16000–32000	20	22.8	3.7	16	16

When the frequencies are arranged on the abscissa of the audiogram in accordance with these findings (32,000 Hz at 9 percent of the distance, 16,000 Hz at 21.3 percent, 8,000 Hz at 33.6 percent, etc.), the scale may be termed the "anatomical frequency scale." The scale as determined in this manner is somewhat different from Koenig's, particularly for the low frequencies (Fig. 3.19).

There is not yet sufficient anatomical and functional data to develop an accurate anatomical frequency scale for human ears; therefore, the Koenig

Fig. 3.19: Koenig's anatomical frequency scale for the cat compared with that based on experimental data.

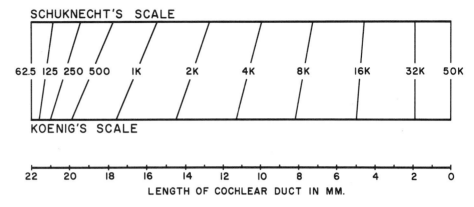

scale is used for the presentation of human data in this book. The lowest frequency having a point of maximum amplitude on the human basilar membrane is taken to be 35 Hz, the highest frequency, 20,000 Hz, and the breaking point between the logarithmic and arithmetic scales as 500 Hz (one octave lower than that used for the cat). The frequencies above 500 Hz are plotted on the logarithmic scale, and those below 500 Hz on the arithmetic scale, so that each 100-cycle interval is equal to the distance between 400 and 500 on the log scale. Utilizing the Koenig method for the frequency range 35 Hz to 20,000 Hz, the locations of the octaves in terms of the percentage of the distance along the basilar membrane as measured from the basal end are shown in Table 3.2.

Table 3.2   Location of Frequency in the Human Cochlea (Koenig Scale)

Frequency	Distance from the basal end in percent of total length
35	0
62.5	1.3
125	4.3
250	10.3
500	21.9
1K	36.6
2K	51.2
4K	65.9
8K	80.6
16K	94.6
20K	100

The anatomical frequency scale, which crowds the lower octaves on the left side of the scale, provides a more realistic presentation of the functional deficit in relation to the spatial distribution and severity of cochlear lesions. In routine clinical testing, little is gained by determining auditory thresholds at each octave below 500 Hz because of the proximity in the cochlea of their points of maximum amplitude and because of the overlap of their fields of excitation at stimulus intensities above threshold.

(g) The fields of excitation

A series of experiments in which correlations were made of cochlear lesions with changes in hearing also has provided evidence on the longitudinal spread of the field of excitation along the cochlear duct as a function of frequency and intensity.

The data for this study came from 21 cat ears from five different experiments (Schuknecht, 1960a). In each case the cochlear lesion was characterized by being of restricted size and having normal receptors on the basal side of the lesion. The audiograms of all of these animals, therefore, demonstrated an ascending slope. The reasoning employed in correlating the data is graphically displayed in Fig. 3.20.

The data were grouped, according to the locations of the cochlear lesions,

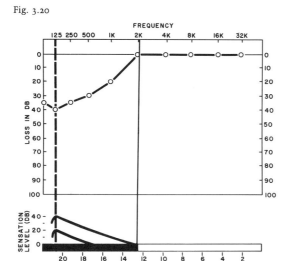

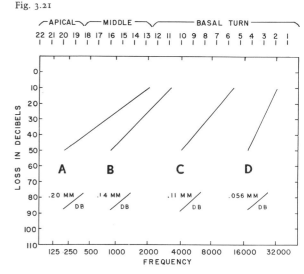

Fig. 3.20: The behavioral audiogram of a cat having a low-frequency hearing loss resulting from an experimentally induced lesion in the apical region of the cochlea (Schuknecht and Neff, 1952). Histological examination of the cochlea revealed a total loss of hair cells from the 12.8 mm region to the apex, which is shown as black filling in the lower chart. Frequency is plotted on the anatomical frequency scale. Resonance curves for 500 Hz have been drawn on the cochlear chart to show the displacement amplitudes on the basilar membrane for sensation levels of 20 and 40 db. The resonance curve for the 20 db stimulus, to which the animal did not respond, lies entirely within the injured zone of the cochlea. The 40 db stimulus, however, to which the animal has responded, has caused displacement of the cochlear duct sufficiently far in the basal direction to reach the responsive hair cells in the 12.8 mm region. Thus, the 125 Hz stimulus tone at an intensity of 40 db has created a displacement pattern on the basilar membrane which has extended from the 21 mm region, which is the point of maximum amplitude for that frequency, to the 13 mm region, a total distance of 8 mm.

Fig. 3.21: Contour lines representing the mean values of data presented in Table 3.3. The ascending lines show the audiometric configuration for lesions in four areas of cat cochleae. The increasing steepness of the slopes from apex to base reflects the increased sharpness of the resonance curves on the basilar membrane. See text for details.

into apical, middle, upper basal, and lower basal regions. For each ear the values were recorded for the lowest frequency and the highest frequency which best described the ascending slope of the audiometric curve. The range usually extended over several octaves for apical lesions and less than an octave for basal lesions (see Table 3.3).

Table 3.3   Spread of Field of Excitation

	Cochlea	Low	High	Thresh. diff.		db/oct.	db/mm	mm/db
	1	125	1K	20		6.6	3.70	.27
	2	125	4K	50		10.0	4.59	.24
	3	250	1K	15		7.5	3.73	.26
	4	250	1K	20		10.0	5.00	.20
Apical	5	250	1K	30		15.0	7.50	.13
	6	250	1K	40		20.0	10.00	.10
	7	250	2K	35		10.1	5.22	.19
	8	250	2K	30		10.0	4.48	.22
	9	250	8K	60		12.0	4.91	.20
					Mean	11.2	5.46	.20
	10	500	1K	30		30.0	13.00	.08
	11	500	4K	60		20.0	7.76	.13
Middle	12	500	16K	70		14.0	5.32	.19
	13	1K	4K	45		22.5	8.30	.12
	14	1K	16K	60		15.0	5.53	.18
	15	2K	8K	35		17.5	6.47	.15
					Mean	19.8	7.78	.14
	16	3K	6K	30		30.0	11.10	.09
Upper basal	17	4K	16K	40		20.0	7.39	.13
	18	4K	16K	45		22.5	8.31	.11
					Mean	24.2	8.93	.11
	19	16K	32K	45		50.0	18.5	.054
Lower basal	20	16K	32K	40		45.0	16.6	.060
	21	18K	32K	45		49.8	18.5	.054
					Mean	30.6	17.8	.056

The mean values for the data are graphically shown in Fig. 3.21. The increasing steepness of the slope, from apex to base, reflects the increased sharpness of the resonance curves along the cochlear duct. For the low frequencies, the data indicate that the field of excitation spreads in the basal direction about 0.2 mm for each decibel increase in stimulus intensity. These values are 0.14 mm/db in the middle turn, 0.11 mm/db in the upper basal turn, and 0.056 mm/db in the lower basal turn. It is quite probable, of course, that the spread of the field of excitation with increasing intensity is not a linear function.

(h) Psychoacoustic manifestations of sensory lesions

The auditory sense organ encompasses all the structures of the cochlear partition exclusive of the nerve endings. Alterations in the inner ear fluids, as well as structural changes in the organ of Corti, stria vascularis, tectorial membrane, Reissner's membrane, and the basilar membrane, may interfere with sensory function.

The cytological elements of importance in the organ of Corti (exclusive of nerve endings) are (1) the hair cells; (2) the supporting cells (pillar cells, Deiters' cells; Hensen's cells, sulcus cells); (3) the tectorial membrane; and (4) the basilar membrane. Animal specimens fixed by arterial perfusion are usually suitably preserved to allow evaluations of morphological change in individual cells; however, human specimens fixed by immersion show greater postmortem autolysis and usually permit only a determination of the presence or absence of cells.

Among the psychoacoustic manifestations which can be measured quantitatively and which are of significance in the diagnosis of sensory lesions are elevation of auditory threshold, loudness recruitment, distortion of pitch, and loss of speech discrimination.

Threshold elevations of sensory etiology may result from several different patterns of pathology, which can often be identified by the configuration of the audiometric curves. Light microscopic studies of both human and animal ears suggest a direct correlation between the loss in hair cell population and the magnitude of the threshold elevation. Meaningful correlations must be based on a consideration of frequency localization and fields of excitation. Ordinarily such correlations are justified only in ears with lesions extending over several millimeters in which the hair cell loss is uniform.

The ears of both animals and humans seem to show that loss of the external hair cells with preservation of internal hair cells results in threshold elevations of about 50 db. A loss of all external and some internal hair cells is associated with hearing losses greater than 50 db. These relationships seem to hold true only for lesions involving frequencies up to 4000 Hz. A loss of external hair cells in the basal end of the cochlea seems to create threshold losses for the involved frequencies which are greater than 50 db.

Except for the possible threshold differences, there is no evidence which suggests special functions for the internal and external hair cells or that the nerve endings can be excited acoustically without hair cells (Schuknecht, 1953b). Complete loss of hair cells consistently causes total deafness. The behavioral studies showing considerable difference in sensitivity of internal and external hair cells are at variance with electrophysiological data on the response characteristics of single cochlear nerve fibers, for Kiang (1965) was unable to find differences in threshold sensitivity of more than 20 db. This discrepancy remains unresolved.

Atrophy of the stria vascularis is an entity described in detail in Chapter 10 J 3, Strial presbycusis. It results in threshold elevations which are nearly equal for all frequencies. In such cochleae there is a normal volume of endolymph, but presumably there is some deficit in strial function which adversely affects the sensitivity of the sense organ throughout the cochlear duct.

Another possible cause for threshold elevation, which remains purely hypothetical because of the lack of supportive studies, is stiffness of the basilar membrane. This condition, as yet unconfirmed, is presented as a possible cause for the descending audiometric pattern and is also discussed in Chapter 10 J 4, Cochlear conductive presbycusis.

The recruitment phenomenon was first described by Fowler (1937) as occurring in patients with "perceptive deafness." By perceptive deafness he meant a threshold elevation for bone conduction. Although he did not differentiate between sensory and neural lesions, it is now quite clear that the phenomenon occurs only when the sense organ is involved and not with pure neural lesions. Simply stated, loudness recruitment means that, with increased stimulus intensity, there is an abnormally rapid rise in loudness sensation so that even though the threshold is elevated, loudness sensation at high stimulus intensities approximates or equals that of the normal ear. Although the precise neurophysiological correlate of loudness is not known, one possibility is that loudness is determined by the magnitude of neural activity, the main variables being the number of nerve fibers excited and the frequency of the impulses within these fibers.

The hair cells are more susceptible to most forms of injury than the supporting cells and cochlear neurons. A large percentage of the hair cells of the organ of Corti may be lost with little or no concomitant degeneration of cochlear neurons. The extent of loss of cochlear neurons seems to parallel the extent of injury suffered by the supporting cells, particularly Deiters' cells and the pillar cells (Figs. 3.22, 3.23). The organ of Corti may be devoid of hair cells but, if the pillar cells and Deiters' cells remain, there may be little or no loss of cochlear neurons. When there is shortening of the height of the pillar arch, or partial collapse of external pillars, some decrease in innervation density may occur. A total loss of pillar cells and Deiters' cells is almost always associated with severe loss of cochlear neurons; however, some morphologically altered neurons usually persist (Fig. 3.24).

The intimate anatomical relationship of the afferent nerve fibers to the pillar cells and Deiters' cells is well known (Spoendlin and Gacek, 1963). The

Fig. 3.22: Photomicrographs showing different degrees of injury to the organ of Corti and cochlear neurons, following experimental head blows (cat). Survival times were three to six months.

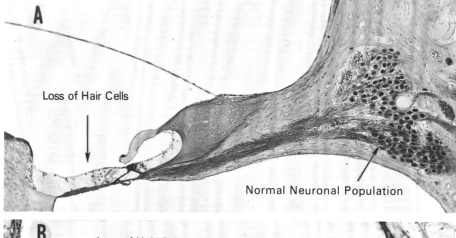

A: There is a loss of external hair cells and some of the Hensen's cells and Deiters' cells. The pillar cells are intact. There is no loss of cochlear neurons.

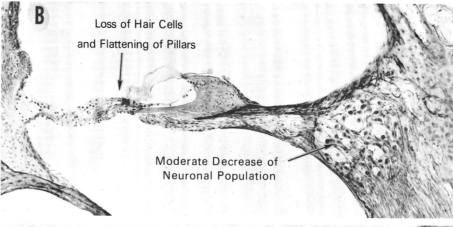

B: There is a severe loss of hair cells and partial collapse of the pillar cells. About 20 percent of the cochlear neurons show swelling and some are missing.

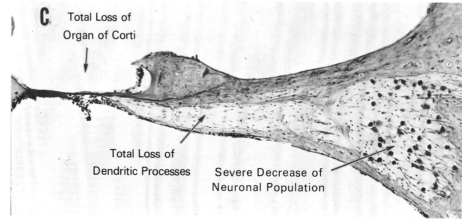

C: The organ of Corti and tectorial membrane are totally missing. About 60 percent of the cochlear neurons are missing and the remainder are devoid of dendritic processes. See also Fig. 3.24.

Fig. 3.23: Chart showing behavioral audiogram and cochlear chart of a cat with a concussion injury produced by a blow to the head. The neuronal population was established by counts of cell density in Rosenthal's canal. The extent of pillar cell injury was based on an arbitrary scale of 10. The graph shows that the site and magnitude of loss of cochlear neurons parallels more closely the extent of injury to the pillar cells than the loss of hair cells.

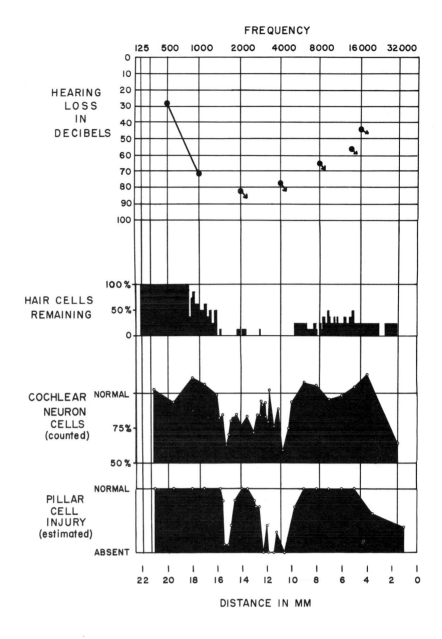

Fig. 3.24: Appearance of the cochlear neurons in a cat five months following total destruction of the organ of Corti by a head blow. About 50 percent of the neurons remain. Each cell body appears to have an axonal but no dendritic process. Many of the cell bodies contain a large clear vacuole and a small chromatin mass at the dendritic pole of the cell. The nuclei are severely pyknotic.

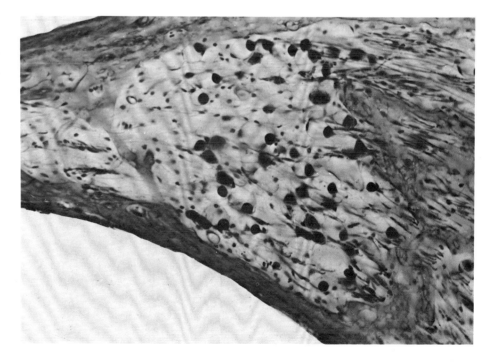

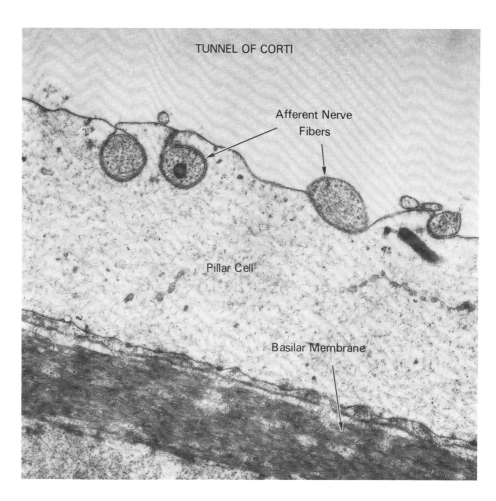

nerve endings at the base of the hair cells are enveloped on their lateral and basal surfaces by the cell bodies of Deiters' cells and are, in fact, attached to them by desmosomes. Furthermore, the nerve fibers as they pass from the hair cells to the habenulae perforatae, frequently lie in invaginations of the cell membranes of the Deiters' and pillar cells (Fig. 3.25).

Neural degeneration occurring secondary to a loss of supporting cells is a manifestation of acquired lesions. In developmental aplasia of the organ of Corti, the nerve fiber population may be normal in spite of severe morphological anomalies, even to the extent of total absence of pillar cells and Deiters' cells (Fig. 3.26).

The pathological correlates for loudness recruitment appear to be (1) a sense organ with a diminished but not absent capability for neural excitation and (2) a population of afferent neurons adequate to relay an intense barrage of neural activity to the higher centers of the auditory system. A model illustrating the recruitment phenomenon is shown in Fig. 3.27. The mechanism by which a sense organ with an elevated response threshold might excite large numbers of fibers at high levels of stimulus intensity is not known. It may be related to an abnormally rapid growth pattern in the microphonic response. Another possibility is that the phenomenon is related in some way to the distribution of afferent nerve fibers within the cochlea. The studies of Lorente de No (1937) and Fernández (1951) illustrate the complexity of afferent innervation in the organ of Corti. Some fibers appear to end only on internal hair cells, others on external hair cells. Possibly some end on both. Many fibers are known to pass for some distance within the internal and external spiral bundles and give collaterals to many hair cells.

The "recruiting" ear has been shown to exhibit a better than normal capability for detecting small increments of intensity change. The interrelationship of the loudness recruitment phenomenon and the decreased intensity difference limen is also illustrated in Fig. 3.27.

Distortion of pitch sensation is a common manifestation of sensory lesions. A pure tone may be heard as noisy, rough, or buzzing. If it is perceived to

Fig. 3.26: When genetically determined structural abnormalities develop in the organ of Corti during embryonic life, the organ of Corti may show marked abnormality in the presence of a normal population of cochlear neurons.

A: A ten-year-old child born deaf. Histological study shows cochleo-saccular aplasia (Scheibe dysplasia). The organ of Corti is incompletely formed, and only remnants of pillar and Deiters' cells are present. The population of cochlear neurons is normal. (Courtesy of Rüedi)

B: Deaf Dalmatian dog (cochleo-saccular aplasia). In spite of severe dysplasia of the structures of the cochlea due to faulty development, the population of cochlear neurons is normal.

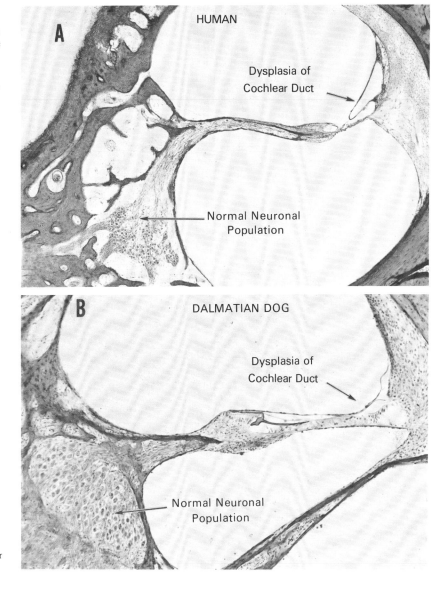

Fig. 3.27: Model demonstrating a possible mechanism for loudness recruitment and the decreased intensity difference limen. On either side of an arbitrary stimulus intensity scale are schematically drawn sets of neurons showing normal populations for both the normal and abnormal cochleae. Let us assume that with increasing stimulus intensity an increasing number of neurons is activated and that at an intensity of 100 db the maximum available number of neurons is activated and loudness sensation is maximum. In our hypothetical model of the cochlea with the sensory lesion, the level at which the first neural unit is excited is at an intensity of 50 db; however, as stimulus intensity is increased, additional neurons are activated at an abnormally rapid rate. Thus, at an intensity of 100 db, the full set of neurons is activated and loudness sensation is equal to that of the normal ear. It also is apparent from a study of the model that a smaller change in stimulus intensity is required in the pathological ear to activate an additional neural unit than in the normal ear, the psychoacoustic manifestation of which is the decreased intensity difference limen.

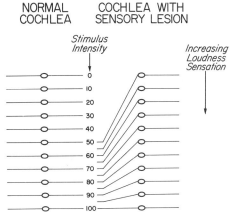

NORMAL COCHLEA   COCHLEA WITH SENSORY LESION

sound as double, as though two tones were being introduced in combination, it is known as monaural diplacusis, and if the pitch is different from that perceived by the normal ear, it is known as binaural diplacusis.

One possible explanation for diplacusis is harmonic distortion, for the ear, like all acoustic instruments, exhibits this phenomenon. The middle and inner ear systems respond unequally to different frequencies; some are transmitted readily while others are enfeebled. When driven at high intensities, the ear will introduce nonlinear distortion into the transmitted sounds. Thus, it is conceivable that a cochlea which has sustained a localized area of injury and hearing loss for a restricted range of frequencies may demonstrate diplacusis because a more responsive area of the cochlea is responding to a harmonic tone introduced by the middle ear or cochlea. Studies by Békésy (1960) and by Wever and Lawrence (1954) have shown frequency distortions to occur at only moderate stimulus intensities, particularly for the low frequencies.

Another theory for altered pitch perception has its basis in the "place" theory of pitch perception. It suggests that a pure tone causes maximal neural excitation at some site along the cochlear duct other than the locus of maximum displacement for that tone. This explanation implies that the locus of maximum displacement is exhibiting an elevated threshold because of a disturbance in sensory function and that more intense neural activity is occurring in an adjacent area which at supra-threshold intensities is included in the field of excitation. This thesis gains support from the study of Davis et al. (1950), who investigated pitch and loudness sensation in human subjects following exposures to pure tones at high intensities. They made the following observations: (1) large degrees of diplacusis were produced only when hear-

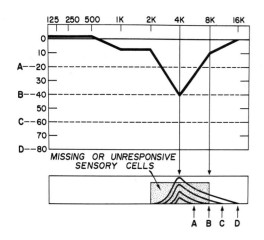

Fig. 3.28: This is a model to explain a possible mechanism for binaural diplacusis. The audiogram shows a 4000 Hz "dip" characteristic of stimulation deafness and typical of the temporary hearing losses produced by Davis et al. (1950). The underlying bar-graph represents the sense organ and the stippled area indicates the area of diminished sensitivity. Curves A, B, C, and D represent displacement amplitudes on the basilar membrane for sensation levels of 20, 40, 60, and 80 db for the 4000 Hz tone. The model shows that at a 20 db sensation level, Curve A, the displacement pattern lies entirely within the unresponsive zone. At 40 db, Curve B, the displacement pattern has moved in the basal direction sufficiently to activate the sensory elements located in the region which is normally most responsive for 8000 Hz and presumably pitch is perceived at a level higher than 4000 Hz. At 60 db, Curve C, the maximum neural activity still occurs at point B and pitch is unchanged from that perceived at the previous 40 db sensation level although loudness is greater. At a level of 80 db, Curve D, the displacement pattern is sufficiently intense to excite sensory units of high threshold in the 4,000 Hz region and (possibly aided by the mechanism of recruitment) pitch is normal for 4,000 Hz. The concept, of course, relegates a strong role to the place theory of pitch perception.

Fig. 3.29: Audiometric findings of a patient with a surgically proven vestibular schwannoma of the left ear. The relatively good pure tone thresholds associated with poor speech discrimination (16 percent) and absence of loudness recruitment are characteristic of a lesion involving the cochlear nerve.

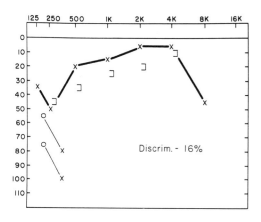

Discrim. - 16%

Fig. 3.30: Surgical approach to the cochlear nerve of the cat. After exposing the superior surface of the petrous bone, the internal auditory canal can be entered from above. After cutting and retracting the facial and vestibular nerves, the cochlear nerve is widely exposed deep within the canal.

ing losses were restricted to a small frequency range; (2) large displacements of pitch were always upward; (3) there was a strong tendency for many different frequencies to sound the same in pitch, with their pitches being displaced upward by varying amounts to the same final pitch; (4) usually, loudness increased while pitch remained constant as the frequency of the test tone was increased at constant intensity; and (5) as the intensity of the test tone was increased, the displacement of pitch decreased (and loudness increased) until finally pitch matched that of the test tone.

Fig. 3.28 depicts a model showing how the place theory of pitch perception and the resonance curves of displacement of the cochlear partition may interact to account for binaural diplacusis.

Loss of speech discrimination is a manifestation of the inability of the cochlea to receive complex acoustic stimuli and code them into patterns of neural activity which are appropriate for the decoding functions of the higher auditory system. For example, an elevation in the threshold of hearing, whether it involves a broad or restricted region of the auditory spectrum, leaves acoustic information unrepresented in the neural patterns. Increasing signal intensity to optimum supra-threshold levels may improve the neural pattern, but abnormalities will persist for several reasons: (1) a loss of sensory cells or cells which have abnormal and different levels of threshold sensitivity will produce abnormal patterns of neural discharge regardless of stimulus levels; (2) the narrowed intensity range to which the sense organ responds produces an abnormal neural pattern which evolves psychologically as loudness recruitment; and (3) acoustic distortion, be it the result of harmonic distortions originating in the middle or inner ear or aberrant response zones along the cochlear partition, produces abnormal neural patterns and diminished discrimination.

(i) Psychoacoustic manifestations of neural lesions

Deficits in the afferent neural system may occur at any level. The psychoacoustic manifestations have been studied most thoroughly in individuals with neoplasms involving the cochlear nerve. The characteristic pattern of dysfunction consists of (1) decreased speech discrimination with preservation of pure tone thresholds (Schuknecht and Woellner, 1953), (2) absence of loudness recruitment (Dix et al., 1948), and (3) abnormal auditory fatigue (Hood, 1950; Hirsh and Ward, 1952; Owens, 1971) (Fig. 3.29). Similar patterns of hear-

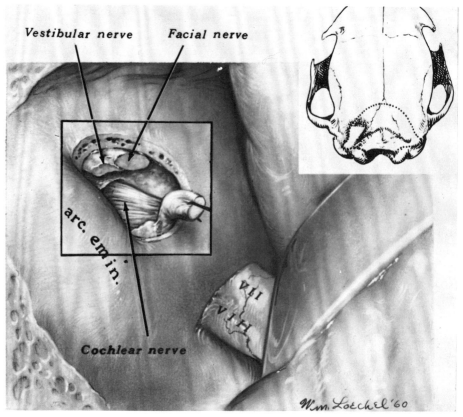

Vestibular nerve   Facial nerve

arc. em. in.

Cochlear nerve

Wm. Loechel '60

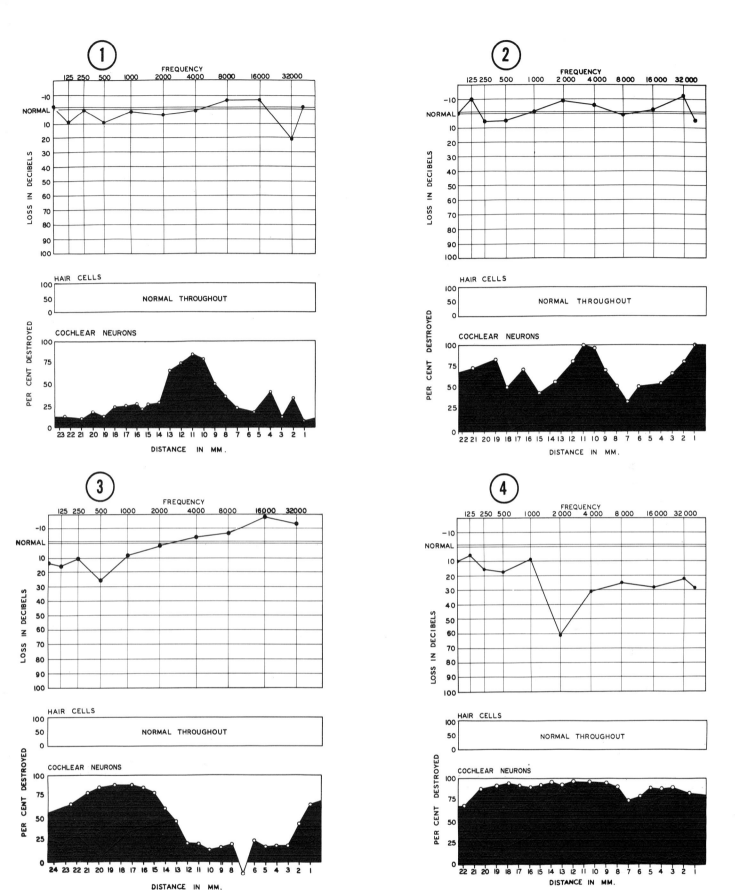

Fig. 3.31: Behavioral audiograms and charts of cochlear pathology for four cats with partial section of the cochlear nerve. The postoperative survival times were three to six months. The black filling represents the percent of cochlear neurons missing as determined by counts on microscopic sections and compared with the mean for normal animals. The charts of Cats #1 and #2 show that normal pure tone thresholds may be retained after extensive loss of cochlear neurons.

ing loss occur in multiple sclerosis (Citron et al., 1963) and in the neural type of presbycusis.

To determine more precisely the effect of loss of cochlear neurons on hearing, Schuknecht and Woellner (1955) performed partial cochlear nerve sections on cats which were behaviorally conditioned for pure tone threshold tests. The nerve was partially sectioned deep in the internal auditory canal by an approach through the superior surface of the petrous bone (Fig. 3.30). The results clearly demonstrated that loss of up to 75 percent of the cochlear neurons to large regions was consistent with normal pure tone thresholds. Greater losses of neurons created moderate threshold elevations (Fig. 3.31).

Fig. 3.32: Graphs showing pure tone audiograms, pitch discrimination limens, and charts of cochlear pathology in two animals with partial sections of the cochlear nerves. Pure tone audiograms were taken periodically until the thresholds were stabilized (30 to 60 days) after which pitch discrimination thresholds were determined behaviorally at 40 db sensation levels. The cat was placed in a double grill box and presented with constantly repeated pure tone pulses at a standard frequency. At random time intervals, a comparison pulse tone of higher frequency was substituted for every other one of the standard pulses, and the cat was conditioned to move across the barrier of the cage when these higher frequency pulses were detected. By gradually decreasing the difference in frequency between the standard and comparison tones, the limits of the animals' frequency discrimination could be determined. Using this procedure, the relative discrimination threshold (that is, the ratio of the just-noticeable difference in frequency to the standard frequency) were obtained at several frequencies. These thresholds were then compared with the thresholds which had been determined previously on normal cats. The cat, whose data appears on the left, showed a loss of about 95 percent of the cochlear neurons in the apical half of the cochlea. This animal had moderate low-frequency hearing loss, but pitch discrimination remained normal. The cat, whose data appear on the right, showed a severe loss of cochlear neurons in the 12 to 17 mm region of the cochlea. The animal showed no change in pure tone thresholds or pitch discrimination. (Courtesy of Elliott)

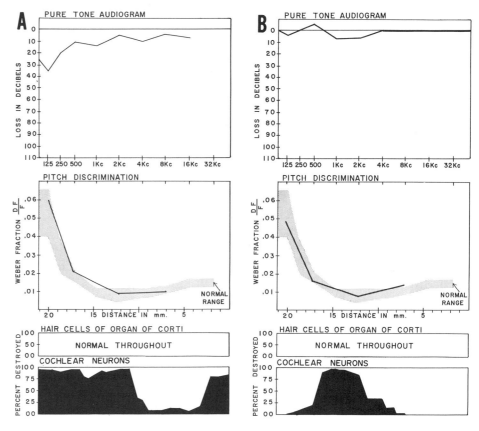

Fig. 3.33: This chart shows the absolute pure tone thresholds as determined for the cat by the behavioral test method (Elliott et al., 1960), and the population density of cochlear neurons (Schuknecht, 1960), both plotted as a function of distance along the cochlear duct. Although it was hypothesized at one time that innervation density might relate directly to threshold sensitivity, this appears now to be clearly incorrect. See text.

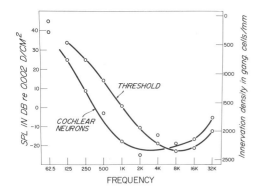

A logical extension of these studies was the determination of the extent to which such lesions affect pitch discrimination (Elliott, 1961). The experiments demonstrated that at the 40 db sensation level, pitch discrimination remained normal in the presence of severe deficits in the population of cochlear neurons (Fig. 3.32). An interpretation of the findings in terms of the place theory of pitch perception indicates that the detection of shift in location of the field of excitation is not impaired so long as some small number of neural units remains spatially distributed along the longitudinal dimension of the sense organ.

These studies show that possibly 25 percent or less of the cochlear neurons is sufficient to transmit the threshold response. This fact mitigates against the concept that auditory threshold is determined by innervation density. Curves showing the relationship of these two functions and originally considered as support for such a hypothesis (Schuknecht, 1960a) must now be considered invalid (Fig. 3.33).

A subject of some importance is the method by which the population of cochlear neurons have been assigned positions along the cochlear duct. Two-dimensional graphic reconstructions were made for both the organ of Corti and spiral ganglion, following which the graphs were superimposed and the ganglion cells assigned positions in that region of the organ of Corti located nearest them. There seems to be some justification for this procedure, because localized injuries to the organ of Corti result in concomitant degeneration of the cochlear neurons located in the adjacent region of Rosenthal's canal.

Among those who have contributed information on cochlear nerve section are Wittmaack, who reported in 1911 that the cochlear nerve could be sectioned in animals without injury to the organ of Corti, and later Kaida in 1931, and Hallpike and Rawdon-Smith in 1934, who confirmed this observation and showed that to prevent degeneration of the membranous labyrinth it was necessary to avoid injury to the labyrinthine artery.

Dandy performed numerous partial sections of the VIIIth cranial nerve for the relief of Ménière's disease. The object, of course, was to cut the vestibular nerves and preserve the cochlear nerve. He reported his results in 1934 and stated that frequently no change in auditory thresholds occurred even if large portions of the cochlear nerve were cut. The hearing losses that did occur were for the high frequencies.

Neff (1947) performed partial sections of the cochlear nerve in conditioned cats and found that severe neural lesions were compatible with normal auditory thresholds. He also found that hearing losses, when produced, were always for high frequencies even though attempts were made to section selectively different portions of the nerve.

It is now quite clear that these authors produced high-frequency hearing losses because they cut that part of the nerve which supplies the basal turn of the cochlea. These fibers pass in the superficial and posterior part of the cochlear nerve trunk and are most vulnerable to the surgeon approaching the nerve through the posterior cranial fossa. The partial nerve sections in the experiment of Schuknecht and Woellner (1955) were made from a superior approach, deep in the internal auditory canal, and did not create selective high-frequency hearing losses.

A summary analysis of the data from both human observations and animal experiments seems to justify the following comments. (1) The earliest manifestation of pure cochlear nerve degeneration is loss of discrimination for complex signals which is manifested clinically as a loss in speech discrimination. (2) More than 75 percent of the cochlear neurons to a particular region of the cochlea may be missing without creating threshold losses for frequencies having their locus of importance in those regions. (3) More than 90 percent of the cochlear neurons may be missing to a particular region of the cochlea without influencing pitch discrimination for frequencies having their displacement patterns in those regions. (4) Loudness recruitment and the decreased intensity difference limen (which are characteristic of sensory lesions) do not occur with pure cochlear nerve lesions.

The concept of cortical deafness has elicited considerable controversy. In 1962 DiCarlo et al. denied the existence of even a single convincing case study showing an unequivocally measured reduction in auditory sensitivity with a clearly demonstrable central nervous system lesion and no demonstrable peripheral lesion. It is quite clear that the cochlea has bilateral cortical representation and that the temporal lobes, particularly the transverse temporal gyri, constitute a major functional unit of the auditory system. It has been well documented that unilateral temporal lobe lesions do not lead to pure tone hearing losses in animals or man (Bunch, 1928; Mettler et al., 1934; Penfield and Evans, 1934; Goldstein et al., 1956). Routine speech discrimination scores also show no abnormalities as the result of such lesions; however, special testing techniques have demonstrated an impairment in ability to localize sound in the contralateral auditory field (Sanchez-Longo et al., 1957) and a deterioration in the discrimination of interrupted, distorted, accelerated, dichotic simultaneous, and time-staggered speech in the contralateral ear (Bocca et al., 1955; Bocca, 1958; Jerger, 1960, 1964; Berlin et al., 1972).

Hearing loss thought to be due to cerebral disease has been reported only in patients with demonstrable or presumed naturally occurring lesions in the posterior parts of both temporal lobes (Mott, 1907; Henschen, 1917; Bramwell, 1927; Misch, 1928; Lemoyne and Mahoudeau, 1959; Hansen and Reske-Nielsen, 1963).

An important documentation for the existence of cortical deafness is the case report by Jerger et al. (1969). Extensive clinical studies indicated that this patient had experienced, at two different points in time, occlusion of the terminal branches of the middle cerebral arteries on each side, resulting in bilateral partial cerebral hemisphere infarction, maximum in the temporal lobes, and producing the clinical picture of cortical deafness. This patient demonstrated essentially normal manual audiometry, right-sided hearing loss by Békésy audiometry, impaired speech understanding for phonetically balanced word lists (worse on the right), bilateral impairment of auditory temporal order, and severe impairment of ability to localize sound. The authors interpreted the poorer performance of the right ear to be due to greater damage to the auditory area of the left temporal lobe.

Experiments on behaviorally trained cats have shown that unilateral ablation of the auditory cortex results in a profound deficit in attending to stimuli on the side contralateral to the lesion (Cranford et al., 1971).

The human cerebral cortex has been mapped according to minor variations in the pattern of gray matter. The auditory cortex of man is located in the superior temporal gyrus along the Sylvian fissure, which corresponds to topographical areas 41, 42, and 22 of Brodmann (1925). Campbell (1905) divided this area into an audito-sensory region (41) thought to be related to auditory perception, and an audito-psychic region (42 and 22) thought to be important for auditory memory. These concepts are not established well enough to justify the consideration of these areas as discrete functional zones.

Further evidence regarding the function of the auditory cortex of man comes from the investigations of Penfield and Rasmussen (1955) who electrically stimulated the cortex during the course of intracranial operations performed under local anesthesia. They found that (1) auditory responses are more numerous in the audito-psychic area and less frequent in the audito-sensory area; (2) electrical stimulation results in a sensation of sound in some patients and of deafness in others; and (3) auditory sensations resulting from cortical stimulation were most often referred to the contralateral ear. They also found that electrical stimulation close to the margins of the Sylvian fissure was more apt to produce a sensation of simple sounds, such as buzzing or ringing, while stimulation away from the fissure was more apt to introduce an element of interpretation of the sound. These observations have not been confirmed and must be interpreted with some degree of caution.

In a series of experiments on behaviorally trained cats, Neff and Yela (1948) found that total bilateral ablation of the cortical projection areas of the auditory systems does not alter the pure tone thresholds. They found that after auditory cortical ablations, cats can respond to (1) the onset of a sound, (2) change in intensity of a stimulus, and (3) change in frequency of a tone; however, they cannot respond to (1) changes in patterns of tones, (2) changes in duration of sounds, or (3) localization of sound in space. In an analysis of these findings Jerison and Neff (1953), Neff (1965), and Trahiotis and Elliott (1970) pointed out that the tasks which can be learned appear to involve the use of new neural units when the stimulus is altered. It is not known whether these tasks are performed by other lower centers or by other parts of the higher centers.

The auditory efferent neural system has not yet been assigned a clear functional role in hearing. It has been suggested that it might be involved in such behavioral phenomena as attention (Galambos, 1960; Maruseva, 1961), detection of signals in noise (Dewson, 1968), or frequency discrimination (Capps and Ades, 1968). The experiments of Galambos (1955, 1956), Desmedt (1960), and Fex (1959, 1962, 1965) suggest that the crossed olivocochlear tracts have an inhibitory function; however, these workers were utilizing stimuli in excess of physiological limits. Fex's studies (1962) on the feedback system of the olivocochlear fibers reveal latencies of 5 to 40 milliseconds, which seem too long for an effective function related to integration of acoustic input. Pfalz (1969) was unable to demonstrate an inhibitory function of the crossed olivocochlear tract utilizing stimuli of physiological magnitudes. Wiederhold and Kiang (1970) found, however, that the discharge rate for single auditory nerve fibers was decreased for tones at the characteristic frequency when the crossed olivocochlear bundle was stimulated. Wiederhold's studies (1970) suggest that stimulation of the crossed olivocochlear bundle most effectively reduces responses to low-level stimuli; however, the functional significance of this finding is not clear.

In human subjects, cutting of the vestibular nerves, including the composite olivochlear bundle, has failed to elicit any alteration in auditory function (House and House, 1964; Fisch and Yasargil, 1968; Fluur and Tovi, 1965).

From a purely anatomical standpoint the efferent system might function as a mechanism for balancing the output from the afferent nerves in two ways: (1) through direct presynaptic inhibitive action on the hair cells and

(2) through post-synaptic inhibition of the dendrites of the cochlear neurons. The widespread ramification of each efferent nerve fiber makes it improbable that they have a more localized effect on a specific part of the cochlea (Wersäll, 1968).

6. AUDIOMETRY

In order to clarify references made elsewhere to audiometric and vestibulo-metric techniques, a brief description of these methods and their usual clinical interpretations is offered here. Although there is no single auditory or vestibular test which indicates the exact location of a lesion in these systems, by utilizing a battery of available tests in combination with the history, otological examination, neurological examination, auditory and vestibular testing, the general area of involvement can be determined. This is intended only as a brief summary, and the reader will need to refer elsewhere for detailed descriptions. The current status of tests for auditory function has been expertly reviewed by Jerger (1968).

Pure tone threshold test. Standard audiometry is performed by a method of limits which consists of presenting pure tones of brief duration to which the patient responds with signals if he hears them. Intensity adjustments are presented in ascending and descending sequences until the threshold for a series of tones has been determined. Normally thresholds are determined for pure tones at octave intervals in a range from 125 Hz to 8,000 Hz. Prior to 1964 American audiometers were calibrated in accordance with threshold values obtained in the United States Public Health Service Survey of 1935-1936. This reference level was accepted by the American Standards Association in 1951 (ASA-51), and was based on responses obtained from nonsophisticated listeners. As this reference level was different from that adopted by other nations where the reference level was related to the thresholds obtained from trained listeners, the International Standards Organization recommended a new reference level, now known as ISO-64 and utilized by most institutions (Davis and Kranz, 1964). In this book all audiograms are plotted according to the ISO-64 audiometric calibration. Tests which were made on audiometers calibrated on the ASA-51 norm have been converted by the recommended conversion factors.

Bone conduction audiometry requires careful masking of the non-test ear (Carhart, 1950; Dirks and Malmquist, 1964). The failure to utilize masking in the testing of bone conduction may result in a false impression of inner ear function, for it has been established that there is less than 5 db attenuation between the two ears for a bone conduction receiver placed on any part of the skull. Refinements in bone conduction testing consist of the use of narrow band masking noise (Zwislocki, 1951), use of insert receivers (Studebaker, 1962), a systematic method for determining optimal masking noise level in the non-test ear (Hood, 1957), and the development of an artificial mastoid for calibration of bone conduction receivers (Weiss, 1960).

Loudness recruitment test. The simplest test for loudness recruitment is the alternate binaural loudness balance test which may be performed when there is a substantial difference between threshold intensity levels of the two ears at the same frequencies. In this test a record is made of the intensity levels required in the normal ear to produce equal loudness sensations to a range of sensation levels in the impaired ear. In the monoaural loudness balance test, similar evaluations are made when there is a substantial difference between the threshold sensitivity levels of two frequencies in the same ear (Jerger and Harford, 1960).

The decreased intensity difference limen which is considered to be another psychoacoustic manifestation of a sensory disorder of the cochlea may be tested by the small increment sensitivity index (SISI) test (Jerger et al., 1959). In this test an evaluation is made of the individual's ability to detect 1 db increments of intensity change for pure tones at sensation levels of 20 db. The decreased intensity difference limen is also readily demonstrated by the semiautomatic audiometer developed by Békésy (1947b). The phenomenon is recorded as a reduction in the amplitudes of the threshold tracings from the normal 8 to 10 db range to a range of 2 to 3 db. Dix et al. (1948) showed that loudness recruitment is characteristically absent in disorders involving the cochlear nerve. Thus direct tests for recruitment, especially the binaural loudness balance test, are of great importance in differentiating sensory from neural lesions.

The frequency increment sensitivity test (FIST) is an audiometric test using incremental frequency variations in a presentation and scoring method analogous to the SISI test. It has the same significance as the SISI test for differentiating sensory from neural lesions (Campbell, 1970).

Auditory fatigue test. Another important test for the identification of neural lesions is based on adaptation to sustained pure tone signals. Lierle and Reger (1955), utilizing a semiautomatic audiometer, demonstrated that a patient with a hearing loss caused by a vestibular schwannoma, when asked to track his threshold for a fixed-frequency pure tone, required increasing intensity levels as a function of time. The test when used on the pure tone audiometer is known as the "tone decay test" (Carhart, 1957).

Tone decay of 35 db or more occurring over a period of one minute is considered to be evidence in favor of a lesion involving the cochlear nerves or nuclei.

Speech reception threshold test. The speech reception threshold test (SRT) consists of determining the intensity level at which 50 percent of spondaic words are correctly heard. The threshold should be approximately equal to the average pure tone level for 500, 1,000 and 2,000 Hz and therefore serves to validate pure tone tests.

Speech discrimination test. The speech discrimination test consists of evaluating the individual's ability to repeat correctly a list of phonetically balanced monosyllabic words presented at comfortable loudness levels. It was first pointed out by Schuknecht and Woellner (1953), and subsequently by Lidén (1954), Walsh and Goodman (1955), and Goodman (1957), that speech discrimination scores are particularly low with lesions involving the cochlear nerve.

Bocca et al. (1955) and Bocca and Calearo (1963) demonstrated that the ability to understand distorted speech was diminished in the contralateral ear of patients with temporal lobe tumor. This group of investigators systematically varied the redundancy of speech messages by means of low-pass filtering, periodic interruption or acceleration of rate of presentation, and variation in message length. They found that any reduction in redundancy produced the desired effect but that low-pass filtering provided the most effective clinical technique for the diagnosis of temporal lobe tumors. Bocca and Calearo (1963) and Jerger (1964) clearly demonstrated that for tests indicating lesions in the higher auditory centers, simple tasks involving tonal phenomena are inadequate and that considerably more complex stimuli are required.

Lidén (1969), in a study of patients with tumors of the brain stem, found abnormal tone decay and tone perversion to be commonly present. Tone perversion is characterized by subjective change in the quality of the pure tone. These tests seem to be negative with lesions of the auditory cortex.

Impedance test. The development of instrumentation for impedance audiometry has resulted in the electromechanical bridge (Zwislocki, 1961; Feldman, 1964) and the electroacoustic bridge (Thomsen, 1955; Terkildsen and Nielsen, 1960; Møller, 1960. The electroacoustic technique is probably the most versatile and permits the recording of three basic components of impedance audiometry: acoustic impedance, tympanometry, and the acoustic reflex threshold.

Tympanometry measures changes in eardrum compliance as air pressure is varied in the external canal, and the acoustic reflex threshold measures changes in impedance resulting from the stapedius reflex. The tests readily differentiate between stapes fixation and ossicular discontinuity (Feldman, 1963; Zwislocki and Feldman, 1969).

Although acoustic impedance values are too variable for accurate diagnosis, the combination of test results yields patterns which are of value in the diagnosis of sensory and neural lesions, particularly in children (Jerger, 1970).

Objective audiometry. Several types of objective hearing tests, that is, hearing tests not requiring a behavioral response of the test subject, are being used with varying degrees of success.

Electrodermal audiometry, also called the psychogalvanic skin response (PGSR) audiometry, measures the electrical resistance or potential or both between the palm and the back of the hand. It is made useful for audiometry by forming a conditioned reflex with sound as the conditioned stimulus.

Electroencephalic audiometry is a method which measures the blocking effect of sound stimulation on the alpha rhythm of the electroencephalic response. The method has proved to be most effective when the patient is tested asleep.

Evoked response audiometry, like electroencephalic audiometry, utilizes responses from scalp electrodes but takes advantage of an average response computer to detect activity in the auditory cortex, which is normally obscured or masked by spontaneous electroencephalic activity.

Impedance audiometry consists of recording the stapedial reflex by measuring alterations in the acoustic impedance of the external auditory canal.

Electrocochlear audiometry is a method by which neural responses of the cochlea are measured by an electrode placed through the tympanic membrane onto the bony wall of the cochlea (Portmann and Aran, 1971), in the external auditory canal (Montandon et al., 1974), or elsewhere (Sohmer and Feinmesser, 1974; Galambos, 1974).

B. THE VESTIBULAR SYSTEM

The vestibular system is one of the major sensory inflows to the postural control apparatus. A mobile or potentially mobile organism requires a highly complex integration of sensory input and motor inflow in order to maintain static and dynamic postural stability. The major sensory inputs are visual, vestibular, kinesthetic, and proprioceptive. The motor output is primarily neuromuscular, but this is modified by so-called "voluntary," extrapyramidal, cerebellar, and other influences. It is well known that vestibular stimulation gives rise to certain motor phenomena, such as ocular movement, rotation of the head on the neck, changes in tonus and positioning of limbs, as well as subjective and autonomic responses.

1. EARLY INVESTIGATIONS

The first serious research on vestibular physiology appears to be that of Flourens (1842) who, in the course of an acoustical study, opened the horizontal canals of the pigeon and noted characteristic head movements. After further studies he noted that the movements occurred in the plane of the involved canal, a finding which later was to form the basis for Ewald's First Law. No note was made of this work for many years until Ménière (1861a, 1861b, 1861c, 1861d), knowing of Flourens' work, related the semicircular canals to a vertiginous syndrome which later was to bear Ménière's name. Crum-Brown (1874), Mach (1875), and Breuer (1891) proposed the theory that excitation of the cristae occurred through movement of the endolymphatic fluid. Several investigators observed that destruction of the peripheral vestibular labyrinth of one ear caused (1) nystagmus to the opposite side, (2) rotation of the head so that the normal ear became uppermost, and (3) rotation of the spine associated with increased extensor tone of the limbs of the opposite side. In 1882 Bechterew demonstrated that if a suitable interval of time was allowed to elapse after unilateral labyrinthectomy so that adjustment could take place, that is, loss of nystagmus and diminution of musclar imbalance, destruction of the opposite ear created an upset similar to that which occurred with the first procedure. He also showed that nystagmus did not occur when both labyrinths were extirpated simultaneously, although there was loss of tonus and weakness of the muscular system.

Further experiments showed that if after recovery from unilateral labyrinectomy the vestibular nuclei were destroyed on the same side, the symptoms of vestibular imbalance recurred. If, after compensation had occurred from destruction of one labyrinth, the opposite labyrinth and the vestibular nuclei of the first side were destroyed together, there was no nystagmus. Also, if, after both labyrinths had been destroyed and adjustment periods had taken place, the vestibular nuclei of one side were destroyed, the typical nystagmus and muscular imbalance occurred again.

In 1892 Ewald, working with pigeons, made important observations which would be known later as Ewald's laws. These laws state that (1) the eyes and head move in the plane of the canal stimulated as well as in the direction of endolymph flow; (2) in the lateral canal a flow of endolymph toward the ampulla (utriculo-petal) causes greater stimulation than flow away from the ampulla (utriculo-fugal); and (3) in the superior and posterior canals a flow of endolymph away from the ampullae causes more stimulation than a flow toward the ampullae.

By injecting ink into the canal system of fish, Steinhausen (1931) and later Dohlman (1938) demonstrated cupular movement and showed that the cupula seals the ampulla hermetically (Fig. 3.34).

2. CELLULAR POLARIZATION AND FUNCTIONAL DIRECTIVITY

The importance of polarization as related to the kinocilium or the centriole was originally demonstrated in the fish by Lowenstein and Wersäll (1959) and in mammals by Wersäll (1961). Wersäll et al. (1965) demonstrated the same to be true of the frog and bird, and Spoendlin (1966), using phase contrast microscopy, described this polarity of the vestibular hair cells in more detail. Numerous subsequent studies have shown that in the lateral canal crista the kinocilium is located on each hair cell on the side which is closest to the utricle, whereas the opposite is true for the superior and posterior canal cristae (see Chapter 2D2b, The vestibular sense organs). This arrangement of the cilia presumably has functional significance. Ewald's law states that utriculo-petal deviation (toward the utricle) of the cupula of the lateral canal evokes a stronger reaction than utriculo-fugal deviation (away from the utricle), whereas for the superior and posterior canals, the opposite is true. Further support for this functional directivity is found in the studies of Lowenstein and Sand (1940), who recorded two types of response characteristics of single neural units of the crista, one with spontaneous activity at rest and the other without. They noted that utriculo-petal stimulation of the lateral canal crista increased the activity of the spontaneously firing units and activated the silent ones. On the other hand, utriculo-fugal stimulation reduced the activity of the spontaneously active units but had no effect on the silent ones. The response pattern was reversed for the cristae of the superior and posterior canals.

Trincker (1957) further confirmed the functional behavior of the cristae in studies on the resting potentials in the ampullae of guinea pigs. He found that utriculo-petal cupular deviation in the lateral canal created a depression of the resting potential, whereas utriculo-fugal deviation increased this potential. The opposite pattern occurred in the superior and posterior ampullae. Thus, deviation of the cupula in the direction of the kinocilium increases neural activity, whereas the opposite effect occurs with a deviation away from the kinocilium.

Numerous investigators have also found consistent patterns of ciliary po-

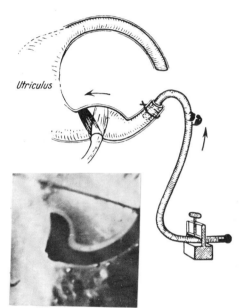

Fig. 3.34: India ink injection of a semicircular canal of the shark showing that the cupula makes an hermetic seal with the ampullary wall. (After Steinhausen and Dohlman)

Utriculus

larization in the hair cells of the maculae (see Chapter 2D2b, The vestibular system). Here the arrangement is related to the striolae. In the macula utriculi the polarization of most cells is toward the striola, that is, kinocilia are located on the side nearest the striola. In the macula sacculi, on the other hand, the main polarization is away from the striola. These findings are in agreement with the electrophysiological studies of Lowenstein and Roberts (1950) on single neural units of the utricle. They found that each single neural unit had a maximum positive and negative response to tilting around a specific horizontal axis, and in the total neural population there were units sensitive to all possible directions of tilt from the horizontal.

Fluur and Mellström (1970a, 1970b) and Fluur (1959, 1970) have demonstrated that the sensory epithelium of the utricle, saccule, and canals have a specific functional organization in relation to the extraocular muscles. Experiments on cats showed that electrical stimulation of specific regions of the maculae activated specific muscles or muscle groups, providing evidence for the functional significance of the directional polarization of the ciliary tufts of the hair cells of the vestibular sense organs.

3. NYSTAGMUS

Various forms of ocular nystagmus are important in the evaluation of vestibular function and malfunction. Defined strictly, ocular nystagmus consists of a reciprocating movement of the eyes having different velocities in the two directions (jerk nystagmus). Since vestibular nystagmus is of the jerk nystagmus variety, the discussion here will be limited to this type. Jerk nystagmus may be horizontal, vertical, oblique, or rotatory, and by convention directionality is indicated by the quick component. Rotatory nystagmus consists of the rotation of the eyeball around an axis drawn perpendicular to the pupillary aperture. By convention, such nystagmus is designated by the direction of rapid movement of the twelve o'clock point of the limbus. Thus the movement for left rotatory nystagmus is clockwise and for right rotatory nystagmus is counterclockwise. Nystagmus may be synchronous for both eyes or asynchronous. Horizontal nystagmus may be further classified into first degree, second degree, and third degree. This is defined in terms of the positions of eye deviation in which nystagmus is seen. Thus right-beating nystagmus present only with eyes deviated 30° to the right is called first degree; if present also on looking straight ahead it is designated as second degree, and if present on looking 30° to the left, it is designated as third degree. It is important to add to these the description of nystagmus which occurs on looking 30° upward or 30° downward. Nystagmus is described as spontaneous if it is present, in the absence of stimulation, with the patient in the erect position. Nystagmus which occurs only in different positions, as described in this Chapter, B4, Vestibulometry, is designated as positional nystagmus. Nystagmus which occurs expectedly as a result of specific stimulations such as rotation, optokinetic stimulation, or caloric stimulation is called induced nystagmus.

It must be understood that the vestibular system and oculomotor system are parts of a complex postural control apparatus. Nystagmus may occur as a result of lesions in the oculomotor system or as the result of lesions in or stimulations of several systems other than the vestibular system. Movement of the visual field, such as occurs when watching a rotating striped drum, is termed optokinetic nystagmus. Stimulation of dorsal cervical roots unilaterally may produce cervical nystagmus. Lesions in the cortical bulbar system may transiently produce a gaze paretic nystagmus. Cerebellar lesions may also transiently produce nystagmus. Neuromuscular weakness in the oculomotor system may produce direction paretic nystagmus. Certain drugs such as Dilantin may produce nystagmus, presumably on a brain stem basis. Congenital nystagmus is a variable form, varying in intensity and direction, and is thought to be on a brain stem basis although no specific locus has been demonstrated pathologically. Nystagmus associated with amblyopia, such as the so-called miner's nystagmus, has been described but seems rare. In the absence of ocular pathology, dissociated or asynchronous nystagmus, such as is found in internuclear opthalmoplegia, and vertical nystagmus are pathognomonic of central nervous system disorders. Spontaneous synchronous horizontal nystagmus may originate in the vestibular labyrinth, nerve, or brain stem.

(a) Vestibular habituation

Abels in 1906 reported that postrotatory nystagmus in man declines after repeated stimulations. Griffith in 1920 and Maxwell et al. (1922) described the same phenomenon in rabbits and pigeons. Dodge (1923) first called it habituation. Dunlap (1925), King (1926), and others demonstrated that the phenomenon could be produced by caloric stimulation as well as by rotation.

Monnier et al. (1970) ascribed four characteristics to habituation. (1) Acquisition of habituation consists of a progressive waning of the response with stimuli repeated many times. Habituation is expressed by a decrease in velocity and frequency of the slow and fast component during per-rotatory acceleration and post-rotatory deceleration (Fernández and Schmidt, 1963). (2) Retention of habituation may last for hours to months depending upon the intensity and duration of the stimulus (McCabe and Gillingham, 1964). (3) Dishabituation is the phenomenon of recovery of the normal reaction. Jouvet and Hernandez-Peon (1957) demonstrated that recovery may be evoked by a long period of rest, a sudden change in intensity or frequency of stimulation, and the association of a concurrent noxious stimulus such as electric shock and anesthesia. (4) Transfer of vestibular habituation is that phenomenon by which repeated thermal stimulation leads to habituation not only of the ear being stimulated but also of the opposite ear (Henriksson et al., 1961).

Presumably habituation is mediated through inhibitory effects generated by cortical and subcortical systems which have not as yet been clearly defined. It has been demonstrated by many authors including Lenzi and Pompeiano (1970) and by Torok (1970) that nystagmus is more vigorous during a high state of arousal. Clinicians have observed from the beginning of vestibular testing that variations in nystagmic responses occur not only between individuals but in the same person on different occasions. For this reason mental alertness is considered to be mandatory during vestibular testing.

McCabe (1960), and subsequently Osterhammel et al. (1970), demonstrated that ballet dancers have much less nystagmus when exposed to high-velocity rotation than normal individuals. Dancers who performed the pirouette or the fouette utilizing the spotting technique demonstrated more habituation than those who did not use this method.

McCabe and Ryu (1969) have shown in animal experiments that unilateral deafferentization of the medial vestibular nucleus results in loss of resting activity of virtually all tonic neurons of both nuclei for three to five days, with recovery of spontaneous activity in the contralateral nucleus in one week and in the ipsilateral nucleus in one month. They demonstrated that when the cerebellum was removed, the period of silence of the contralateral medial vestibular nucleus following unilateral deafferentization was reduced to a few hours. They interpreted this observation as indicating that the cerebellum exhibits an inhibitory effect on the vestibular nuclei.

Fernández et al. (1959), in an experiment on cats, demonstrated that destruction of the nodulus of the cerebellum resulted in positional nystagmus in certain positions of the animal, suggesting that it acts as an inhibitor of the vestibulo-ocular reflex arc. Proctor and Fernández (1963) showed that the acquisition, retention, and transfer of habituation occurred as readily in cats that were blindfolded as in those permitted vision. Fernández and Riesco-MacClure (1963), in a study using human subjects, found that there is no habituation phenomenon for the optokinetic response.

Vestibular threshold values are the smallest specific stimulations which will produce a vestibular reflex or sensation. In general, the threshold values of the vestibular system for various mammals are of the same order of magnitude when the same technique is utilized. Oosterveld (1970) studied the effect of different gravitational conditions on vestibular stimulation. He found that an increase in gravity of about 2g produced during air flight, reduced both amplitude and duration of postrotatory nystagmus by 50 percent, 3g reduced the nystagmus by 70 percent, and 4.8g eliminated it completely.

Several investigators (Jackson and Sears, 1966; Kellogg and Graybiel, 1967) have determined that weightlessness achieved during parabolic flight completely suppresses caloric nystagmus.

(b) The labyrinthine fistula phenomenon

The labyrinthine fistula phenomenon develops as a consequence of a defect in the bony wall of one of the semicircular canals. The most frequent cause of bone resorption resulting in fistula formation is keratoma (cholesteatoma) of the mastoid. It is also a common clinical finding in congenital syphilis (see Chapter 5A4, Keratoma, and 5E2, Congenital syphilis).

A fistula is often manifested clinically by vertigo on sneezing, straining, blowing the nose, sudden head movements, Valsalva maneuver or by manipulations of the auricle.

The common test procedure for a labyrinthine fistula consists of applying positive or negative pressure to the external auditory canal, utilizing either a politzer bag with an adapter fitted to the ear canal or a Siegle's otoscope. Characteristically, the response is greater with negative than with positive pressure.

Vertigo is produced when movement of the soft tissue bridging the fistula displaces endolymphatic fluid, with resultant cupular deflection (Fig. 3.35).

It is usual for the fistula phenomenon to be present following surgical fenestration of the lateral semicircular canal and occasionally occurs after the introduction of a prosthesis in the oval window in the stapedectomy operation for otosclerosis. In the latter instance eye deviation is presumably caused either by massive fluid displacements or by contact of the prosthesis with some part of the membranous labyrinth.

(c) The Tullio phenomenon

The Tullio phenomenon consists of vertigo and nystagmus on exposure to high-intensity acoustic stimuli and is an indication of a fistula in the bony wall of the semicircular canals. It seems to occur only in the presence of an intact tympanic membrane and ossicular chain, suggesting that only under these conditions will inner ear fluid movement be sufficiently large to incite a vestibular response (Fig. 3.36). The response is most sensitive to low-frequency sounds and is usually readily elicited by the Bárány noise apparatus. The most common disorder giving rise to the Tullio phenomenon is congenital syphilis, although rarely it may occur as a result of bone resorption in association with chronic suppurative disease and keratoma.

Fig. 3.35: Labyrinthine fistula phenomenon. When positive or negative pressure is transmitted to a fistula of the bony wall of a semicircular canal, endolymph is moved across the ampulla. The resultant cupular movement causes nystagmus and vertigo.

Fig. 3.36: The Tullio phenomenon. When a high-intensity sound stimulus is directed into an ear with a bony fistula of a semicircular canal, endolymph movements across the ampulla may cause nystagmus and vertigo. The phenomenon is most readily evoked by low-frequency stimuli, which cause greater amplitudes of fluid displacement than high frequency stimuli. It usually occurs only in the presence of an intact ossicular mechanism. The phenomenon is most commonly observed in congenital syphilitic disease of the bony labyrinth.

Fig. 3.35

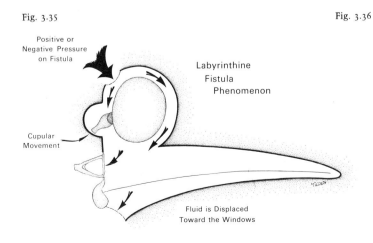

Positive or Negative Pressure on Fistula

Cupular Movement

Labyrinthine Fistula Phenomenon

Fluid is Displaced Toward the Windows

Fig. 3.36

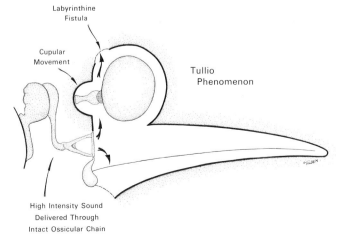

Labyrinthine Fistula

Cupular Movement

Tullio Phenomenon

High Intensity Sound Delivered Through Intact Ossicular Chain

(d) Oscillopsia

Oscillopsia is an optic illusory movement of a viewed stationary object (Bender, 1965). Symptoms need not be associated with nystagmus. It appears to be caused by a failure to prevent movement of the retinal image during fixation on a stationary object while the head is in movement. Patients with this symptom complain of blurring of the field of vision when walking, riding in an automobile, or on certain other head movements. A descriptive term sometimes used for the symptom is "jumbling of the panorama."

Keeney and Roseman (1966) and Cogan (1968) state that the lesions responsible for oscillopsia are commonly in the posterior fossa or brain stem. Farmer and Morris (1964) reported oscillopsia in a patient with unilateral loss of vestibular function from a keratoma of the cerebellopontine angle. Maw (1971) reported the findings on ten patients with oscillopsia, all of whom complained of the symptom when walking and during sudden head movements. None exhibited spontaneous or positional nystagmus; six showed a loss of caloric responses in both ears and four in one ear. Schuknecht (1957) found the symptom to be a common manifestation of streptomycin ototoxicity. In these patients the phenomenon subsided over a period of months after the administration of streptomycin had been discontinued. It would appear that the cause for slipping of the retinal image associated with head movements is due to a lesion involving the vestibular-ocular pathways and that it is most common with bilateral lesions.

Maw (1971) found that neither vestibular sedatives, nor tranquilizers or head exercises brought any noticeable improvement in the symptoms. Some patients noted, however, that wearing thick soft rubber heels minimized the distressing illusory movement of the surroundings when walking.

(e) Positional alcoholic nystagmus

Aschan et al. (1956, 1964) demonstrated that alcohol provokes positional nystagmus. About thirty minutes after the consumption of one or two normal-size alcoholic drinks, the patient exhibits a nystagmus in the direction of gaze (Phase I) and about 1½ hours later the nystagmus reverses direction (Phase II). One average alcoholic drink produces a reaction which can be measured nystagmographically for approximately eleven hours following intake. Weightlessness eliminates positional alcoholic nystagmus (Oosterveld, 1970). Money (1974) has presented convincing evidence that alcoholic nystagmus is caused by an alteration in specific gravity of the cupulae as the result of infiltration of these structures with alcohol.

(f) Cerebral disequilibrium

Bauer and Leidler (1911), and later Dusser de Barenne and de Kleyn (1923), demonstrated that removal of one cerebral hemisphere of the rabbit produced a preponderance of induced vestibular nystagmus toward the side of the lesion. Carmichael et al. (1954, 1961) tested human subjects with unilateral cerebral lesions by the bithermal caloric test and found that lesions in the frontal and parietal lobes as well as in the anterior part of the temporal lobe were associated with normal caloric responses. On the other hand, lesions localized in the posterior part of the temporal lobe produced a marked directional preponderance of caloric nystagmus to the side of the lesion. It was pointed out that this response occurred only with the eyes fixed in forward gaze. Hakas and Kornhüber (1959) found that if the eyes were permitted to first assume a resting position, for example, with eyes closed, the directional preponderance is abolished.

There appears to be no specific clinical manifestation associated with this asymmetry in vestibulo-ocular control.

(g) Cervical vertigo

Numerous clinicians have reported that vertigo of a transient and episodic nature can be caused by disorders of the cervical region. De Kleyn and Nieuwenhuyse (1927) and Ryan and Cope (1955) have suggested that certain neck movements might result in interference with blood supply to the vestibular system. Others (Maspetiol et al., 1954; Decker et al., 1960) proposed that dysfunction of the cervical sympathetic nervous system is responsible for disequilibrium from neck movements. Hinoki and Terayama (1966) and Philipszoon and Bos (1963) have demonstrated head and eye nystagmus from neck torsion. Igarashi et al. (1969), working with the squirrel monkey, showed that injecting lidocaine into the deep neck muscles produced temporary disequilibrium, and that section of the upper cervical dorsal roots produced more severe and persistent disequilibrium. They interpreted their findings to indicate that deep neck proprioceptors are essential for the maintenance of dynamic equilibrium.

A study of these reports and others, however, fails to reveal conclusive evidence that cervical lesions are either a frequent or important cause of vertigo. It seems probable that vertigo associated with head movement is more frequently caused by lesions in the vestibular sense organs.

4. VESTIBULOMETRY

While nystagmus, particularly spontaneous nystagmus, is always pathological, it is of variable significance. The assessment of the vestibular contribution to such a finding can be made only by keeping the other possible factors in mind. Within these limitations, however, the assessment of nystagmus induced by vestibular stimulation becomes a powerful tool for assessing vestibular function.

The current commonly used tests of vestibular function consist of examination of the eyes for spontaneous nystagmus, calorically induced nystagmus, and positional nystagmus. Galvanic stimulation has been used sporadically for many years, but at the present time the results seem too unreliable to be clinically useful.

Rotational tests have been used widely in the past, but the main shortcoming is that they stimulate both ears simultaneously, making impossible the determination as to which side is defective. Two forms of tests have been used, the Bárány rotation of ten full turns in twenty seconds, in which the duration of the postrotatory nystagmus is measured, and, more recently, a short turning test in which provoked nystagmus merely indicates the presence of a lesion in the vestibular system.

Spontaneous vestibular nystagmus and induced caloric nystagmus are principally expressions of semicircular canal activity. There are currently no simple clinical tests for assessing the functional integrity of the utricular and saccular maculae. Whereas the role of the saccule is uncertain, the utricle seems clearly involved in postural control mechanisms. It is sensitive omnidirectionally to linear accelerations, although the sensitivity may well not be identical in all directions. The force of gravity, of course, is a form of linear acceleration. Stimulation of the utricle may produce ocular deviations although it is uncertain whether it can produce nystagmus. The ocular counterrolling test assesses some dimension of macular function but is currently too cumbersome and complex for routine clinical use (Miller and Graybiel, 1962; Miller, 1962).

Caloric tests. Caloric tests of the vestibular apparatus are performed with the head positioned so that the lateral semicircular canal is vertical. With the patient in the sitting position this is accomplished by tilting the head backward to an angle of 60° from the vertical plane (Fig. 3.37). With the patient in the supine position this is achieved by elevating the head 30° from the horizontal plane. By irrigating the external auditory canal with fluid at a temperature different from normal body temperature, a temperature gradient is established which produces cooling or heating of the portion of the lateral semicircular canal nearest the middle ear. The temperature gradient pro-

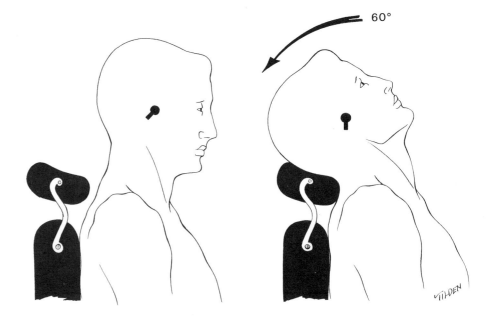

Fig. 3.37: When the caloric test is performed with the test subject in the sitting position, the head is tilted backward at an angle of about 60 degrees to bring the lateral semicircular canal into the vertical plane.

60°

duced in the semicircular canal is thought to produce a convection current in the canal, causing movement of the cupula. A stimulus at a temperature below body temperature (cold caloric test) produces a posteriorly moving current which normally induces a contralaterally beating nystagmus (Fig. 3.38). A hot caloric stimulus produces ipsilaterally beating nystagmus. Irrigating each ear alternately with hot and cold caloric stimulation thus provides a measure of the relative responsivity of each ear compared to the other, plus a comparison of right-beating nystagmus to left-beating nystagmus.

There is substantial disagreement as to whether duration, slow phase velocity, fast phase velocity, frequency, or total amplitude represents the most valid or useful measures of response. There is also considerable disagreement as to whether such measurements should be made with eyes closed or eyes opened. Correlational analyses have shown that reduced vestibular response as measured by duration with eyes open or by slow phase velocity with eyes closed are in reasonably good agreement. The other measures, particularly those relating to directional preponderance, do not show significant correlation, and their interpretation is therefore not as clear, except to indicate abnormality.

A variety of so-called minimal caloric tests have also been advocated using

Fig. 3.38: Cold water injected into the external auditory canal creates a downward convection current in the endolymph of the canal, with utriculo-fugal (away from the utricle) movement of the cupula. The eyes move in the plane of the canal and in the same direction as endolymph flow, and the direction of the quick component of the nystagmus is toward the opposite side.

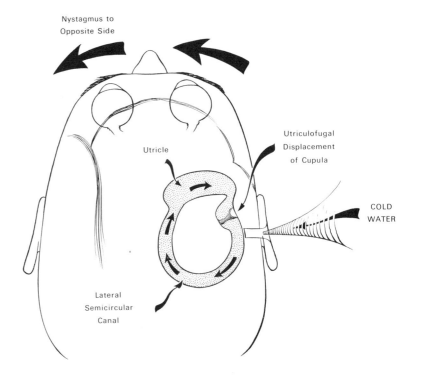

Nystagmus to Opposite Side

Utriculofugal Displacement of Cupula

Utricle

COLD WATER

Lateral Semicircular Canal

from 2 to 20 ml of water, ranging in temperature from ice water to cold tap water. The Kobrak minimal caloric test, slightly modified, is used by the author as a routine office procedure. Illuminated Frenzel glasses (20 diopters) are strapped to the head, and in a darkened room the eyes are observed for spontaneous nystagmus in the straight-ahead and right and left lateral gaze positions. With the patient in the sitting position, the head is tilted backward to an angle of 60°, and caloric irrigation is performed on the first ear by injecting 5 cc of water at 80°F directly against the tympanic membrane through a 20-gauge needle during a period of ten seconds. With the eyes in forward gaze the duration of nystagmus is timed in seconds, recording from the moment of completion of irrigation until the end of nystagmoid movement. After a rest period of one minute or longer an identical test is performed on the second ear. If an ear gives no response to water at 80°F, the test is repeated with 5 cc of ice water. Normal response times vary considerably with individual differences in vestibular sensitivity; however, the reactions of the two ears should be symmetrical. Most responses to 80°F water fall within a range of one to three minutes, the average being one minute forty seconds.

An asymmetry of response of thirty seconds or more, when recorded by a sophisticated observer, is an indication of abnormality and demonstrates either a diminished response on the less reactive side or directional preponderance toward the side of longest response. Directional preponderance can sometimes be detected during the pre-test examination for spontaneous nystagmus and consists of conjugate deviation of the eyes, when at rest without fixation, toward the side which on testing gives the lesser response. In the presence of spontaneous nystagmus 5 cc of hot water at 118°F may be used in the ear opposite to the direction of nystagmus. This test is somewhat painful, however, so that the bithermal test (Hallpike, 1956) is usually preferable when hot caloric testing is required. The ice water caloric test should not be used initially because nausea, vomiting, sweating, pallor, or syncope may occur in individuals who exhibit a highly reactive vestibular response.

In 1942 Fitzgerald and Hallpike described the bithermal procedure for performing the caloric test which has subsequently received wide usage. The test is performed with the patient lying comfortably on a couch with his head raised 30° above the horizontal. Each ear canal is irrigated in turn for forty seconds with warm water at a temperature of 44°C and cold water at 30°C. These temperatures have remained the most commonly used; however, some clinicians prefer to irrigate for thirty seconds so as to reduce the automatic side-effects of stimulation. It is possible also to use hot and cold air at these temperatures but the technique is technically more difficult.

Normal standards of bithermal caloric techniques depend on the particular measures and conditions used. For example, Hallpike, measuring the duration of nystagmus with eyes open, found that a difference between ears of forty seconds or more or a directional preponderance of forty seconds or more was significant. Durations with eyes closed required a difference of sixty seconds for reduced vestibular response and ninety seconds for directional preponderance to be significant. Slow phase velocity differences may be taken as either absolute or percentage differences, and the limits of normal differ for eyes open and eyes closed.

Directional preponderance means simply that bithermal testing yields a greater response in one direction than the other. Thus an individual exhibiting right directional preponderance will have a longer nystagmic response with cold water in the left ear and with hot water in the right ear. It seems to depend upon the extent to which the resting position or zero setting of the eyes coincides with the straight-ahead line of gaze in which the caloric tests are performed (Hallpike, 1967). Thus, if the zero setting of the eyes coincides with the straight-ahead position as in the normal, there will be no directional preponderance. This abnormal setting of the eyes to one side or the other of the straight-ahead position is presumably due to asymmetry of tonus in the extraocular muscles and may be due to either a peripheral or central vestibular lesion.

Hallpike (1967) has demonstrated that nystagmus which is enhanced by the elimination of fixation is most likely due to a lesion of the semicircular canals. On the other hand, nystagmus which is increased by fixation is most likely due to a lesion of the central nervous system. This latter type has been called fixation nystagmus by Holmes (1917) and gaze nystagmus by Kestenbaum (1946). Because it does not depend upon a visual mechanism, as implied by the words fixation and gaze but is probably due to the presence of conjugate deviation, Hallpike prefers to call it central or deviation-maintenance nystagmus. Carmichael et al. (1965) have shown that deviation-maintenance nystagmus is most likely caused by lesions involving the more caudal part of the vestibular nuclear complex. These lesions cause tonus asymmetry and conjugate deviation of the eyes, thus resulting in nystagmus on forward gaze in accordance with Alexander's law, which states that nystagmus is enhanced by voluntary deviation in the direction of the rapid component and decreased in the opposite direction.

A reduced vestibular response indicates abnormality in the vestibular labyrinth, nerve, or vestibular nuclei. Directional preponderance indicates a lesion somewhere in the system without specifying the locus more precisely. The occurrence of a perverted response to caloric irrigation, i.e., the occurrence of vertical or oblique nystagmus, is considered to be indicative of a brain stem lesion. If the nystagmic response is better with eyes opened than with eyes closed, a brain stem lesion is implied also. Unusually prolonged responses to caloric stimulation are thought to indicate a loss of central inhibition rather than a hyperactivity of the peripheral mechanism per se.

Electronystagmography. Electronystagmography, a technique by which eye movements are graphically recorded, is a useful tool in the evaluation of vestibular disorders. Ordinarily the method consists of placing electrodes at the external canthi of the eyes if the recording is monocular (Rubin, 1968). This provides a measure of horizontal eye movement. Vertical eye movement may be recorded similarly by placing electrodes at the eyebrow and below the lower lid margin. Because the eye normally has a steady potential between the cornea and retina or choroid, the eye acts like an electrical bipole, movements of which produce differential polarities at the recording electrodes. With this method, eye movements and positions may be recorded with eyes open in light or darkness or with eyes closed.

Another method currently used for recording eye movements, known as electric nystagmography, consists of directing a light beam onto the eye and recording the changes in intensity of reflected light which occur with eye movements (Torok et al., 1951). The method is limited to recording with eyes open. If an infrared light source is used, it is possible to record with eyes open in darkness without providing a fixation point for the eye. Both of these techniques have the advantage of permitting a permanent record of eye movement and a more precise measurement of nystagmic duration, amplitude, velocity, and frequency. It should be noted that purely rotatory nystagmus is not recordable by electronystagmographic techniques.

The advantage of electronystagmography over direct observation of eye movements is increased sensitivity. It is known, for example, that weak nystagmus may be consciously or unconsciously suppressed during fixation with the eyes open. In such cases electronystagmography has the advantage of recording nystagmus with the eyes closed. Clinical studies have shown electronystagmography to be capable of demonstrating nystagmus, which was not evident by direct observation, in such conditions as Ménière's disease and mild alcoholic intoxication and after administration of certain drugs. The technique also permits the recording of mild degrees of positional nystagmus which would otherwise escape direct observation. Electronystagmography may also be used with the caloric test and as such provides an important refinement in the evaluation of vestibular function. Most authorities (Stahle, 1966) believe that the intensity of the reaction is more important than the duration of the reaction to caloric stimulation. This is determined by measuring the speed of the slow phase of eye movement. Electronystagmography also permits a more accurate evaluation of caloric responses in patients who have spontaneous nystagmus (Aschan et al., 1956).

Positional nystagmus. Routine positional testing is usually performed by bringing the patient from the erect sitting position backward into the supine position with the head hanging over the edge of the table, returning to the upright position, turning the head to the right and bringing the patient into the supine position again, and finally to the upright position again. The sequence is then repeated with the head turned to the left. This may be done with eyes open in light or darkness and with eyes closed. It has been determined that both spontaneous and positional nystagmus are seen twice as often with illuminated Frenzel spectacles as with the naked eye examination and ten to twenty times as often with eyes closed (utilizing electronystagmography) as with the naked eye examination (Weiss, personal communication). Consequently, electronystagmography is an important adjunct for eliciting vestibular abnormalities.

The most commonly utilized classification for positional nystagmus is that proposed by Aschan et al. (1956), which is a modification of the one suggested by Nylén (1950). Type I positional nystagmus is persistent and direction changing; type II is persistent and direction fixed; and type III is transient and may be either direction-changing or direction-fixed. Persistent refers to the continuation of nystagmus for over one minute. Types I and II are of central origin twice as often as of peripheral origin (Nylén, 1931; Aschan et al., 1956; Hallpike, 1967) while the reverse holds for type III. Vertical nystagmus is almost always of central origin, up-beating usually implicating the brain stem and down-beating usually implicating a midline cerebellar lesion. One particular type of positional nystagmus appears to be caused by deposits on the cupula of the posterior semicircular canal and is described in Chapter 12B, Cupulolithiasis.

C. THE FLUID SYSTEM

The inner ear has two fluid systems which have distinctly different chemical compositions and functional significance (Fig. 3.39). The endolymphatic system contains fluid having a high potassium and low sodium concentration and bathes the gelatinous structures (tectorial, otolithic, and cupular membranes) which overlie the sense organs. The perilymphatic system has an electrolyte composition similar to that of cerebrospinal fluid, low potassium and high sodium concentration, and constitutes a medium which is satisfactory for neural excitation and synaptic activity.

The vestibular and auditory sense organs operate on hydrodynamic prin-

Fig. 3.39: Schematic drawing showing the general configuration and relationship of the endolymphatic and perilymphatic systems.

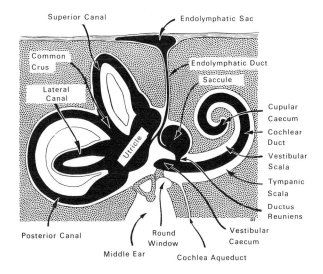

Superior Canal

Endolymphatic Sac

Common Crus

Endolymphatic Duct

Saccule

Lateral Canal

Cupular Caecum

Cochlear Duct

Vestibular Scala

Tympanic Scala

Ductus Reuniens

Posterior Canal

Round Window

Vestibular Caecum

Middle Ear

Cochlea Aqueduct

Fig. 3.40: Dark cells of the crista ampullaris of the opossum. A light photomicrograph is shown above and a corresponding electron micrograph below. Note the marginal position of the nuclei in the dark cells. The pigmented cells beneath the dark cells are melanocytes. The dark cells contain numerous vacuolar spaces in the apical cytoplasm and show numerous plasma membrane infoldings at their bases. (Courtesy of Kimura)

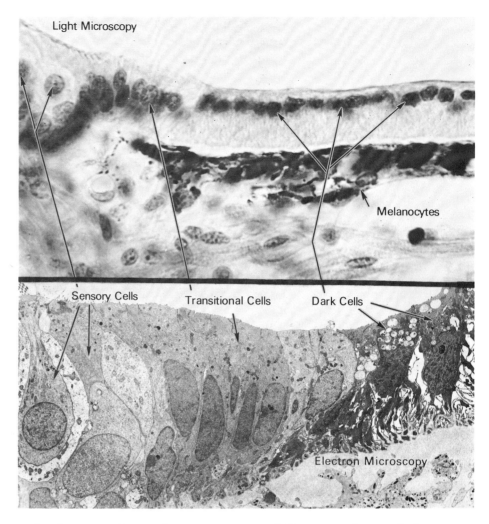

ciples; however, the mechanisms are quite different. In the vestibular system the sensory epithelium remains fixed and the stimulus for excitation consists of movement of the overlying gelatinous structure, whereas in the auditory system, the sensory epithelium moves with the overlying gelatinous structure. The cytoarchitecture of the organ of Corti is loosely structured to permit this movement without mechanical or frictional injury to the cells. Consequently, there are perilymphatic fluid spaces within the organ of Corti (tunnel of Corti, spaces of Nuel).

The areas of secretion and resorption of the fluids are not yet clearly defined, nor are the mechanisms by which the volumetric, chemical, and electrical values are maintained. On a morphological basis it seems probable that endolymph is secreted in the cochlea by cells of the stria vascularis and in the vestibular labyrinth by the dark cell areas (Kimura et al., 1963; Kimura, 1969) (Fig. 3.40). The areas of absorption of endolymph are less obvious but the endolymphatic sac almost certainly plays some role in this regard. It seems probable that the perilymph is derived, in part at least, from cerebrospinal fluid and reaches the inner ear via the cochlear aqueduct or modiolus and may be resorbed in the spiral ligament.

Another possible source for the perilymph is the blood vessels of the inner ear. It has been shown that when the cochlear aqueduct is blocked, the concentrations in the perilymph of sodium, potassium, and glucose remain unchanged. Total protein increases temporarily and then returns to normal levels (Silverstein et al., 1969). Some insight into the functional significance of endolymph and perilymph can be gained by observing the changes occurring in induced and spontaneous inner ear disorders (Schuknecht, 1970).

1. ALTERATIONS IN STAINING AND VOLUME OF ENDOLYMPH

Several specimens in the temporal bone collection at the Massachusetts

Eye and Ear Infirmary have shown selective staining of the endolymph of either the pars superior (utricle and canals) or pars inferior (cochlea and saccule), suggesting a physiologic independence of these two systems (Schuknecht and McNeill, 1966). Eosinophilic staining of the fluid of the pars inferior, including the endolymphatic duct and sac occurred in the ear of a patient with aplasia of the Mundini type (Fig. 3.41). On the other hand, the fluid of the pars superior was stained selectively with eosin in an ear with endolymphatic hydrops due to Ménière's disease (Fig. 3.42). In several animals in which the superior vestibular nerve was cut, the fluid of the pars superior stained with eosin, thus demonstrating the effectiveness of the utriculo-endolymphatic valve in preventing a flow of endolymph from the pars superior (Fig. 3.43). Fluctuation in the volume of endolymph of the pars superior, such as might occur if the utriculo-endolymphatic valve did not exist, might allow deformation of the ampullary walls and interference with the motion mechanics of the cupulae.

Ears with severe agenesis or degeneration of the striae vasculares uniformly show decrease in the volumes of endolymph in the cochleae and sacculi. Atrophy of the stria has been observed in both animal and human subjects and may either be developmental or acquired in origin (Schuknecht et al., 1965). Inherited agenesis or early degeneration of the cochlea and saccule has been shown to occur in many mammals, including man (Scheibe, 1891–1892), Dalmatian dogs (Hudson and Ruben, 1962), albino cats (Wilson and Kane, 1959), waltzing guinea pigs (Lurie, 1939), and mice (Lurie, 1942). The characteristic changes consist of atrophy of the organ of Corti and the stria vascularis, displacement of Reissner's membrane onto the remaining structure of the organ of Corti, and collapse of the saccular wall onto an atrophic saccular macula. The volume of endolymph is greatly reduced. The utricle and semicircular canals appear normal in these ears, suggesting that the pars superior and pars inferior function independently for the secretion and absorption of endolymph.

An increase in the volume of endolymph is known to occur in a variety of disorders, including bacterial inflammatory reactions, Ménière's disease, and congenital syphilis. The distention is most severe in the pars inferior, possibly because Reissner's membrane and the saccular wall are more yielding than the walls of the utricle and semicircular canals.

Bacterial infections of the perilymphatic system incite leukocytic infiltration, followed by endolymphatic hydrops and eventually severe destruction of the membranous labyrinth. A less severe inflammatory reaction, such as that produced by bacterial toxins without actual bacterial invasion, may cause varying degrees of endolymphatic hydrops, often without any permanent morphological changes in the sense organs and is known as toxic labyrinthitis (see Chapter 5 A 10, Labyrinthitis). In inflammatory hydrops the increased endolymph volume is maintained after the inflammatory reaction has subsided. The hydrops does not recede or progress. Presumably the mechanisms which control endolymph secretion and resorption are reestablished with the membranes remaining in their newly acquired positions. This condition, which may be termed nonprogressive endolymphatic hydrops, does not cause episodic vertigo.

Progressive endolymphatic hydrops, on the other hand, is a manifestation of Ménière's disease, congenital syphilis, and possibly other disorders. It is characterized by episodic vertigo and fluctuating hearing loss presumably as a consequence of ruptures of the walls of the membranous labyrinth, resulting in potassium intoxication of the perilymphatic spaces (see Chapter 12A, Ménière's Disease).

Endolymphatic hydrops is characteristically absent in Paget's disease and otosclerosis, as well as in viral labyrinthitis associated with mumps, measles, and upper respiratory tract infection. Presumably these disorders produce degenerative change without inciting an inflammatory response.

Fig. 3.41: This human ear with mild Mundini type developmental hypoplasia exhibits acidophilic staining of the endolymph of the pars inferior (cochlea, saccule), as well as the endolymphatic duct and sac. There is a large anomalous saccular duct.

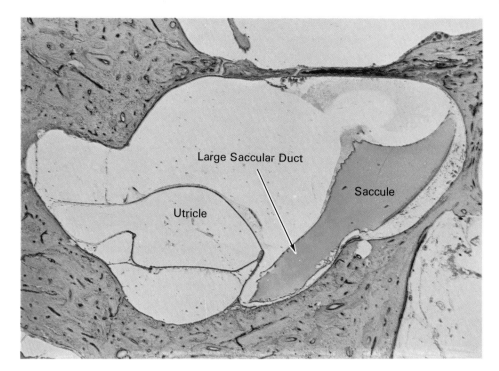

Fig. 3.42: The ear of this patient with Ménière's disease has a greatly distended saccule which fills the vestibule and displaces the utricle posteriorly. The utriculo-endolymphatic valve is compressed. The endolymph of the pars superior (utricle and semicircular canals) takes a deeply acidophilic stain.

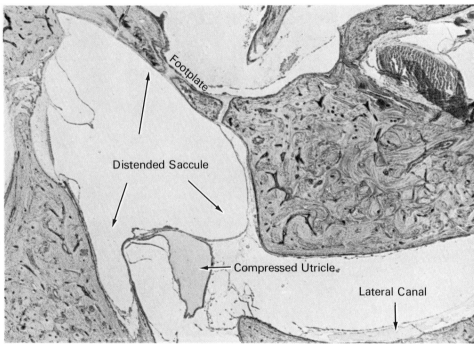

Fig. 3.43: Staining of the endolymph of the pars superior (utricle and semicircular canals) of a cat following section of the superior division of the vestibular nerve and the anterior vestibular artery. The utriculo-endolymphatic valve appears to have effectively maintained separation of the fluid of the pars superior from pars inferior.

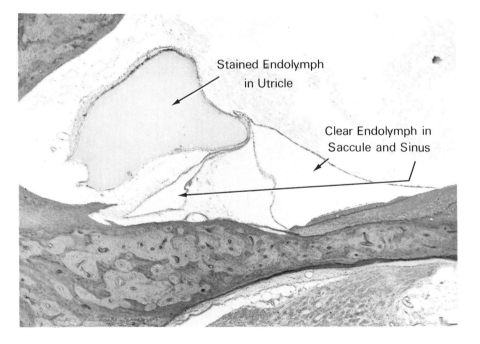

Guild (1927) suggested that the endolymphatic sac may play an important role in the normal metabolic activity of the inner ear. Subsequently evidence has provided support for this concept. Dye or pigment injected into the cochlea has been observed to accumulate in the endolymphatic sac (Guild, 1927; Yamakawa, 1929; Altmann and Waltner, 1950; Engström and Hjorth, 1951; Rudert, 1969), and silver particles concentrate in macrophages in the lumen of the endolymphatic sac 24 hours after injection into the cochlear duct (Lundquist et al., 1964a, 1964b; Lundquist, 1965). Electron microscopic studies have revealed the greatest pinocytotic activity to exist in the intermediate portion of the sac where the lining membrane has numerous infoldings similar to those of cells involved in fluid transport in the kidney, submaxillary gland, and ciliary body. High concentrations of total protein and lactic and malic dehydrogenase were found in the sac (Silverstein, 1966a, 1966b). The lining cells of the intermediate portion of the endolymphatic sac contain enzymes which catalyze important metabolic processes (Ishii et al., 1966). The injection of radioactive carbon-labeled foreign protein into the endolymph with visualization by autoradiography shows phagocytosis of these materials in free-floating cells as well as in the lining membrane of the sac (Ishii et al., 1966). These observations are in general agreement with the idea that endolymph flows from the inner ear to the endolymphatic sac where proteins are phagocytized and/or transported via the lining epithelial cells into the perivascular connective tissue.

Experimental studies in cats have shown that the morphology and fluid volume of the sac is not altered by blocking the vestibular end of the endolymphatic duct or by producing a chronic chemical irritation of the dural surface of the sac (Schuknecht and Seifi, 1963).

McNally (1926) destroyed the endolymphatic sac in rabbits and found no changes in the membranous labyrinth. In 1947 Lindsay demonstrated mild endolymphatic hydrops in two of four monkeys with postoperative survival times of one to three months in which the endolymphatic sac and duct had been destroyed; however, it could not be determined with certainty that this apparent slight increase in endolymph volume was more than that which might be caused by histological artifact. In 1952 Lindsay et al. repeated the experiments in cats with survival times of about three months, and although there were mild degrees of hydrops in several animals, the lack of satisfactory controls resulted again in inconclusive findings. Behavioral audiograms showed these same animals to have normal pure tone thresholds (Schuknecht and Kimura, 1953).

Naito in 1950 and Kimura and Schuknecht in 1965 demonstrated that endolymphatic hydrops could be produced consistently by obstructing the endolymphatic duct in guinea pigs. In further studies, Kimura (1967) found that the volume of the scala media increased an average of 38 percent during the first 24 hours after obstruction and was slowly progressive over a period of several months (Fig. 3.44). The saccule always showed dilatation and often was in contact with the footplate of the stapes. In most specimens the utricle was slightly dilated; however, the semicircular canals appeared normal. In some cases there was degeneration of the hair cells and cochlear neurons, particularly in the apical turns. These changes occurred as early as one month after obstruction and increased as a function of survival time. In several cochleae there was degeneration of neurons without reduction of hair cell populations in the corresponding areas. Some showed degeneration of the striae vasculares, but this was always limited to their apical regions. The vestibular hair cells and neurons appeared normal.

Schuknecht et al. (1968b) performed a similar experiment in which the endolymphatic sacs of the left ears of fifteen cats were destroyed surgically. After survival times of six months to three years, twelve were found to have endolymphatic hydrops (Fig. 3.45). Four control ears, which were subjected to sham operations, and eighteen opposite ears failed to show endolymphatic

Fig. 3.44: Endolymphatic hydrops associated with severe degeneration of the stria vascularis, organ of Corti, and cochlear neurons two months following surgical obstruction of the endolymphatic duct in the guinea pig. (Courtesy of Kimura)

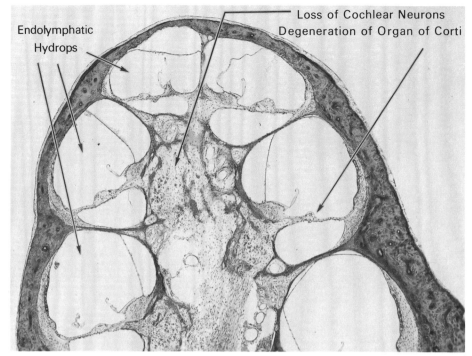

Fig. 3.45: Endolymphatic hydrops in the cat three years following surgical destruction of the endolymphatic sac. There is loss of cochlear neurons in the apical region. All other structures are normal. (Schuknecht et al., 1968b)

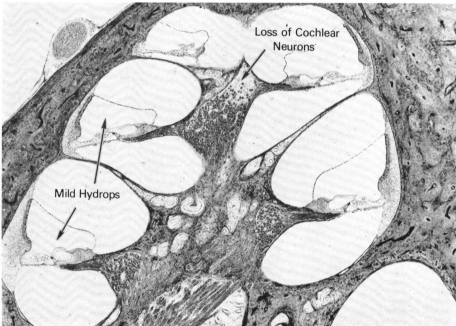

Fig. 3.46: Mild endolymphatic hydrops associated with loss of hair cells and cochlear neurons in the apical region of the cochlea three years following destruction of the endolymphatic sac in the cat.

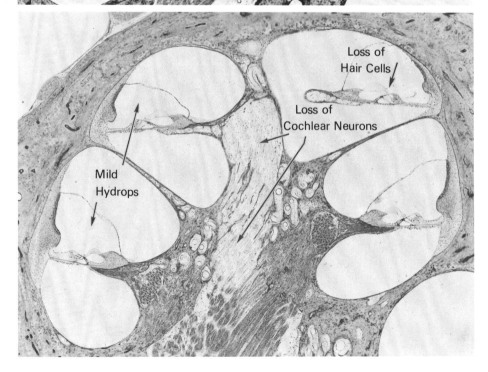

hydrops. Three of four animals with postoperative survival times of 2¼ to 3 years also had atrophic changes in the organs of Corti and cochlear neurons, most severe in the apical regions (Fig. 3.46). Beal (1968) observed diminished cochlear microphonic responses following destruction of the endolymphatic sacs of cats and rabbits. The rabbits also demonstrated a loss of vestibular function. Histological studies showed mild cochlear hydrops in the cats and severe cochlear and vestibular hydrops in the rabbits.

The accumulated evidence indicates that the endolymphatic sac functions as a metabolically active filter for the endolymphatic system and that a loss of this function results in a progressive increase in the volume of endolymph. The first changes consist of distention of the most yielding membranes (Reissner's membrane and the saccular wall), and this is followed by more diffuse distortion of the membranous labyrinth. More prolonged loss of function of the endolymphatic sac sometimes causes degeneration of the organ of Corti and cochlear neurons which tends to be more severe in the apical region. It seems probable that loss of function of the endolymphatic sac is the cause for Ménière's disease (see Chapter 12A, Ménière's Disease).

3. FUNCTION OF THE COCHLEAR AQUEDUCT

The cochlear aqueduct is a bony channel connecting the scala tympani of the basal turn with the subarachnoid space of the posterior cranial cavity. In man the lumen is usually very small but in exceptional ears it may be widely patent (Figs. 3.47, 3.48). In animals such as the dog, cat, guinea pig, and rabbit

Fig. 3.47: This photomicrograph shows a human cochlear aqueduct with an exceptionally large lumen.

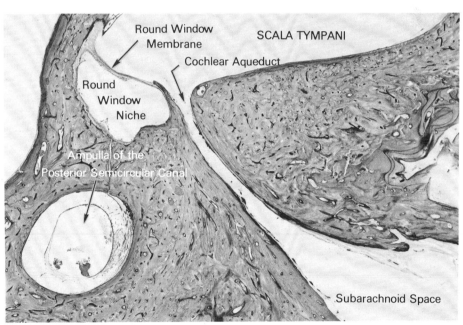

Fig. 3.48: Photomicrograph shows a large patent cochlear aqueduct in the ear of a newborn infant.

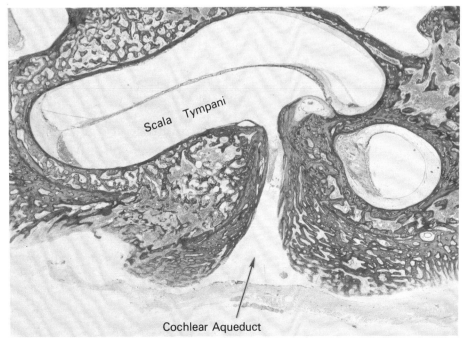

it is an open channel establishing a free communication between the peri-lymphatic and subarachnoid spaces. Within the aqueduct there is a loose net-work of fibrous tissue continuous with the arachnoid.

Experiments designed to produce information on flow through the aque-duct have given variable results. Waltner (1948) and Altmann and Waltner (1950) injected avian erythrocytes into the subarachnoid space of rabbits and found them trapped in the meshwork of the cochlear aqueducts but not in the inner ears.

Schuknecht and Seifi (1963) performed a similar experiment on cats and found after survival times of 15 minutes to 72 hours that not only were avian erythrocytes caught in the meshwork of the cochlear aqueducts but great numbers of them passed through the aqueducts into the inner ears (Fig. 3.49). Under the conditions of the experiment it was quite clear that the cochlear aqueduct of the cat will pass small particulate matter and, furthermore, that a current of cerebrospinal fluid normally flows from the subarachnoid space into the inner ear.

Fig. 3.49: Avian erythrocytes are seen in the scala tympani of the basal turn of the coch-lea (cat). Washed avian erythrocytes were in-jected into the subarachnoid space of the posterior cranial fossa, and the animal was sacrificed by arterial perfusion twelve hours later.

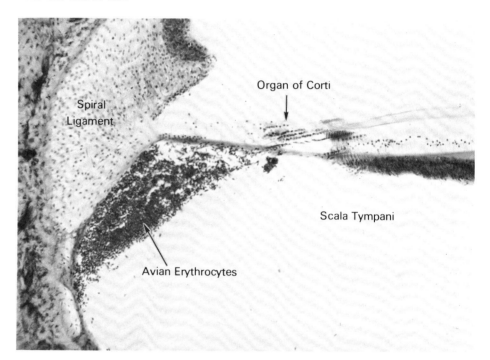

Uyama (1933) obstructed the cochlear aqueducts of rabbits with sarcoma transplants and with dry catgut and observed mild endolymphatic hydrops. Schuknecht and Kimura (1953) blocked the cochlear aqueducts of cats util-izing bone wax and bone dust and found that the animals maintained normal auditory thresholds and had normal appearing inner ears after survival times as long as one year.

Perlman and Lindsay (1939) studied the inner ears of individuals who died of acute meningitis or subarachnoid hemorrhage and found that leukocytes and red blood cells could pass through the cochlear aqueduct to reach the scalae tympanii in some ears. Further evidence concerning the patency of the human cochlear aqueduct comes from temporal bone studies of patients hav-ing had spontaneous subarachnoid hemorrhage (Holden and Schuknect, 1968). Only ears with large caliber aqueducts showed blood cells in the coch-leae. Ears with small aqueducts, on the other hand, had blood cells extending into the internal auditory canals, modioli, and osseous spiral laminae sug-gesting that an interchange between cerebrospinal fluid and perilymph may occur by this route in these ears.

Palva (1970), in a study of the cochlear aqueducts of six infants, found the the average length to be 3.5 mm (average adult 6.2 mm) and the diameters to be at least 150 micra at their narrowest points, 0.5 to 1 mm from the scala tympani. He noted that erythocytes passed readily through the aqueducts of these infants.

These observations on human and animal ears indicate that cerebrospinal

Fig. 3.50: Photomicrograph of three cat cochleae showing openings (arrows) of the perilymph canaliculae in the tympanic laminae of the osseous spiral laminae. Stain was deposited in these channels in the course of an experiment on localization of acetylcholinesterase.

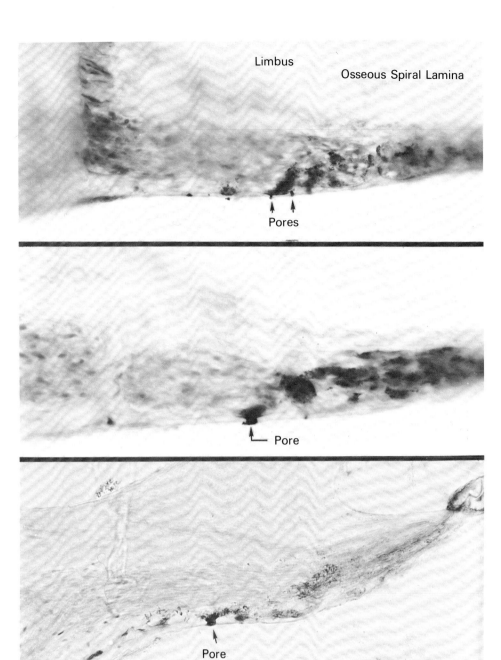

fluid and perilymph normally communicate via the cochlear aqueduct. Blocking the cochlear aqueduct, on the other hand, appears to have no adverse effect on inner ear morphology or function (Kimura et al., 1974).

4. THE PERILYMPH CANALICULAE

The cochlea of the cat has been shown to possess a system of channels which connect the scala tympani with the fluid spaces surrounding the organ of Corti. The discovery was made during an experiment designed to study the localization of acetylcholinesterase in the inner ears of cats (Schuknecht, 1959, 1960b, 1970; Schuknecht and Seifi, 1963) utilizing the histochemical method of Koelle (Koelle and Friedenwald, 1949; Koelle, 1950, 1951). The method results in deposition of copper sulphide in areas containing acetylcholinesterase. Perilymphatic canaliculae in the osseous spiral laminae were demonstrated in all 27 cochleae treated in this manner. The experiment by Sando et al. (1971) in which a carbon particle suspension was injected into the subarachnoid space of guinea pigs supported the concept of a fluid communication between the scala tympani and organ of Corti via the osseous spiral lamina.

The channels begin as a series of very small openings, canaliculi perforantes (Lim, 1970, 1973), in the tympanic shelf of the osseous spiral lamina (Fig. 3.50). They vary from 1.72 microns to 5.16 microns (average 3.24 microns) and are located approximately 0.2 mm from the habenula perforata in

Fig. 3.51A: Scanning electron micrograph showing openings on the surface of the osseous spiral lamina which faces the scala tympani (chinchilla). (Courtesy of Lim)

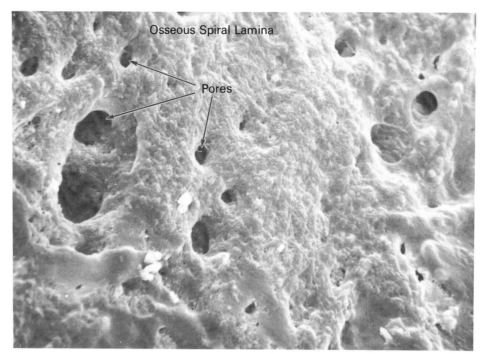

Osseous Spiral Lamina

Pores

Fig. 3.51B: Scanning electron micrograph of osseous spiral lamina of the guinea pig showing perilymphatic pores (P) and canaliculi perforates (arrows). (Courtesy of Takahara)

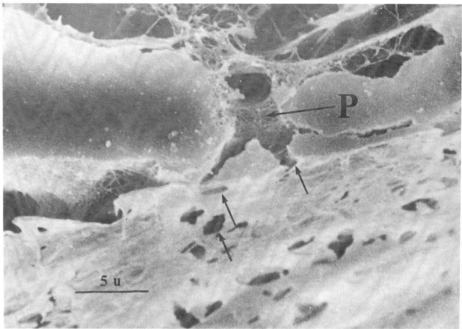

P

5 u

a spiral distribution throughout all three turns of the cochlea. These openings in the osseous spiral lamina have been observed by scanning electron microscope in the chinchilla by Lim (1973) (Fig. 3.51A) and in the guinea pig by Tanaka et al. (1973) (Fig. 3.51B). The canaliculae lead to fluid channels which immediately widen and coalesce to form pools around the nerve fibers. The channels then pass within the osseous spiral lamina with the nerve fibers to reach the habenulae perforatae and the organ of Corti (Fig. 3.52). This system of channels appears to be the main route by which perilymph reaches the organ of Corti to provide electrolyte concentrations suitable for neural excitation and transmission.

Masuda et al. (1971) injected inulin-methoxy-H[3] into the scala tympani of the guinea pig and found large amounts of the substance in the habanulae perforatae and tunnel of Corti and concluded that the habenulae perforatae are one of the main communication routes to the organ of Corti. They also found the substance in the intercellular spaces of Claudius' cells, Hensen's cells, the reticular lamina and inner sulcus cells and absence of the substance on the surface of these cells. They concluded from these observations that the epithelial cells, with the zonula occludens of their intercellular spaces, effectively separate the endolymphatic space from the scala tympani. The close

Fig. 3.52: Photomicrographs of cat cochleae in which stain (copper sulfide) precipitated along the course of the perilymph canaliculae and channels. These channels extend from openings in the tympanic plate of the osseous spiral lamina through the habenulae perforatae to the organ of Corti, thus bathing the neural and sensory cells with perilymph, which has electrolyte concentrations suitable for neural excitation and transmission.

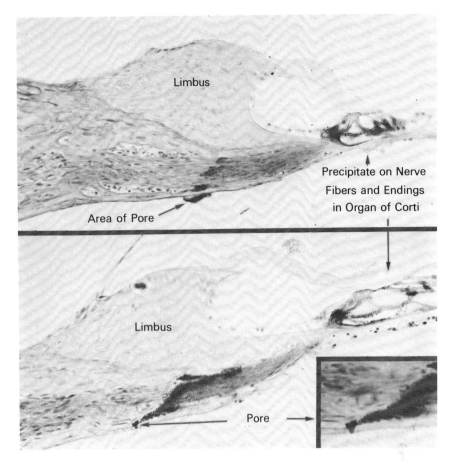

relationship of the scala tympani to the spaces of the organ of Corti was demonstrated by Tasaki and Fernández (1952), who found that cochlear microphonic responses and action potentials were abolished when artificial endolymph was perfused into the scala tympani but not when perfused into the scala vestibuli.

Further evidence that the tunnel of Corti and spaces of Nuel contain perilymph is found in two human ears (Schuknecht, 1970), one with stained endolymph and the other with stained precipitate in the perilymph (Figs. 3.53, 3.54). The findings show the tunnel of Corti to be free of endolymph in one ear and to contain perilymph in the other. Furthermore, both ears indicate the presence of endolymph in the inner sulcus and within the tectorial membrane.

5. ENDOLYMPH-PERILYMPH FISTULAE

A histological study of the cochleae of behaviorally conditioned cats with surgically induced ruptures of the cochlear ducts has revealed four ears with permanent endolymph-perilymph fistulae (Schuknecht and Seifi, 1963). In all cochleae there was destruction of the sensory and neural structures at the site of the fistulae, and generally the loss of auditory thresholds reflected the severity and spatial distribution of these lesions. There were no unexplained hearing losses which could be attributed to the endolymph fistulae (Figs. 3.55, 3.56). These findings were in agreement with those of Lawrence (1966b) and suggest that the biochemical and bioelectric properties of the cochlear duct can be maintained a few millimeters distant from a fistula.

6. CHEMISTRY OF THE INNER EAR FLUIDS

Biochemistry and molecular biology have developed into sciences of increasing importance in the understanding of disease processes. Studies on the chemistry of labyrinthine fluids are providing a better understanding of the physiological mechanisms involved in hearing and hopefully will provide knowledge leading to therapy of certain types of deafness (Paparella, 1970).

Fig. 3.53: Same ear as in Fig. 3.41, showing acidophilic stain of the endolymph of the cochlea. The fluid of the inner sulcus and within the tectorial membrane is stained. The tunnel of Corti and Nuel's spaces are not stained and presumably contain perilymph. There is an artifactual separation of the external sulcus cells from the spiral ligament.

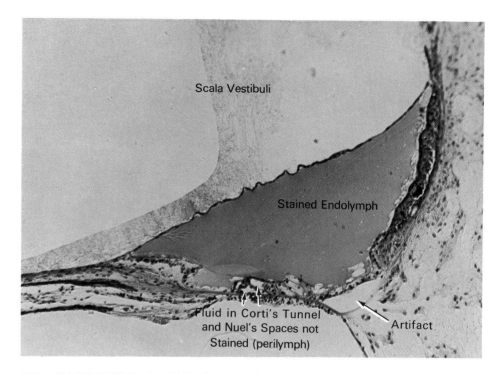

Fig. 3.54: Stained precipitate in the perilymphatic spaces of the inner ear of a newborn infant. Note that precipitate exists in the tunnel of Corti and Nuel's spaces. (Courtesy of Rutledge)

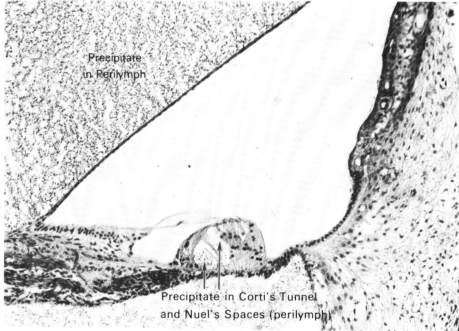

Fig. 3.55: Surgically created fistula of the cochlear duct of a cat. A needle was passed through the round window membrane into the osseous spiral lamina perforating the limbus and tearing Reissner's membrane to create a permanent fistula in the 5 mm region. Survival time after surgery was three months. See Fig. 3.56.

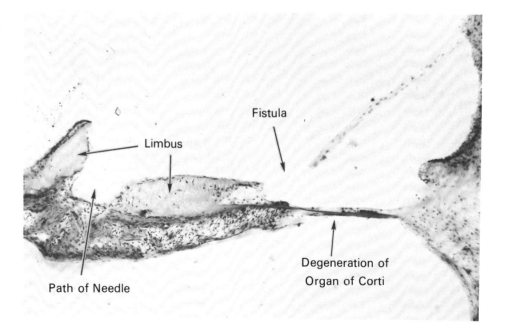

(a) Methods of analysis

Sodium and Postassium: Sodium and potassium can be determined simultaneously, using a microflame photometer as described by Müller (1958), modified by Giebisch et al. (1964), and recently automated. This method requires a volume of sample in the magnitude of one-half microliter diluted to 200 microliters with lithium standard. The glass pipets in which the inner ear fluid samples are collected, sorted, and measured are known to release sodium and potassium ions when in contact with a solution. By measuring sodium and potassium ion standards, an appropriate correction factor is obtained and applied to the unknown sample determinants.

Protein: Total protein may be determined by the folin phenol reaction (Lowry et al., 1951). The fluid samples are first treated with a solution of 0.5 percent copper sulfate and 1 percent sodium tartrate (100 microliters). After ten minutes, the folin phenol reagent diluted 1:1 (10 microliters) is added, followed immediately by vigorous vortex mixing. Standard solutions are prepared with bovine serum albumin (1 mg per ml) and treated in the same fashion. After 30 minutes, the optical density at 750 microns is measured in the Zeiss spectrophotometer.

Immunoelectrophoretic and immunodiffusion techniques may be used to further identify serum proteins. These methods have been used by Chevance et al. (1960) and Palva and Raunio (1967) on postmortem specimens and by Silverstein (1971) on patients with otological diseases.

Malic Dehydrogenase (MDH): Malic dehydrogenase is an aerobic enzyme that catalyzes the reversible dehydrogenation of malate to oxaloacetate, the latter being an important decomposition product of the energy producing citric acid cycle. The standard method of Boehringer may be adapted to a microanalytical technique. To a quartz cuvette (1 cm light path) is added: 100 microliters at a 4.2×10^{-2} molar laspartate in 0.1 molar phosphate buffer (pH 7.4), 2 microliters of a 6.2 molar keto glutarate sodium, and 2 microliters of glutamic oxaloacetic transaminase. After five minutes, a measured quantity of the sample to be analyzed (e.g. 0.3 to 1 microliter) is added to the cuvette. The change in optical density is measured over a five-minute period in a spectrophotometer at 340μ. The activity of MDH is calculated in international milliunits per milliliter.

Lactic Dehydrogenase (LDH): Lactic dehydrogenase is an enzyme which, using reduced diphosphopyridine nucleotide as the hydrogen carrier, catalyzes the reduction of pyruvate to lactate. A microanalytical technique may

Fig. 3.56: Same ear as in Fig. 3.55. Behavioral audiogram and chart of cochlear pathology for an ear with a fistula in the 5 mm area of the cochlear duct. It appears that the fistula has not significantly impaired pure tone thresholds for frequencies having their principal locus of activity elsewhere in the cochlear duct.

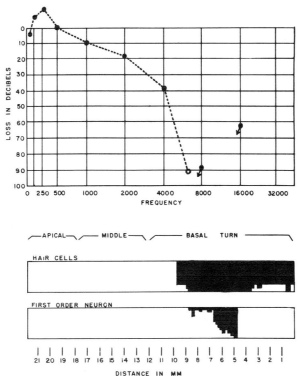

be adapted from the standard clinical method of Boehringer. To a quartz cuvette (1 cm light path) is added: 100 microliters of a 3.1 x 10^{-4} molar pyruvate in 0.05 molar phosphate buffer (pH. 7.5), 2 microliters of a 2 x 10^{-3} molar reduced diphosphopyridine nucleotide solution, and 1 microliter of the sample to be analyzed. The change in optical density is measured at 340 μ in a spectrophotometer. The activity of LDH is also calculated in international milliunits per milliliter.

Glucose: True glucose is determined by adapting the enzymatic test kit of Boehringer to a microanalytical technique. This method is based on the work of Huggett and Nixon (1957). Glucose oxidase is used to catalyze the oxidation of B-D glucose to gluconolactone which, with water, forms gluconic acid and hydrogen peroxide. The latter substance with peroxidase oxidizes o-dianisidine which is converted into a reddish brown dye. The amount of dye is determined colormetrically at 436 μ. The volume of glucose reagent used is 100 microliters to which the unknown sample of glucose standard is added. The concentration of glucose is calculated by comparison with the values obtained from the glucose standard.

(b) Method of fluid collection

Fluid may be collected from the vestibule with a micropipette introduced through a fistula in the footplate (Figs. 3.57, 3.58). About 2 to 5 microliters of fluid can be acquired by capillary attraction, sometimes aided by gentle aspiration. The removal of fluid from the scala tympani of the basal turn of the cochlea may be accomplished by introducing the pipette through the round window membrane. Access to the human round window requires the prior removal of the bony margin of the niche. Fluid may be acquired from a semicircular canal after bony fistulization of the canal.

Fig. 3.57: This drawing shows the surgical technique for acquiring fluid from the vestibule of the human ear. The middle ear is exposed by elevating the posterior part of the tympanic membrane and an adjacent collar of canal wall skin. The mucous membrane is removed from the footplate. All bleeding is controlled, and the area is thoroughly dried with an aspiration tube. A small opening is made in the center of the footplate and fluid is aspirated with a micropipet. The pipet is introduced no more than ½ mm into the vestibule.

Fig. 3.58: This stapes was removed during the course of a labyrinthectomy operation for Ménière's disease. It shows the fistula that was made in the footplate for removal of fluid as a diagnostic test at the time of surgery.

Fig. 3.58

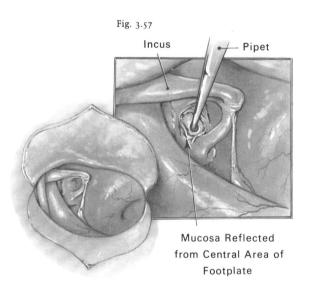

Fig. 3.57

Incus — Pipet

Mucosa Reflected from Central Area of Footplate

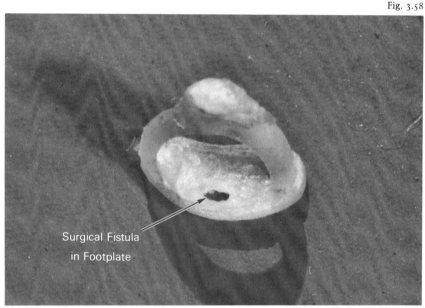

Surgical Fistula in Footplate

(c) Concentrations in cat and man

Normal. The concentrations for several substances in the normal living cat are shown in Fig. 3.59 (Silverstein, 1966b). The values for K$^+$ and Na$^+$ are given in mEq/L, protein and glucose in mg% and LDH and MDH in international units. Chemical values have been determined for the human ear for fluid removed from the vestibule, the scala tympani of the basal turn and from the lateral semicircular canal in both the living and dead conditions (Silverstein and Schuknecht, 1966; Schuknecht et al., 1968a).

Otosclerosis. The values for sodium, potassium, and protein in fluid removed from the vestibule of ears with otosclerosis are similar to that for normal perilymph of the cat. Wullstein et al. (1960) and Schindler et al. (1965), however, found the protein concentrations of ears with otosclerosis to be slightly elevated.

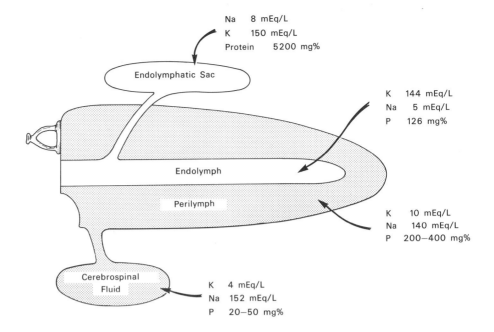

Fig. 3.59: Mean values for K+, Na+, and total protein for endolymph of the cochlear duct and endolymphatic sac, for perilymph and for cerebrospinal fluid (cat). The values for K+ and Na+ are expressed in mEq/L, and protein in mg/100 ml.

The mean values for these substances in otosclerotic ears are as follows:

Sodium: 142 mEq/L
Potassium: 7 mEq/L
Protein: 223 mg%

Ménière's disease. Fluid removed from the vestibule of patients undergoing labyrinthectomy for Ménière's disease reveals concentrations of sodium, potassium, and protein which are slightly greater than those of normal endolymph for the cat. The mean values are shown below:

Sodium: 29 mEq/L
Potassium: 165 mEq/L
Protein: 215 mg%

The explanation for the presence of endolymph in the vestibule in Ménière's disease is provided by histological studies and by observations made during surgical procedures which consistently show either a dilated saccule or herniated cochlear duct in contact with the footplate of the stapes (see Chapter 12A, Ménière's Disease). The analysis of fluid taken from the scala tympani through the round window membrane in patients with Ménière's disease reveals values which are normal for perilymph.

Vestibular schwannoma. The removal of perilymph from the lateral semicircular canal or vestibule of ears with vestibular schwannoma has revealed greatly increased protein but normal perilymph values for potassium and sodium. This may occur in association with normal protein concentrations in the cerebrospinal fluid. The increased concentration of protein probably accounts for the granular acidophilic-staining precipitate which is frequently observed by light microscopy in the perilymphatic spaces of such ears. The mean values for fluid from the vestibules of ears with vestibular schwannomas are as follows:

Sodium: 149 mEq/L
Potassium: 13 mEq/L
Protein: 1800 mg%

Utilizing immunoelectrophoretic and immunodiffusion techniques, Silverstein (1971) identified 14 protein fractions in the perilymph of ears with vestibular schwannoma and pointed out the similarity to the pattern of proteins existing in blood serum.

After death the perilymph sodium concentration decreases slowly, appearing to stabilize approximately 300 minutes postmortem while the potassium concentration rises slowly from approximately 10 mEq/L to 40 mEq/L. The

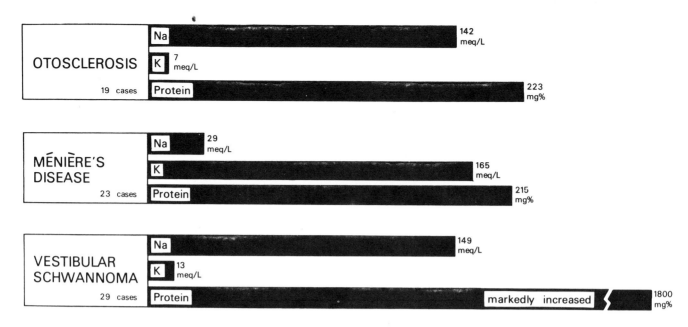

Fig. 3.60: This graph shows mean concentrations of sodium, potassium, and protein as found in inner ear fluid samples from the vestibules of patients with typical clinical manifestations of otosclerosis, Ménière's disease, and vestibular schwannoma. (Courtesy of Silverstein)

endolymph sodium concentration elevates rapidly while the potassium concentration decreases rapidly so that the values equalize at approximately 150 minutes postmortem. Meaningful evaluations of electrolyte concentrations must therefore be made during life or very soon after death. There appears to be a gradual decrease in the perilymph glucose as a function of time after death; however, there is a wide variation which may depend in part upon the nutritional and disease state of the individual. The protein concentration does not appear to change significantly with postmortem time lapse (Silverstein and Griffin, 1970a). Suga et al. (1970), using cation-sensitive glass electrodes, observed that intense acoustic stimulation increased the sodium and decreased the potassium concentrations of endolymph.

The chemical analysis of inner ear fluid may be used as a diagnostic aid for the differentiation of Ménière's disease from vestibular schwannoma and to provide confirmative evidence of Ménière's disease (Silverstein and Griffin, 1970b) (Fig. 3.60).

D. THE VASCULAR SYSTEM

A rich cholinergic nerve supply accompanies the basilar and anterior inferior cerebellar arteries but does not extend to the labyrinthine arteries (Fig. 3.61).

It has been demonstrated by Terayama et al. (1965, 1966, 1968) and by Spoendlin and Lichtensteiger (1967) that the arteries, arterioles, and some of the veins of the internal auditory canal and modiolus are supplied by sympathetic fibers arising in the cranial cervical ganglia, reaching the ear via the internal carotid nerves. They also showed a rich sympathetic nerve supply to the small blood vessels in the cochlear nerve trunk, Rosenthal's canal, and osseous spiral lamina. No sympathetic vascular innervation could be found in the vessels in the stria vascularis, spiral ligament, limbus, or to the vascular arcades on the scala tympani surface of the basilar membrane and osseous spiral lamina. These studies utilized fluorescent histochemical techniques which stain primary catacholamines (Falck et al., 1962).

Perlman and Kimura (1955) found that neither cutting the cervical trunk at the stellate ganglion nor electrical stimulation of the stellate ganglion, cervical trunks, superior cervical ganglion, vertebral artery, basilar artery, or inferior cerebellar artery produced any visible changes in the caliber of the blood vessels or in blood flow in the stria vascularis. In contrast, stimulation of the stellate ganglion and cervical sympathetic trunk produced prompt slowing and eventual arrest of blood flow through the vessels in the mucosa of the middle ear. While sympathetic stimulation causes no change in the

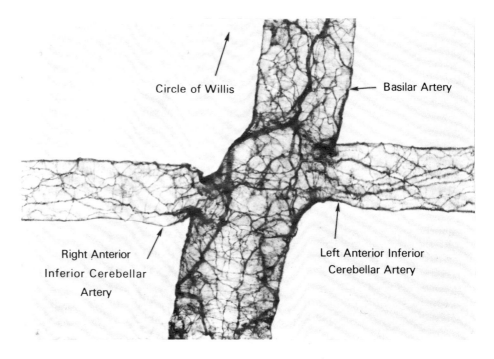

caliber of the vessels of the stria vascularis, it does cause an increase in the velocity of blood flow (Nomura, 1961).

Nomura (1962) and Perlman et al. (1963) demonstrated that the intravenous injection of pressor agents (adrenaline, noradrenaline) failed to alter the caliber of the strial vessels but did cause an increase in blood flow which generally paralleled the increase in carotid blood pressure. Hypothermia caused no change in the caliber of blood vessels of the stria vascularis, although flow rate decreased (Perlman et al., 1959a). Perlman and Kimura (1962) demonstrated that strong acoustic stimulation (120 db) failed to cause a change in caliber of strial vessels although microphonic response was greatly reduced. An increase in blood flow rate was measured after intense stimulation (135 to 153 db) when microphonic response was further impaired or permanently abolished.

More recently, Perlman and Yamada (1967) have demonstrated an autoregulation mechanism of strial blood flow. By producing graded abrupt decreases in carotid pressure, they noted immediate corresponding reduction of blood flow in the capillaries of the stria vascularis which persisted for about 30 seconds but returned to normal within 60 to 120 seconds while carotid pressure remained low. When the pressure was permitted to return to normal, after a period of lowered carotid pressure, there was a supernormal strial flow for 60 to 80 seconds followed by a return to normal. Hypocapnia produced by hyperventilation reduced strial flow rates without significant change in blood pressure. Hypercarbia and hypoxia increased strial flow rate.

These findings suggest that intravascular pressure, as well as arterial oxygen and carbon dioxide tension, affects the smooth muscles of cochlear resistance vessels and indicate that cochlear blood flow is adjusted to psysiological stresses so that function can be sustained.

Perlman et al. (1959b) performed experiments in which the blood supply to the inner ear was temporarily interrupted by pressure on the labyrinthine artery. They found the bioelectric potentials of the inner ear to be greatly reduced within 60 seconds after complete interruption of blood supply and showed that these functions may return to normal even after eight minutes of complete obstruction. Interruption of blood flow for more than 30 minutes resulted in permanent loss of electrical responses, although blood flow in the stria vascularis returned to normal even after one hour of arterial obstruction. They noted that the magnitude of histological changes was directly related to the duration of arterial blockage. Obstruction for five minutes or more produced scattered degenerative changes which were more severe in the cochlea than in the vestibular labyrinth. Within the cochlea, the hair cells, cells of the limbus, and cochlear neurons were principally involved. The external hair cells were more susceptible to injury than the internal hair cells and supporting cells. The stria vascularis and spiral ligament showed only minimal changes to even prolonged arterial obstruction. Arterial obstruction for an hour was required to produce morphological changes in the vestibular sense organs, and these consisted primarily of loss of hair cells.

Perlman and Kimura (1957) also studied the effects of interruption of the inferior cochlear vein and its tributaries. Within 24 hours after venous obstruction there was loss of external hair cells; however, the internal hair cells were more resistant, and only scattered areas of degeneration were found after 48 hours of blockage. The stria vascularis was particularly susceptible, showing first dilatation of capillaries and edema of the epithelium and, after a few hours, hemorrhage into the strial tissue, followed by degeneration. Bleeding occurred into the scala tympani from the collecting venules. Changes in the saccule and utricle paralleled those in the organ of Corti, and again the hair cells were most vulnerable. Hemorrhage was rarely seen within the utricle or saccule but extensive hemorrhages often occurred in the perilymphatic mesh-work around the utricle.

Permanent interruption of arterial supply by coagulating the labyrinthine artery produced more rapid and more profound changes in the labyrinth than venous obstruction. Within thirty minutes the external hair cells began to degenerate, followed in a few hours by the internal hair cells and supporting cells. Eventually there was severe degeneration of the entire organ of Corti and vestibular sense organs. The vessels of the stria vascularis remained filled with blood; however, the strial tissue proceeded to degenerate rapidly, becoming detached in four hours. At the end of 17 hours the entire organ of Corti and stria were reduced to cellular fragments in the cochlear duct. The spiral ligament and limbus degenerated less rapidly but progressed to complete degeneration. The cochlear neurons showed reduction of Nissl substance and pyknosis within a few hours, and degeneration progressed to disappearance of cochlear neurons in eight to fourteen days. Alterations of the vestibular labyrinth paralleled those of the cochlea. By the end of one week fibrosis had begun in the perilymphatic spaces, particularly in the scala tympani near the round window, finally leading to ossification within the labyrinthine spaces.

The absence of hemorrhage after arterial obstruction is in striking contrast to the severe hemorrhages that followed venous obstruction; however, subsequent fibrosis and ossification were more severe and extensive after arterial obstruction. In none of the ears subjected to venous or arterial obstruction was there evidence of endolymphatic hydrops.

Alford et al. (1965) and Igarashi et al. (1969) created peripheral vascular lesions in the inner ear by injecting sterile styrene divinylbenzene copolymer beads into the vertebral arteries of dogs. They demonstrated patchy areas of degeneration in the spiral ligament, stria vascularis, organ of Corti, limbus, vestibular sense organs, etc. The lesions generally correlated well with the location of the beads. The pathology of the organ of Corti was not closely related to the severity of the changes in the stria vascularis. Because degeneration of the cochlear neurons paralleled that of the organ of Corti both in spatial distribution and severity, it is probable that these changes were secondary to organ of Corti injury (see Chapter 9A2, secondary degeneration of the cochlear neurons). In the vestibular system the most commonly involved structures were the macula sacculi and crista of the posterior semicircular canal. Engström and Wersäll (1953), Lawrence (1965), Kikuchi and Hilding (1967) have suggested that the nutritional supply of the organ of Corti comes from the arcade of spiral vessels beneath the basilar membrane; however, Alford et al. (1965) and Igarashi et al. (1969) could not establish an anatomical relationship between organ of Corti lesions and the location of copolymer beads in these vessels.

Kimura (unpublished data) ligated the anterior inferior cerebellar artery in four cats, obtaining a total destruction of the inner ear in three, and a loss of cochlear hair cells and neurons, most severe in the apical region, in one. He was unable to produce pathological changes in the inner ear by ligating the basilar artery. Neff and Kiang (unpublished data) produced total loss of cochlear neurons in the middle and apical turns in two cats following cautery of the anterior inferior cerebellar artery. One of these animals exhibited a hearing loss more severe for the low tones. Bernstein and Silverstein (1966) ligated the anterior inferior cerebellar artery and its branches in twenty-one cats and found three with sensory lesions restricted to the apical regions of the cochleae.

The tendency for vascular deficiency to cause lesions in the apical region of the cochlea is well documented, but the pathophysiological mechanism is not clear (see Chapter 12D, Apical Lesions of the Cochlea).

References

Abels, H., 1906: Über Nachempfindungen im Gebiete des kinästhetischen und statichen Sinnes. Ein Beitrag zur Lèhre vom Bewegungsschwindel (Drehschwindel). Z. Psychol. u. Physiol. d. Sinnesborg. 42:268.

Alford, B., Shaver, E., Rosenberg, J., and Guilford, F., 1965: Physiologic and histopathologic effects of microembolism of of the auditory artery. Ann. Otol. Rhinol. Laryng. 74:728.

Allen, G., 1967: Abnormal patency of the eustachian tube; a complication of oral contraception. J. Amer. Med. Asssn. 200:412.

Allen, G., and Fernández, C., 1960: The mechanism of bone conduction. Ann. Otol. Rhinol. Laryng. 69:5.

Altmann, F., and Waltner, J., 1950: Further investigations on the Physiology of labyrinthine fluids. Ann. Otol. Rhinol. Laryng. 59:657.

Aschan, G., 1961: The pathogenesis of positional nystagmus. Acta oto-laryng. Suppl. 159:90.

Aschan, G., Bergstedt, M., and Goldberg, M., 1964: Positional alcohol nystagmus in patients with unilateral and bilateral labyrinthine destructions. Confin. neurol. 24:80.

Aschan, G., Bergstedt, M., Goldberg, M., and Laurell, L., 1956: Positional nystagmus in man during and after alcohol intoxication. Quart. J. Stud. Alcohol. 17:381.

Aschan, G., Bergstedt, M., and Stahle, J., 1956: Nystagmography, recording of nystagmus in clinical neuro-otological examinations. Acta oto-laryng. Suppl. 129:1.

Aubry, M., and Giraud, J., 1943: Etude audiométrique du signe de Gellé. Ann. oto-laryng., Paris 61:137.

Bárány, E., 1938: A contribution to the physiology of bone conduction. Acta oto-laryng. Suppl. 26:1.

Bauer, J., and Leidler, R., 1911: Ueber den Einfluss der Ausschaltung verschiedener Hirnabschite auf die vestibularen Augenreflexe. Arb. neurol. Inst. Univ. Wein, Leipzig and Vienna. 19:155.

Baxter, A., 1970: Personal communication.

Beal, D., 1968: Effect of endolymphatic sac ablation in the rabbit and cat. Acta oto-laryng. 66:333.

Bechterew, W., 1882: Ergebnisse der Durchschneidung des N. acusticus, Nebst Erörterung der Bedeutung der semicirculären Canäle für das Körpergleichgewicht. Arch. ges. Phys. des Menschen und der Thiere. 30:312.

Békésy, G. von, 1932: Zur Theorie des Hörens bei der Schallaufnahme durch Knochenleitung. Ann. Physik. 13:111.

Békésy, G. von, 1936: Fortschritte der Hörphysiologie. Z. tech. Physik. 12:522.

Békésy, G. von, 1941: Über die Schallausbreitung bei Knochenleitung. Z. Hals-Nas.-Ohrenheilk. 47:430.

Békésy, G. von, 1944: Über die mechanische Frequenzanalyse in der Schnecke verschiedener Tiere. Akustische Z. 9:3.

Békésy, G. von, 1947a: The variation of phase along the basilar membrane with sinusoidal vibrations. J. Acoust. Soc. Amer. 19:452.

Békésy, G. von, 1947b: A new audiometer. Acta oto-laryng. 35:411.

Békésy, G. von, 1953: Shearing microphonics produced by vibrations near the inner and outer hair cells. J. Acoust. Soc. Amer. 25:786.

Békésy, G. von, 1960: Experiments in Hearing. Translated and edited by E. G. Wever. McGraw-Hill, New York.

Békésy, G. von, 1967: Sensory Inhibition. Princeton University Press, Princeton, N.J.

Békésy, G. von, and Rosenblith, W., 1951: The mechanical properties of the ear, in S. S. Stevens Handbook of Experimental Psychology. pp. 1075–1115. John Wilely and Sons, Inc., New York.

Bender, M., 1965: Oscillopsia. Arch. Neurol. 13:204.

Berlin, C., Lowe-Bell, S., Jannetta, P., and Kline, D., 1972: Central auditory deficits after temporal lobectomy. Arch. Otolaryng. 96:4.

Bernstein, J., and Silverstein, H., 1966: Anterior cerebellar and labyrinthine arteries, a study in the cat. Arch. Otolaryng. 83:422.

Bing, A., 1891: Ein neuer Stimmgabelversuch. Beitrag zur Differential-Diagnose ker Krankheiten des mechanischen Schalleitungs und nervösen Hörapparates. Wien. med. Blätter, 41.

Bluestone, C., 1971: Eustachian tube obstruction in the infant with cleft palate. Ann. Otol. Rhinol. Laryng. Suppl. 2, 80:1.

Bocca, E., 1958: Clinical aspects of cortical deafness. Laryngoscope 68:301.

Bocca, E., and Calearo, C., 1963: Central hearing processes. Modern Development in Audiology. J. Jerger, Editor, Academic Press Inc., New York.

Bocca, E., Calearo, C., Cassinari, V., and Migliavacca, F., 1955: Testing "cortical" hearing in temporal lobe tumours. Acta oto-laryng. 45:289.

Bosher, S., and Warren, R., 1968: Observations on the electrochemistry of the cochlear endolymph of the rat: a quantitative study of its electrical potential and ionic composition as determined by means of flame spectrophotometry. Proc. Roy. Soc. B 171:227.

Bramwell, E., 1927: Case of cortical deafness. Brain 50:579.

Breuer, J., 1891: Ueber die Function der Otolithenapparate. Arch. ges. Physiol. 48:195.

Brodmann, K., 1909–1925: Vergleichende lokalisationslehre der Grosshirnrinde in irhren prinzipien Dargestellt auf grand des Zellenbaues. J. A. Barth, Leipzig.

Bunch, C., 1928: Auditory acuity after removal of the entire right cerebral hemisphere. J. Amer. Med. Assn. 90:2102.

Campbell, A., 1905: Histological Studies on the Localization of Cerebral Function. Cambridge University Press, Cambridge, England.

Campbell, I., Jr., 1970: The frequency increment sensitivity test. Acta oto-laryng. 70:371.

Capps, M., and Ades, H., 1968: Auditory frequency discrimination after transection of the olivocochlear bundle in squirrel monkeys. Exp. Neurol. 21:147.

Carhart, R., 1950: Clinical application of bone conduction audiometry. Arch. Otolaryng. 51:798.

Carhart, R., 1957: Clinical determination of abnormal auditory adaptation. Arch. Otolaryng. 65:32.

Carmichael, E., Dix, M., and Hallpike, C., 1954: Lesions of cerebral hemispheres and their effects upon optokinetic and caloric nystagmus. Brain 77:345.

Carmichael, E., Dix, M., Hallpike, C., and Hood, J., 1961: Some further observations upon the effect of unilateral cerebral lesions on caloric and rotational nystagmus. Brain 84:571.

Carmichael, E., Dix, M., and Hallpike, C., 1965: Observations upon the neurological mechanism of directional preponderance of caloric nystagmus resulting from vascular lesions of the brain-stem. Brain 88:51.

Chevance, L., Galli, A., Jeanmarie, J., 1960: Immuno-electrophoretic study of the human perilymph. Acta oto-laryng. 52:41.

Citron, L., Dix, M., Hallpike, C., and Hood, J., 1963: A recent clinico-pathological study of cochlear nerve degeneration resulting from tumor pressure and disseminated sclerosis, with particular reference to the finding of normal threshold sensitivity for pure tones. Acta oto-laryng. 56:330.

Cogan, D., 1968: Down beat nystagmus. Arch. Ophthal. 80:757.

Compere, W., Jr., 1958: Tympanic cavity clearance studies. Trans. Amer. Acad. Ophthal. Otolaryng. 62:444.

Cranford, J., Ravizza, R., Diamond, I. and Whitfield, I., 1971: Unilateral ablation of the auditory cortex in the cat impairs complex sound localization. Science 172:286.

Crum-Brown, A., 1874: One the sense of rotation and the anatomy and physiology of the semicircular canals of the internal ear. J. Anat. Physiol. 8:327.

Dandy, W., 1934: Effects on hearing after subtotal section of cochlear branch of auditory nerve. Bull. Johns Hopk. Hosp. 55:240.

Dankbaar, W., 1970: The diagnostic value of Gellé's test. Acta oto-laryng. 69:266.

Davis, H., 1960: Mechanism of excitation of auditory nerve impulses. Neural Mechanisms of the Auditory and Vestibular Systems. Edited by G. Rasmussen and W. Windle, Charles C. Thomas, Springfield, Ill. Chap. II.

Davis, H., Gernandt, B., Riesco-MacClure, J., and Covell, W., 1949: Aural microphonics in the cochlea of the guinea pig. J. Acoust. Soc. Amer. 21:502.

Davis, H., and Kranz, F., 1964: The international standard reference zero for pure tone audiometers and its relation to the evaluation of impairment of hearing. J. Speech Res. 7:7.

Davis, H., Morgan, C., Hawkins, J., Jr., Galambos, R., and Smith, F., 1950: Temporary deafness following exposure to loud tones and noise. Acta oto-laryng. Suppl. 88.

Decker, H., Rohr, H., and Unterharnscheidt, F., 1960: The influence of traumatic cervical root avulsion on the auditory and labyrinth apparatus. Excerpta med. 12:293.

Desmedt, J., 1960: Neurophysiological mechanisms controlling acoustic input, in Neural Mechanisms of the Auditory and Vestibular Systems. Edited by G. Rasmussen and W. Windle, Charles C. Thomas, Springfield, Ill. Chap. II, p. 152.

Dewson, J., III, 1968: Efferent olivocochlear bundle: Some relationships to stimulus discrimination in noise. J. Neurophysiol. 31:122.

Diamant, M., 1940: Otitis and pneumatisation of the mastoid bone, A clinical-statistical analysis. Acta oto-laryng. Suppl. 41:149.

DiCarlo, L., Kendall, D., and Goldstein, R., 1962: Diagnostic procedures for auditory disorders in children. Folia phoniat. 14:206.

Dirks, D., and Malmquist, C., 1964: Changes in bone-conduction thresholds produced by masking in the non-test ear. J. Speech Res. 7:271.

Dishoeck, H. van, 1937: Das Pneumophon. Arch. Ohr. Nas.-Kehlk-Heilk. 144:53.

Dix, M., Hallpike, C., and Hood, J., 1948: Observations upon the loudness recruitment phenomenon, with especial reference to the differential diagnosis of disorders of the internal ear and VIIIth nerve. J. Laryng. 62:671.

Dodge, R., 1923: Habituation to rotation. J. Exp. Psychol. 6:1.

Dohlman, G., 1938: On the mechanism and transformation into nystagmus on stimulation of the semicircular canals. Acta oto-laryng. 26:425.

Drettner, B., and Ekvall, L., 1970: Chronic obstruction of the eustachian tube treated with a tympano-maxillary shunt. Acta oto-laryng. Suppl. 263:29.

Dunlap, K., 1925: Adaptation of nystagmus to repeated caloric stimulation in rabbits. J. Comp. Psychol. 5:485.

Dusser de Barenne, J., and Kleyn, A. de, 1923: Ueber vestibuläre Augenreflexe. V. Vestibularuntersuchungen nach Ausschaltung einer Grossliernhemisphäre beinn Kaninchen. Arch. Ophtal. Berl. 111:374.

Duvall, A., III, Flock, Å., and Wersäll, J., 1966: The ultrastructure of the sensory hairs and associated organelles of the cochlear inner hair cell, with reference to directional sensitivity. J. Cell. Biol. 29:497.

Ekvall, L., 1970: Eustachian tube function in tympanoplasty, clinical aspects. Acta oto-laryng. Suppl. 263:33.

Eldredge, D., and Miller, J., 1971: Physiology of hearing. Ann. Rev. Physiol. 33:281.

Elliott, D., 1961: The effect of sensorineural lesions on pitch discrimination in cats. Ann. Otol. Rhinol. Laryng. 70:582.

Elliott, D., Stein, L., and Harrison, J., 1960: Determination of absolute-intensity thresholds and frequency-difference thresholds in cats. J. Acoust. Soc. Amer. 32:380.

Engström, H., and Hjorth, S., 1951: On the distribution and localization of injected dyes in the labyrinth of the guinea pig. Acta oto-laryng. Suppl. 95:149.

Engström, H., and Wersäll, J., 1953: Is there a special nutritive cellular system around the hair cells in the organ of Corti? Ann. Otol. Rhinol. Laryng. 62:507.

Ewald, J., 1892: Physiologische Untersuchungen uber des Endorgan des Nervus Octavus. J. F. Bergmann, Wiesbaden.

Ewald, J., 1898: Ueber eine neue Hörtheorie. Wien. klin. Wschr. 11:721.

Falck, B., Hillarp, N., Thieme, G., and Torp, A., 1962: Flourescence of catecholamines and related compounds condensed with formaldehyde. J. Histochem. Cytochem. 10:348.

Farmer, T., and Morris, C., 1964: Oscillopsia in association with cerebellopontine angle cholesteatoma. Neurology 14:973.

Feldman, A., 1963: Acoustic impedance measurements at the eardrum as an aid to diagnosis. J. Speech Res. 6:315.

Feldman, A., 1964: Acoustic impedance measurement as a clinical procedure. Int. Aud. 3:156.

Fernández, C., 1951: The innervation of the cochlea (guinea pig). Laryngoscope 61:1152.

Fernández, C., Lindsay, J., and Alzate, R., 1959: Postural nystagmus due to localized cerebellar lesions in the cat. Acta oto-laryng. 50:287.

Fernández, C., and Riesco-MacClure, J., 1963: Studies on habituation of vestibular reflexes. V., The optokinetic nystagmus. Ann. Otol. Rhinol. Laryng. 72:336.

Fernández, C., and Schmidt, R., 1963: Studies in habituation of vestibular reflexes. III. A revision. Aerospace med. 34:311.

Fex, J., 1959: Augmentation of cochlear microphonic by stimulation of efferent fibres to the cochlea. Acta oto-laryng. 50:540.

Fex, J., 1962: Auditory activity in centrifugal and centripetal fibres in cat. Acta physiol. scand. Suppl. 55:189.

Fex, J., 1965: Auditory activity in uncrossed centrifugal cochlear fibres in cat. A study of a feedback system, II. Acta physiol. scand. 64:43.

Fisch, U., and Yasargil, M., 1968: Transtemporale, extra-pyramidale Eingriffe am inneren Gehörgang. Pract. oto-rhino-laryng. 30:377.

Fitzgerald, G., and Hallpike, C., 1942: Studies in human vestibular function; observations on the directional preponderance of caloric nystagmus resulting from cerebral lesions. Brain 65:115.

Flisberg, K., 1966: Ventilatory studies on the eustachian tube. Acta oto-laryng. Suppl. 219:1.

Flisberg, K., and Ingelstedt, S., 1970: Middle-ear mechanics in patulous tube cases. Acta oto-laryng. 263:18.

Flisberg, K., Ingelstedt, S., and Örtegren, U., 1963: On the function of middle ear and eustachian tube. Acta oto-laryng. Suppl. 182:1.

Flock, Å., Kimura, R., Lundquist, P., and Wersäll, J., 1962: Morphological basis of directional sensitivity of the outer hair cells in the organ of Corti. J. Acoust. Soc. Amer. 34:1351.

Flourens, P., 1842: Recherches expérimentales sur les propriétés et les fonctions due système nerveux 2°3 d., Paris.

Fluur, E., 1959: Influences of semicircular ducts on extraocular muscles. Acta oto-laryng. Suppl. 149:1.

Fluur, E., 1970: The interaction between the utricle and the saccule. Acta oto-laryng. 69:17.

Fluur, E., and Mellström, A., 1970a: Utricular stimulation and oculomotor reactions. Laryngoscope 80:1701.

Fluur, E., and Mellström, A., 1970b: Saccular stimulation and oculomotor reactions. Laryngoscope 80:1713.

Fluur, E., and Tovi, D., 1965: Microscopic intracranial section of the vestibular nerve in Ménière's disease. Acta oto-laryng. 59:604.

Fowler, E., 1937: Measuring the sensation of loudness: A new approach to the physiology of hearing and the functional and differential diagnostic tests. Arch. Otolaryng. 26:514.

Fumagalli, Z., 1949: Ricerche morfologiche sull'apparato di transmissione del suono. Arch ital. Otol. Suppl. 60:1.

Galambos, R., 1955: Suppression of auditory nerve activity by stimulation of efferent fibers to the cochlea. Fed. Proc. 14:53.

Galambos, R., 1956: Supression of auditory nerve activity by stimulation of efferent fibers to cochlea. J. Neurophysiol. 19:424.

Galambos, R., 1960: Studies of the auditory system with implanted electrodes. In Neural Mechanisms of the Auditory and Vestibular Systems. Edited by G. Rasmussen and W. Windle. Charles C. Thomas, Springfield, Ill. Chap. X, p. 137.

Galambos, R., 1974: Brainstem evoked response audiometry. In press.

Gellé, M., 1885: Valeur de l'epreuve des pressions centripètes? Est-ce par inhibition? Ann. mal. oreil. larynx. 11:63.

Giebisch, G., Klose, R., and Windhager, E., 1964: Micropuncture study of hypertonic sodium chloride loading in the rat. Amer. J. Physiol. 206:687.

Goldstein, R., Goodman, A., and King, R., 1956: Hearing and speech in infantile hemiplegia before and after left hemispherectomy. Neurology 6:869.

Goodman, A., 1957: Some relations between auditory function and intracranial lesions with particular reference to lesions of the cerebellopontine angle. Laryngoscope 67:987.

Graham, M., 1963: A longitudinal study of ear disease and hearing loss in patients with cleft lips and palates. Trans. Amer. Acad. Ophthal. Otolaryng. 67:213.

Griffith, C., 1920: The organic effects of repeated bodily rotation. J. Exp. Psychol. 3:15.

Guild, S., 1927: The circulation of endolymph. Amer. J. Anat. 39:57.

Guinan, J., and Peake, W., 1967: Middle-ear characteristics of anesthetized cats. J. Acoust. Soc. Amer. 41:1237.

Hakas, P. and Kornhuber, H., 1959: Der vestibuläre Nystagmus bei Grosshirnläsionen des Menschen. Arch. Psychiat. Nervenkr. 200:19.

Hallpike, C., 1956: The caloric tests. J. Laryng. 70:15.

Hallpike, C., 1967: Some types of ocular nystagmus and their neurological mechanisms. Proc. Roy. Soc. Med. 60:1043.

Hallpike, C., and Rawdon-Smith, A., 1934: The "Wever and Bray Phenomenon." A study of the electrical response in the cochlea with especial reference to its origin. J. Physiol. 81:395.

Handl, K., 1959: Zur vegetativen Versorgung den menschlichen Tube. Arch. Ohr. Nas.-Kehlk-Heilk. 175:482.

Hansen, C., and Reske-Nielsen, E., 1963: Central hearing loss in a patient with glioblastoma: Neuropathological analysis of a case. Arch. Otolaryng. 77:461.

Helmholtz, H., 1863: Die Lehre von den Tonempfindungen als physiologische Grundlage für die Theorie der Musik. 1st ed. Vieweg Verlag, Brunswick, Germany.

Henriksson, N., Kohut, R., and Fernández, C., 1961: Studies on habituation of vestibular reflexes. Acta oto-laryng. 53:333.

Henschen, S., 1917: Über die Hörspähre. J. Psychol. Neurol. 22:19.

Herzog, H., and Krainz, W., 1926: Das Knochenleitungsproblem. Z. Hals-Nas.-Ohrenheilk. 15:300.

Hind, J., and Schuknecht, H., 1954: A cortical test of auditory function in experimentally deafened cats. J. Acoust. Soc. Amer. 26:89.

Hinoki, M., and Terayama, K., 1966: Physiological role of neck muscles in the occurrence of optic eye nystagmus. Acta oto-laryng. 62:157.

Hirsch, I., and Ward, W., 1952: Recovery of the auditory threshold after strong acoustic stimulation. J. Acoust. Soc. Amer. 24:131.

Holborow, C., 1962a: Deafness associated with cleft palate. J. Laryng. 76:762.

Holborow, C., 1962b: Conductive deafness associated with the cleft-palate deformity. Proc. Roy. Soc. Med. 55:305.

Holden, H., and Schuknecht, H., 1968: Distribution pattern of blood in the inner ear following spontaneous subarachnoid hemorrhage. J. Laryng. 82:321.

Holmes, G., 1917: The symptoms of acute cerebellar injuries due to gunshot injuries. Brain 40:461.

Holmgren, G., 1934: Recherches expérimentales sur les fonctions de la trompe d'eustache. Communication prealable. Acta oto-laryng. 20:381.

Holmquist, J., 1968: The role of the eustachian tube in myringoplasty. Acta oto-larng. 66:289.

Holmquist, J., 1970: Middle ear ventilation in chronic otitis media. Arch. Otolaryng. 92:617.

Hood, J., 1950: Auditory adaptation and its relationship to clinical tests of auditory function. Proc. Roy Soc. Med. 43:1129.

Hood, J., 1957: The principles and practice of bone conduction audiometry: a review of the present position. Proc. Roy. Soc. Med. 50:689.

House, H., and House, W., 1964: Monograph transtemporal bone microsurgical removal of acoustic neuromas. I. Introduction and pathology. Historical review and problems of acoustic neuroma. Arch. Otolaryng. 80:601.

House, W., Glasscock, M., and Miles, J., 1969: Eustachian tuboplasty. Laryngoscope 79:1765.

Hudson, W., and Ruben, R., 1962: Hereditary deafness in the Dalmatian dog. Arch. Otolaryng. 75:213.

Huggett, A., and Nixon, D., 1957: Enzymic determination of blood glucose. Biochem. J. (Proc. Biochem. Soc.) 66:12P.

Huizing, E., 1960: Bone conduction: The influence of the middle ear. Acta oto-laryng. Suppl. 155:1.

Hurst, C., 1895: A new theory of hearing. Trans. Liverpool Biol. Soc. 9:351.

Igarashi, M., Alford, B., Konishi, S., Shaver, E., and Guilford, F., 1969: Functional and histopathological correlations after microembolism of the peripheral labyrinthine artery in the dog. Laryngoscope 79:603.

Igarashi, M., Watanabe, T., and Maxian, P., 1969: Role of neck proprioceptors for the maintenance of dynamic bodily equilibrium in the squirrel monkey. Laryngoscope 79:1713.

Ingelstedt, S., 1964: Chronic adhesive otitis: Analysis of some predisposing factors. Acta oto-laryng. Suppl. 188:19.

Ingelstedt, S., and Örtegren, U., 1963: Qualitative testing of eustachian tube function. Acta-oto-laryng. Suppl. 182:7.

Ishii, T., 1971: Acetlycholinesterase activity in the perivascular nerve plexus of the basilar and labyrinthine arteries, Acta oto-laryng. 72:281.

Ishii, T., Silverstein, H. and Balogh, K., Jr., 1966: Metabolic activities of the endolymphatic sac. Acta oto-laryng. 62:61.

Ishii, T., Takahashi, T., and Balogh, K., Jr., 1969: Glycogen in the inner ear after acoustic stimulation: A light and electron microscopic study. Acta oto-laryng. 67:573.

Iurato, S., 1967: Submicroscopic Structure of the Inner Ear. Ed. S. Iurato, 59–106, 174. Pergamon Press, London.

Jackson, M., and Sears, C., 1966: Effect of weightlessness upon the normal nystagmic reaction. Aerospace Med. 37/7:719.

Jago, J., 1867: The functions of the tympanum. Brit. For. Med. Chir. Rev. 39:175.

Jerger, J., 1960: Observations on auditory behavior in lesions of the central auditory pathways. Arch. Otolaryng. 71:797.

Jerger, J., 1964: Auditory tests for disorders of the central auditory mechanism, in Neurological Aspects of Auditory and Vestibular Disorders, Edited by W. S. Fields and B.R. Alford. Charles C. Thomas, Springfield, Ill., p. 77.

Jerger, J., 1968: Review of diagnostic audiometry. Ann. Otol. Rhinol. Laryng. 77:1042.

Jerger, J., 1970: Clinical experience with impedance audiometry. Arch. Otolaryng. 92:311.

Jerger, J., and Harford, E., 1960: Alternate and simultaneous binaural balancing of pure tones. J. Speech Res. 3:15.

Jerger, J., Shedd, J., and Harford, E., 1959: On the detection of extremely small changes in sound intensity. Arch. Otolaryng. 69:200.

Jerger, J., Weikers, N., Sharbrough, F., III, and Jerger, S., 1969: Bilateral lesions of the temporal lobe. A case study. Acta oto-laryng. Suppl. 258:1.

Jerison, H., and Neff, W., 1953: Effect of cortical ablation in the monkey on discrimination of auditory patterns. Fed. Proc. 12:73.

Johansen, H., 1948: Relation of audiograms to the impedance formula. Acta oto-laryng. Suppl. 74:65.

Jouvet, M., and Hernandez-Peon, R., 1957: Mecanisme neurophysiologies concernant l'habituation, l'attention et le conditionnement. Electroenceph. clin. Neurophysiol. Suppl. 6:39.

Kaida, Y., 1931: Ueber das Verhalten des inneren Ohres nach Stammläsion des N. acusticus. Jap. J. Med. Sci. Tr. 1:237.

Kato, T., 1913: Zur Physiologie der Binnenmuskeln des Ohres. Pflügers Arch. ges. Physiol. 150:569.

Keeney, A., and Roseman, E., 1966: Acquired, vertical illusory movement of the environment. Amer. J. Ophthal. 61:118.

Kellogg, R., and Graybiel, A., 1967: Lack of response to thermal stimulation of the semicircular canals in the weightless phase of parabolic flight. Aerospace med. 38/5:487.

Kestenbaum, A., 1946: Nystagmus. In Clinical Methods of Neuro-ophthalmologic Examination. Grune & Stratton, New York. Chap. VIII, p. 216.

Kiang, N., 1965: Discharge Patterns of Single Fibers in the Cat's Auditory Nerve. Research Monograph No. 35, M.I.T. Press, Cambridge, Mass.

Kikuchi, K., and Hilding, D., 1967: The spiral vessel and stria vascularis in Shaker-1 mice. Acta oto-laryng. 63:395.

Kimura, R.: Unpublished data.

Kimura, R., 1967: Experimental blockage of the endolymphatic duct and sac and its effect on the inner ear of the guinea pig. Ann. Otol. Rhinol. Laryng. 76:664.

Kimura, R., 1969: Distribution, structure, and function of dark cells in the vestibular labyrinth. Ann. Otol. Rhinol. Laryng. 78:542.

Kimura, R., Lundquist, P-G., and Wersäll, J., 1963: Secretory epithelial linings in the ampullae of the guinea pig labyrinth. Acta oto-laryng. 57:517.

Kimura, R., and Schuknecht, H., 1965: Membranous hydrops in the inner ear of the guinea pig after obliteration of the endolymphatic sac. Pract. oto-rhino-laryng. 27:343.

Kimura, R., Schuknecht, H., and Ota, C., 1974: Blockage of the cochlear aqueduct. Acta oto-laryng. 77:1.

King, B., 1926: The influence of repeated rotations on decerebrate and on blinded squabs. J. Comp. Psychol. 6:399.

Kirikae, I., 1960: The Structure and Function of the Middle Ear. University of Tokyo Press.

Kirikae, I., 1969: Physiopathology of the middle ear. Refresher Audiovisual course. University of Tokyo Press.

Kleyn, A. de, and Nieuwenhuyse, P., 1927. Schwendelanfalle und Nystagmus bei einer bestimmten Stellung des Kapfes. Acta oto-laryng. 11:115.

Klockhoff, I., 1961: Middle ear muscle reflexes in man. Acta oto-laryng. Suppl. 164:1.

Klockhoff, I., and Anderson, H., 1959: Recording of the stapedius reflex elicited by cutaneous stimulation. Acta oto-laryng. 50:451.

Kobrak, H., 1930: Zur Physiologie der Binnenmuskeln des Ohres. Beitr. Anat. Ohr. 28:138; 29:383.

Kobrak, H., 1959: The Middle Ear. University of Chicago Press.

Koelle, G., 1950: The histochemical differentiation of types of cholinesterases and their localizations in tissues of the cat. J. Pharmacol. Exp. Ther. 100:158.

Koelle, G., 1951: The elimination of enzymatic diffusion artifacts in the histochemical localization of cholinesterases and a survey of their cellular distributions. J. pharmacol. Exp. Ther. 103:153.

Koelle, G., and Friedenwald, J., 1949: A histochemical method for localizing cholinesterase activity. Proc. Soc. Exp. Biol. 70:617.

Koenig, W., 1949: A new frequency scale for acoustic measurements. Bell Laboratory Record, p. 299.

Konishi, T., and Kelsey, E., 1968: Effect of tetrodotoxin and procaine on cochlear potentials. J. Acoust. Soc. Amer. 43:471.

Konishi, T., Kelsey, E., and Singleton, G., 1966: Effects of chemical alteration in the endolymph on the cochlear potentials. Acta oto-laryng. 62:393.

Kuijpers, W., van der Vleuten, A., and Bonting, S., 1967: Cochlear function and sodium and potassium activated adenosine triphosphatase. Science 157:949.

Lawrence, M., 1965: Fluid balance in the inner ear. Ann. Otol. Rhinol. Laryng. 74:486.

Lawrence, M., 1966a: Effects of interference with terminal blood supply on organ of Corti. Laryngoscope 76:1318.

Lawrence, M., 1966b: Histological evidence for localized radial flow of endolymph. Arch. Otolaryng. 83:406.

Lemoyne, J., and Mahoudeau, D., 1959: A propos d'un cas d'agnosie auditive pure avec surdité corticale associée à une dysphonie fonctionnelle. Ann. Otol. Rhinol. Laryng. 76:293.

Lenzi, G., and Pompeiano, O., 1970: Orthodromic transmission of VIIIth nerve volleys through the vestibular nuclei during sleep. Adv. Oto-Rhino-Laryng. Edited by L. Rüedi, S. Karger, Basel, Switzlerland.

Lidén, G., 1954: Speech audiometry: An experimental and clinical study with Swedish language material. Acta otolaryng. Suppl. 114:1.

Lidén, G., 1969: The scope and application of current audiometric tests. J. Laryng. 83:507.

Lierle, D., and Reger, S., 1955: Experimentally induced temporary threshold shifts in ears with impaired hearing. Ann. Otol. Rhinol. Laryng. 64:263.

Lim, D., 1970: Surface ultrastructure of the cochlear perilymphatic space. J. Laryng. 84:413.

Lim, D., 1973: Personal communication.

Lindsay, J., 1943: Eustachian tube function and deafness. Minn. Med. 26:250.

Lindsay, J., 1947: Effect of obliteration of the endolymphatic sac and duct in the monkey. Arch. Otolaryng. 45:1.

Lindsay, J., Schuknecht, H., Neff, W., and Kimura, R., 1952: Obliteration of the endolymphatic sac and the cochlear aqueduct. Ann. Otol. Rhinol. Laryng. 61:697.

Lindsay, W., LeMesurier, A., and Farmer, A., 1962: A study of the speech results of a large series of cleft palate patients. Plast. Reconstr. Surg. 29:273.

Lorente de No, R., 1937: Symposium. The neural mechanism of hearing. I. Anatomy and physiology. (b) The sensory endings in the cochlea. Laryngoscope 47:373.

Lowenstein, O., and Roberts, T., 1950: The equilibrium function of the otolith organs of the thornback ray (Raja clavata). J. Physiol. 110:392.

Lowenstein, O., and Sand, A., 1940: The mechanism of the semicircular canal. A study of the responses of single fibre preparations to angular accelerations and to rotation at constant speed. Proc. Roy. Soc. B. 129:256.

Lowenstein, O., and Wersäll, J., 1959: A functional interpretation of the electron microscopic structure of the sensory hairs in the cristae of the elasmobranch Raja clavata in terms of directional sensitivity. Nature 184:1807.

Lowry, O., Rosebrough, N., Farr, A., and Randall, R., 1951: Protein measurement with the folin phenol reagent. J. biol. Chem. 193:265.

Lundquist, P.-G., 1965: The endolymphatic duct and sac in the guinea pig. Acta otolaryng. Suppl. 201:1.

Lundquist, P.-G., Kimura, R., and Wersäll, J., 1964a: Ultrastructural organization of the epithelial lining in the endolymphatic duct and sac in the guinea pig. Acta oto-laryng. 57:65.

Lundquist, P.-G., Kimura, R., and Wersäll, J., 1964b: Experiments in endolymph circulation. Acta oto-laryng. Suppl. 188:198.

Lurie, M., 1939: Studies of waltzing guinea pigs. Laryngoscope 49:558.

Lurie, M., 1942: The degeneration and absorption of the organ of Corti in animals. Ann. Otol. Rhinol. Laryng. 51:712.

Lüscher, E., 1930: Über eine neue Methode zur Untersuchung des Gehörsorganes zu physiologischen und diagnostischen Zwecken mit Hilfe des Interferens-Otoscopes. Arch. Ohr. Nas.-Kehlk-Heilk. 3:186.

Mach, E., 1875: Grundlinien der Lehre von den Bewegungsempfindungen. Wilhelm Englemann, Liepzig.

MacKinnon, D., 1970: Relationship of preoperative eustachian tube function to myringoplasty. Acta oto-laryng. 69:100.

Maruseva, A., 1961: The electrophysiological expression of changes in the function of the auditory system in the presence of the orientation response. Fiziol. Ž. (SSSR) 5:542.

Maspétriol, R., Chardin, and Millard, 1954: Vertigo during the course of a posterior cervical sympathetic syndrome cured by vertebral neurotomy. Excerpta med. 7:312.

Masters, F., Bingham, H., and Robinson, D., 1960: The prevention and treatment of hearing loss in the cleft palate child. Plast. Reconstr. Surg. 25:503.

Masuda, Y., Sando, I., and Hemenway, W., 1971: Perilymphatic communication routes in guinea pig cochlea. Arch. Otolaryng. 94:240.

Matschinsky, F., and Thalmann, R., 1967: Quantitative histochemistry of microscopic structures of the cochlea: II. Ischemic alterations of levels of glycolytic intermediates and cofactors in the organ of Corti and stria vascularis. Ann. Otol. Rhinol. Laryng. 76:638.

Maw, A., 1971: Bobbing oscillopsia. Ann. Otol. Rhinol. Laryng. 80:233.

Maxwell, S., Burke, U., and Reston, C., 1922: The effect of repeated rotation on the duration of after-nystagmus in the rabbit. Amer. J. Physiol. 58:432.

McCabe, B., 1960: Vestibular suppression in figure skaters. Trans. Amer. Acad. Opthal. Otolaryng. 64:264.

McCabe, B., and Gillingham, K., 1964: The mechanism of vestibular suppression. Ann. Otol. Rhinol. Laryng. 73:816.

McCabe, B., and Ryu, J., 1969: Experiments on vestibular compensation. Laryngoscope 79:1728.

McNally, W., 1926: Experiments on the saccus endolymphaticus in the rabbit. J. Laryng. 41:349.

Ménière, P., 1861a: Report and commentary. Gaz med. Paris 16:55.

Ménière, P. 1861b: Auricular pathology. Gaz. med. Paris 16:88.

Ménière, P., 1861c: Medical correspondence. Gaz. med. Paris 16:239.

Ménière, P., 1861d: Auricular pathology. Gaz: med. Paris 16:597.

Mettler, F., Finch, G., Girden, E., and Culler, E., 1934: Acoustic value of the several components of the auditory pathway. Brain 57:475.

Metz, O., 1946: The acoustic impedance measured on normal and pathological ears. Acta oto-laryng. Suppl. 63:1.

Metz, O., 1951: Studies on the contraction of the tympanic muscles as indicated by changes in the impedance of the ear. Acta oto-laryng. 39:397.

Miller, E., 1962: Counterrolling of the human eyes produced by head tilt with respect to gravity. Acta oto-laryng. 54:479.

Miller, E., and Graybiel, A., 1962: A comparison of ocular counterrolling movements between normal persons and deaf subjects with bilateral labyrinthine defects. U.S. Naval School of Aviation Medicine Research Report 68:1.

Miller, G., 1965: Eustachian tubal function in normal and diseased ears. Arch. Otolaryng. 81:41.

Misch, W., 1928: Uber kortikale Taubheit. Z. ges. Neurol. Psychiat. 115:567.

Møller, A., 1958: Intra-aural muscle contraction in man, examined by measuring acoustic impedance of the ear. Laryngoscope 68:48.

Møller, A., 1960: Improved technique for detailed measurements of the middle ear impedance. J. Acoust. Soc. Amer. 32:250.

Møller, A., 1961: Network model of the middle ear. J. Acoust. Soc. Amer. 33:168.

Møller, A., 1972: Coding of sounds in lower levels of the auditory system. Quart. Rev. Biophys. 5:59.

Money, K., 1974: Motion sickness. The vestibular system (Symposium at University of Chicago). In press.

Monnier, M., Belin, I., and Polc, P., 1970: Facilitation, inhibition and habituation of the vestibular responses. Adv. Oto-Rhino-Laryng. Edited by L. Rüedi. 17:28, S. Karger, Basel.

Montandon, P., Shepard, N., Marr, E., Peake, W., and Kiang, N., 1974: Auditory nerve potentials from ear canals of patients with otologic problems. In press.

Mott, F., 1907: Bilateral lesion of the auditory cortical center: complete deafness and aphasia. Brit. Med. J. 2:310.

Müller, P., 1958: Experiments on current flow and ionic movement on single myelinated nerve fibers. Exp. Cell Res. Suppl. 5:118.

Naito, T., 1950: Experimental studies on Ménière's disease. Jap. J. Otol. Tokyo 53:19.

Nakai, Y., and Hilding, D., 1967: Adenosine triphosphatase distribution in the organ of Corti. Acta oto-laryng. 64:477.

Neff, W., 1947: The effects of partial section of the auditory nerve. J. Comp. Physiol. Psychol. 40:203.

Neff, W., 1965: Auditory discriminations affected by cortical ablations. International Symposium on Sensorineural Processes and Disorders, Henry Ford Hospital, ed. A. Graham, Little, Brown, Boston, p. 201.

Neff, W., and Kiang, N.: Personal communication.

Neff, W., and Yela, M., 1948: Function of the auditory cortex. The localization of sound in space. Amer. J. Psychol. 3:243.

Nomura, Y., 1961: Capillary permeability of the cochlea. An experimental study. Ann. Otol. Rhinol. Laryng. 70:81.

Nomura, Y., 1962: Observations on the microcirculation of the cochlea. Ann. Otol. Rhinol. Laryng. 70:1037.

Nylén, C., 1931: Clinical study on positional nystagmus in cases of brain tumour. Acta oto-laryng. Suppl. 15.

Nylén C., 1950: Positional nystagmus. J. Laryng. 64:295.

Odoi, H., Proud, G., and Toledo, P., 1971: Effects of pterygoid hamulotomy upon eustachian tube function. Laryngoscope 81:1242.

Okamoto, M., Sato, M., and Kirikae, I., 1954: Studies of the acoustic reflex. Part II. Experimental studies on the function of the tensor tympani muscle. Ann. Otol. Rhinol. Laryng. 63:950.

Onchi, Y., 1954: The blocked bone conduction test for differential diagnosis. Ann. Otol. Rhinol. Laryng. 63:81.

Oosterveld, W., 1970: Effect of gravity on

positional alcohol nystagmus. Aerospace med. 41:557.

Osterhammel, P., Terkildsen, K., and Zilstorff, K., 1970: Vestibular habituation in ballet dancers. Adv. Oto-Rhino-Laryng. 17:158.

Owens, E., 1971: Audiologic evaluation in cochlear versus retrocochlear lesions. Acta oto-laryng. Suppl. 283.

Palva, A., and Kärjä, J., 1970: Eustachian-tube patency in chronic ears, pre-operative evaluation correlated to postoperative results. Acta oto-laryng. 263:25.

Palva, T., 1970: Cochlear aqueduct in infants. Acta oto-laryng. 70:83.

Palva, T., and Raunio, V., 1967: Disc electrophoretic studies of human perilymph and endolymph. Acta oto-laryng. 63:128.

Paparella, M., 1970: Biochemical Mechanisms in Hearing and Deafness. Edited by M. Paparella. Charles C. Thomas, Springfield, Ill.

Penfield, W., and Evans, J., 1934: Functional defects produced by cerebral lobectomies. Res. Publ. Ass. Nerv. Ment. Dis. 13:352.

Penfield, W., and Rasmussen, G., 1955: The Cerebral Cortex of Man. Macmillan, New York.

Perlman, H., 1939: The eustachian tube: Abnormal patency and normal physiologic state. Arch. Otolaryng. 30:212.

Perlman, H., 1943: Quantitative tubal function. Arch. Otolaryng. 38:453.

Perlman, H., 1960: The place of the middle ear muscle reflex in auditory research. Arch. Otolaryng. 72:201.

Perlman, H., and Kimura, R., 1955: Observations of the living blood vessels of the cochlea. Ann. Otol. Rhinol. Laryng. 64:1176.

Perlman, H., and Kimura, R., 1957: Experimental obstruction of venous drainage and arterial supply of the inner ear. Ann. Otol. Rhinol. Laryng. 66:537.

Perlman, H., and Kimura, R., 1962: Cochlear blood flow in acoustic trauma. Acta oto-laryng. 54:99.

Perlman, H., Kimura, R., and Butler, R., 1959a: Cochlear blood flow during hypothermia. Ann. Otol. Rhinol. Laryng. 68:803.

Perlman, H., Kimura, R., and Fernández, C., 1959b: Experiments on temporary obstruction of the internal auditory artery. Laryngoscope 69:591.

Perlman, H., and Lindsay, J., 1939: Relation of the internal ear spaces to the meninges. Arch. Otolaryng. 29:12.

Perlman, H., Tsunoo, M., and Spence, A., 1963: Cochlear blood flow and function: Effect of pressor agents. Acta oto-laryng. 56:587.

Perlman, H., and Yamada, S., 1967: Autoregulation of strial blood flow. Affect of increased expiratory resistance: Hyperventilation. NASA Third Symp. Vest. Organ 152:289.

Pfalz, R., 1969: Absence of a function for the crossed olivocochlear bundle under physiological conditions. Arch. Ohr.-Nas.-Kehlk.-Heilk. 193:89.

Philipszoon, A., and Bos, J., 1963: Neck torsion nystagmus. Pract. oto-rhino-laryng. (Basel) 25:339.

Pichler, H., und Bornschein, H., 1957: Audiometrischer Nachweis nichtakustisch ausgelöster Reflexkontraktionen der Intraauralmuskulatur. Acta oto-laryng. 48:498.

Pitman, L., 1929: The open eustachian tube. Arch Otolaryng. 9:494.

Portmann, M., and Aran, J., 1971: Electrocochleography. Laryngoscope 81:899.

Proctor, L., and Fernández, C., 1963: Studies

on habituation of vestibular reflexes. Acta oto-laryng. 56:500.

Pulec, J., 1967: Abnormally patent eustachian tubes: Treatment with injection of polytetrafluoroethylene (teflon) paste. Laryngoscope 77:1543.

Pulec, J., and Hahn, F., Jr., 1970: The abnormally patulous eustachian tube. Otolaryng. Clinics of North America. p. 131.

Pulec, J., and Simonton, K., 1964: Abnormal patency of the eustachian tube: Report on 41 cases. Laryngoscope 74:267.

Reiner, C., and Pulec, J., 1969: Experimental production of otitis media. Ann. Otol. Rhinol. Laryng. 78:880.

Reitjö, A., 1914: Beiträge zur Physiologie der Knochenleitung. Verh. deutsch. otol. Ges. 23:268.

Rich, A., 1920: A physiological study of the eustachian tube and its related muscles. Johns Hopkins Hosp. Bull. 31:206.

Rogers, R., Kirchner, F., and Proud, G., 1962: The evaluation of eustachian tubal function by flourescent dye studies. Laryngoscope 72:456.

Rubin, W., 1968: Nystagmography: Terminology, technique, and instrumentation. Arch. Otolaryng. 87:266.

Rudert, H., 1969: Experimentelle Untersuchungen zur Resorption der Endolymphe im Innenohr des Meerschweinchens. Arch. klin. exp. Ohr.-Nas.-Kehlk.-Heilk. 193:138.

Rundcrantz, H., 1969: Posture and eustachian tube function. Acta oto-laryng. 68:279.

Runge, H., 1923: Über die Lehre von der Knochenleitung und über einen neuen Versuch zu ihrem weiteren Ausbau. Z. Hals-Nas.-Ohrenheilk. 5:306.

Ryan, G., and Cope, S., 1955: Cervical vertigo. Lancet 2:1355.

Sade, J., 1966: Middle ear mucosa. Arch. Otolaryng. 84:137.

Sanchez-Longo, L., Forster, F., and Auth, T., 1957: A clinical test for sound localization and its applications. Neurology 7:655.

Sando, I., Masuda, Y., Wood, R., II, and Hemenway, W., 1971: Perilymphatic communication routes in guinea pig cochlea. Ann. Otol. Rhinol. Laryng. 80:826.

Sato, I., 1939: Experimentelle Untersuchengen über die Flimmerbewegungen in der Tuba eustachii. Zbl. Hals-Nas.-Ohrenheilk. 31:687.

Scheibe, A., 1891–1892: Ein Fall von Taubstummheit mit Acusticusatrophie und Bilungsanomalien in haütigen Labyrinth beiderseits. Z. Ohrenheilk. 22:11.

Schindler, K., Schnieder, E., and Wullstein, H., 1965: Vergleichende Bestimmung einiger Elektrolyte und organischer Substanzen in der Perilymphe otosklerosekranker Patienten. Acta oto-laryng. 59:309.

Schuknecht, H., 1953a: Techniques for study of cochlear function and pathology in experimental animals: Development of the anatomical frequency scale for the cat. Arch. Otolaryng. 58:377.

Schuknecht, H., 1953b: Lesions of the organ of Corti. Trans. Amer. Acad. Ophthal. Otolaryng. 57:366.

Schuknecht, H., 1957: Ablation therapy in the management of Ménière's disease. Acta oto-laryng. Suppl. 132:42.

Schuknecht, H., 1959: Discussion. Trans. Amer. Acad. Ophthal. Otolaryng. 47:112.

Schuknecht, H., 1960a: Neuroanatomical correlates of auditory sensitivity and pitch discrimination in the cat, in Neural Mechanisms of the Auditory and Vestibular Systems. Edited by G. L. Rasmus-

sen and W. Windle. Charles C. Thomas, Springfield, Ill. Chap. VI, p. 76.

Schuknecht, H., 1960b: Discusion on pp. 94–95 in Neural Mechanisms of the Auditory and Vestibular Systems, Edited by G. L. Rasmussen and W. Windle. Charles C. Thomas, Springfield, Ill.

Schuknecht, H., 1970: Pathophysiology of the fluid systems of the inner ear. In Contributions to Sensory Physiology, ed. W. D. Neff. 4:75–93. Academic Press, New York

Schuknecht, H., Chasin, W., and Kurkjian, J., 1966: Stereoscopic Atlas of Mastoidotympanoplastic Surgery. C. V. Mosby, St. Louis, Missouri.

Schuknecht, H., Igarashi, M., and Gacek, R., 1965: The pathological types of cochleo-saccular degeneration. Acta oto-laryng. 59:154.

Schuknecht, H., and Kimura, R., 1953: Functional and histological findings after obliteration of the periotic duct and endolymphatic sac in sound conditioned cats. Laryngoscope 63:1170.

Schuknecht, H., and McNeill, R., 1966: Light microscopic observations on the pathology of endolymph. J. Laryng. 80:1.

Schuknecht, H., and Neff, W., 1952: Hearing losses after apical lesions in the cochlea. Acta oto-laryng. 42:263.

Schuknecht, H., Griffin, W., Jr., Davies, G., and Silverstein, H., 1968a: Chemical evaluation of inner ear fluid as a diagnostic aid. Acta oto-laryng. 65:169.

Schuknecht, H., Northrop, C., and Igarashi, M., 1968b: Cochlear pathology after destruction of the endolymphatic sac in the cat. Acta oto-laryng. 65:479.

Schuknecht, H., and El Seifi, A., 1963: Experimental observations on the fluid physiology of the inner ear. Ann. Otol. Rhinol. Laryng. 72:687.

Schuknecht, H., and Sutton, S., 1953: Hearing losses after experimental lesions in basal coil of cochlea. Arch. Otolaryng. 57:129.

Schuknecht, H., and Woellner, R., 1953: Hearing losses following partial section of the cochlear nerve. Laryngoscope 63:441.

Schuknecht, H., and Woellner, R., 1955: An experimental and clinical study of deafness from lesions of the cochlear nerve. J. Laryng. 69:75.

Schwartze, H., 1864: Respiratorische Bewegung des Trommelfelles. Arch. Ohr. Nas.-Kehlk.-Heilk. 1:139.

Shambaugh, G., 1938: Continuously open eustachian tube. Arch. Otolaryng. 27:420.

Shambaugh, G., Jr., 1967: Surgery of the Ear. 2nd ed. W. B. Saunders, Philadelphia, Pa.

Sharp, M., 1970: The manometric investigation of tubal function with reference to myringoplasty results. J. Laryng. 84:545.

Siedentop, K., Tardy, M., and Hamilton, L., 1968: Eustachian tube function. Arch. Otolaryng. 88:386.

Silverstein, H., 1966a: Biochemical and physiologic studies of the endolymphatic sac in the cat. Laryngoscope 76:498.

Silverstein, H., 1966b: Biochemical studies of the inner ear fluids in the cat. Ann. Otol. Rhinol. Laryng. 75:48.

Silverstein, H., 1971: Inner ear fluid proteins in acoustic neuroma, Ménière's disease and otosclerosis. Ann. Otol. Rhinol. Laryng. 80:27.

Silverstein, H., Davies, D., and Griffin, W., Jr., 1969: Cochlear aqueduct obstruction changes in perilymph biochemistry. Ann. Otol. Rhinol. Laryng. 78:532.

Silverstein, H., and Griffin, W., Jr., 1970a: Comparison of inner ear fluids in the antemortem and postmortem state of the cat. Ann. Otol. Rhinol. Laryng. 79:178.

Silverstein, H., and Griffin, W., Jr., 1970b: Diagnostic labyrinthotomy in otologic disorders. Arch. Otolaryng. 91:414.

Silverstein, H., Miller, G., Jr., and Lindeman, R., 1966: Eustachian tube dysfunction as a cause for chronic secretory otitis in children. Laryngoscope 76:259.

Silverstein, H., and Schuknecht, H., 1966: Biochemical studies of inner ear fluid in man. Arch. Otolaryng. 84:395.

Sohmer, H., and Feinmesser, M., 1974: Electrocochleography in clinical-audiological diagnosis. Arch. Oto-Rhino-Laryng. 206:91.

Sokolovski, A., 1973: The protective action of the stapedius muscle in noise-induced hearing loss in cats. Arch. Ohr. Nas.-Kehlk.-Heilk. 203:289.

Spoendlin, H., 1966: Ultrastructure of the vestibular sense organ, in The Vestibular System and Its Diseases, Edited by R. J. Wolfson. University of Pennsylvania Press, Philadelphia, p. 39.

Spoendlin, H., and Gacek, R., 1963: Electronmicroscopic study of the efferent and afferent innervation of the organ of Corti in the cat. Ann. Otol. Rhinol. Laryng. 72:660.

Spoendlin, H., and Lichtensteiger, W., 1967: The sympathetic nerve supply to the inner ear. Arch. Ohr. Nas.-Kehlk-Heilk. 189:346.

Stahle, J., 1966: Electronystagmography—Its value as a diagnostic tool. In The Vestibular System and Its Diseases. Edited by R. J. Wolfson. University of Pennsylvania Press, Philadelphia, p. 267.

Steinhausen, W., 1931: Über den Nachweis der Bewegung der Capula in der intakten Bogengangsampulle des Labyrinthes bei der natürlichen rotatorischen und calorischen Reizung. Pflügers Arch. ges. Physiol. 228:322.

Studebaker, G., 1962: On masking in bone-conduction testing. J. Speech Res. 5:215.

Suga, F., Nakashima, T., and Snow, J., Jr., 1970: Sodium and potassium ions in endolymph: In vivo measurements with glass microelectrodes. Arch. Otolaryng. 91:37–43.

Sutton, S., and Schuknecht, H., 1954: Regional hearing losses from induced cochlear injuries in experimental animals. Ann. Otol. Rhinol. Laryng. 63:727.

Tanaka, T., Kosaka, N., Takiguchi, T., Aoki, T., and Takahara, S., 1973: Observation on the cochlea with SEM. In Scanning Electron Microscopy. Part III. Proceedings of the Workshop on Scanning Electron Microscopy in Pathology, IIT (Illinois Institute of Technology) Research Institute, Chicago, Ill. 60616. (April).

Tasaki, I., Davis, H., and Eldredge, D., 1954: Exploration of cochlear potentials in guinea pig with a microelectrode. J. Acoust. Soc. Amer. 26:765.

Tasaki, I., Davis, H., and Legouix, J., 1952: The space-time pattern of the cochlear microphonics (guinea pig), as recorded by differential electrodes. J. Acoust. Soc. Amer. 24:502.

Tasaki, I., and Fernández, C., 1952: Modification of cochlear microphonics and action potentials by KCl solution and by direct currents. J. Neurophysiol. 15:497.

Tasaki, I., and Spyropoulos, C., 1952: Stria vascularis as source of endocochlear potential. J. Neurophysiol. 22:149.

Terayama, Y., Holz, E., and Beck, C., 1965: Fluoreszenzmikroskopischer Nachweis adrenergischer Fasern in der Meerschweinchenschnecke. Mschr. Ohrenheilk. 99:513.

Terayama, Y., Holz, E., and Beck, C., 1966: Adrenergic innervation of the cochlea. Ann. Otol. Rhinol. Laryng. 75:69.

Terayama, Y., Yamamoto, K., and Sakamoto, T., 1968: Electron microscopic observations on the postganglionic sympathetic fibers in the guinea pig cochlea. Ann. Otol. Rhinol. Laryng. 77:1152.

Terkildsen, K., and Nielsen, S., 1960: An electroacoustic impedance measuring bridge for clinical use. Arch. Otolaryng. 72:339.

Thalmann, I., Matschinsky, F., and Thalmann, R., 1970: Quantitative study of selected enzymes involved in energy metabolism of the cochlear duct. Ann. Otol. Rhinol. Laryng. 79:12.

Thomsen, K., 1955: Employment of impedance measurements in otologic and otoneurologic diagnostics. Acta oto-laryng. 45:159.

Tonndorf, J., 1966: Bone conduction. Studies in experimental animals. A collection of seven papers. Acta oto-laryng. Suppl. 213:1.

Tonndorf, J., and Khanna, S., 1970: The role of the tympanic membrane in middle ear transmission. Ann. Otol. Rhinol. Laryng. 79:743.

Torok, N., 1970: The effects of arousal upon vestibular nystagmus. Adv. Oto-Rhino-Laryng. p. 76. Edited by L. Rüedi, S. Karger, Basel.

Torok, N., Guillemin, V., and Barnothy, J., 1951: Photoelectric nystagmography. Ann. Otol. Rhinol. Laryng. 60:917.

Trahiotis, C., and Elliott, D., 1970: Extension of the Neff neural model to situations demanding discrimination among complex stimuli. J. Acoust. Soc. Amer. 47:1116.

Trincker, D., 1957: Permanent potentials in the semicircular canal system of the guinea pig and their changes in experimental cupula leads. Pflügers Arch. ges. Physiol. 264:351.

Tröger, J., 1930: Die Schallaufnahme durch das äussere. Ohr. Physik. Z. 31:26.

Uyama, Y., 1933: Histopathologische Veränderungen am Innenohre, bedingt durch den experimentellen Verschluss des Aqueductus Cochleae, Okayama Igakkai Zasshi 45:1128.

Vosteen, K.-H., 1970: Passive and active transport in the inner ear. Arch. klin. exp. Ohr.-Nas.-Kehlk.-Heilk. 195:226.

Walsh, T., and Goodman, A., 1955: Speech discrimination in central auditory lesions. Laryngoscope 65:1.

Waltner, J., 1948: Barrier membrane of the cochlear aqueduct. Arch. Otolaryng. 47:656.

Weber, E., 1834: De pulsu, resorptione auditu et tactu. De utilitate cochleae in organo auditus. Lipsiae.

Weiss, A.: Personal communication.

Weiss, E., 1960: An air damped artificial mastoid. J. Acoust. Soc. Amer. 32:1582.

Wersäll, J., 1961: Vestibular receptor cells in fish and mammals. Acta oto-laryng. Suppl. 163:25.

Wersäll, J., 1968: Efferent innervation of the inner ear, in Structure and Functions of Inhibitory Neuronal Mechanisms. (Proceedings of the Fourth International Meeting of Neurobiologists). Pergamon Press, New York.

Wersäll, J., Flock, Å., and Lundquist, P-G., 1965: Structural basis for directional sensitivity in cochlear and vestibular sensory receptors. Cold Spring Harbor Symposia on Quantitative Biology. 30:115.

Wersäll, R., 1958: The tympanic muscles and their reflexes. Acta oto-laryng. Suppl. 139.

Westergaard, O., 1970: Tubal function in patients with chronic secretory otitis media. Acta oto-laryng. 263:23.

Wever, E., and Bray, C., 1936: The nature of acoustic response: The relation between sound intensity and the magnitude of responses in the cochlea. J. exper. Psychol. 19:129.

Wever, E., and Lawrence, M., 1954: Physiological Acoustics. Princeton University Press, Princeton, N.J.

Wever, E., and Smith, K., 1944: The problem of stimulation deafness, cochlear impairment as a function of tonal frequency. J. exper. Psychol. 34:239.

Wiederhold, M., 1970: Variations in the effects of electric stimulation of the crossed olivocochlear bundle on cat single auditory-nerve-fibre responses to tone bursts. J. Acoust. Soc. Amer. 48:966.

Weiderhold, M., and Kiang, N., 1970: Effects of electric stimulation of the crossed olivocochlear bundle on single auditory-nerve fibers in the cat. J. Acoust. Soc. Amer. 48:950.

Wilson, T., and Kane, F., 1959: Congenital deafness in white cats. Acta oto-laryng. 50:269.

Wittmaack, K., 1911: Ueber sekundäre Degenerationen im inneren Ohre nach Akustikustammverletzungen. Verh. dtsch. otol. Ges. 20:289.

Wullstein, H., Kley, W., Rauch, S., und Köstlin, A., 1960: Zur Biochemie der Perilymphe operierter Otosklerosen. Z. Laryng. Rhinol. 39:665.

Yamakawa, K., 1929: Die Wirkung der arsenigen Säure auf das Ohr. Arch. Ohr.Nas.-Kehlk.-Heilk. 123:238.

Yules, R., 1970: Hearing in cleft palate patients. Arch. Otolaryng. 91:319.

Zöllner, F., 1963: Therapy of the eustachian tube. Arch. Otolaryng. 78:394.

Zwislocki, J., 1951: Eine verbesserte vertäubungsmethode für die audiometrie. Acta oto-laryng. 39:338.

Zwislocki, J., 1957a: Some measurements of the impedance at the eardrum. J. Acoust. Soc. Amer. 29:349.

Zwislocki, J., 1957b: Some impedance measurements on normal and pathological ears. J. Acoust. Soc. Amer. 29:1312.

Zwislocki, J., 1961: Acoustic measurement of the middle ear function. Ann. Otol. Rhinol. Laryng. 70:599.

Zwislocki, J., and Feldman, A., 1969: Acoustic impedance of pathological ears. Technical Report LSC-S-5, Laboratory for Sensory Communication. Syracuse University, New York.

4 Developmental Defects

The formulation of a logical and all-inclusive classification for deafness from developmental defects is not a simple matter. Recent intense interest in developmental defects is creating a rapidly accumulating body of knowledge so that any current description will soon be incomplete.

The term *congenital*, as applied to deafness, implies existence at birth and carries no etiologic significance. Deafness that is present at birth is *hereditary* if the causal factors were present in the zygote (fertilized egg), and it is *acquired* if the causal factors were not present in the zygote but were obtained during development in the uterus.

A. HEREDITARY SENSORINEURAL DEAFNESS

The incidence of hereditary sensorineural deafness is not definitely known but probably occurs in about one in four thousand live births. Considering all cases of congenital deafness, including rubella, birth injury, and erythroblastosis, about one-third to one-half appear to be due to hereditary factors.

Brown (1967), in an analysis of several sets of data including Fraser's (1964) study of 2,355 English special school children, suggests that about 25 percent of childhood deafness can be attributed to identifiable prenatal or postnatal disease or trauma, 18 percent to undiagnosed disease or genetic factors, 15 percent to simple autosomal dominant genes, 40 percent to simple autosomal recessive genes, and 2 percent to sex-linked genes.

Danish et al. (1963) studied 490 students at the Pennsylvania School for the Deaf and estimated that 31 percent developed deafness after birth, 17.6 percent had congenital nonhereditary deafness, and 51.4 percent had congenital hereditary deafness. Arnvig (1954) determined that hereditary deafness accounted for 28.5 percent of deafness in Danish children. Barton et al. (1962) stated that 25 percent of the children in the Deaf School at Durham and Northumberland had hereditary deafness. Of 102 cases of congenital deafness at the Clark School for the Deaf (Hopkins, 1954), 36 were determined to be hereditary, 12 due to rubella, 4 to erythroblastosis, 1 to birth injury, and 49 unknown. In a study of 348 children exhibiting deafness, Ruben and Rozycki (1970) found that 20 percent were caused by genetic disease.

Environment often has a profound effect on the severity with which a genetic disorder expresses itself. Often heredity and environment interact strongly, and only in special cases is it possible to differentiate these etiologic factors clearly. The manifestations and pathology of a disorder of genetic etiology may be indistinguishable from that of environmental origin.

Hereditary factors vary greatly in the severity of their effect, and this effect is referred to as variability in "specificity." The frequency with which a genetic abnormality is manifested among those who possess the gene or genes involved is a statistical concept referred to as "penetrance." The severity of a disorder, in a particular individual, is termed "expressivity." These concepts have been well defined only in a few types of hereditary deafness, a good example being Waardenbërg's syndrome.

Although there is great variability in the expression of inherited disorders, it is useful in studying inherited deafness to describe dominant and recessive types (Figs. 4.1 and 4.2). Among the types of genetic deafness occurring alone, congenital and nonprogressive deafness is usually recessive, whereas acquired or familial progressive deafness is usually dominant. The classification appearing in Table 4.1 is a modified version of the one devised by Proctor and Proctor (1967). It is based on a consideration of both clinical features with the main types being dominant and recessive, and both occurring with or without associated defects in other organs. The classification is not intended to be complete. There are many other syndromes which include deafness but most of them are so rare that they do not constitute an important otological entity.

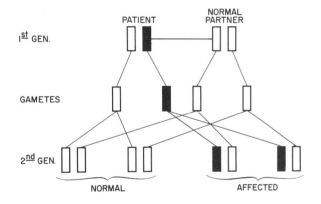

Fig. 4.1: Diagram illustrating the dominant mode of transmission of a disease. One pair of chromosomes is shown for each individual, with the black chromosome carrying the defective gene. Half the children of an affected patient are diseased.

Table 4.1 Hereditary Sensorineural Deafness

1. Dominant hereditary sensorineural deafness
   a) Hereditary sensorineural deafness occurring alone
      1) Dominant congenital severe deafness
      2) High tone deafness
   b) Inborn errors of metabolism and deafness
      1) Tietz's syndrome; albinism and deafness, abnormality of tyrosine metabolism (Tietz, 1963)
      2) Waardenbërg's syndrome; partial albinism and deafness, 1 percent of hereditary deafness, abnormality of tyrosine metabolism (Waardenbërg, 1951)
      3) Schafer's syndrome; hereditary mental retardation, prolinemia and deafness, abnormality of proline metabolism (Schafer et al., 1962)
      4) Hereditary mental retardation, homocystinemia, and deafness; abnormality of methionine metabolism (Nelson, 1964)
   c) Nephropathies and deafness
      1) Alport's syndrome; hereditary nephritis and deafness, 1 percent of hereditary deafness
      2) Muckle and Well's syndrome; hereditary nephritis, urticaria, amyloidosis, and deafness (Muckle and Wells, 1962)
      3) Herrmann's syndrome; hereditary nephritis, mental retardation, epilepsy, diabetes, and dominant nerve deafness (Herrmann et al., 1964)
   d) Ectodermal defects and deafness
      1) Ectodermal dysplasia; anhidrosis, and deafness (Marshall, 1958)
      2) Von Recklinghausen's disease, localized; bilateral vestibular schwannomas and deafness (Gardner and Turner, 1940)
   e) Degenerative diseases of the nervous system and deafness
      1) Huntington's chorea and deafness
2. Recessive hereditary nerve deafness
   a) Hereditary recessive sensorineural deafness without associated defects (possibly 50 percent of recessive hereditary deafness)

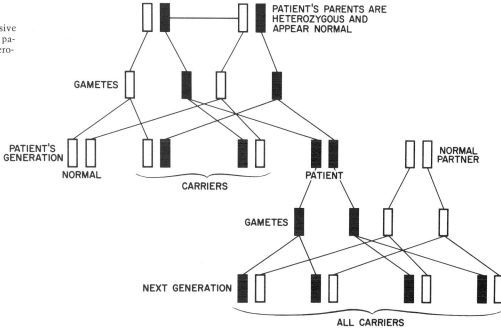

Fig. 4.2: Diagram to illustrate the recessive mode of transmission of a disease. The patient's parents are both unaffected heterozygotes, as are all of his children.

1) Recessive congenital severe deafness
2) High frequency deafness
3) Mid frequency deafness
b) Inborn errors of metabolism and deafness
    1) Albinism and deafness (Ziprowski and Adam, 1964; Margolis, 1962)
    2) Hurler's syndrome or gargoylism; lipo-chondrodystrophy, abnormality of mucopolysaccharide metabolism
    3) Morquio's disease and deafness; osteochondrodystrophy, abnormality of mucopolysaccharide metabolism
    4) Onychodystrophy and deafness (Feinmesser and Zelig, 1961); abnormality of mucopolysaccharide metabolism
    5) Tay-Sachs' disease; amaurotic familial idiocy and deafness, ganglioside lipidoses (Jampel and Quaglio, 1964)
    6) Wilson's disease; hepatolenticular degeneration and deafness
    7) Hypophosphatasia; decreased mineralization of bone, decreased alkaline phosphatase activity
    8) Hereditary hyperphosphatasia; skeletal deformities, dwarfism, deafness, elevated alkaline and acid phosphatase activity
c) Degenerative disease of the nervous system and deafness
    1) Friedreich's ataxia; spinocerebellar ataxia and deafness
    2) Schilder's disease; subcortical encephalopathy and deafness (Lichtenstein and Rosenbluth, 1956)
    3) Unverricht's epilepsy; myoclonic epilepsy and deafness (Latham and Munro, 1938)
d) Congenital heart disease and deafness
    1) Jervell and Lange-Nielsen syndrome; EKG abnormalities and deafness
    2) Lewis' syndrome; congenital pulmonary stenosis and deafness (Lewis et al., 1958)
e) Endocrine system disorders and deafness
    1) Pendred's syndrome; nonendemic goiter and deafness (10 percent of hereditary deafness)
f) Diseases of the eye and deafness
    1) Usher's syndrome; retinitis pigmentosa and deafness (10 percent of hereditary deafness)
    2) Cockayne's syndrome; retinitis pigmentosa, mental retardation, dwarfism, and deafness
    3) Alstrom's syndrome; retinitis pigmentosa, obesity,

diabetes mellitus, and deafness (Alstrom et al., 1959)

4) Laurence-Moon-Bardet-Biedle syndrome; retinitis pigmentosa, mental retardation, obesity, polydactyly, hypogonadism, and deafness (Burn, 1950)

5) Refsum's syndrome; retinitis pigmentosa, polyneuritis, ichthyosis, and deafness (Refsum, 1946; Prior, 1964)

6) Norrie's disease; retinal pseudotumor, mental retardation, and deafness (Warburg, 1963)

7) Leber's disease; juvenile optic atrophy and deafness (François, 1961)

8) Fehr's dystrophy and deafness (Moro and Amidei, 1957)

1. DOMINANT HEREDITARY SENSORINEURAL DEAFNESS

About 10 percent of hereditary sensorineural deafness is of the dominant type. If one parent carries the affected gene the incidence of involvement of the offspring is about 50 percent; however, the incidence may be modified by such factors as penetrance and sex linkage.

a. *Dominant congenital severe deafness*

Individuals with this disorder are severely deaf from birth and have no associated abnormalities (Fay, 1898; Konigsmark, 1971). Caloric responses are usually normal. Pathological studies from well-documented cases are lacking, although Altmann's (1950) case, a 22-year-old deaf mute woman, might represent such a case. The temporal bones of this individual exhibited dysplasia of the organs of Corti and saccules (Scheibe dysplasia).

b. *High-tone deafness*

Martensson (1960), as well as Dolowitz and Stephens (1961) and more recently Teig (1968) have described a type of high-tone deafness which is due to a single dominant gene with complete penetrance. The deafness may be present at birth or have its onset at any age. The hearing loss is worse for high frequencies and is progressive. The histopathological change appears to be atrophy of the organ of Corti and cochlear neurons, most severe in the basal turn. Huizing et al. (1966) studied the hearing losses in a family of 335 members in five generations and found an autosomal dominant mode of inheritance with complete penetrance. In their cases the deafness was bilateral and symmetrical and in the beginning was most severe for high frequencies. It was progressive during the first three decades of life, reaching a loss of 60 to 70 db, after which progression was less rapid. Recruitment was positive as tested by the SISI test, thus implicating a sensory lesion.

Goodhill (1950) has classified hereditary high-tone deafness into infantile and adult types; however, it seems probable that the age of onset is a continuum from birth to old age and encompasses many of those pathological types of progressive deafness, now termed presbycusis. The audiograms of a young mother and her three female children, showing a dominant sex-linked hereditary deafness, are shown in Fig. 4.3.

c. *Tietz's syndrome*

Tietz (1963) described this disorder as a dominant autosomal hereditary syndrome, characterized by profound deafness with albinism. In contrast to Waardenbërg's syndrome, there is generalized rather than localized loss of pigment. The eyebrows are absent and the irides are blue. Because photophobia and nystagmus are absent, it is not true albinism.

d. *Waardenbërg's syndrome (white forelock, heterochromia iridis, deafness)*

Waardenbërg (1951) first described this syndrome after finding 12 cases among 840 severely deaf patients in five Dutch institutions. The characteristic features were (1) lateral displacement of the medial canthae and lacrimal

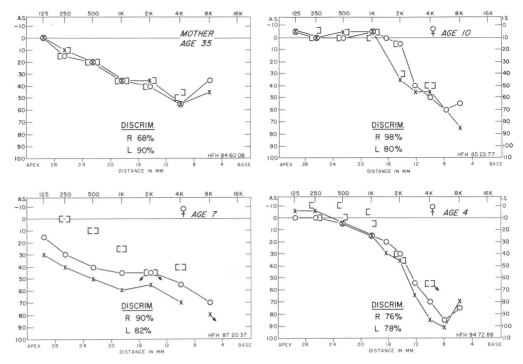

Fig. 4.3: Recessive hereditary sensorineural deafness in mother and three daughters. The seven-year-old child had a superimposed conductive hearing loss due to seromucinous otitis media. Over a five-year observation period there was no progression of the loss of hearing of these individuals.

punctae; (2) hyperplastic high nasal root; (3) hyperplasia of the medial portions of the eyebrows; (4) partial or total heterochromia iridis; (5) sensorineural deafness, bilateral or unilateral; and (6) circumscribed albinism of the frontal head hair (white forelock).

Wildervanck (1957) described a mitigated form of the syndrome in three children having only severe sensorineural deafness and heterochromia iridis.

Heterochromia iridis may consist of one blue eye and one brown eye or mixed pigmentation in one or both eyes. A white forelock may or may not be present. It should be noted that the white forelock without deafness is not a rare phenomenon. It has occurred in the family of Percy Dukes of Northumberland for over 500 years.

Fisch (1959) observed that the upper eyelid of individuals with Waardenbërg's syndrome approximates the medial margin of the cornea and should not be confused with the prominent epicanthic fold of the Mongolian eye. He observed three distinctive audiometric patterns: (1) almost total deafness with some slight residual hearing for the low frequencies; (2) moderate deafness, most severe for the low frequencies with normal hearing for 6,000 Hz and 8,000 Hz; and (3) unilateral deafness, usually with near normal hearing in one ear and moderate hearing loss in the other. In his patients the most frequent combination of findings was deafness, eyelid deformity, and deep blue eyes. The combination of all signs of the syndrome was rare. Fisch also acquired the temporal bones of a profoundly deaf 3½-year-old girl with partial heterochromia iridis and typical eyelid deformity. Examination revealed atrophy of the organ of Corti, stria vascularis, and cochlear neurons.

In a study of the disorder in a family traced back for four generations, Marcus (1968) found frequent abnormalities of vestibular response and radiographic evidence of inner ear anomalies.

Reed (1967) has described several other syndromes of hereditary deafness with dermatological manifestations, including pili torti (twisted hair) with deafness (Bjornstad, 1965).

(e) Alport's syndrome (nephritis and deafness)

Dickinson (1875) referred to three generations of a family in which 11 of 17 members had albuminaria with several dying prematurely of nephritis. No mention was made of deafness.

Guthrie (1902) investigated a family that was later restudied by Kendall and Hurst (1912), then again by Hurst (1923), and finally by Alport (1927). It was Alport who pointed out the high incidence of sensorineural deafness in those individuals who were afflicted with "hereditary, familial, congenital, hemorrhagic nephritis."

Perkoff et al. (1951) reported a clinical study of hereditary interstitial pyelonephritis with progressive renal insufficiency only in the males. Of eight males who died of the disease, six had sensorineural deafness. Their study was important for it permitted a genetic analysis based on data from 232 descendants of a single person. It appeared that the trait was transmitted by an incompletely sex-linked dominant gene. Other reports of kidney disease associated with deafness have been made by Reyersback and Butler (1954), Sohar (1956), Sturtz and Burke (1956), Goldbloom et al. (1957), Robin et al. (1957), and Whalen et al. (1961).

The mode of inheritance of this syndrome remains somewhat uncertain, for although it tends to be much more severe in males, its manifestations occur more frequently in females. The disease probably appears initially as a mutation. Perkoff et al. (1951), who conducted the first large-scale family study of this syndrome, felt that the trait followed the pattern of a dominant, partially sex-linked gene. Graham (1959) presented an alternative theory to explain the apparent greater prevalence in females, suggesting that the trait was a sex-linked dominant one, and that some heterozygous males died early in intrauterine life. Shaw and Glover (1961) and Cohen et al. (1961), noting that partial sex-linkage had not been shown to occur in mammals, proposed a preferential segregation of chromosomes during meiosis, the chromosome bearing the defective gene being selected to pass into the functional gamete in association with the X-chromosome.

While deafness and renal disease are the principal abnormalities of this syndrome, a number of other lesions have been described. Ocular manifestations are common and consist chiefly of lens abnormalities such as cataracts, anterior lenticonus, and spherophakia, but myopia and rupture of the lens capsule have also been described (Sohar, 1956; Arnott et al., 1966). Isolated cases of associated abnormalities in the skeletal system, skin, and central nervous system have been reported, but are seen so infrequently that they probably represent unrelated disease.

Of recent interest has been the discovery of abnormal metabolism of lipids and amino acids. Elevation of the serum lipids, especially of the B-lipoproteins, has been reported by Dubach et al. (1966) in a small number of cases. Abnormal amino acids have been found in the serum and urine in some individuals (Efron, 1965). The primary defect appears to be a deficiency of proline oxidase, an enzyme necessary for the degradative metabolism of the amino acid L-proline (Kopelman et al., 1964). Thus proline appears in elevated levels in the serum of affected patients. Aminoaciduria has also been noted, involving proline, hydroxyproline, and glycine. The mechanism appears to be an excessive amount of proline in the plasma to be filtered, combined with impaired tubular reabsorption of hydroxyproline and glycine (Schafer et al., 1962). These apparent abnormalities of lipid and amino acid metabolism have occurred only in a minority of cases, even among members of an affected family, and their significance requires further investigation.

The histopathological findings in the kidneys are those of a "mixed" nephritis with alternating areas of severe tubular atrophy and tubular dilation combined with patchy glomerulonephritis. Lipid-laden foam cells, derived from tubular epithelial cells occurring in rows and nests, occupy the lower renal cortex (Krickstein et al., 1966).

Males usually die before the age of 30 of the renal disease. Females usually have a less severe form of the disease manifested only by recurring albuminaria, and life expectancy is normal.

The auditory disorder consists of a slowly progressive bilateral sensorineural hearing loss affecting the entire frequency range, somewhat worse for high frequencies and often first noted about the age of 10. The loss may become seriously handicapping to those who survive beyond the age of 20.

Miller et al. (1970) found that these patients consistently show high SISI

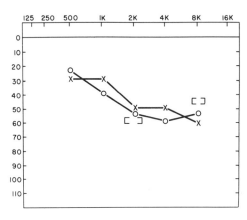

Fig. 4.4: Alport's syndrome. Audiogram of a male who died of familial nephritis at the age of 24. He was one of six siblings, three males and three females, of which four showed familial nephritis. See Fig. 4.5.

Fig. 4.5: Alport's syndrome. Same case as Fig. 4.4. The cochlea appears normal except for a dense basophilic deposit in the spiral ligament adjacent to the stria vascularis throughout the basal turn. This deposit was found in both temporal bones. Because such deposits have not been observed in temporal bones of other cases of Alport's syndrome, it probably represents an alteration that is secondary to some primary pathology which has not yet been detected by light microscopic study.

scores, type II Békésy tracings, and normal tone decay, all of which point toward a sensory disorder. They also found decreased vestibular responses which with successive increases in thermic stimuli exhibited vestibular recruitment, suggesting a sensory disorder of the vestibular system.

Histological studies of temporal bones of individuals with Alport's syndrome have failed to reveal a consistent pathological change. Among the changes described are loss of cochlear neurons, atrophy of the spiral ligaments, and loss of hair cells (Gregg and Becker, 1963; Dubach et al., 1966; Winter et al., 1968; Schreiner, 1968; Crawfurd and Toghill, 1968; Fujita and Hayden, 1969; Meyers and Tyler, 1972; Ruby and Schuknecht, 1974). Other isolated findings include a single case of endolymphatic hydrops (Fujita and Hayden, 1969), partial degeneration of the stria vascularis (Gregg and Becker, 1963), and deposits of a basophilic staining material in the substrial zone of the spiral ligament (Ruby and Schuknecht, 1974) (Figs. 4.4, 4.5).

Because these changes are not found consistently in the cochleae of individuals with Alport's syndrome, they probably represent secondary alterations—that is, secondary to some primary pathology which has eluded detection by light microscopy.

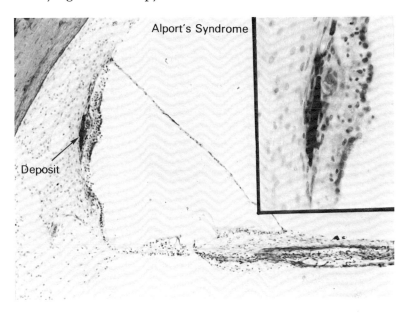

Alport's Syndrome

Deposit

2. RECESSIVE HEREDITARY SENSORINEURAL DEAFNESS

About 90 percent of inherited sensorineural deafness is of the recessive type. Both parents must be carriers of the gene, and according to mendelian law, only 25 percent of the offspring will be affected. For this reason there often is no family history of deafness, making the hereditary origin difficult to establish. It is more common in consanguineous marriages. At the Clark School for the Deaf, cousin marriages were present in 8 percent of all deaf children, while the incidence in the population at large is only 0.2 percent (Hopkins, 1954).

Recessive sensorineural deafness without associated defects is very common and may be either static or progressive. The hearing loss is usually equal in both ears.

a. Recessive congenital severe deafness

Individuals with this disorder have severe, often total loss of hearing as the result of recessive transmission (Hopkins and Guilder, 1949; Stevenson and Cheeseman, 1956; Konigsmark, 1971). About 20 to 40 percent of all cases of early total deafness appear to be of autosomal recessive origin (Sank, 1963; Fraser, 1972).

One study showed caloric tests of vestibular function to be normal (Mengel et al., 1969). Several different genes are obviously involved in producing the same phenotype of congenital deafness, for paired deaf parents with pedigrees for autosomal recessive deafness may have normal hearing children (Lehmann, 1950; Stevenson and Cheeseman, 1956).

Studies on the temporal bones of individuals presumed to have recessive hereditary severe deafness have shown severe atrophy of the structures of the cochlear duct and moderate loss of cochlear neurons (Nager, 1925; Gray and Nelson, 1926).

b. High-tone deafness

This type of loss may be present at birth or begin in early childhood and is slowly progressive, often resulting in severe deafness in old age. The histopathological changes consist of atrophy of the organ of Corti and cochlear neurons, most severe in the basal end of the cochlea (Crowe et al., 1934).

c. Mid-tone deafness

Patients with mid-tone deafness have audiometric patterns showing bilateral symmetrical V-shaped or basin-shaped patterns. Speech discrimination usually is relatively good considering the magnitude of threshold elevation, and the hearing loss is not progressive (Fig. 4.6). There are no reported temporal bone studies from such individuals.

d. Albinism and deafness

The generalized form of albinism associated with deafness is inherited as an autosomal recessive trait. There is fair skin, fine silky hair, absence of pigment in the iris, sclera, and fundus, refractive errors, nystagmus, photophobia, and strabismus, as well as sensorineural deafness of varying severity.

Partial albinism and deafness (Ziprowski et al., 1962) and piebaldness and deafness (Reed, 1967) occur by sex-linked inheritance.

e. Hurler's syndrome (Gargoylism); (skeletal deformity, mental deficiency, blindness, hepatomegaly, splenomegaly, deafness)

Hurler (1920) first fully described this disorder, recognizing its hereditary feature, and considering it to be a skeletal growth disturbance. The disease begins in early childhood, causing skeletal deformity, failure of mental development, corneal opacities, enlargement of the liver and spleen, and sometimes deafness. It is an autosomal recessive hereditary disorder of mucopolysaccharide metabolism with production, storage, and urinary excretion of chrondroitin sulfate (B) and heparitin sulfate and cerebral storage of three gangliosides, GM_3, GM_2 and GM_1. MacBrinn et al. (1969) have found a deficiency of B-galactosidase in these patients. When sex-linked (X-chromosomal recessive) it is termed Hunter's syndrome. Deafness usually is more severe in Hunter's than in Hurler's syndrome (Gorlin and Sedano, 1968).

The head may be large, the forehead low and covered with fine hair, the nasal bridge sunken, and the nostrils flared. The interocular distance is increased; the ears set low and far back on the head. The tongue is large and thick and the teeth widely separated and poorly formed. The abdomen is usually protuberant because of an enlarged liver and spleen. There is retardation in the development of motor skills and, during the first two or three years of life, the cornea begins to cloud with progressive loss of vision. Because of failure to develop normal stature, the individual remains dwarfed (Zellweger et al., 1952). Deafness, when present, is usually mild and of the combined sensorineural and conductive type. The conductive component is due in part to seromucinous otitis media secondary to malfunction of the eustachian tube (Fig. 4.7).

Zechner and Altmann (1968) studied the temporal bones from a 19-year-old boy and reported finding thick middle ear mucosa containing many large cells with foamy cytoplasm which was PAS positive (gargoyle cells).

f. Hypophosphatasia

Hypophosphatasia, named by Rathbun in 1948, is a rare genetically deter-

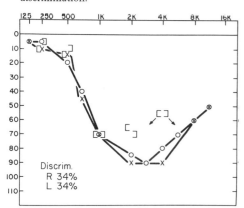

Fig. 4.6: Severe midfrequency congenital hearing loss (basin-shaped audiogram). This case with a severe threshold loss shows a moderately severe loss of speech discrimination. Individuals showing less severe threshold losses characteristically exhibit excellent speech discrimination.

mined metabolic disease characterized by decreased mineralization of bone, lowered serum and tissue alkaline phosphatase activity, and increased urinary excretion of phosphoethanolamine.

Nomura and Mori (1968) reported the temporal bone findings in a full-term infant, born to consanguinous parents, who died one hour after birth. The skeleton was soft, and decalcification was not necessary for temporal bone sectioning. The bone was similar to that of rickets, consisting of acidophilic osteoid tissue and bone marrow which contained many lymphocytes. The membranous labyrinth appeared normal. There was a dense, homogeneously staining area within the spiral ligament beneath the stria vascularis, throughout the upper basal turns. The areas were PAS-positive, stained blue with Azan, showed no metachromasia with toluidine blue, and were iron-negative with Hale's colloid stain. This material was interpreted to be either an area of hyaline degeneration or calcification. There appears to be no clear explanation for this deposit (Fig. 4.8).

g. Hyperphosphatasia

Hereditary hyperphosphatasia is a rare disorder characterized by progressive skeletal deformities which become apparent in the second or third year of life resulting in dwarfing and cranial nerve involvement, severe progressive

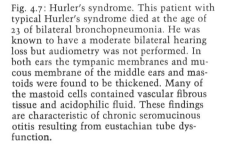

Fig. 4.7: Hurler's syndrome. This patient with typical Hurler's syndrome died at the age of 23 of bilateral bronchopneumonia. He was known to have a moderate bilateral hearing loss but audiometry was not performed. In both ears the tympanic membranes and mucous membrane of the middle ears and mastoids were found to be thickened. Many of the mastoid cells contained vascular fibrous tissue and acidophilic fluid. These findings are characteristic of chronic seromucinous otitis resulting from eustachian tube dysfunction.

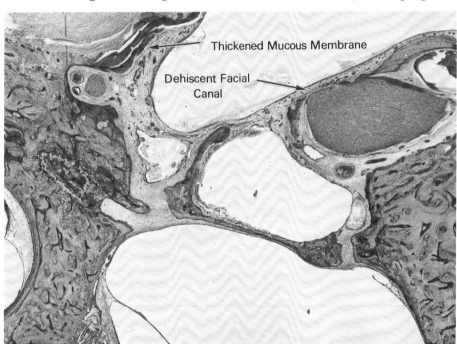

Thickened Mucous Membrane

Dehiscent Facial Canal

Fig. 4.8: Hypophosphatasia in an infant. A dense PAS positive deposit is found within the spiral ligament beneath the stria vascularis (Courtesy of Nomura)

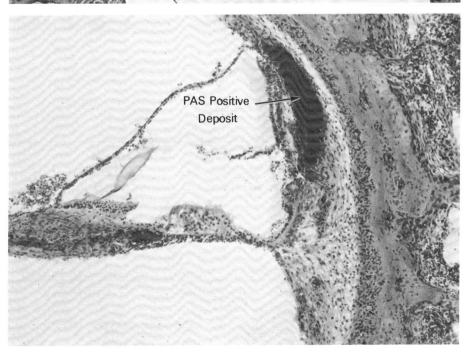

PAS Positive Deposit

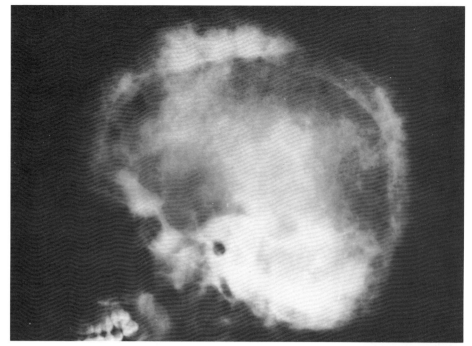

Fig. 4.9: Hyperphosphatasia in a 19-year-old girl. The diffuse "cotton balling" of the skull resembles changes seen in Paget's disease. She had a progressive hearing loss from the age of 14, and when tested at the age of 19 had bone conduction thresholds of about 20 db and air conduction thresholds of 70 to 80 db. (Courtesy of Thompson, Jr.)

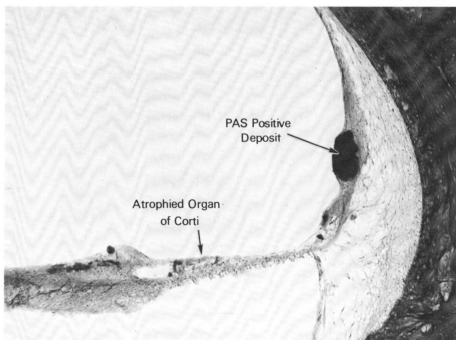

PAS Positive
Deposit

Atrophied Organ
of Corti

Fig. 4.10: Syndrome of Jervell—Lange-Nielsen. This female patient was profoundly deaf from birth and at the age of 18 months began having attacks of syncope. She had about two attacks per year until age 4, after which they became more frequent. ECG revealed prolongation of the Q-T interval. She died during a syncopal attack at the age of 12. Examination of the temporal bones reveals atrophy of the auditory and vestibular sense organs. There are large PAS positive deposits in the membranous labyrinth, particularly in the stria vascularis. (Courtesy of I. Friedmann)

combined deafness, and elevated serum concentrations of alkaline and acid phosphatase with normal concentrations of calcium and phosphorus. It is apparently transmitted as an autosomal recessive trait. Thompson et al. (1969) demonstrated in these cases a rapid turnover of lamellar bone with a failure to lay down compact cortical bone. The etiology of the deafness is not known as no temporal bone studies have been made (Fig. 4.9).

h. *Jervell–Lange-Nielsen syndrome (cardiac conduction anomaly and deafness*

Jervell and Lange-Nielsen (1957) first reported a syndrome observed in four children of a family of six in Scandinavia, characterized by congenital deafness, syncopal attacks, prolonged Q-T interval in the ECG, and sudden death occurring early in life. In none of these cases could the usual causes for prolonged Q-T interval be demonstrated.

In the decade following the first case report, 19 additional cases have been described. The hearts of several of these patients have shown abnormal fibrosis, infarction, hemorrhage, and degeneration of fibers of the sinu-atrial node (Fraser et al. 1964).

Studies of the temporal bones of three patients were made by Friedmann et al. (1966, 1968). They found atrophy of the organ of Corti, spiral ganglion, and cristae, and large PAS-positive hyaline deposits throughout the membranous labyrinths, particularly in the striae vasculares and cristae (Fig. 4.10). The incidence of this disorder in Britain is estimated to be three or four cases per million births.

i. Pendred's syndrome (sporadic goiter and deafness)

Pendred (1896) first reported the combination of goiter and deafness in two sisters. The deafness was severe and had been present since infancy, and the goiters were first noted at about the age of 13. One sister was mentally deficient, and both had normal body builds. Brain (1927) discovered 12 individuals who were deaf from birth and developed goiters in childhood. Deraemaeker (1956), Thieme (1957), and Elman (1958) described similar findings in single families. Fraser et al. (1961) reported the findings in 113 individuals from 72 families.

Present evidence favors the view that the goiter is a response to an enzymatic defect in the thyroid. Many patients with Pendred's syndrome who have undergone partial thyroidectomy have subsequently developed recurrent goiter.

Deafness is bilateral and sensorineural in type with a greater loss of hearing for the high frequencies. Nilsson et al. (1964) demonstrated recruitment in some patients suggesting that the lesion is in the cochlea. They found that thyroid function was characterized by a defect in the organic binding of iodine as shown by decreased radioactivity over the thyroid following administration of perchlorate in the radio-iodine test. On treatment with thyroxin, the goiter diminished in all of their patients and disappeared in some.

Illum et al. (1972) defined Pendred's syndrome as a triad consisting of congenital sensorineural hearing loss, goiter, and an abnormal perchlorate test. By polytomographic roentgenography, they found that seven of fourteen cases exhibited the Mundini type of otic dysplasia.

The incidence of Pendred's syndrome in Sweden has been estimated at one in 50,000 school children. The syndrome occurs as a recessive inherited disease. Studies show a high incidence of various thyroid disorders among relatives in previous generations suggesting a predisposition to thyroid disease in presumed heterozygotes.

There are no temporal bone reports on patients with Pendred's syndrome.

j. Usher's syndrome (retinitis pigmentosa and deafness)

Although von Graefe (1858) was the first to describe this syndrome, it is usually termed Usher's syndrome because Usher (1914) presented a more extensive study of this disorder. His report of 69 cases of retinitis pigmentosa revealed 11 with profound deafness and 19 with some degree of hearing loss. The most extensive study to date is that of Hallgren (1959) who reported the findings of 177 affected individuals and geneologically traced 5,327 ancestors.

Retinitis pigmentosa is usually diagnosed about the age of ten years because of a suspicion of night blindness or contraction of the fields of vision. The loss of vision is progressive, and about one-half of the patients reaching the age of 50 are totally blind.

The hearing loss is of the sensorineural type (Vernon, 1969; McLeod et al., 1971) (Fig. 4.11). It is present at birth and often first discovered between the ages of 1 and 2 years. In Sweden the overall incidence of the syndrome is about 3 in 100,000 accounting for about 3 percent of all congenitally deaf individuals. About 85 percent of affected individuals eventually become totally deaf and the remainder have varying degrees of hearing loss (Hallgren, 1959).

Vestibulo-cerebellar ataxia is present in a high percentage of those who have severe deafness. The ataxia is described as a falling gait suggestive of alcoholic intoxication. There are no spastic signs and no other cerebellar signs. Caloric responses are diminished in most patients with gait disturbances, but are normal in those with only partial hearing loss and no gait disturbances

Fig. 4.11: Usher's syndrome (retinitis pigmentosa and deafness). Audiogram of a 29-year-old man with progressive deafness and blindness.

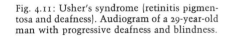
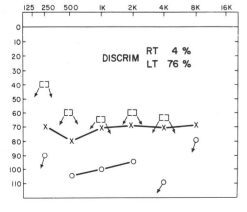

(Wagemann, 1960–1961). Spontaneous nystagmus was present in 7 percent of Hallgren's patients. The ataxia and the nystagmus probably are due to the combined loss of vestibular function and blindness. Hallgren found mental retardation in 23.8 percent and psychosis (usually paranoid reaction) in 23 percent.

Wagemann (1960–1961) also found diminished or absent caloric responses and sensorineural hearing losses which were worse for the high frequencies.

Kloepfer et al. (1966) studied hereditary hearing impairment in a three-parish area of Louisiana and found severe hearing impairment in 114 of 485 clinically tested individuals of which 44 had retinitis pigmentosa. They found the syndrome to be the result of an autosomal recessive gene defect with 100 percent penetrance.

No informative temporal bone studies have been made in these cases to date.

k. Cockayne's syndrome (dwarfism, retinal atrophy, deafness)

Cockayne (1936, 1946) has described a syndrome of dwarfism with retinal atrophy and deafness. The condition has its onset during the second year of life after a normal infancy.

Characteristics of the syndrome include dwarfism with kyphosis and ankylosis, disproportionately long extremeties and large hands and feet, a lack of subcutaneous fat of the face with prognathism, sunken eyes and thin nose giving a prematurely senile appearance, mental deficiency, sensitivity of skin to sunlight with pigmentation and scarring, retinal degeneration with pigmentation, optic atrophy, cataract, cold blue extremities, unsteady gait, thickened skull bones, carious teeth, and hearing loss (MacDonald et al., 1960).

Neill and Dingwall (1950) found a similar condition in two brothers who had, in addition, coarse tremor, enlargement of the liver and spleen, prominent ears, arteriosclerosis, intracranial calcification, and poor pupillary response to mydriatrics.

This syndrome differs from progeria because of its familial incidence, the presence of mental retardation and retinal pigmentation, and normal values for serum lipids and cholesterol.

Civantos (1963) described the trisomy F. chromosome in one patient but Windmiller et al. (1963) found a normal karyo-type in a case of Cockayne's syndrome.

No temporal bone studies have been made. The hearing loss is bilateral, sensorineural, and progressive.

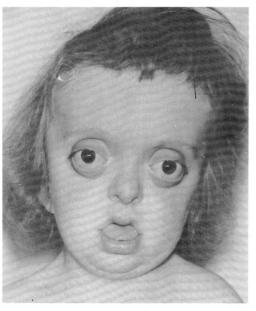

Fig. 4.12: Six-year-old female child with Crouzon's syndrome. Note exophthalmos, hypertelorism, and underveloped maxillae. She had an IQ of 110 and a 60 db purely conductive hearing loss. (Courtesy of Baldwin)

B. HEREDITARY DEAFNESS, PREDOMINANTLY CONDUCTIVE, OCCURRING IN SYNDROMES

There are many inherited syndromes in which deafness, predominantly conductive, occurs in combination with other characteristic developmental defects. These syndromes usually are identified by the name of the individual who provided the first complete description of the disorder and recognized it as an entity.

1. CROUZON'S SYNDROME (CRANIO-FACIAL DYSOSTOSIS)

Crouzon's syndrome, Crouzon, (1912) is characterized by exophthalmos, divergent squint, under-developed maxillae, deformity around the sagittal suture and bregma, short upper lip, hypertelorism, parrot-beak nose, and deafness (Fig. 4.12). It appears to be transmitted as a dominant character with a heterozygous genetic pattern (Lake and Kuppinger, 1950).

The deafness is usually of the conductive type due to anomalies of the middle ear and atresia of the external auditory canal (Wiegand, 1954). Attempts to widen the natural suture lines of the skull by surgical measures have met with some success (King, 1942).

The temporal bone findings were first reported by Nager (1936) and the characteristic features were described in detail in a recent report by Baldwin (1968) (Figs. 4.13, 4.14).

2. KLIPPEL-FEIL SYNDROME *

Klippel and Feil in 1912 described a syndrome characterized by congenital fusion of two or more cervical vertebrae and manifested by shortening of the neck, a low hair line posteriorly, and restricted movement of the head and neck. Other anomalies which may occur are high scapulae, spina bifida, facial asymmetry, torticollis, cervical rib, meningocele, cleft palate, vascular and pulmonary anomalies, and deafness. Galladeau (1936) described 20 cases of which 18 were female and 30 percent were deaf mutes. McLay and Maran (1969) reported the findings in three patients, two of whom had profound unilateral deafness and one profound bilateral deafness. Examination of one temporal bone of the individual with bilateral deafness revealed deformed ankylosed ossicles and a vestigial inner ear having a rudimentary cystic cavity representing the cochlea and only one incomplete semicircular canal.

Fig. 4.13: Photomicrograph of the temporal bone of a two-year-old child with Crouzon's syndrome. The tympanic membrane is missing, and the medial part of the external auditory canal is obliterated with fibrous tissue. The mucous membrane is thickened, and the oval window is narrowed. The stapes has dense crura bent anteriorly and a small fibrous intercrural space. The malleus and incus were found to be ankylosed to the lateral epitympanic wall. The membranous labyrinth is normal. Reported by Nager (1936). (Courtesy of Rüedi)

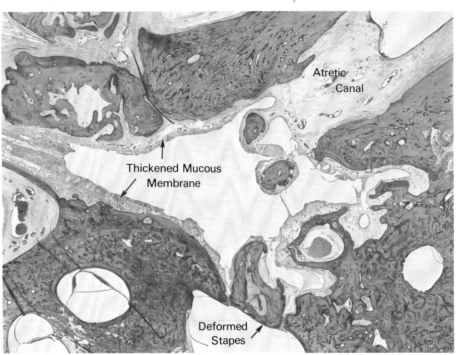

Fig. 4.14: This view shows the oval window area in an infant, age three weeks, with Crouzon's syndrome. The stapes is bent anteriorly, and the posterior wall of the middle ear is displaced anteriorly. Reported by Nager (1936). (Courtesy of Rüedi)

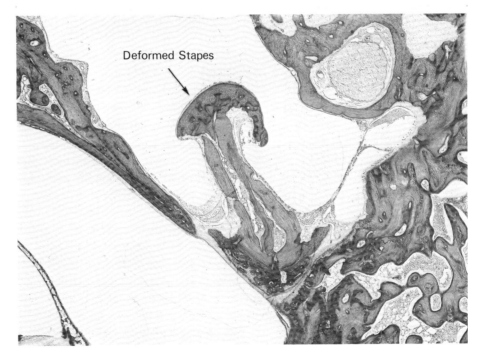

3. MARFAN'S SYNDROME (ARACHNODACTYLY, ECTOPIA LENTIS, DEAFNESS)

Marfan in 1896 described a syndrome consisting of arachnodactyly (sometimes also scoliosis, pigeon breast, flat feet, hammer toe, doliococephaly, high arched palate), ectopia lentis (dislocation of the lens), hypotonic muscles and laxity of joints, anomalies of the heart and lungs, and deafness.

The hearing loss may be of the conductive type due to mesodermal anomalies characterized by large soft auricles without cartilaginous support (Ganther, 1927; Everberg, 1959). Others have reported an associated sensorineural deafness (Brock, 1929; Schilling, 1936).

Kelemen (1965) studied the temporal bones of an 11-month-old infant with Marfan's syndrome and found normal inner ear structures.

Death is usually due to cardiac complications, particularly aortic dilatation, dissection, and rupture, and involvement of the aortic and mitral valves. The average age at the time of death is 32 years (Murdoch et al., 1972).

4. FRANCESCHETTI, TREACHER COLLINS SYNDROME (MANDIBULO-FACIAL DYSOSTOSIS)

A London ophthalmologist, G. A. Berry (1888) first described three patients having congenital defects of the lower eyelids, and two years later, his colleague, E. Treacher Collins (1900) described cases having, in addition, defective development of the malar bones. It was the Swiss physicians, Franceschetti and Zwahlen (1944) who first fully described the syndrome of mandibulo-facial dysostosis.

Among the explanations for the cause of the syndrome have been poor nutrition, intra-uterine abuse, irradiation, faulty chromosomes, drugs, and pressure on the fetus (Mall, 1917; Granrud, 1953; Herberts, 1962; Snyder, 1956).

The familial occurrence has been well established (McKenzie, 1958; Brohm and Kluska, 1947), and it seems most logical that the syndrome is an arrest in development most likely transmitted as an irregular dominant gene and affecting the embryo between the fifth and ninth month of gestation. It would seem reasonable to consider the syndrome as an independent genotypic entity which follows the irregular dominant form of transmission. Brohm and Kluska (1947) and Harrison (1957) showed intrafamilial variability with increasing severity in succeeding generations.

Whereas Mann (1943) has stated that the syndrome is due to retardation of differentiation of the maxillary mesoderm, this explanation is not sufficiently inclusive to account for all features of the syndrome. Harrison (1957) has pointed out, for example, that the syndrome involves not only the maxillary process but also the mandibular and hyoid arches as manifested by the occasional occurrences of cleft lip and palate and stapedial abnormalities. The most significant abnormalities, however, are due to congenital deformities arising from structures of the first branchial arch or Meckel's cartilage. Some have divided the syndrome into various classifications, depending upon the number of abnormalities and their severity. A profile view of these individuals reveals a diminished fronto-nasal angle, receding mandible, and relatively prognathic maxilla creating a fish or bird-like appearance. The most striking feature affecting the eyes is the antimongoloid slant or obliquity of the palpebral fissure, and notching at the junction of the middle and lateral thirds of the lower eyelids. The lower lid is thin and atrophic with underdeveloped or absent orbicularis oculi muscle, and occasionally the punctum is lacking. The arrested development of the zygoma together with faulty development of the maxilla accounts for the defective lower margins of the orbit. The mandible is hypoplastic, though this feature may be lacking in incomplete cases. Developmental defects which affect the maxilla consist of small or absent antra and a high arched or cleft palate. There may be an abnormal growth of hair from the temporal area toward the cheeks. In addition, some cases exhibit blind fistulae midway between the corners of the mouth and the auricles. The nose may be large with a short columella, small lateral cartilages, narrow external nares, and bulbous tip. The teeth may be anomalous in number and position. Although the general appearance of the patients with the syndrome suggests that they are mentally retarded, such is not the case.

The auricle may be completely missing, rudimentary, or normal. When there is hypoplasia of the mandible, the auricles often are located more inferiorly. The external auditory canal may be normal but usually it is stenotic or atretic, and when the tympanic membrane is present, it is usually abnormal in shape. More often the medial part of the external auditory canal is replaced by a plate of bone, and the middle ear space is small and contains a deformed and ankylosed malleus and a fused incudomalleal articulation. Fernandez and Ronis (1964), Holborow (1961), Herberts (1962), and McKenzie (1958) all found abnormalities of the stapes. The mastoid often is poorly pneumatized and the facial nerve may pursue an anomalous course. Associated anomalies of the vestibular labyrinth are frequent. Absence of canals has been reported by Herberts (1962), Livingstone (1959), and Harrison (1957). Sando et al. (1968) reported the histological findings in an infant with the fully developed syndrome. In addition to atresia of the external auditory canals and middle ear anomalies, they found in one ear an enlarged utricle and absence of the lateral semicircular canal. The cochleae were normal. Ruben et al. (1969) reported the histological findings in a patient with associated renal abnormalities.

The results of surgery for the correction of deafness have been variable. The correction of atresia with a small or absent middle ear space presents major surgical problems. Improvement in hearing can be achieved in carefully selected patients and consists of creating an external auditory canal and establishing a sound transmission system via either the oval window or a surgical fenestra of the lateral semicircular canal. The difficulties of surgical correction have been described by Gill (1969) and Schuknecht (1974).

5. PIERRE ROBIN SYNDROME

This syndrome is characterized by cleft palate, micrognathia and glossoptosis, as well as anomalies of the heart, blood vessels, skeletal system, eyes and ears. About 20 percent of the patients exhibit severe mental retardation. At birth the facies is striking, showing a small symmetrically receded mandible producing an "Andy Gump" appearance. Respiratory difficulty is obvious from the beginning as the tongue without support falls downward and backward to obstruct the airway. These individuals have low-set ears, deformed pinna, and conductive hearing loss (Smith and Stowe, 1961). The syndrome occurs in about one in thirty thousand live births and is thought to be inherited as an autosomal dominant with variable penetrance.

6. OTHER HEREDITARY DISORDERS CAUSING CONDUCTIVE DEAFNESS

Osteopetrosis (Albers-Schonberg disease, marble bone disease) is a rare bone disorder of otologic interest because of the high incidence of facial paralysis and hearing loss. It occurs in both a clinically benign dominantly inherited form and in a malignant recessively inherited form. (See Chapter 10E Osteopetrosis)

Otosclerosis is a common disease of the bony labyrinth causing hearing loss due to fixation of the stapes. The evidence favors an autosomal dominant inheritance with variable expressivity (Morrison and Bundey, 1970). (See Chapter 10A Otosclerosis)

Osteogenesis imperfecta is characterized by blue sclerae, fragile bones, and deafness transmitted as an autosomal dominant character with extreme variation in genetic expressivity. The lesion of the bony labyrinth appears identical to that of otosclerosis. (See Chapter 10C Osteogenesis imperfecta)

C. DEAFNESS CAUSED BY NOXIOUS PRENATAL INFLUENCES

There has been intensive study in recent years on noxious prenatal influences which cause birth defects. The discussion which follows is limited in scope but includes several well-known causes of congenital deafness.

1. MATERNAL RUBELLA

In 1941 Gregg reported the occurrence of congenital cataracts in infants born to mothers having rubella during early pregnancy. Subsequently, numerous studies have shown that maternal rubella may cause many congenital defects including cataracts, patent ductus arteriosus and other cardiovascular defects, hearing loss, microcephaly, dental defects, and a general stunting of growth and development. Swan et al. (1943) first reported deafness from maternal rubella, and subsequently Carruthers (1945) described 116 patients with severe deafness out of 147 having congenital defects following maternal rubella. Hiller (1950) found 32 cases of maternal rubella deafness among 42 congenitally deaf children in Tasmania.

Barr and Lundström (1961) elicited a history of maternal rubella in 12 percent of 752 deaf children in Sweden. Typically these children exhibited hearing losses characterized by rather flat audiometric patterns. The degree of hearing loss usually differed considerably in the two ears. Of approximately 220,000 children born in Sweden in 1951 and 1952, .07 percent had severe hearing loss, whereas in children with histories of maternal rubella 4 to 8 percent had severe hearing loss.

In an outbreak of rubella in Taiwan in 1957, 25 percent of pregnant women had births with tragic outcomes attributable to the disease (Grayston et al., 1967). Monif et al. (1966) showed that defects may occur with maternal rubella in the second trimester as well as in the first and isolated the rubella virus from the products of conception. Auditory deficits occurred in 6 of 27 live-born children of mothers having rubella in the first and second trimester. Karmody (1968, 1969) demonstrated a great increase in congenital deafness in Trinidad occurring during an epidemic in 1960 and 1961, and suggested that many resulted from asymptomatic maternal infections.

Schall et al. (1951), in a study of 4½ month-old fetuses from mothers having maternal rubella in the first trimester, found evidence of hemorrhage but no definite abnormality of the cochlear ducts. Nager (1952), Lindsay et al. (1953), Hemenway et al. (1969) and Lindsay (1973a, 1973b) have found cochleo-saccular aplasia to be the cause of the sensorineural hearing loss

Fig. 4.15: Maternal rubella. The organ of Corti is slightly flattened, and the hair cells are missing. The tectorial membrane is rounded, retracted into the inner sulcus and partially encapsulated. (Courtesy of Sando)

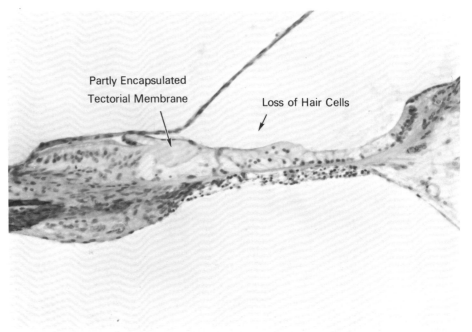

Partly Encapsulated Tectorial Membrane

Loss of Hair Cells

(Fig. 4.15). Middle ear anomalies are less frequent. In a histological study of the temporal bones of an infant with the rubella syndrome, Sando and Wood (1971) found an anomalous stapes having a thickened capitulum and crura and cartilaginous fixation of the footplate.

Major progress is being made toward the development of a live attenuated rubella virus vaccine (Weibel et al., 1969; Hilleman et al., 1968), and control of this problem appears imminent (Bordley and Hardy, 1969; Sever, 1973).

2. BIRTH INJURIES

The role which birth injuries play in the causation of deafness has not yet been clearly determined. It has long been suspected that auditory disorders at the time of birth may be caused by prematurity, prolonged gestation, prolonged labor, difficult labor, Caesarian delivery, breech delivery, placenta previa, toxemia of pregnancy, the use of sedatives and anesthetic drugs during labor, and asphyxia neonatorum. Vernon (1967a) found that 17 percent of deaf school-age children were premature and that the lower the birth weight of a premature child the greater is the probability of deafness.

In a study of 161 severely handicapped children, Barr and Klockhoff (1959) found 17 percent with hearing defects. Among children with cerebral palsy, the incidence was 10.5 percent in the spastic group and 68 percent in the athetoid group. The hearing losses were of the sensorineural type, but the location of the lesions was not precisely determined. The relationship of difficult labor to auditory disorders in young children has been mentioned by Myklebust (1954), Windle et al. (1944), Doll et al. (1932), Moloy (1942) and Strauss and Werner (1943). Zonderman (1959) found that prematurity, traumatic labor, and cyanosis at birth occurred in 15 percent of 328 congenitally deaf children. Many of these authors believe the auditory damage is caused by anoxia.

Although the incidence of hearing loss is higher in children born of difficult or complicated births of prematurity, a causal relationship has not been clearly established. The cochlea and auditory pathways actually appear to be less susceptible to anoxic injury than the neopallium. For example, deafness is not a complication of severe anoxic states in adults suffering nonfatal cardiac arrest or suffocation, even though severe brain injury may have occurred.

3. HYPERBILIRUBINEMIA (ERYTHROBLASTOSIS FETALIS)

The principal manifestations in erythroblastosis fetalis are hemolytic anemia, icterus, hydrops, deafness, and encephalopathy. The latter manifestation is the most serious in that there may be mental retardation, emotional instability, muscular spasticity of the extrapyramidal type, choreoathetosis, and convulsive seizures. Vernon (1967b) found that over 70 percent of children with deafness of this cause have multiple handicaps and that psychodiagnostic measures revealed a high incidence of central nervous system dysfunction. The principal etiology of the syndrome has been found to be maternal Rh incompatibility (mother, Rh negative; child, Rh positive). Occasionally an incompatibility of the A or B factors may also cause erythroblastosis. Severe systemic hemolysis results in an intense concentration of circulating bilirubin.

In 1875, Orth noted the association of severe jaundice in newborn infants with yellow pigmentation of the basal ganglia, and in 1904 Schmorl proposed the term *kernicterus*. In 1932, Diamond et al. came to the conclusion that diffuse edema of the fetus, familial icterus gravis neonatorum, and anemia of the newborn were expressions of the same pathologic process and represented an entity which subsequently has been known as erythroblastosis fetalis. In 1940 Landsteiner and Wiener discovered the rhesus factor which provided the basis for a better understanding of the etiology of this disorder.

Coquette (1944) first observed deaf mutism in a child with rigidity of the lower extremities following icterus gravis. Goodhill (1950) studied congenitally deaf children of Rh negative mothers and proposed that kernicterus resulted in injury to the cochlea or auditory neural pathways. Asher (1952) studied 63 cases of athetosis and found a history of neonatal jaundice in 34 and Rh iso-immunization in 22. There were hearing losses in 24 of the 34 jaundiced infants. The hearing losses were bilateral, sensorineural, and most severe for the high frequencies. By contrast, hearing losses were found in only four of the 18 non-jaundiced athetoid children. Dublin (1951) studied the brains of seven newborn infants having erythroblastosis fetalis and showed that the golden pigment, which was best seen in frozen sections, was not bilirubin because it failed to turn green when reduced in formaldehyde solution. He believed anoxia to be the cause of cerebral injury because the distribution of lesions appeared to be the same as that of other anoxic disorders such as asphyxia from carbon monoxide toxicity. Both Dublin (1951) and Gerrard (1952) described degenerative changes in the auditory neural pathways of individuals with icterus who died in the neonatal period. Kelemen (1956) examined the temporal bones of a three-day-old newborn infant who died from erythroblastosis fetalis but was unable to detect any specific changes which might be related to the disorder.

Based on audiometric findings, the auditory lesion must quite clearly be located in the cochlea, for the audiometric patterns consistently exhibit the characteristics of sensory lesions (author's observations, unpublished data). (Fig. 4.16)

Methods of prophylaxis and improved management of neonatal hyperbilirubinemia has almost eliminated this disorder as a cause of deafness. Maternal Rh antibody formation can be reduced by administration in the immediate postpartum period of an immunoglobulin G obtained from the plasma of highly sensitized Rh negative donors. During pregnancy, suspect mothers can be monitored for antibody titers, and in the presence of rising titers an amniocentesis and spectrophotometric evaluation of the level of bilirubin-like pigment can be done. If the level is high, early parturition or intra-uterine transfusions may be performed. For a fully developed reaction in the newborn, the treatment consists of exchange transfusions using low titer O-negative donor blood. The most widely accepted indication for exchange transfusion is a serum bilirubin level above 20 mg per 100 ml (Comley and Wood, 1968; Lucey, 1968; Freda and Bowe, 1969).

4. DRUGS

a. Thalidomide malformations

The teratogenic effects of drugs has become a matter of great concern, particularly since the catastrophic reactions to the tranquilizing drug, thalidomide, became apparent in 1962. The suspicion that thalidomide might be responsible for congenital anomalies as a consequence of ingestion of the drug by pregnant mothers was first reported by Lenz and Knapp (1962). The critical period when thalidomide ingestion by the mother may cause anom-

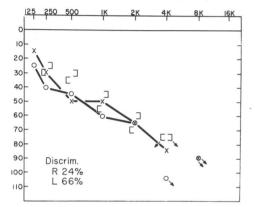

Fig. 4.16: Neonatal hyperbilirubinemia. Audiogram of a 21-year-old man who was born of an Rh negative mother and Rh positive father and was extremely jaundiced at birth with high serum bilirubin levels. He required several transfusions. He was apathetic and had episodic motor spasms as an infant. He exhibited delayed motor development, sitting at 12 months and walking at two years. First speech was noted at 3½ years, and his IQ was 72. The first child of his family died prematurely, and a later sibling had hydrocephalus.

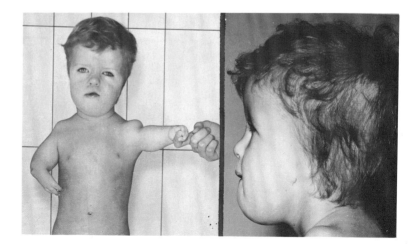

Fig. 4.17: Teratogenic drug induced (thalidomide) anomalies. This male was born in 1960 of a woman who ingested thalidomide during the first month of pregnancy. The child has upper limb phocomelia and abscence of auricles and auditory canals. Roentgenograms show deformed ossicles and labyrinths. Examination revealed total right facial palsy and partial left facial palsy, bilateral palatal paralysis, bilateral abducens nerve paralysis, and right oculomotor nerve paralysis. Tests revealed total absence of auditory and vestibular function. (Courtesy of Barr)

alies is generally between the 37th and 50th days after the last menstruation. In Sweden, the use of the drug for three years resulted in the birth of at least 150 abnormal children.

In addition to ectromelia (hypoplasia or aplasia of one or more limbs) (Fig. 4.17), thalidomide may produce malformations of the intestinal tract, urinary tract, heart, and ears. In 1963, Miehlke and Partsch reported the findings in 13 patients with deformities of the ears and paralyses of the facial and ab-ducens nerves. In 1964, d'Avignon and Barr reported on the otological find-ings in 100 of these children who were surviving at the time. They found all degrees of malformation of the auricles, external auditory canals, and middle ears and losses of auditory and vestibular function varying from mild to complete. In a histological study, Jorgensen et al. (1964) found total laby-rinthine aplasia in an infant born of a mother who received thalidomide dur-ing the first month of pregnancy. There was no trace of cavitation in the temporal bone or of differentiation of the labyrinthine capsule. The cochlear, vestibular, and facial nerves were totally missing. (See Chapter 6E, Thalido-mide Ototoxicity)

Livingstone (1965) found 75 percent of patients with ear deformities due to thalidomide to be satisfactory candidates for surgical reconstruction.

b. Quinine

The ingestion of quinine in malarial therapeutic doses by the mother dur-ing pregnancy may create profound deafness in the child while having no effect on the mother. Clinical studies of one family revealed that three chil-dren, whose gestation period occurred when their mother was taking quinine, showed severe bilateral deafness, whereas two other siblings, whose gestation occurred during periods of nonmedication, had normal hearing (author's ob-servation, unpublished data). A similar tragic family history was reported by Hart and Naunton (1963) in which case the mother had been treated with chloroquine phosphate. (See Chapter 6B, Quinine and Chloroquin Oto-toxicity)

5. CRETINISM

Cretinism was originally described as incorporating three salient features: (1) retarded body growth, (2) retarded mental development, and (3) combined (conductive and sensorineural) deafness.

This condition was found to exist in populations located in certain geo-graphic areas, accounting for the term endemic cretinism. Recently an en-demic goiter area in India was studied by Raman and Beierwaltes (1959), who found that, of 48 individuals, 21 had goiters, 17 had severe sensorineural deaf-ness, and 10 were mentally defective. The protein-bound-iodine levels were no lower than for other inhabitants of the village. Most individuals were small in stature.

In Northern Ireland, where neither congenital deafness nor goiter is en-demic, the prevalence of deaf mutism is 0.3 per 1000 inhabitants. On the other hand, in the Alps, Himalayas, and Andes, the prevalence of severe con-genital deafness is 20 per 1000 inhabitants, these areas being known as areas of endemic goiter. It appears that some endemic goiter areas are accompanied by a high prevalence of deafness, while others are not.

Endemic cretinism should not be confused with two sporadic syndromes to which the name "cretinism" has also been applied. These two syndromes are not associated with deafness. One is termed sporadic goiter cretinism in which a goiter is present and a congenital defect exists in the enzymatic proc-esses of the thyroid gland. The other is sporadic non-goiter cretinism, in which there is total failure of the thyroid to develop during fetal life, or the presence of only a small fragment of thyroid at the base of the tongue. Be-cause thyroid replacement therapy is successful in the management of these patients, these two syndromes can be attributed to hypothyroidism alone.

Severe sensorineural deafness in cretins seems to be associated with abnormality of the thyroid gland because it is found in areas where goiter is quite prevalent and because some of the features of endemic cretinism can be attributed to hypothyroidism. Nonetheless, the deafness cannot be the result of hypothyroidism operating during postnatal life, because it does not occur in sporadic cretins. It is possible that the auditory anomalies are due to hypothyroidism during fetal life where a goiterous mother with a low iodine intake would take needed iodine from the fetus. A genetic etiology seems ruled out as there is a case on record of endemic cretins who married and produced a normal child. The temporal bone pathology has been described by Nager (1926) (Figs. 4.18, 4.19, 4.20).

D. VARIFORM ANOMALIES

1. EXTERNAL AND MIDDLE EAR

a. Anomalies of the auricle

Auricular deformities and aplasias may occur in all degrees, from simple outstanding (prominent) ears due to absence of the antihelix, to severe aplasia (microtia). The more severe aplasias are often associated with atresia of the external auditory canal and sometimes are associated with middle ear anomalies (Wolff, 1964). Potter (1937) described malformations of the auricle occurring as a dominant hereditary trait through five generations in 92 individuals.

Pre-auricular appendages are small tags, sometimes containing a piece of cartilage, usually lying anterior to the auricle at the level of the supratragal incisura and often continuous with the anterior margin of the helix. The mode of heredity is dominant. Presumably, the pre-auricular appendages arise by excessive growth from the mandibular arch or by abnormal growth of skin covering the tubercles of the margin of this arch.

The *auricular pit* usually is located anterior to the auricle close to the anterior border of the ascending limb of the helix. It is not connected with the tympanic cavity, and its walls are microscopically ectodermal and of cutaneous character (Congdon et al., 1932). The pit probably arises from the ectodermal groove between the first and second visceral arches. Another theory proposes that the pit arises by failure of fusion of the tubercles of the margin of the first arch (Streeter, 1922). The pit may descend as far as the level of the inferior border of the tragus. It may contain glandular structures and often becomes infected, requiring surgical excision. Wildervanck (1962) described a family in which three generations had outstanding ears with auricular pits and pre-auricular appendages. Conductive deafness, presumably due to middle ear anomalies, was present in some of the patients.

b. Congenital aural atresia

Congenital atresia of the external auditory canal may be unilateral or bilateral and may occur alone or as part of a more complex syndrome. Altmann (1955) has made a study of the anatomical features in 59 temporal bones with this anomaly and developed the following classification:

> TYPE I (mild): A mild case is characterized by a small external auditory canal. The tympanic bone is hypoplastic and somewhat misshapen, and the tympanic membrane is smaller than normal. The tympanic cavity may be normal in size or small, and the middle ear structures may show malformations of varying degree. Squamous epithelium can be trapped medial to a bony or fibrous atresia of the external auditory canal, leading to cholesteatoma. Unless the condition becomes manifest and surgically corrected, the middle ear is invaded and infection usually ensues. (Author's personal experience; also Hoenk et al., 1969).

Fig. 4.18: Cretin, age 43. There is narrowing of the anteroposterior diameter of the middle ear cleft. The posterior wall of the middle ear is displaced anteriorly and is in contact with the incudostapedial joint, a characteristic deformity in cretins. The sensory and neural elements of the inner ear are normal. (Courtesy of Rüedi)

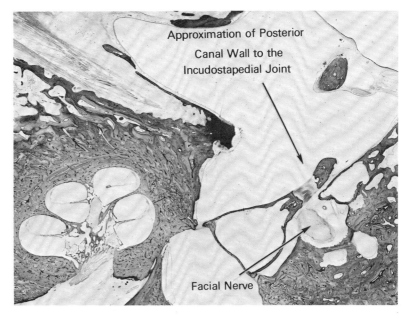

Fig. 4.19: Cretin, age 72. A characteristic finding in the cretin ear is failure of development of the round window niche. It appears as a narrow cleft filled with fibrous tissue. In this ear the organ of Corti and cochlear neurons are severely degenerated. (Courtesy of Rüedi)

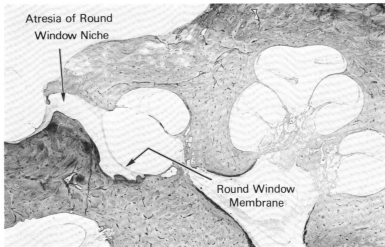

Fig. 4.20: Fixation of the anterior margin of the footplate in an endemic cretin. (Courtesy of Rüedi)

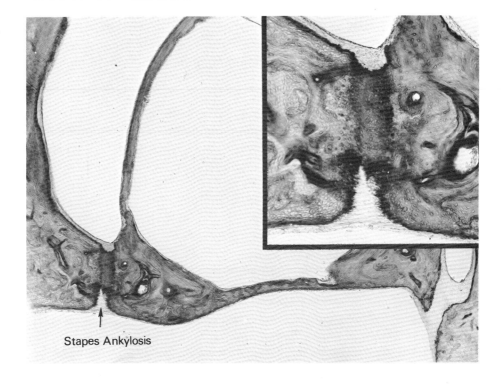

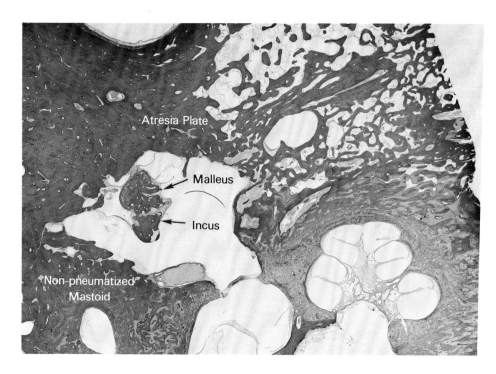

Fig. 4.21: Congenital atresia of the external auditory canal in a 64-year-old male. There is a large bony atresia plate, a small middle ear space, and a nonpneumatized mastoid. (Courtesy of Rüedi)

TYPE II (medium): The external auditory canal is absent, the tympanic cavity is diminished in size, and its contents deformed in varying degrees. The lateral wall of the tympanic cavity consists of an "atresia plate" which is either completely or partly osseous (Fig. 4.21). The tympanic bone, if present, is deformed and plate-like. Sometimes it contains, at its center, a layer of connective tissue which is continuous with the connective tissue occupying the place of the missing external auditory canal. The malleus is fixed and the incudomalleal articulation is fused (Fig. 4.22).

TYPE III (severe): The external auditory canal is absent, and the tympanic cavity is either very small or missing.

Congenital atresia exists in certain animals, such as the Norwegian sheep (Mohr, 1952–1953). The condition has been produced in newborn rats by injecting aqueous trypan blue solution into pregnant mothers on the 7th and 8th day of pregnancy (Gillman et al., 1948).

c. Persistent stapedial artery

About the fifth week of fetal life, the primordial tissues of the stapes area begin to form, and it is then that the stapedial artery is first seen in the obturator foramen of the stapes. The stapes anlage tissue appears to fold, thus changing the rounded lobe of stapes tissue into a ring-like structure. During the third month of fetal life the stapedial artery normally disappears in human ears. The artery arises from the internal carotid and after passing through the obturator foramen of the stapes it turns anteriorly and ends by branching into the supra-orbital, infra-orbital, and mandibular arteries which accompany the three divisions of the trigeminal nerve. Subsequently, an anastomotic branch develops between the external carotid and stapedial artery where it divides, and this anastomosis later becomes the internal maxillary artery. The incidence of occurrence of persistent stapedial artery apparently is about one in five thousand to ten thousand (House and Patterson, 1964; Scheer, 1968), and when it occurs, may be associated with other abnormalities (Altmann, 1957; Kelemen, 1958; Maran, 1965) (Fig. 4.23).

The persistent stapedial artery should not be confused with the small artery which normally is present on the footplate of the adult stapes (Davies, 1967).

d. Anomalies of the ossicles

Hough (1963) believes that the body of the incus and the head of the mal-

Fig. 4.22: Malleus and incus removed during the course of surgical reconstruction of the ear of a 21-year-old female with type II congenital aural atresia. The long and short processes of the incus are shorter than normal, the incudomalleal articulation is fused, the head of the malleus is deformed and was found to abut the atresia plate. The lateral process and manubrium of the malleus are missing.

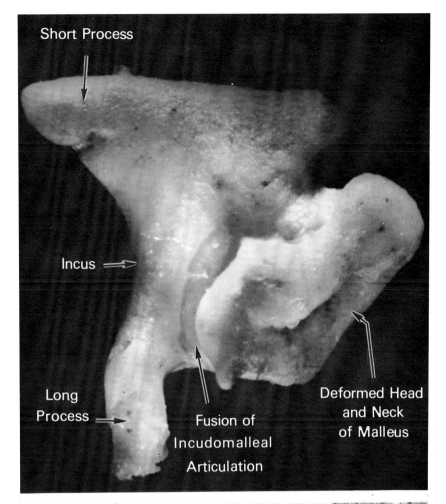

Fig. 4.23: Persistent stapedial artery in an 84-year-old patient. A coincident and probably unrelated condition was profound deafness from birth as the result of otitic labyrinthitis. A higher magnification of the stapedial artery is seen in the lower view.

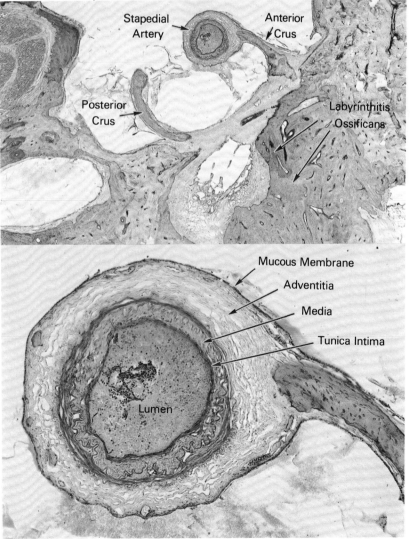

Fig. 4.24: Malleus ankylosis as an incidental autopsy finding in a 53-year-old male. No local inflammatory reaction or bone disease is evident. A higher magnification of the area of bony ankylosis is seen in the lower view.

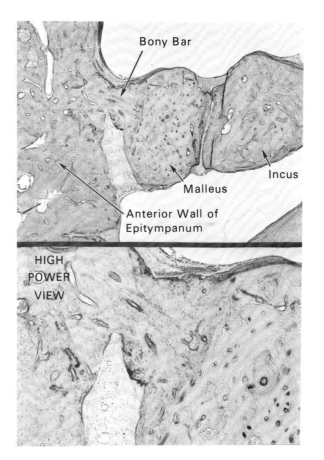

Fig. 4.25: Vertical section showing fibrous fixation of the head of the malleus to the superior wall of the epitympanum (tegmen tympani). The pars tensa shows extensive post-inflammatory pathology, there being a thick fibrous marginal ridge, a superior replacement membrane, and a large inferior perforation. Audiometric studies at the age of 79 revealed a combined sensorineural and conductive hearing loss in this ear. The findings in the opposite ear were nearly identical but without malleus fixation. The histological appearance does not provide a certain determination as to whether the malleus fixation is the result of inflammatory osteogenesis or a developmental defect. Same ear as Fig. 4.30. (Female, age 87)

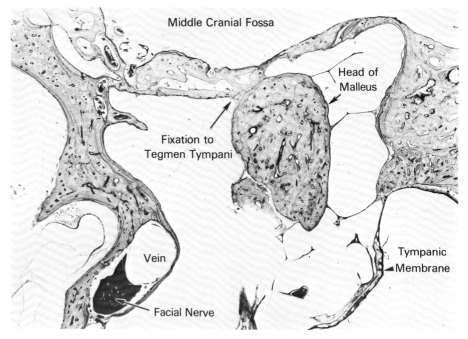

leus are derived from the first branchial arch, whereas the long process of the incus, manubrium of the malleus, capitulum and crural arches of the stapes are derived from the mesenchyme of the second branchial arch as well as the bridge of tissue between the two arches. Thus, the upper part of the ossicular chain is related to the first arch and the lower part to the second arch. This accounts for many of the malformations involving the ossicles.

Abnormal development of the superior part of the ossicular structures may result in fusion of the head of the malleus with the body of the incus, fixation of the head of the malleus to the epitympanic wall (Figs. 4.24, 4.25), and fixation of the short process of the incus to the incudal fossa.

Many cases of fixation of the head of the malleus have been reported (Ritter, 1971), some of which have been in conjunction with stapedial fixation

Fig. 4.26: Malleus fixation in a 60-year-old female who coincidentally had stapes fixation due to otosclerosis. There is a bar of bone fixing the head of the malleus to the anterior epitympanic wall. The cytoarchitecture of this bone is identical to that of the epitympanic wall. There is no evidence of inflammatory reaction, otosclerosis, Paget's disease, or other acquired bony disorder involving the malleus or epitympanic wall.

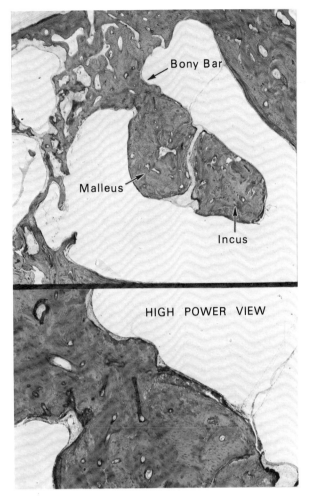

due to otosclerosis (Powers et al., 1967; Sleeckx et al., 1967; Guilford and Anson, 1967) (Fig. 4.26). Davies (1968) has shown that in normal temporal bones an anterior epitympanic bony spur usually is in close approximation to the head of the malleus. This spur is independent of the anterior process of the malleus and anterior malleal ligament. Goodhill (1966a, 1966b) has described techniques for the surgical management of the fixed malleus. He gives no indication as to whether his cases were congenital, hereditary, or acquired.

House (1956) presented three cases in which the short process of the incus was fixed in the incudal fossa. He pointed out that minor congenital abnormalities of the ossicular chain can be differentiated from otosclerosis by the history of conductive hearing loss existing in early childhood, lack of progression of the hearing loss, and a flat audiometric pattern. Abnormal development of the caudal part of the ossicular anlage may result in triple bony union of the manubrium of the malleus, long process of the incus, and head of the stapes.

The mesenchymal anlage cells of the long process of the incus normally grow toward the stapedial ring and fuse with the head of the stapes, thus forming the incudostapedial joint. The most common anomaly in this area consists of aplasia of the long process of the incus and the head of the stapes, occurring occasionally in association with aplasia of the manubrium of the malleus (Hough, 1963).

In the development of the bony labyrinth, precartilaginous cells develop into a hard, bony otic capsule, except in the vicinity of the stapes where exceptional cells are predestined to mold into the stapes footplate, termed the "stapedial lamina" by Anson and Bast (1959). Thus, the stapes footplate is histologically continuous with the marginal cartilaginous vestibular window and it is through the thinning out and specific differentiation of a marginal zone that the annular ligament is formed and the footplate becomes a separate mobile structure. By improper differentiation of the precartilaginous rest

Fig. 4.27: This patient had a 15 to 20 db conductive hearing loss in the right ear. Histological study shows cartilaginous fixation of the posterior margin of the footplate and is presumed to be of congenital origin.

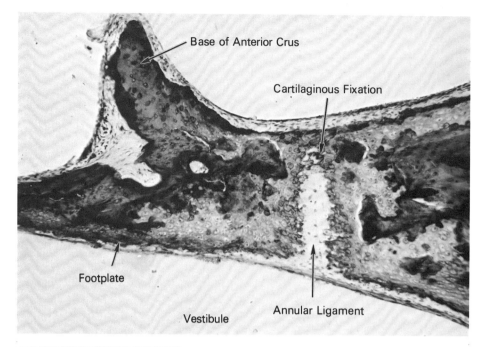

Fig. 4.28: This patient reported having a hearing loss in his left ear for as long as he could remember. He died at the age of 30 of renal failure. Histological studies of the left ear reveal the footplate to be fixed in the oval window by incomplete formation of the stapediovestibular joint. Except in a small posterior region, the footplate blends into the bony labyrinthine wall and is ankylosed to the facial canal by a continuum of lamellar bone. See Fig. 4.29.

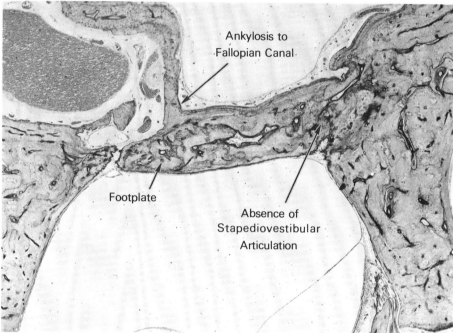

Fig. 4.29: Same ear as Fig. 4.28. The capitulum is well developed; however, the crural arch has been replaced by a thick column of bone which terminates in short thick crura. These crura contact the promontory inferior to the oval window and do not come in contact with the footplate.

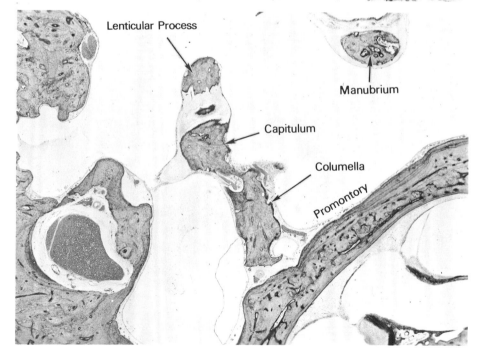

cells it is possible for osseous fixation of the footplate to occur, resulting in congenital stapes fixation (Figs. 4.27, 4.28, 4.29).

House et al. (1958) reported on 23 cases of congenital stapes footplate fixation discovered during surgical exploration of the middle ear. Lindsay et al. (1960) described a case with bilateral anomalies of the labyrinthine capsules in which there was solid bony ankylosis of the stapedial footplates without evidence of otosclerosis. Gerhardt and Otto (1970) found stapes malformations in 8 of 1000 patients undergoing surgery for conductive hearing loss and found that the reconstructive procedures now used for otosclerosis are quite successful in these cases. In 16 patients with congenital middle ear deform- ities which were subjected to surgical correction, Scheer (1967) found six with small mobile footplates and crurae which were replaced by columellae and three with normal-appearing fixed footplates.

Nakamura and Sando (1966) found three ears with congenital absence of the stapes and oval window, two of which also had absence of the round window. Total lack of differentiation of the footplate of the stapes has also been reported by Tabor (1961).

Congenital absence of the stapedial tendon is not uncommon, being found in about 1 percent of all ears operated on by Hough (1958) and 0.5 percent by Gerhardt and Otto (1970).

e. Anomalous internal carotid artery

The internal carotid artery may assume an anomalous course and enter the middle ear in the hypotympanum, then turn forward beneath the oval window to reach its normal position anterolateral to the cochlea. The patient may complain of pulsating tinnitus, and a bruit is often heard in the external auditory canal. Otoscopy reveals a reddish mass medial to the inferior part of the tympanic membrane. The nature of the mass is readily established by carotid angiography (Goldman et al., 1971), and by polytomographic roentgenograms (Ruggles and Reed, 1972).

f. Anomalies of the venous system

The veins which traverse the middle ear are more variable in size and course than are the arteries. Most of the veins are small and serve as one or more vena communicans accompanying the arteries. The most common anatomical variant is a large vein within the fallopian canal (Fig. 4.30).

It is not uncommon for the jugular bulb to lie in a superior position, placing it in juxtaposition with the tympanic membrane and round window niche (see Chapter 2A4, The Vascular System; Fig. 2.19). It may reach the manubrium to create a conductive hearing loss (author's observation, unpublished data).

The lateral venous sinus, like the other cranial venous sinuses, usually lies within split layers of the dura and presents a prominent bulge into the posterior part of the mastoid. Its location and size, however, is extremely variable. It may lie in an anterior position adjacent to the posterior aspect of the bony labyrinth, and in this position may interfere with surgical access to the endolymphatic sac (Fig. 4.31).

g. Salivary gland choristoma

Salivary gland choristoma of the middle ear in association with ossicular anomalies has been reported by Noguera and Haase (1964) and Caplinger and Hora (1967). A choristoma is a mass of tissue which is histologically normal for an organ but is located in an abnormal site in the body. Choristomas may be diagnosed by biopsy; they may be so large that removal is not possible without risk of injury to the facial nerve (Taylor and Martin, 1961; Steffen and House, 1962).

h. Anomalies of the muscles of the middle ear

Anomalous muscle is found in about .05 percent of temporal bones (Wright

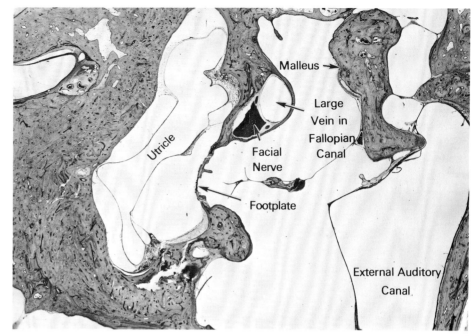

Fig. 4.30: Vertical section showing a large vein accompanying the facial nerve in the fallopian canal. Same ear as Fig. 4.25. (Female, age 87)

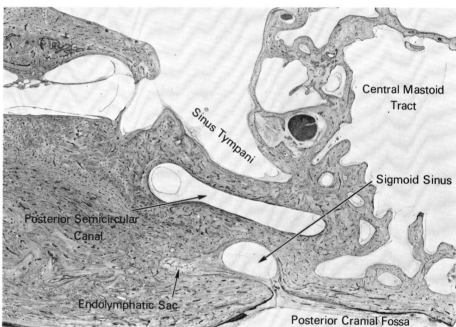

Fig. 4.31: Both temporal bones of this 40-year-old woman showed the lateral venous sinuses to pursue a course within the petrous bones.

and Etholm, 1973). The most common abnormality is small bundles of ectopic striated muscle located near the geniculate ganglion and along the course of the tympanic segment of the facial nerve (Fig. 4.32). Other abnormalities consist of bifurcated or duplicated tensor tympani or stapedius muscles and absence of the stapedius muscle.

i. Anomalies of the facial nerve

The occasional abnormal route of the facial nerve in the temporal bone has been the bane of the otologist since the advent of surgery in this region. Minor deviations in the course of the nerve (Fig. 4.33) and dehiscences of the fallopian canal occur in over 50 percent of temporal bones (Baxter, 1971) and should not be considered to be anomalies (see Chapter 2C, Facial Nerve). A nerve which herniates abruptly out of its fallopian canal is a particularly serious surgical hazard (Johnsson and Kingsley, 1970), particularly in the presence of hyperplastic mucous membrane, granulation tissue, or cholesteatoma. The geniculate ganglion may be widely exposed at the facial hiatus in the floor of the middle cranial fossa where it may be injured during surgery in this area (Dandy, 1929). Hall et al. (1969) found the ganglion exposed to the middle cranial fossa in 15 percent of 100 temporal bones. In the mastoid segment (oval window to stylomastoid foramen) the nerve occasionally pursues

Fig. 4.32: Anomalous ectopic striated muscle located adjacent to the tympanic segment of the facial nerve. The area in inset in upper view is shown at higher magnification in the lower view.

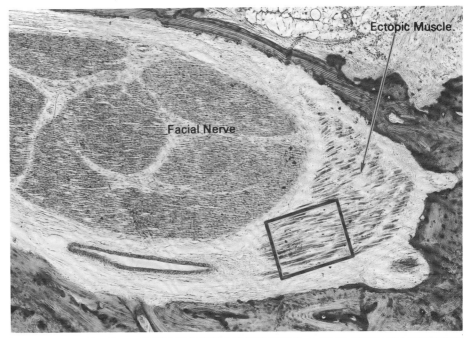

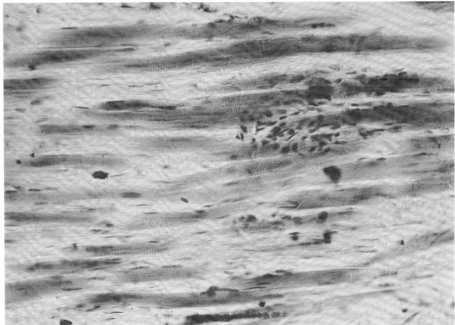

Fig. 4.33: This view shows a common anatomical variant of the facial nerve. In its intratemporal course the nerve divides into two bundles which take separate courses around a space containing fluid to join again in the region of the geniculate ganglion.

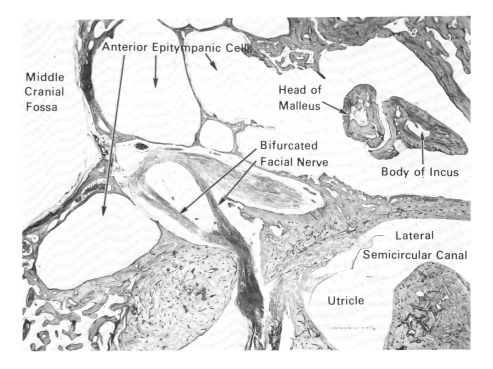

Fig. 4.34: Anomaly of the osseous spiral lamina. This patient had several congenital malformations among which were bicornuate uterus, spina bifida of the thoracic region, and fusion of the second and third cervical vertebrae. She experienced a slowly progressive bilateral sensorineural hearing loss and died at the age of 45 of nephrosclerosis. Chromosomal studies were normal. Histological studies show severe loss of cochlear neurons in the basal turns of both ears. Throughout a large part of the basal turn of the left ear there are dehiscences in the osseous spiral lamina as shown in this graphic reconstruction. See also Fig. 4.35.

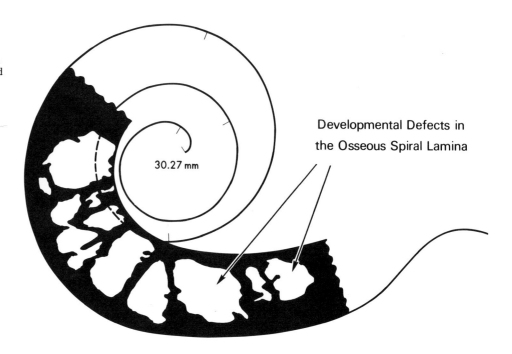

Developmental Defects in the Osseous Spiral Lamina

Fig. 4.35: Anomaly of the osseous spiral lamina (same ear as Fig. 4.34). Photomicrographs show the defects in the osseous spiral lamina and loss of cochlear neurons in the basal turn.

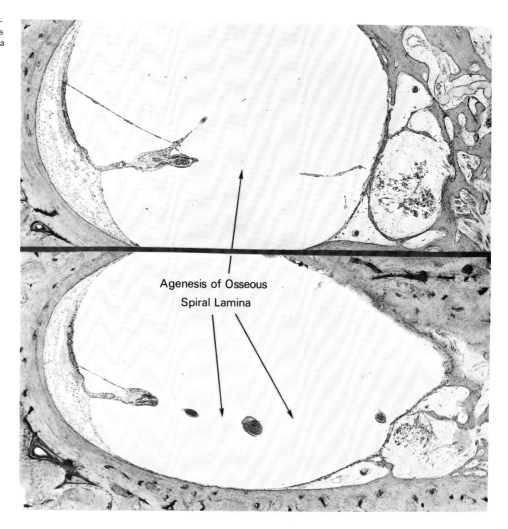

Agenesis of Osseous Spiral Lamina

a course posterior to its normal position and in unusual cases may lie near the sigmoid sinus (Kettel, 1959; Wright et al., 1967). Glasscock (1971) has observed a sharp anterior curvature of the nerve in the region of exit of the chorda tympani. The mastoid segment of the nerve may bifurcate into 2 or 3 bundles, which may reunite before reaching the stylomastoid foramen (Botman and Jonkees, 1955; Miehlke, 1965). The nerve may cross the middle ear by passing between the oval and round windows (Durcan et al., 1967; Gerlach and Cope, 1963; Shambaugh, 1967) and in rare instances it may pass over the promontory anterior to both windows (Fowler, 1961; Dickinson et al., 1968).

2. INNER EAR

Minor anomalies of the inner ear are compatible with normal auditory and vestibular function; however, more extensive anomalies appear to be characterized by progressive hearing loss during life, and is assumed to be an expression of genetically defective protoplasm with early cellular decay.

a. *Osseous spiral lamina and semicircular canals*

Malformations of the osseous spiral lamina may occur as part of a more extensive deformity (Mundini dysplasia, trisomy dysplasia) or as an isolated cochlear finding (Figs. 4.34, 4.35).

The spiral lamina develops in the early stages of fetal life as the result of differentiation of scalae tympani and vestibuli, and ossification occurs in the twenty-third week. The spiral lamina and interscalar septum develop almost simultaneously. Presumably defects in the spiral lamina are caused by excessive resorption of mesenchymal tissue during cavity formation of the scalae, a mechanism which Guild (1929) believed was responsible for the scala communis defect.

Abnormalities of the semicircular canals presumably are due to interruption in differentiation at about the 6–7 mm stage of fetal development. Siebenmann (cited by Altmann, 1950) stated that gross malformation of the semicircular canals can occur with or without other anomalies, the most frequently involved being the lateral canal. According to Altmann (1953), mild malformations of the pars superior may be found as an isolated condition, whereas more severe malformations are associated with changes in the pars inferior. He also stated that malformations of the semicircular canals can occur with congenital aural atresia.

Sidman et al. (1965) found *Twirler* mice to have small or absent lateral canals, absent otoliths, uneven outlines of the vertical canals, and normal cochleae. *Waltzer-type* mice are known to have abnormalities involving the lateral and posterior canals, but never the superior canals or cochleae. In *Zigzag* mice, one or both of the lateral canals are reduced in size, malformed or absent. In *Fidget* mice, the semicircular canals are abortive or absent, and the cristae of the lateral canals are always absent, although the cochleae develop

b. *Scala communis*

Scala communis cochleae is a dehiscence of the partition separating the turns of the cochlea. It has been termed "scala communis" by Alexander (1904), "cloaca" by Nager (1907), and "interscalar septum defect" by Altmann (1953). It usually occurs between the middle and apical turns. A study of 375 temporal bones in the collection of the Massachusetts Eye and Ear Infirmary reveals scala communis to be present in 7 ears. It commonly occurs in the Mundini deformity of the cochlea or in association with other congenital defects such as anencephaly (Agazzi, 1946; Altmann, 1947), hydrocephalus (Altmann, 1964), and trisomy dysplasias (see Section E3, this chapter). Guild (1929) assumed that the etiology was excessive resorption of mesenchymal tissues beyond normal limits during the stage of cavity formation of the scalae vestibuli and tympani, and he regarded it as a phase of mesenchymal development which had proceeded beyond its usual limits (over-differentiation). Polvogt and Crowe (1937) reported five cases of scala communis (four scalae unilateral and one bilateral) without hearing impairment. Bast and Anson (1949) stated that the bony partition between the first and second turns develops at about the twenty-second week of embryonic life and is complete in all turns by the twenty-fourth or twenty-fifth week.

3. PETROUS BONE

a. *Anencephaly*

Anencephaly is a common malformation in man as well as animals. It is characterized by defective development of the vault of the skull and brain. A comprehensive study of the changes occurring in such temporal bones was presented by Agazzi (1946) and by Wolff and Maniglia (1967). There appears to be a higher incidence of anencephaly among the Irish than other ethnic groups. The petrous bone in these cases is shorter and thicker with a narrow internal auditory canal. The cochlear neuronal population is diminished and sometimes missing, and there is a reduction in the number of cochlear turns.

Otocephaly constitutes a group of cephalic abnormalities described by Altmann (1957) which occur only rarely in man but more often in certain animals such as sheep, cattle, dogs, guinea pigs, mice, and rabbits.

b. *Primary keratoma (cholesteatoma)*

Primary keratoma of the temporal bone is an epidermoid cystic growth arising from congenital rests of keratinizing squamous epithelium. Secondary keratomas, on the other hand, are caused by invasion of the temporal bone by keratinizing squamous epithelium from the external auditory canal and are discussed in Chapter 5A4, Keratoma.

Primary keratomas may be classified as to the site of origin: (1) petrous apex area, (2) middle ear and mastoid area, and (3) external auditory canal. The primary keratomas of the petrous apex area usually first become symptomatic between the ages of 35 and 55. Cawthorne and Griffith (1961) found facial weakness to be the presenting symptom in eight of nine cases. The bony labyrinth is frequently eroded, and there is loss of auditory and vestibular function. As the mass of exfoliated keratin enlarges it may invade the internal auditory canal or the middle ear and may eventually reach the external auditory canal. Encroachment on the cerebellopontine angle is common, occurring in 53 of 142 cases reported by Mahoney (1936). If infection occurs, there is sudden onset of pain and suppurative discharge.

Surgical exploration of uninfected primary keratoma characteristically reveals a flaky, odorless mass having a sheen which has led to the term "pearly tumor". Small lesions may be removed completely with primary closure of the operative site; however, more commonly the size and location preclude complete removal (House and Doyle, 1962). In some cases the cavity can be exteriorized to the external auditory canal.

When the site of origin is in the middle ear and mastoid, the usual presenting symptom is hearing loss in childhood (Peron and Schuknecht, 1975). Examination often reveals a whitish mass behind an intact tympanic membrane (Derlacki and Clemis, 1965; Derlacki et al., 1968). These lesions lead to destruction of the ossicles; however, early detection may permit complete removal and reconstruction of the sound-transmitting system. If large or infected, more extensive surgery may be required and exteriorization may be necessary.

Primary keratoma of the external auditory canal usually occurs medial to an atretic membranous canal, and occasionally medial to a bony atresia plate (Hoenk et al., 1969). Embryologically the external auditory canal develops by canalization of a solid cord of epithelium. The canalization occurs from medial to lateral, and it is obvious that arrest in development might result in atresia with an epithelialized canal medial to it. The symptoms are pain and swelling in the location of the ear canal in a child with congenital atresia. Early surgical intervention is required to prevent destruction of the tympanic membrane and ossicles.

E. MORPHOLOGICAL PATTERNS OF INNER EAR DYSPLASIA

Dysplasia (incomplete or aberrant development) of the inner ear may be inherited, sporadic, or the result of chromosomal aberrations. Characteristically, both ears are involved but not always to the same extent. Inner ear dysplasias may be classified simply into the Scheibe, Mundini, and trisomy types. Other types which have been mentioned (Cawthorne and Hinchcliffe, 1957; Ormerod, 1960) are the Bing Siebenmann type (normal bony labyrinth and underdeveloped membranous labyrinth) and the Alexander type (familial high tone deafness with presumed underdevelopment of the basal turn). These latter types are so inadequately documented, both clinically and pathologically, that they cannot be considered as established forms of dysplasia. Furthermore, the Michel dysplasia (Michel, 1863), which is characterized by complete failure of development of the inner ear, is so rare that it is of little otological significance.

1. SCHEIBE DYSPLASIA (COCHLEO-SACCULAR DYPLASIA)

This type of dysplasia (Scheibe, 1892) involves only the phylogenetically newer part of the inner ear, the cochlea and the saccule (Fisch, 1959). The utricle and semicircular canals are histologically and functionally normal. Characteristically, the stria vascularis shows areas of aplasia alternating with regions of hyperplasia and gross deformity (Lindsay, 1973b). Reissner's membrane usually is collapsed and lying on the stria and on a rudimentary organ of Corti. The tectorial membrane often has a rounded appearance and lies in the internal sulcus. The supporting elements of the organ of Corti are distorted and collapsed, and hair cells are sparse or missing (Figs. 4.36, 4.37, 4.38). The appearance is similar to that occurring in inherited deafness in some animals, e.g. Dalmatian dogs. The wall of the saccule usually is collapsed and lying on an atrophic sensory epithelium and deformed otolithic membrane (Fig. 4.39). The cochlear neurons may be normal and remain so until late in life.

2. MUNDINI DYSPLASIA (DYSPLASIA OF BONY AND MEMBRANOUS LABYRINTH)

This inner ear deformity was first described by Mundini (1791) and then by Alexander (1904) and Siebenmann (1950). Ormerod (1960) defined the condition as a "flattened cochlea with development of the basal coil only, and with a comparable underdevelopment of the vestibular structures".

Less severe deformities than those described originally by these authors might also be appropriately classified as the Mundini anomaly (Beal et al., 1967). Altmann (1950) characterized the Mundini dysplasia as a flattened bony cochlear capsule with a normal scalar arrangement only in the basal turn, and an underdeveloped bony structure in the apical part of the cochlea (defective interscalar septum, modiolus, and osseous spiral lamina), reduction in the number of cochlear turns, and dilated saccule and endolymphatic duct system (Figs. 4.40, 4.41). He also stated that the "extent of the changes in the stria vascularis, organ of Corti, spiral ganglion cells, and the other parts of the cochlearis system determined the degree of hearing loss, and that clinically, malformation of the Mundini-type might therefore show complete deafness or only partial loss of hearing".

Fig. 4.36: This full-term infant with bilateral Scheibe dysplasia was born of deaf-mute parents and died ten hours after birth. In the basal turn the stria vascularis forms multiple layers between the spiral ligament and partly collapsed Reissner's membrane. In other areas the stria vascularis is missing. A few hair cells can be identified. The tectorial membrane has a rounded shape and is lying in the internal sulcus. The population of cochlear neurons is normal. The macula of the saccule is aplastic, and the saccular wall is collapsed onto the macula. The utricle and semicircular canals appear normal. (Courtesy of Rüedi)

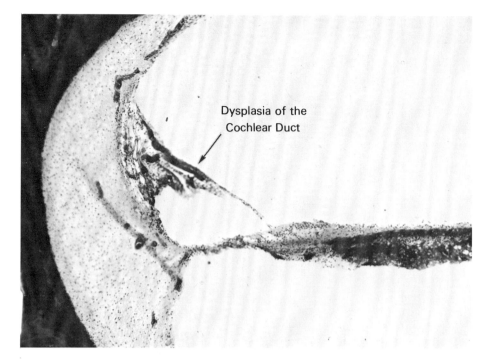

Fig. 4.37: This child was known to have been profoundly deaf from birth and died at the age of ten of peritonitis following appendicitis. Both ears show severe aplasia of the structures of the cochlear duct and saccule, typical of Scheibe dysplasia. The utricle and semicircular canals are normal. The organ of Corti consists of a flattened mound of cells containing remnants of pillars and undifferentiated cells. Reissner's membrane is depressed onto the stria vascularis and organ of Corti so as to obliterate the endolymphatic space. In some areas the stria vascularis is atrophied and in others it is hyperplastic. The tectorial membrane has a spherical shape and lies in the internal sulcus. There is a slight loss of cochlear neurons in the basal turn. (Courtesy of Rüedi)

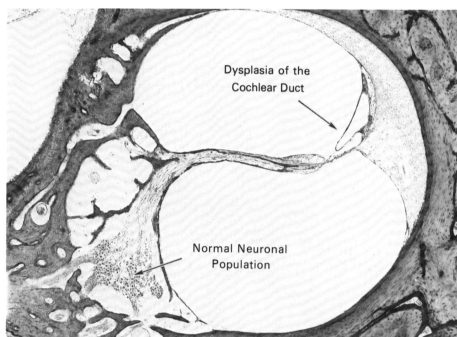

Fig. 4.38: This patient was known to have been deaf since birth and died at the age of 66. Both ears show severe aplasia of the structures of the cochlear duct and saccule, typical of Scheibe dysplasia. The utricle and semicircular canals appear normal. The stria vascularis appears as an irregular mass of strial tissue in the region of the spiral prominence. Reissner's membrane is atrophied and lies on the stria vascularis and limbus, thus obliterating much of the endolymphatic space. The organ of Corti is missing in some areas and in others consists of a mound of undifferentiated cells. The tectorial membrane lies in the inner sulcus. There is a loss of about 75 percent of the cochlear neurons throughout the cochlea. See Fig. 4.39. (Courtesy of Rüedi)

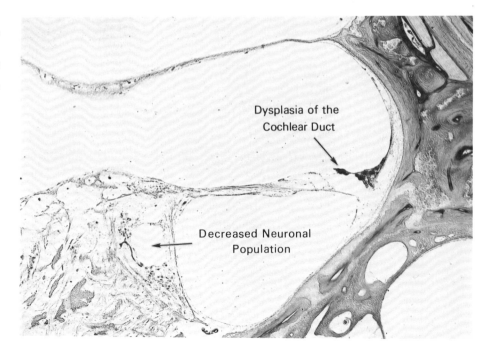

Fig. 4:39: Same case as Fig. 4.38. This view of the vestibule shows the normal utricular macula and the aplastic saccular macula, typical of Scheibe dysplasia. (Courtesy of Rüedi)

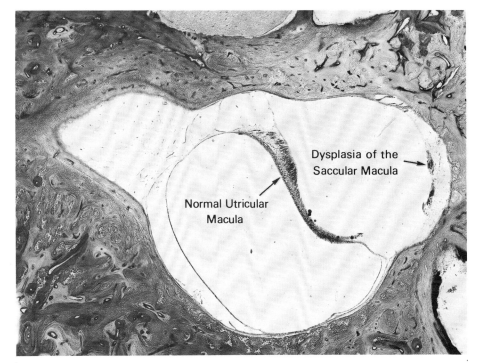

Fig. 4.40: Mundini dysplasia (dysplasia of the bony and membranous labyrinths). The cochlea consists of 1½ turns and shows multiple anomalies, including absent interscalar partitions, vestigial modiolus, and deformed structures of the cochlear duct. The vestibular system consists of a large vestibule with deformed semicircular canals and sense organs. Reported by Fraser (1927). (Courtesy of Rüedi)

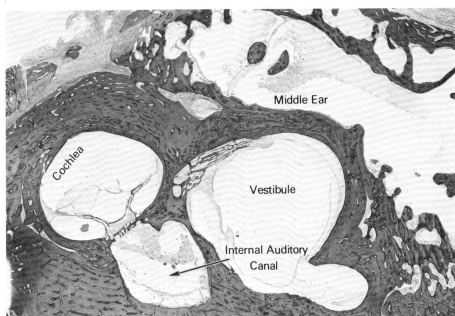

Fig. 4.41: Severe bilateral Mundini dysplasia was present in this woman, who was born profoundly deaf and died at the age of 85. Her father and mother had normal hearing as did her only daughter and brother. The cochlea is a round space with a rudimentary modiolus, and deformed osseous spiral lamina. Only remnants of stria vascularis and spiral ligament are present, and the organ of Corti is a small mound of epithelial cells with no hair cells. A few cochlear neurons are seen in a small bony canal at the base of the osseous spiral lamina. The utricle and saccule are large and occupy the greater portion of a large vestibule. The semicircular canals are deformed, and the cristae are aplastic and without hair cells. The cochlea is in wide communication with the vestibule. The endolymphatic sac occupies a large round space adjacent to the crus commune. In the opposite ear the endolymphatic duct and sac are missing.

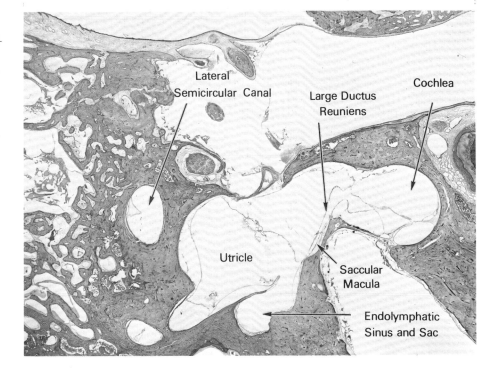

Polvogt and Crowe (1937) described the findings in two cases with normal hearing and anomalies of the bony structures in the apical portion of the modiolus. They also reported one case in which the cochlea had only two turns, but normal hearing. Murakami and Schuknecht (1968) examined the temporal bones of a patient who exhibited a bilateral symmetrical progressive hearing loss beginning in middle age, and found cochleae measuring 24 mm in length with typical Mundini dysplasia (Figs. 4.42, 4.43, 4.44). Paparella and El Fiky (1972) found an ear with Mundini anomaly to have complete absence of the three semicircular canals, the utricle, and the vestibular nerves.

Valvasorri et al. (1969) and Illum (1972) have shown that the Mundini anomaly is clearly evident on polytomographic radiography. Montgomery (1973) and Biggers et al. (1973) have shown that the Mundini dysplasia may lead to spontaneous cerebrospinal otorrhea via a fistula in the oval window. The pathway from the subarachnoid space to the inner ear apparently is the cochlear aqueduct.

Fig. 4.43

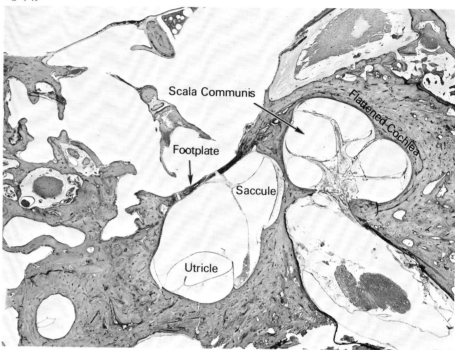

Fig. 4.42: This woman first complained of hearing loss at the age of 47. Audiometric tests performed on five occasions during the next 25 years showed a bilateral slowly progressive sensorineural hearing loss characterized by flat audiometric patterns. Speech discrimination scores deteriorated progressively and were finally recorded at 32 percent on the left and 20 percent on the right. She died at the age of 73. The ears show similar pathological changes. In the right ear (shown here) there is a severe loss of cochlear neurons and hair cells in the basal 10 mm of the cochleae and partial loss in the remainder of the cochleae. Both ears show small areas of atrophy of the stria vascularis in the apical regions. See Figs. 4.43 and 4.44.

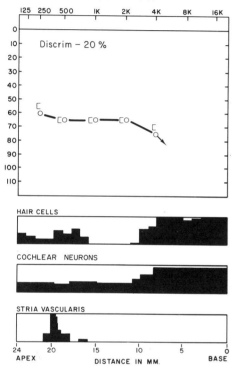

Fig. 4.43: For history see 4.42. This midmodiolar section of the right ear shows a somewhat flattened cochlea with a missing interscalar septum in the apical region. Graphic reconstruction shows a small second turn and a widened apical turn with the cochlear ducts measuring 24 mm in length (normal is 32 mm). The saccule, saccular duct, endolymphatic duct, and endolymphatic sac are enlarged. The vestibular sense organs and nerves appear normal. The opposite ear shows nearly identical anomalies.

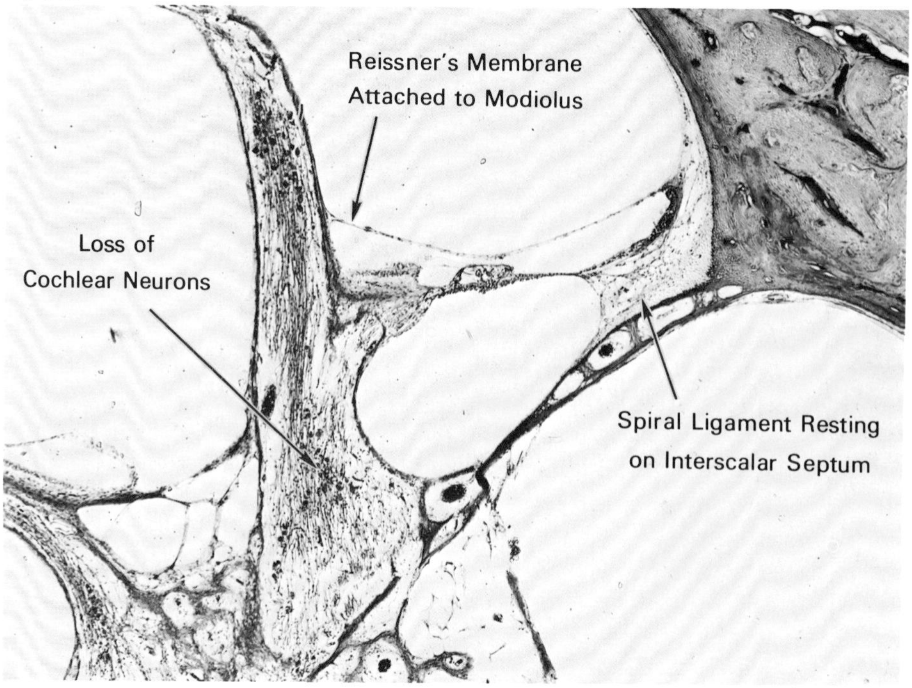

Fig. 4.44: Same case as Figs. 4.42 and 4.43. Middle turn of the right ear. The osseous spiral lamina is narrow, Reissner's membrane is attached to the bony wall of the modiolus, and the spiral ligament rests partly on the interscalar septum.

Fig. 4.44

The discovery of an extra chromosome as the cause of Mongoloidism by Lejeune et al. (1959) and by Jacobs et al. (1959) initiated studies in a new field of genetics. A genetic principle was established, namely, that the normal number of genes must be present in balanced number to produce a normal zygote. Deviations from the normal number (aneuploides) may lead to serious alterations of the phenotype. Normally, all euploid cells have 46 paired chromosomes, except for gametes (ova and sperm) which have 23 chromosomes. If during meiotic division the segregation of chromosomes of a pair does not take place (nondysjunction), both homologous chromosomes may migrate to one and the same daughter cell (Zellweger, 1965). The result, therefore, is an eneuploid gamete with 24 chromosomes. If fertilization occurs with a normal gamete of the other sex, a zygote with 47 chromosomes is formed.

All ovogonia are laid down in the second half of the embryonal period and remain in a prophase-like condition (dictyotene) until years later when ovulation occurs. It seems that during this long period something happens to prevent proper segregation during subsequent stages of meiosis. Trisomies are known to occur more often in offspring of older mothers, presumably because the incidence of nondysjunction is directly related to the duration of dictyotene.

Anomalies may also occur when the chromosomes are normal in number but abnormal in structure. Translocation consists of the transfer of the segment of one chromosome to a different site of the same chromosome, or more often to a different chromosome. When translocation is balanced, that is, the correct quantity of chromosomal substance is present, the individual is phenotypically normal; however, anomalies such as mongolism may result from unbalanced translocation. Fragmentation consists of the translocation of small fragments of a chromosome. The fragments may be introduced into the middle part of another chromosome. The deletion of the short arms of a B group chromosome results in the syndrome *le cri du chat* (cry of the cat) (Lejeune et al., 1963). Children so afflicted have a peculiar cry which resembles the meow of a cat. The laryngeal anomalies have been described by Ward et al. (1968). These individuals also manifest hypertelorism, antimongoloid eye, low-set ears, microcephaly, astigmatism, and hypoplasia of the external auditory canals.

The clinical symptomatology of sex chromosomal aneuploidies, such as Turner's syndrome (ovarian dysgenesis), Klinefelter's syndrome (testicular dysgenesis), and trisomy X (superfemales), is less severe than that of the autosomal aneuploides and does not present otological anomalies.

The most familiar autosomal aneuploides is that of chromosome 21 (trisome 21) which causes mongolism, the incidence of which approximately one in six hundred live births. About half die before reaching the age of five. Ear anomalies are not part of the mongolism syndrome.

The trisomies of the larger chromosomes of groups D (13, 14, 15) and E (17, 18) occur less frequently but are more disastrous. Infants afflicted with either of these aberrations fail to thrive and die within a few weeks or months. The clinical signs and symptoms of trisomy D and trisomy E are quite similar, although cleft lip and palate and malformations of the eye are more common in trisomy D.

a. Trisomy 13 (D₁)

Among the anomalies frequently found in individuals with trisomy 13 are low-set ears, poorly differentiated pinna, pre-auricular tags, absence of external auditory canal, absence of middle ear, cleft lip and/or palate, micrognathia, microphthalmia, iris coloboma, cataracts, retrolental membrane, anophthalmia, retinal dysplasia, hypoplasia or aplasia of optic nerve, and facial capillary hemangiomata (Zellweger, 1965) (Fig. 4.45).

Histological studies have revealed a variety of anomalies of the inner ears of individuals with trisomy 13 (Kos et al., 1966; Black et al., 1971; Maniglia et al., 1970). Among the alterations observed were (1) aplasia of the organ of Corti and stria vascularis; (2) displacement and encapsulation of the tectorial membrane; (3) collapsed cochlear duct with Reissner's membrane lying on the organ of Corti; (4) collapsed saccular wall; (5) incomplete development of the saccular macula and its otolithic membrane; (6) communicating scalae; (7) underdeveloped modiolus; and (8) large patent cochlear aqueduct (Figs. 4.46, 4.47, 4.48, 4.49).

b. Trisomy 18

Some of the abnormalities observed in trisomy 18 are low-set ears, poorly differentiated pinna, absence of the external auditory canal, micrognathia, high palate, cleft lip and/or palate, ptosis of eyelids, microstomia, choanal atresia, slanting eyes, microphthalmia, iris coloboma, glaucoma, and optic atrophy.

The morphological alterations observed by Kos et al. (1966) in the temporal bones of an infant with trisomy 18 (E) were deformed ossicles, bifurcated ten-

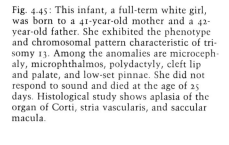

Fig. 4.45: This infant, a full-term white girl, was born to a 41-year-old mother and a 42-year-old father. She exhibited the phenotype and chromosomal pattern characteristic of trisomy 13. Among the anomalies are microcephaly, microphthalmos, polydactyly, cleft lip and palate, and low-set pinnae. She did not respond to sound and died at the age of 25 days. Histological study shows aplasia of the organ of Corti, stria vascularis, and saccular macula.

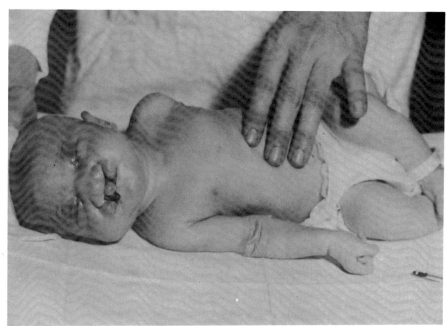

Fig. 4.46: Trisomy 13. This white boy was born of a 40-year-old mother who died in childbirth. He exhibited microcephaly, low-set deformed pinnae, microphthalmia, corneal opacities, flat occiput, and rocker-bottomed feet. He failed to respond to sound and he died at the age of three months. Histological study shows the modiolus is incompletely developed and most of the cochlear neurons lie within the internal auditory canal. The interscalar septum between the basal and middle turn is partly missing, and the stria vascularis is aplastic and cystic. See Figs. 4.47, 4.48, and 4.49.

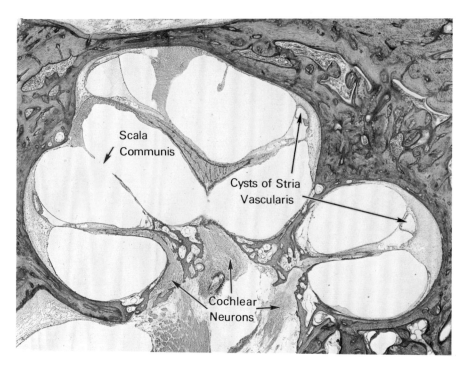

Scala Communis

Cysts of Stria Vascularis

Cochlear Neurons

Fig. 4.47: Trisomy 13. Same case as Figs. 4.46, 4.48, and 4.49. This view shows an underdeveloped cystic stria vascularis. The tectorial membrane appears deformed and incompletely developed. The hair cell population of the organ of Corti is normal.

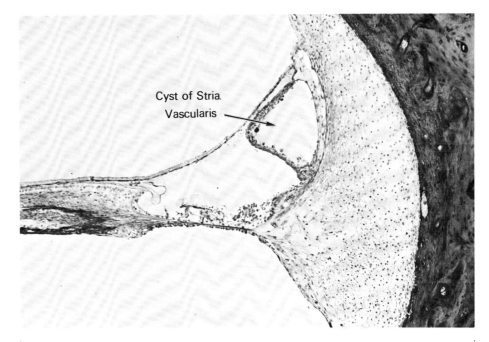

Fig. 4.48: Trisomy 13. Same case as Figs. 4.46, 4.47, and 4.49. The saccular wall is collapsed and lying upon an underdeveloped otolithic membrane and sensory epithelium.

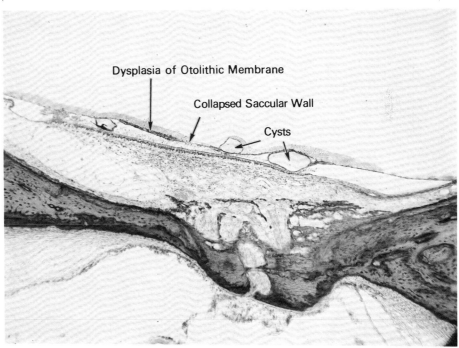

Fig. 4.49: Trisomy 13. Same case as Figs. 4.46, 4.47, and 4.48. This view shows a widely patent cochlear aqueduct.

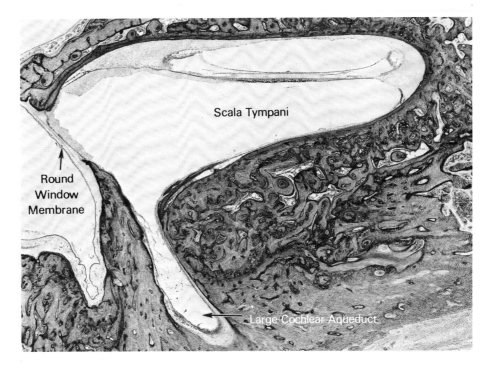

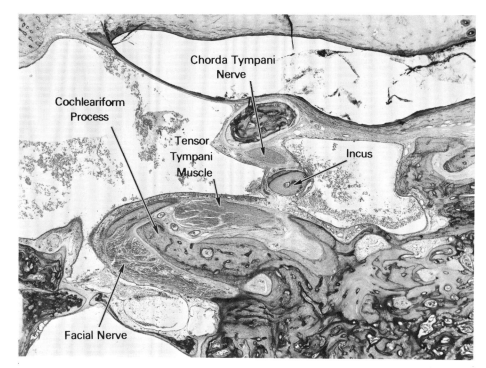

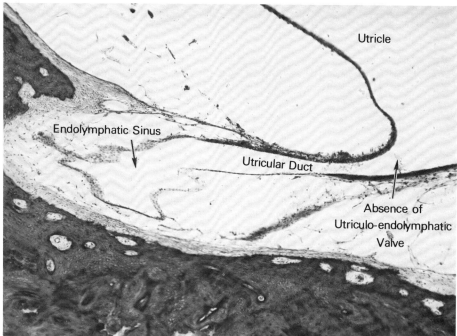

sor tympani muscle, incomplete development of the modiolus, near total absence of cochlear neurons, absence of the utriculo-endolymphatic valve, communicating scalae, and underdeveloped stria vascularis (Figs. 4.50, 4.51).

F. HEREDITARY DEAFNESS IN ANIMALS

Hereditary deafness seems to occur in all species of mammals. It is often associated with pigmentary disorders and frequently follows the true Mendelian patterns of inheritance. The correlation of morphological changes with the bioelectric, enzymatic, and biochemical properties of these ears promises to be a fruitful area for future investigation.

1. SHAKER MOUSE

This strain of mouse exhibits motor disturbances and deafness. It became known as the Japanese dancing mouse and was used by them as a source of entertainment for their children. The adult shaker mouse exhibits a general restlessness; some run in circles part of the time, and most of them exhibit choreic movements of the head in the form of rapid, repeated upward jerk-ings. Lord and Gates (1934), as well as Schaff (1938), observed that the young animals responded to sound but that deafness developed around 22 days of age. Mikaelian and Ruben (1964) demonstrated that this mouse never de-velops a normal eighth nerve potential or a normal range of cochlear poten-tials, and that cochlear potentials are at a maximum at 17 days and then decrease. In some animals they found the cochlear microphonic potentials and VIIIth nerve action potentials, as recorded from the round window mem-brane, to be absent at 19 days, when the cochlea and cochlear neurons still appeared histologically normal. Gruneberg et al. (1940) found inner ear de-velopment to be normal to the twelfth day after which there was progressive degeneration of the structures of the cochlear duct. By 100 days the changes had spread to the apical turn and, by this time, there was also degeneration of the cochlear neurons. Wever (1965) noted the following progression of events: (1) degenerative change in the hair cells and large extraneous cells in the tunnel of Corti; (2) disappearance of the external hair cells; and (3) dis-appearance of the pillar cells and other supporting elements.

Three theories have been advanced as to the nature of cochlear degenera-tion in the shaker mouse: (1) inherited organ weakness (Gruneberg et al., 1940); (2) vascular insufficiency following atrophy of the spiral vessel (also Gruneberg et al., 1940); and (3) degeneration secondary to unrestrained growth of supporting cells (Wever, 1965).

Kikuchi and Hilding (1965) in electron microscopic studies showed that the normal mouse cochlea is not fully developed until twelve days after birth, and that in the shaker-1 mouse, degeneration of the organ of Corti began on the twelfth day and progressed rapidly. Sidman et al. (1965) have compiled a listing of over 30 strains of inner ear mutant mice. Among the interesting names given some of these mutants are: Dancer, Twirler, Gyro, Jerker, Pirou-ette, Spinner, Waltzer, Whirler, Quinky, Shaker, Dervish, Dreher, and Fidget.

2. WALTZING GUINEA PIG

The waltzing guinea pig tends to run in circles and is deaf. The circling begins very soon after birth and becomes pronounced on the third to the fifth day. The animal tends to throw the head backward with a trembling or tremor of the head. The circling may be in either direction, and, when the guinea pigs are excited, will last for considerable periods of time. The animals are retarded in growth but may live to the age of 4 or 5 years, while continu-ing to show all the circling characteristics present at birth (Ibsen and Risty, 1929). The inheritance follows a simple Mendelian recessive characteristic. It is necessary to breed the waltzer with normal animals and then re-breed the hybrid with waltzers to reproduce the strain. Lurie (1941) found that adult waltzers have normal vestibular sense organs and normal vestibular nuclei, and believed that the circling phenomenon was due to central neural abnor-malities. Unborn animals resulting from the mating of waltzing guinea pigs were examined ten days before delivery and were found to have normal organs of Corti, cochlear neurons, and vestibular sense organs. By the fifth to the tenth day after birth, the organ of Corti had begun to degenerate, first in the upper basal and lower middle turns and then in the entire cochlea. De-generation occured in the following sequence: external hair cells, internal hair cells, external pillar cells, internal pillar cells, and the remaining sup-porting structures. Neural degeneration appeared to follow degenerative change of the sense organ.

Ernstson (1971), utilizing electron microscopy, found that the cochlea of the waltzing guinea pig exhibited coalescence of stereocilia and protrusions from the cuticular plate at the time of birth. With increasing age the hair cells vacuolized, the plasma membrane ruptured and cytoplasmic debris was ex-truded into the endolymphatic space. He suggested that this might be caused by an "error of metabolism" occurring as a genetic aberration.

Fig. 4.52: Deaf Dalmatian dog. There is dysplasia
of the stria vascularis, organ of Corti, and tectorial membrane. There is collapse of the
cochlear duct. The population of cochlear
neurons is normal. The saccular macula of
this ear is also underdeveloped, completing
the histologic characteristics of Scheibe
dysplasia.

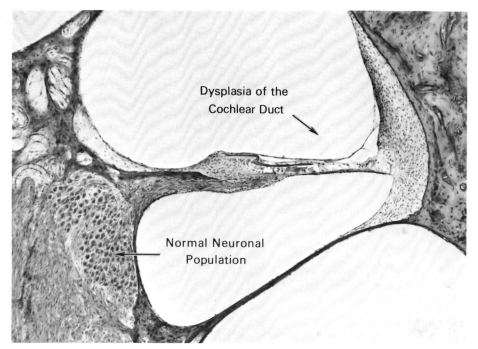

Fig. 4.53: Deaf cocker spaniel. There is incomplete development of the structures of the
cochlear duct and saccule. The cochlear neurons appear normal. See also Fig. 4.54.

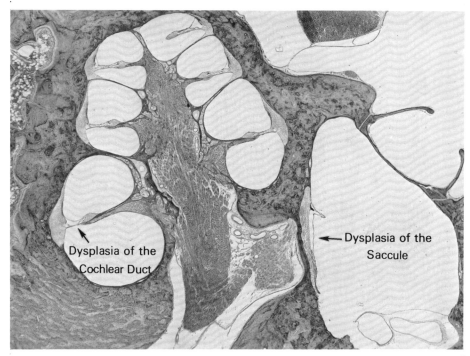

Fig. 4.54: Deaf cocker spaniel. Same ear as Fig.
4.54. There is dysplasia of the organ of Corti
and stria vascularis associated with collapse
of the cochlear duct. The cochlear neurons
appear normal.

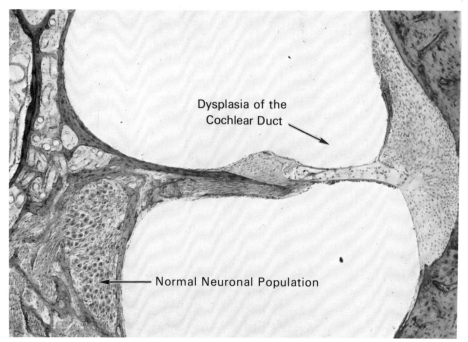

3. SCHEIBE DYSPLASIA IN THE DOG

In histological studies on deaf Dalmatian dogs, Rawitz (1896) and Lurie (1942) found aplasia of the structures of the cochlear duct and saccule, characteristic of the Scheibe type dysplasia (Fig. 4.52). Hughson et al. (1936) and subsequently Hudson and Ruben (1962) found that these deaf animals failed to exhibit electrical responses from round window electrodes in response to pure tone stimuli and clicks. Anderson et al. (1968) found that the deafness was not caused by a dominant or recessive gene with complete penetration, but by a sex-linked gene with varying expressivity. They showed some animals to be totally deaf and others to have flat or basin-shaped audiometric patterns. There was a tendency for the degeneration to be more severe in the middle part of the cochlear duct. The changes were most severe for the external hair cells, and early degenerative changes were evident by electron microscopy when light microscopy showed a normal organ of Corti.

Other strains of dogs which have been found to exhibit hereditary deafness are the collie, Norwegian dunker hound, great Dane, dachshund, fox hound, bull terrier, cocker spaniel, Shetland sheep dog, and old English sheep dog (Figs. 4.53, 4.54). The deafness occurs more frequently in animals that have marbled or mottled coats, tempered throughout with white hairs, and the most striking anomalies occur in homozygous merled matings.

4. PALLID MOUSE

The recessive mutant "pallid" mouse was first described by Roberts in 1931. He noted the pink eye and pale coat color which the mutant produces. Lyon (1951, 1953) noted that some pallid mice showed defects in postural reflexes two to three days after birth. She found that the pallid mice which failed to respond to position change, lacked otoliths in both ears and that those with a normal response always possessed otoliths in at least one ear. Animals with asymmetrical posture showed asymmetry of the otolith defect and tilted the affected side of the head upward. In ears lacking otoliths, the gelatinous layer of the otolith matrix appeared at the normal time and was normal in amount, position, and staining reaction; however, birefringence to calcium salts did not appear. There was hydrops of the cochlear duct, saccule, and endolymphatic duct, and absence of pigment in the stria vascularis. An interesting observation was that animals with otoliths in only one saccule possessed an asymmetrical resting posture, suggesting that the saccule affects posture in these mice. This is in conflict with findings in other experiments, which have failed to establish any change in posture or reflexes after destruction of the saccule (rabbit–Versteegh, 1927; several vertebrates–Lowenstein, 1936; frogs and elasmobranchs–Ashcroft and Hallpike, 1934).

5. THE DEAF WHITE CAT

Darwin (1859) reported that white cats with blue irides were invariably deaf; however, Tait (1883) found that, although deafness was confined to cats having white coats, its incidence was not firmly related to iris color. Przibram (1907) found that cats with heterochromia iridis characteristically exhibited hearing defects limited to the side of the blue iris. Whiting in 1918 pointed out the significant relationship between pigment abnormality in the eye and deafness.

More recently, Bosher and Hallpike (1965) studied the histological features, development, and pathogenesis of inner ear degeneration in 57 kittens bred from four female and two male cats with white coats. They found the inner ears to be normal until the fourth to sixth day of postnatal life, at which time histological abnormalities first appeared. The degenerative change was confined to the cochlea and saccule. They demonstrated progressive degeneration of the organ of Corti and atrophy of the stria vascularis. They interpreted folds in Reissner's membrane to be the result of fluctuations in the volume of endolymph. The utricle and semicircular canals were normal. An analysis of the genetic data indicated that the white coat color and inner ear degeneration was due to a single dominant gene, the penetrance for the white coat color being complete and that for the inner ear degeneration being 80 percent. It was interesting to note that the inner ear degenerative change was unilateral in several animals. Wilson and Kane (1959), studying white cats, also noted unilateral cochlear involvement in some cases and postulated that the changes could be the result of failure in endolymph formation. Howe (1935), as well as Bosher and Hallpike (1965), found minimal secondary neural degeneration in spite of severe atrophic changes in the organ of Corti.

References

Agazzi, C., 1946: Les Altérations de l'oreille dans l'anencéphalie. Pract. oto-rhino-laryng. 8:114.

Alexander, G., 1904: Zur Pathologie und pathologischen Anatomie der kongenitalen Taubheit. Arch. Ohr Nas.-Kehlk-Heilk. 61:183.

Alport, A., 1927: Hereditary familial congenital haemorrhagic nephritis. Brit. Med. J. 1:504.

Alstrom, C., Hallgren, B., Nilsson, L., and Asander, H., 1959: Retinal degeneration ocmbined with obesity, diabetes mellitus and neurogenous deafness. Acta psychiat. scand. Suppl. 129:1.

Altmann, F., 1947: Anomalies of the internal carotid artery and its branches; their embryological and comparative anatomical significance. Report of a new case of persistent stapedial artery in man. Laryngoscope 57:313.

Altmann, F., 1950: Histologic picture of inherited nerve deafness in man and animals. Arch. Otolaryng. 51:852.

Altmann, F., 1953: Malformations, anomalies, and vestigial structures of the inner ear. Arch. Otolaryng. 57:591.

Altmann, F., 1955: Congenital atresia of the ear in man and animals. Ann. Otol. Rhinol. Laryng. 64:824.

Altmann, F., 1957: The ear in severe malformations of the head. Arch. Otolaryng. 66:7.

Altmann, F., 1964: The inner ear in genetically determined deafness. Acta oto-laryng. Suppl. 187:1.

Anderson, H., Henricson, B., Lundquist, P.-G., Wedenberg, E., and Wersäll, J., 1968: Genetic hearing impairment in the Dalmatian dog. Acta oto-laryng. Suppl. 232:1.

Anson, B., and Bast, T., 1959: Development of the stapes of the human ear. Bull. Northwestern University Medical School 33:44.

Arnott, E., Crawfurd, M., and Toghill, P., 1966: Anterior lenticonus and Alport's syndrome. Brit. J. Ophthal. 50:390.

Arnvig, J., 1954: Causes of deafness among pupils of state schools for deaf during 1952–1953. Ugeskr. Laeg. 116:449.

Ashcroft, D., and Hallpike, C., 1934: On the function of the saccule. J. Laryng. 49:450.

Asher, P., 1952: A study of 63 cases of athetosis with special reference to hearing defects. Arch. Dis. Childh. 27:475.

d'Avignon, M., and Barr, B., 1964: Ear abnormalities and cranial nerve palsies in thalidomide children. Arch. Otolaryng. 80:136.

Baldwin, J., 1968: Dysostosis craniofacialis of Crouzon. Laryngoscope 78:1660.

Barr, B., and Klockhoff, I., 1959: Cerebral palsy and hearing impairment. Nord. Med. 62:1512.

Barr, B., and Lundström, R., 1961: Deafness following maternal rubella. Acta oto-laryng. 53:413.

Barton, M., Court, S., and Walker, W., 1962: Causes of severe deafness in school children in Northumberland and Durham. Brit. Med. J. 1:351.

Bast, T., and Anson, B., 1949: The Temporal Bone and the Ear. Charles C. Thomas, Springfield, Ill.

Baxter, A., 1971: Dehiscence of the fallopian canal. An anatomical study. J. Laryng. 85:587.

Beal, D., Davey, P., and Lindsay, J., 1967: Inner ear pathology of congenital deafness. Arch. Otolaryng. 85:134.

Berry, G., 1888: Note on congenital defect (coloboma) of lower lid. Roy. London Ophthal. Hosp. Rep. 12:255.

Biggers, W., Howell, N., Fischer, N., Himadi, G., 1973: Congenital ear anomalies associated with otic meningitis. Arch. Otolaryng. 97:399.

Bjornstad, R., 1965: Pili torti and sensori-neural loss of hearing. Read before the meeting of the Combined Scandinavian Dermatological Association, Copenhagen.

Black, F., Sando, I., Wagner, J., and Hemenway, W., 1971: Middle and inner ear abnormalities, 13–15 (D$_1$) trisomy. Arch. Otolaryng. 93:615.

Bordley, J., and Hardy, J., 1969: Laboratory and clinical observations on prenatal rubella. Ann. Otol. Rhinol. Laryng. 78:917.

Bosher, S., and Hallpike, C., 1965: Observations on the histological features, development and pathogenesis of the inner ear degeneration of the deaf white cat. Proc. Roy. Soc. Med. 162:147.

Botman, J., and Jongkees, L., 1955: Endo-temporal branching of the facial nerve. Acta oto-laryng. 45:111.

Brain, W., 1927: Heredity in simple goitre. Quart. J. Med. 20:303.

Brock, B., 1929: Weiterer Beitrag zur Lehre von der Arachnodaktylie. Z. Kinderheilk. 47:702.

Brohm, F., and Kluska, V., 1947: Mendibulofacial dysostosis (Franceschetti Zwahlen). Lék. Listy 2:329.

Brown, K., 1967: The genetics of childhood deafness, in Deafness in Childhood, p. 177. Ed. F. McConnell and P. Ward. Vanderbilt University Press, Nashville, Tenn.

Burn, R., 1950: Deafness and Laurence-Moon-Biedl syndrome. Brit. J. Ophthal. 34:65.

Caplinger, C., and Hora, J., 1967: Middle ear choristoma with absent oval window: A report of one case. Arch. Otolaryng. 85:365.

Carruthers, D., 1945: Congenital deafmutism as sequela of rubella-like maternal infection during pregnancy. Méd. J. Austr. 1:315.

Cawthorne, T., and Griffith, A., 1961: Primary cholesteatomata of the temporal bone. Arch. Otolaryng. 73:252.

Cawthorne, T., and Hinchcliffe, R., 1957: Familial perceptive deafnesses. Pract. oto-rhino-laryng. 19:69.

Civantos, F., 1963: Human chromosomal abnormalities. Bull. Tulane Med. Fac. 20:241.

Cockayne, E., 1936: Dwarfism with retinal atrophy and deafness. Arch. Dis. Childh. 11:1.

Cockayne, E., 1946: Dwarfism with retinal atrophy and deafness. Arch. Dis. Childh. 21:52.

Cohen, M., Cassady, G., and Hanna, B., 1961: A genetic study of hereditary renal dysfunction with associated deafness. Amer. J. hum. Genet. 13:379.

Collins, E. Treacher, 1900: Case with symmetrical congenital notches in the outer part of each lower lid and defective development of the malar bones. Trans. Ophthal. Soc. U. K. 20:190.

Comley, A., and Wood, B., 1968: Albumin administration in exchange transfusion for hyperbilirubinaemia. Arch. Dis. Childh. 43:151.

Congdon, E., Rowhanavongse, S., and Varamisara, P., 1932: Human congenital auricular and juxta-auricular fossae sinuses and scars (including so-called aural and auricular fistulae) and bearing of their anatomy upon theories of their genesis. Amer. J. Anat. 51:439.

Coquette, M., 1944: Les sequelles neurologiques tardives de l'ictere nubleiaire. Ann. Pediat. 163:83.

Crawfurd, M., and Toghill, P., 1968: Alport's syndrome of hereditary nephritis and deafness. Quart. J. Med. 37:563.

Crouzon, O., 1912: Dysostose cranio-faciale hereditare. Bull. et Mem. Soc. Med. des Hosp. Paris 33:545.

Crowe, S., Guild, S., and Polvogt, L., 1934: Observations on pathology of high-tone deafness. Bull. Johns Hopkins Hosp. 54:315.

Dandy, W., 1929: An operation for the cure of tic douloureux: Partial section of the sensory root at the pons. Arch. Surg. 18:687.

Danish, J., Tillson, J., and Levitan, M., 1963: Multiple anomalies in congenitally deaf children. Eugen. Quart. 10:12.

Darwin, C., 1859: On the Origin of Species. 1st ed., Murray, London.

Davies, D., 1967: Persistent stapedial artery: a temporal bone report. J. Laryng. 81:649.

Davies, D., 1968: Malleus fixation. J. Laryng. 82:331.

Deraemaeker, R., 1956: Congenital deafness and goiter. Amer. J. Hum. Genet. 8:253.

Derlacki, E., and Clemis, J., 1965: Congenital cholesteatoma of the middle ear and mastoid. Ann. Otol. Rhinol. Laryng. 74:706.

Derlacki, E., Harrison, W., and Clemis, J., 1968: Congenital cholesteatoma of the middle ear and mastoid: A second report presenting seven additional cases. Laryngoscope 78:1050.

Diamond, L., Blackfan, K., and Baty, J., 1932: Erythroblastosis fetalis and its association with universal edema of the fetus, icterus gravis neonatorum and anemia of the newborn. J. Pediat. 1:269.

Dickinson, J., Srisomboon, P., and Kamerer, D., 1968: Congenital anomaly of the facial nerve. Arch. Otolaryng. 88:357.

Dickinson, W., 1875: Diseases of the Kidney and Urinary Derangements. p. 379. Longmans, Green, London.

Doll, E., Phelps, W., and Melcher, R., 1932: Mental Deficiency Due to Birth Injuries, p. 1. Macmillan, New York.

Dolowitz, D., and Stephens, F., 1961: Hereditary nerve deafness. Ann. Otol. Rhinol. Laryng. 70:851.

Dubach, U., Minder, F., and Antener, I., 1966: Familial nephropathy and deafness: First observation of a family and close relatives in Switzerland. Helv. med. Acta 33:36.

Dublin, W., 1951: Neurologic lesions of erythroblastosis fetalis in relation to nuclear deafness. Amer. J. Clin. Path. 21:935.

Durcan, D., Shea, J., and Sleeckx, J., 1967: Bifurcation of the facial nerve. Arch. Otolaryng. 86:619.

Efron, M., 1965: Familial hyperprolinemia. New Eng. J. Med. 272:1243.

Elman, D., 1958: Familial association of nerve deafness with nodular goiter and thyroid carcinoma. New Eng. J. Med. 259:219.

Ernstson, S., 1971: Cochlear morphology in a strain of the waltzing guinea pig. Acta oto-laryng. 71:469.

Everberg, G., 1959: Marfan's syndrome associated with hearing defects: Report of a case in one of a pair of twins. Acta paediat. 48:70.

Fay, E., 1898: Marriages of the deaf in America: An inquiry concerning the results of marriages of the deaf in America, chap VII. Volta Bureau, Washington, D.C.

Feinmesser, M., and Zelig, S., 1961: Congenital deafness associated with onychodystrophy. Arch. Otolaryng. 74:507.

Fernandez, A., and Ronis, M., 1964: The Treacher-Collins syndrome. Arch. Otolaryng. 80:505.

Fisch, L., 1959: Deafness as part of an hereditary syndrome. J. Laryng. 73:355.

Fowler, E., Jr., 1961: Variations in the temporal bone course of the facial nerve. Laryngscope 71:937.

Franceschetti, A., and Zwahlen, P., 1944: Un syndrome nouveau: la dysostose mandibulo-faciale. Bull. schweiz. Akad. med. Wiss. 1:60.

Francois, J., 1961: Heredity in Ophthalmology. C. V. Mosby Co., St. Louis.

Fraser, G., 1964: A study of causes of deafness amongst 2,355 children in special schools. In Research into Deafness in Children, ed. L. Fisch, Blackwell, Oxford.

Fraser, G., Froggatt, P., and James, T., 1964: Congenital deafness associated with elec-trocardiographic abnormalities, fainting attacks and sudden death: A recessive syndrome. Quart. J. Med. 33:361.

Fraser, G., Morgans, M., and Trotter, W., 1961: Sporadic goitre with congenital deafness (Pendred's syndrome). In Advances in Thyroid Research. Trans. 4th International Goitre Conference, p. 19. Edited by R. Pitt-Rivers. Pergamon Press, Oxford.

Fraser, J., 1927: A case of congenital deafness with malformation of the bony and membranous labyrinths on both sides. Proc. Roy. Soc. Med. 20:475.

Freda, V., and Bowe, E., 1969: Hemolytic disease due to Rh sensitization. In Current Therapy, p. 245. Edited by H. Conn. W. B. Saunders, Philadelphia, Pa.

Friedmann, I., Fraser, G., and Froggatt, P., 1966: Pathology of the ear in the cardio-auditory syndrome of Jervell and Lange-Nielsen (Recessive deafness with electrocardiographic abnormalities). J. Laryng. 80:451.

Friedmann, I., Fraser, G., and Froggatt, P., 1968: Pathology of the ear in the cardio-auditory syndrome of Jervell and Lange-Nielsen. J. Laryng. 82:883.

Fujita, S., and Hayden, R., 1969: Alport's syndrome. Temporal bone report. Arch. Otolaryng. 90:453.

Galladeau, J., 1936: Malformations congenitales associees au syndrome de Klippel-Feil. These, Paris.

Ganther, R., 1927: Ein Beitrag zur Arachnodaskytlie. Z. Kinderheilk. 43:724.

Gardner, W., and Turner, O., 1940: Bilateral acoustic neurofibromas. Arch. Neurol. 44:76.

Gerhardt, H.-J., and Otto, H.-D., 1970: Steigbügelmissbildungen. Acta oto-laryng. 70:35.

Gerlach, J., and Cope, D., 1963: An anomaly of the intrapetrous portion of the facial nerve. Bull. School of Medicine, University of Maryland 48:27.

Gerrard, J., 1952: Nuclear jaundice and deafness. J. Laryng. 66:39.

Gill, N., 1969: Congenital atresia of the ear: A review of the surgical findings in 83 cases. J. Laryng. 83:551.

Gillman, J., Gilbert, C., and Gillman, T., 1948: Preliminary report on hydrocephalus, spina bifida and other congenital anomalies in rat produced by trypan blue; significance of these results in interpretation of congenital malformations following maternal rubella. South afr. J. med. Sci. 13:47.

Glasscock, M., 3rd, 1971: Unusual facial nerve problems. Laryngoscope 81:669.

Goldbloom, R., Fraser, F., Waugh, D., Aronovitch, M., and Wiglesworth, F., 1957: Hereditary renal disease associated with nerve deafness and ocular lesions. Pediatrics 20:241.

Goldman, N., Singleton, G., and Holly, E., 1971: Aberrant internal carotid artery. Presenting as a mass in the middle ear. Arch. Otolaryng. 94:269.

Goodhill, V., 1950: The nerve-deaf child: significance of Rh, maternal rubella and other etiologic factors. Ann. Otol. Rhinol. Laryng. 59:1123.

Goodhill, V., 1966a: External conductive hypacusis and the fixed malleus syndrome. Acta oto-laryng. Suppl. 217:1.

Goodhill, V., 1966b: The fixed malleus syndrome. Trans. Amer. Acad. Ophthal. Otolaryng. 70:370.

Gorlin, J., and Sedano, H., 1968: Hurler's and Hunter's syndromes. Mod. Med. 36:116.

Graefe, A. von, 1858: Exceptionelles Verhalten des Gesichtfeldes bei Pigmente-nartung der Netzhaut. Arch. Ophth. 4:250.

Graham, J., 1959: Hereditary chronic kidney disease: An alternative to partial sex-linkage in the Utah kindred. Amer. J. Hum. Genet. 11:333.

Granrud, H., 1953: On the etiology of dysostosis mandibulo-facialis. Acta Paediat. 42:499.

Gray, A., and Nelson, S., 1926: The pathological conditions found in a case of deaf-mutism. Proc. Roy. Soc. Med. 19:7.

Grayston, J., Peng, J-Y., and Lee, G., 1967: Congenital abnormalities following gestational rubella in Chinese. J. Amer. Med. Assn. 202:1.

Gregg, J., and Becker, S., 1963: Concomitant progressive deafness, chronic nephritis, and ocular lens disease. Arch. Ophthal. 69:293.

Gregg, N., 1941: Congenital cataract following German measles in the mother. Trans. Ophthal. Soc. Aust. 3:35.

Gruneberg, H., Hallpike, C., and Ledoux, A., 1940: Observations on the structure, development, and electrical reactions of the internal ear of the Shaker-1 mouse (Mus musculus). Proc. Roy. Soc. [B], 129:154.

Guild, S., 1929: A case of bilateral scala communis cochleae uncomplicated by other defects: an embryological interpretation of this and associated anomalies. Anat. Rec. 42:19.

Guilford, F., and Anson, B., 1967: Osseous fixation of the malleus. Trans. Amer. Acad. Ophthal. Otolaryng. 71:398.

Guthrie, L., 1902: "Idiopathic" or congenital hereditary and family haematuria. Lancet 1:1243.

Hall, G., Pulec, J., and Rhoton, A., Jr., 1969: Geniculate ganglion anatomy for the otologist. Arch. Otolaryng. 90:568.

Hallgren, B., 1959: Retinitis pigmentosa combined with congenital deafness with vestibulo-cerebellar ataxia and mental abnormality in a proportion of cases. A clinical and genetico-statistical study. Acta psychiat. scand. Suppl. 138:1.

Harrison, M., 1957: The Treacher Collins-Franceschetti syndrome. J. Laryng. 71:597.

Hart, C., and Naunton, R., 1963: The ototoxicity of chloroquin phosphate. Arch. Otolaryng. 80:407.

Hemenway, W., Sando, I., and McChesney, D., 1969: Temporal bone pathology following maternal rubella. Arch. Ohr. Nas.-Kehlk-Heilk. 193:287.

Herberts, G., 1962: Otological observations on the "Treacher Collins Syndrome." Acta oto-laryng. 54:457.

Herrmann, C., Jr., Aguilar, M., and Sacks, O., 1964: Hereditary photomyoclonus associated with diabetes mellitus, deafness, nephropathy and cerebral dysfunction. Neurology 14:212.

Hilleman, M., Buynak, E., Weibel, R., and Stokes, J., 1968: Live, attenuated rubella-virus vaccine. New Eng. J. Med. 279:300.

Hiller, B., 1950: Rubella congenital inner-ear deafness. J. Laryng. 64:399.

Hoenk, B., McCabe, B., and Anson, B., 1969: Cholesteatoma auris behind a bony atresia plate. Arch. Otolaryng. 89:470.

Holborow, C., 1961: Deafness and the Treacher Collins syndrome. J. Laryng. 75:978.

Hopkins, L., 1954: Heredity and deafness. Eugen. Quart. 1:193.

Hopkins, L., and Guilder, R., 1949: Clarke school studies concerning the heredity of deafness. Edwards Bros., Inc., Mass.

Hough, J., 1958: Malformations and anatomical variations seen in the middle ear during the operation for mobilization of the stapes. Laryngoscope 68:1337.

Hough, J., 1963: Congenital malformations of the middle ear. Arch. Otolaryng. 78:335.

House, H., 1956: Diagnostic aspects of congenital ossicular fixation. Trans. Amer. Acad. Ophthal. Otolaryng. 60:787.

House, W., and Doyle, J., 1962: Early diagnosis and removal of primary cholesteatoma causing pressure to the VIIIth nerve. Laryngoscope 72:1053.

House, H., House, W., and Hildyard, V., 1958: Congenital stapes footplate fixation. Laryngoscope 68:1389.

House, H., and Patterson, M., 1964: Persistent stapedial artery: Report of two cases. Trans. Amer. Acad. Ophthal. Otolaryng. 68:644.

Howe, H., 1935: The reaction of the cochlear nerve to destruction of its end organs. A study of deaf albino cats. J. Comp. Neurol. 62:73.

Hudson, W., and Ruben, R., 1962: Hereditary deafness in the Dalmatian dog. Arch. Otolaryng. 75:213.

Hughson, W., Thompson, E., and Witting, E., 1936: An experimental study of bone conduction. Ann. Otol. Rhinol. Laryng. 45:844.

Huizing, E., Bolhuis, A. van, and Odenthal, D., 1966: Studies on progressive hereditary perceptive deafness in a family of 335 members. Acta oto-laryng. 61:35, 161.

Hurler, G., 1920: Ueber einen Typ multipler Abartgungen, vorwiegend am Skelettsystem. Z. Kinderheilk. 24:220.

Hurst, A., 1923: Hereditary familial congenital haemorrhagic nephritis. Guy's Hosp. Rep. 73:368.

Ibsen, H., and Risty, K., 1929: A new character in guinea pigs, waltzing. Anat. Rec. 44:294.

Illum, P., 1972: The Mondini type of cochlear malformation: a survey of the literature. Arch. Otolaryng. 96:305.

Illum, P., Kiaer, H., Hvidberg-Hansen, J., and Søndergaard, G., 1972: Fifteen cases of Pendred's syndrome: congenital deafness and sporadic goiter. Arch. Otolaryng. 96:297.

Jacobs, P., Baikie, A., Court Brown, W., and Strong, J., 1959: The somatic chromosomes in mongolism. Lancet 1:710.

Jampel, R. and Quaglio, N., 1964: Eye movements in Tay-Sachs disease. Neurology 14:1013.

Jervell, A., and Lange-Nielsen, F., 1957: Congenital deaf-mutism, functional heart disease with prolongation of the Q-T interval and sudden death. Amer. Heart J. 54:59.

Johnsson, L-G., and Kingsley, T., 1970: Herniation of the facial nerve in the middle ear. Arch. Otolaryng. 91:598.

Jørgensen, M., Kristensen, H., and Buch, N., 1964: Thalidomide-induced aplasia of the inner ear. J. Laryng. 78:1095.

Karmody, C., 1968: Subclinical maternal rubella and congenital deafness. New Eng. J. Med. 278:809.

Karmody, C., 1969: Asymptomatic maternal rubella and congenital deafness. Arch. Otolaryng. 89:720.

Kelemen, G., 1956: Erythroblastosis fetalis. Arch. Otolaryng. 63:392.

Keleman, G., 1958: Arteria stapedia, in bilateral persistence Arch. Otolaryng. 67:668.

Kelemen, G., 1965: Marfan's syndrome and hearing organ. Acta oto-laryng. 59:23.

Kendall, G., and Hurst, A., 1912: Hereditary familial congenital hemorrhagic nephritis. Guy's Hosp. Rep. 66:137.

Kettel, K., 1959: Peripheral facial palsy: Pathology and surgery. Copenhagen, p. 341.

Kikuchi, K., and Hilding, D., 1965: The development of the organ of Corti in the mouse. Acta oto-laryng. 60:207.

King, J., 1942: Oxycephaly. Ann. Surg. 115:488.

Klippel, M., and Feil, A., 1912: Un cas d'absence des vertebres cervicales. Nouvelle Iconographic de la Salpetriere. 25:223.

Kloepfer, H., Laguaite, J., and McLaurin, J., 1966: The hereditary syndrome of congenital deafness and retinitis pigmentosa (Usher's syndrome). Laryngoscope 76:850.

Konigsmark, B., 1971: Hereditary congenital severe deafness syndromes. Ann. Otol. Rhinol. Laryng. 80:269.

Kopelman, H., Asatoor, A., and Milne, A., 1964: Hyperprolinaemia and hereditary nephritis. Lancet 2:1075.

Kos, A., Schuknecht, H., and Singer, J., 1966: Temporal bone studies in 13–15 and 18 trisomy syndromes. Arch. Otolaryng. 83:439.

Krickstein, H., Gloor, F., and Balogh, K., Jr., 1966: Renal pathology in hereditary nephritis with nerve deafness. Arch. Path. 82:506.

Lake, M., and Kuppinger, J., 1950: Craniofacial dysostosis (Crouzon's disease). Arch. Ophthal. 44:37.

Landsteiner, K., and Wiener, A., 1940: An agglutinable factor in human blood recognized by immune sera for Rhesus blood. Proc. Soc. Exp. Biol. 43:223.

Latham, A., and Munro, T., 1938: Familial myoclonus epilepsy associated with deaf-mutism in a family showing other psychobiological abnormalities. Ann. Eugen. 8:166.

Lehmann, W., 1950: Ein weiterer Beitrag zur Frage der heterogenie der recessiven Taubstummheit. Z. menschl. vereb. Konstit Lehre 29:825.

Lejeune, J., Gautier, M., and Turpin, R., 1959: Etudes des chromosomes somatiques de neuf enfants mongoliens. C. R. Acad. Sci. 248:1721.

Lejeune, J., Lafourcade, J., Berger, R., Zialatte, J., Boeswillwald, M., Seringe, P., Turpin, R., 1963: Trois cas de délétion partielle du bras court d'un chromosome 5. C. R. Hebdomadaires des Séminaires Acad. Sci. 257:3098.

Lenz, W., and Knapp, R., 1962: Die thalidomide Embryopathie. Dtsch. med. Wschr. 87:1232.

Lewis, S., Sonnenblick, B., Gilbert, L., and Biber, D., 1958: Familial pulmonary stenosis and deaf-mutism: Clinical and genetic considerations. Amer. Heart J. 55:458.

Lichtenstein, B., and Rosenbluth, P., 1956: Schilder's disease with melanoderma. J. Neuropath. Exp. Neurol. 15:229.

Lindsay, J., 1973a: Profound childhood deafness: inner ear pathology. Ann. Otol. Rhinol. Laryng. Suppl. 5.

Lindsay, J., 1973b: Histopathology of deafness due to postnatal viral disease. Arch. Otolaryng. 98:258.

Lindsay, J., Caruthers, D., Hemenway, W., and Harrison, S., 1953: Inner ear pathology following maternal rubella. Ann. Otol. Rhinol. Laryng. 62:1201.

Lindsay, J., Sanders, S., and Nager, G., 1960: Histopathologic observations in so-called congenital fixation of the stapedial footplate. Laryngoscope 70:1587.

Livingstone, G., 1959: The establishment of sound conduction in congenital deformities of the external ear. J. Laryng. 73:231.

Livingstone, G., 1965: Congenital ear abnormalities due to thalidomide. Proc. Roy. Soc. Med. 58:493.

Lord, E., and Gates, W., 1934: Shaker, a new mutation of the house mouse (Mus musculus). Amer. Naturalist 68:435.

Lowenstein, O., 1936: The equilibrium function of the vertebrate labyrinth. Biol. Rev. 1:113.

Lucey, J., 1968: The future demise of exchange transfusions for neonatal hyperbilirubinema. Dev. Med. Child Neurol. 10:521.

Lurie, M., 1941: The waltzing (circling) guinea pig. Ann. Otol. Rhinol. Laryng. 50:113.

Lurie, M., 1942: Degeneration and absorption of the organ of Corti in animals. Ann. Otol. Rhinol. Laryng. 51:712.

Lyon, M., 1951: Hereditary absence of otoliths in house mouse. J. Physiol. 114:410.

Lyon, M., 1953: Absence of otoliths in the mouse: an effect of the pallid mutant. J. Genet. 51:638.

MacBrinn, M., Okada, S., Woollacott, M., Patel, V., Ho, M., Tappel, A., and O'Brien, J., 1969: Beta-galactosidase deficiency in the Hurler syndrome. New. Eng. J. Med. 281:338.

MacDonald, W., Fitch, K., and Lewis, I., 1960: Cockayne's syndrome. An heredofamilial disorder of growth and development. Pediatrics 25:997.

Mahoney, M., 1936: Die Epidermoide des Zentralnervensiptems. Z. Neurol. Psychiat. 155:463.

Mall, F., 1917: On the frequency of localized anomalies in human embryos. Amer. J. Anat. 22:27.

Maniglia, A., Wolff, D., and Herques, A., 1970: Congenital deafness in 13–15 trisomy syndrome. Arch. Otolaryng. 92:181.

Mann, I., 1943: Deficiency of the malar bones with defect of the lower lids. Brit. J. Ophthal. 27:13.

Maran, A., 1965: Persistent stapedial artery. J. Laryng. 79:971.

Marcus, R., 1968: Vestibular function and additional findings in Waardenburg's syndrome. Acta oto-laryng. Suppl. 229:1.

Marfan, A., 1896: Un cas de déformation congénitale des quatre membres, plus pronouncée aux extremeteés, caracteriseé par l'allongement des os avec un certain degré d'amincissement. Bull. Soc. méd. Hôp. Paris. 3:220.

Margolis, E., 1962: A new hereditary syndrome: sex-linked deaf-mutism associated with total ablinism. Acta genet. 12:12.

Marshall, D., 1958: Ectodermal dysplasia. Report of kindred with ocular abnormalities and hearing defect. Amer. J. Ophthal. 45:143.

Mårtensson, B., 1960: Dominant hereditary nerve deafness. Acta oto-laryng. 52:270.

McKenzie, J., 1958: The first arch syndrome. Arch. Dis. Childh. 33:477.

McLay, K., and Maran, A., 1969: Deafness and Klippel-Feil syndrome. J. Laryng. 83:175.

McLeod, A., McConnell, F., Sweeney, A., Cooper, M., and Nance, W., 1971: Clinical variation in Usher's syndrome. Arch. Otolaryng. 94:321.

Mengel, M., Konigsmark, B., and McKusick, V., 1969: Two types of congenital recessive deafness. Eye, Ear, Nose, Throat Monthly 48:301.

Michel, E., 1863: Memoire sur les anomalies congenitales de l'oreille interne. Gaz. med. France 3:55.

Miehlke, A., 1965: Anatomy and clinical aspects of the facial nerve. Arch. Otolaryng. 81:444.

Miehlke, A., and Partsch, C., 1963:

Ohrmissbildung, Facialis-und Abducenslähmung als Syndrom der Thalidomidschädigung. Arch. Ohr. Nas.-Kehlk-Heilk. 181:154.

Mikaelian, D., and Ruben, R., 1964: Hearing degeneration in Shaker-1 mouse. Arch. Otolaryng. 80:418.

Miller, G., Joseph, D., Cozad, R., and McCabe, B., 1970: Alport's syndrome. Arch. Otolaryng. 92:419.

Mohr, O., 1952–53: Letalfaktoren bei Haustieren. Zuchtungskunde 4:1.

Moloy, H., 1942: Studies on head molding during labor. Amer. J. Obstet. Gynec. 44:762.

Monif, G., Hardy, J., and Sever, J., 1966: Studies in congenital rubella, Baltimore, 1964–1965. I. Epidemiologic and Virologic. Bull. Johns Hopkins Hosp. 118:85.

Montgomery, W., 1973: Personal communication.

Moro, F., and Amidei, B., 1957: Speckled corneal dystrophy (Fehr's corneal dystrophy) associated with deafness and stammering. Ann. Ottal. 83:30.

Morrison, A., and Bundey, S., 1970: The inheritance of otosclerosis. J. Laryng. 84:921.

Muckle, T., and Wells, M., 1962: Urticaria, deafness and amyloidosis: A new heredofamilial syndrome. Quart. J. Med. 31:235.

Mundini, C., 1791: Anatomia surdi nedi sectio. De Bononiensi Scientiarum et Artium Instituto Atque Academia Commentarii, Boniensi 7:28, 419.

Murakami, Y., and Schuknecht, H., 1968: Unusual congenital anomalies in the inner ear. Arch. Otolaryng. 87:335.

Murdoch, J., Walker, B., Halpern, B., Kuzma, J., and McKusick, V., 1972: Life expectancy and causes of death in the Marfan syndrome. New Eng. J. Med. 286:804.

Myers, G., and Tyler, H., 1972: The etiology of deafness in Alport's syndrome. Arch. Otolaryng. 96:333.

Myklebust, H., 1954: Auditory Disorders in Children–A Manual for a Differential Diagnosis. Grune and Stratton, New York.

Nager, F., 1907: Beitrage zur Histologie der erworbenen Taubstummheit. Z. Ohrenheilk. 54:217.

Nager, F., 1925: Missbildungen der schnecke und hörvermögen. Z. Hals-Nas.-Ohrenheilk. 11:149.

Nager, F., 1926: Die Beziehungen des endemischen Kretinismus zum Gehörörgan. In: Handbuch der Hals-Nasen-Ohrenheilkunde, p. 637. Ed. Denker und Kahler. Band 6. Verlag Springer, Berlin.

Nager, F., 1936: L'oreille dans la maladie de Crouzon. Extrait du Bulletin de l'Academie de Médicine. 116:349.

Nager, F., 1952: Histologische Ohruntersuchungen bei Kindern nach mütterlicher Rubella. Pract. oto-rhino-laryng. 14:337.

Nakamura, S., and Sando, I., 1966: Congenital absence of the oval window. Arch. Otolaryng. 84:131.

Neill, C., and Dingwall, M., 1950: A syndrome resembling progeria: a review of two cases. Arch. Dis. Childh. 25:213.

Nelson, W., 1964: Textbook of Pediatrics. 8th ed. Edited by W. E. Nelson. W. B. Saunders, Philadelphia, Pa.

Nilsson, L., Borgfors, N., Gamstorp, I., Holst, H., and Liden, G., 1964: Nonendemic goitre and deafness. Acta paediat. 53:117.

Noguera, J., and Haase, F., 1964: Congenital ossicular defects with a normal auditory canal: its surgical treatment. Eye, Ear, Nose, Throat Monthly 43:37.

Nomura, Y., and Mori, W., 1968: Hypo-phosphatasia. Histopathology of human temporal bones. J. Laryng. 82:1129.

Ormerod, F., 1960: The pathology of congenital deafness. J. Laryng. 74:919.

Orth, J., 1875: Uber das Vorkommen von Bilirubinkrystallen bei neugeborenen Kindern. Arch. Path. Anat. 63:447.

Paparella, M., and ElFiky, F., 1972: Mondini's deafness. Arch. Otolaryng. 95:134.

Pendred, V., 1896: Deaf-mutism and goitre. Lancet 2:532.

Perkoff, G., Stephens, F., Dolowitz, D., and Tyler, F., 1951: A clinical study of hereditary interstitial pyelonephritis. Arch. intern. Med. 88: 191.

Peron, D., and Schuknecht, H., 1975: Bilateral congenital cholesteotomata of the middle ears in association with other anomalies. In press.

Polvogt, L., and Crowe, S., 1937: Anomalies of the cochlea in patients with normal hearing. Ann. Otol. Rhinol. Laryng. 46:579.

Potter, E., 1937: Hereditary ear malformations transmitted through five generations. J. Hered. 28:255.

Powers, W., Sheehy, J., and House, H., 1967: The fixed malleus head. Arch. Otolaryng. 85:177.

Prior, I., 1964: Refsum syndrome or heredopathia atactica polyneuritiformis. New Zealand Med. J. 63:322.

Proctor, C., and Proctor, B., 1967: Understanding hereditary nerve deafness. Arch. Otolaryng. 85:23.

Przibram, H., 1907: Vererbungsversuche über asymmetrische Augenfärbung bei Angorakatzen. Arch. Entwcklngsmechr. Organ. Leipz. 25:260.

Raman, G., and Beierwaltes, W., 1959: Correlation of goiter, deaf mutism, and mental retardation with serum thyroid hormone levels in noncretinous inhabitants of a severe endemic goiter area in India. J. clin. Endocrin. 19:228.

Rathbun, J., 1948: "Hypophosphatasia." A new developmental anomaly. Amer. J. Dis. Child. 75:822.

Rawitz, B., 1896: Gehörorgan und Gehirn eines weisson Hundes mit blauen Augen. Morphol. Arb. (Jena) 6:545.

Reed, W., 1967: Congenital cutaneous diseases associated with central nervous disorders. Postgrad. Med. 41:527.

Refsum, S., 1946: Heredopathia atactica polyneuritiformis. Acta psychiat. scand. Suppl. 38:1.

Reyersbach, G., and Butler, A., 1954: Congenital hereditary hematuria. New Eng. J. Med. 251:377.

Ritter, F., 1971: The histopathology of the congenital fixed malleus syndrome. Laryngoscope 81:1304.

Roberts, E., 1931: Abstract: A new mutation in the house mouse (Mus musculus). Science 74:569.

Robin, E., Gardner, F., and Levine, S., 1957: Hereditary factors in chronic Bright's disease: A study of two affected kindreds. Trans. Assn. Amer. Physicians. 70:140.

Ruben, R., and Rozycki, D., 1970: Clinical aspects of genetic deafness. The Neurotology Group at Amer. Acad. Ophthal. Otolaryng.

Ruben, R., Toriyama, M., Dische, M., Bransilver, B., and Daly, J., 1969: External and middle ear malformations associated with mandibulo-facial dysostosis and renal abnormalities: a case report. Ann. Otol. Rhinol. Laryng. 78:605.

Ruby, R., and Schuknecht, H., 1972: Temporal bone pathology in Alport's syndrome. In press.

Ruggles, R., and Reed, R., 1972: Symposium on ear surgery. V. Treatment of aberrant carotid arteries in the middle ear: a report of two cases. Laryngoscope 82:1199.

Sando, I., Hemenway, W., and Morgan, W., 1968: Histopathology of the temporal bones in mandibulofacial dysostosis (Treacher Collins syndrome). Trans. Amer. Acad. Ophthal. Otolaryng. 72:913.

Sando, I., and Wood, R., II, 1971: Congenital middle ear anomalies. Otolaryng. Clin. N. Amer. 4:291.

Sank, D., 1963: Genetic aspects of early total deafness. In Family and Mental Health Problems in a Deaf Population. p. 28. Edited by J. Rainer, K. Altshuler, and F. Kallmann, State Psychiatric Institute, New York.

Schafer, I., Scriver, C., and Efron, M., 1962: Familial hyperprolinemia, cerebral dysfunction and renal anomalies occurring in a family with hereditary nephropathy and deafness. New Eng. J. Med. 267:51.

Schaff, W., 1938: Vergleichende Untersuchungen über das verhalten normaler und hirnkranker (hyperkinetischer) Mause. Arch. ges. Psychol. 102:210.

Schall, L., Lurie, M., and Kelemen, G., 1951: Embryonic hearing organs after maternal rubella. Laryngoscope 61:99.

Scheer, A., 1967: Correction of congenital middle ear deformities. Arch. Otolaryng. 85:269.

Scheer, A., 1968: Personal communication.

Scheibe, A., 1892: A case of deaf-mutism with auditory atrophy and anomalies of development in the membranous labyrinth of both ears. Arch. Otolaryng. 11:12.

Schilling, V., 1936: Striae distensae als hypophysaris Symptom bei basophilen Vorderlappenadenoma und bei Arachnodaktylie mit Hypophysentumor. Med. Welt. 10:183.

Schmorl, C., 1904: Zur Kenntniss des Ikterus neonatorum, insbesondere der dabei auftretenden Gehirnveranderungen. Verh. dtsch. Ges. Path. 15:109.

Schreiner, L., 1968: Klinische und histologische Untersuchungen zum Alport-Syndrom. Arch. Ohr.Nas.-Kehlk-Heilk. 191:618.

Schuknecht, H., 1972: Unpublished data.

Schuknecht, H., 1974: Surgery for congenital atresia. Arch. Otolaryng. In press.

Sever, J., 1973: Present status of vaccines for rubella. Arch. Otolaryng. 98:265.

Shambaugh, G., Jr., 1967: Surgery of the Ear. 2nd ed., p. 571. W. B. Saunders, Philadelphia, Pa.

Shaw, R., and Glover, R., 1961: Abnormal segregation in hereditary renal disease with deafness. Amer. J. Hum. Genet. 13:89.

Sidman, R., Green, M., and Appel, S., 1965: Catalog of the Neurological Mutants of the Mouse. Harvard University Press, Cambridge, Mass.

Siebenmann, F., cited by Altmann, F., 1950: Histologic picture of inherited nerve deafness in man and animals. Arch. Otolaryng. 51:852.

Sleeckx, J., Shea, J., and Pitzer, F., 1967: Epitympanic ossicular fixation. Arch. Otolaryng. 85:619.

Smith, J., and Stowe, F., 1961: The Pierre Robin syndrome (glossoptosis, micrognathia, cleft palate): A review of 39 cases with emphasis on associated ocular lesions. Pediatrics 27:128.

Snyder, C., 1956: Bilateral facial agenesis (Treacher Collins syndrome). Amer. J. Surg. 92:81.

Sohar, E., 1956: Renal disease, inner ear

deafness, and ocular changes; new heredofamilial syndrome. Arch. intern. Med. 97:627.

Steffen, T., and House, W., 1962: Salivary gland choristoma of the middle ear. Arch. Otolaryng. 76:74.

Stevenson, A., and Cheeseman, E., 1956: Hereditary deaf-mutism, with particular reference to Northern Ireland. Ann. Hum. Genet. 20:177.

Strauss, A., and Werner, H., 1943: Comparative psychopathology of the brain-injured child and the traumatic brain-injured adult. Amer. J. Psychiat. 99:835.

Streeter, G., 1922: Development of the auricle in the human embryo. Contrib. Embryol. Carnegie Inst. 14:111.

Sturtz, G., and Burke, E., 1956: Hereditary hematuria, nephropathy and deafness. New Eng. J. Med. 254:1123.

Swan, C., Tostevin, A., Moore, B., Mayo, H., and Black, G., 1943: Congenital defects in infants following infectious diseases during pregnancy, with special reference to relationship between German measles and cataract, deaf-mutism, heart disease and microcephaly, and to period of pregnancy in which occurrence of rubella is followed by congenital abnormalities. Méd. J. Austr. 2:201.

Tabor, J., 1961: Absence of the oval window. Arch. Otolaryng. 74:515.

Tait, L., 1883: Note on deafness in white cats. Nature 29:164.

Taylor, G., and Martin, H., 1961: Salivary gland tissue in the middle ear. Arch. Otolaryng. 73:651.

Teig, E., 1968: Hereditary progressive deafness in a family of 72 patients. Acta oto-laryng. 65:365.

Thieme, E., 1957: A report of the occurrence of deaf-mutism and goiter in four of six siblings of a North American family. Ann. Surg. 146:941.

Thompson, R., Gaull, G., Horwitz, S., and Schenk, R., 1969: Hereditary hyperphosphatasia. Studies of three siblings. Amer. J. Med. 47:209.

Tietz, W., 1963: A syndrome of deaf-mutism associated with albinism showing dominant autosomal inheritance. Amer. J. Hum. Genet. 15:259.

Usher, C., 1914: On the inheritance of retinitis pigmentosa, with notes of case.

Roy. London Ophth. Hosp. Rep. 19:130.

Valvasorri, G., Naunton, R., and Lindsay, J., 1969: Inner ear anomalies: clinical and histopathological considerations. Ann. Otol. Rhinol. Laryng. 78:929.

Vernon, M., 1967a: Prematurity and deafness: the magnitude and nature of the problem among deaf children. Exceptional Children 33:289.

Vernon, M., 1967b: Rh factor and deafness: the problem, its psychological, physical and educational manifestations. Exceptional Children 34:5.

Vernon, M., 1969: Usher's syndrome: Deafness and progressive blindness. J. Chron. Dis. 22:133.

Versteegh, C., 1927: Ergebnisse partieller Labyrinthexstirpation bei Kaninchen. Acta oto-laryng. 11:393.

Waardenburg, P., 1951: A new syndrome combining developmental anomalies of the eyelids, eyebrows, and nose root with pigmentary defects of the iris and head hair and with congenital deafness. Amer. J. Hum. Genet. 3:195.

Wagemann, W., 1960–1961: Zur Kenntnis des Usher-Syndroms, einer Sonderform recessiver Labyrinthschädigungen. Hals-Nas.-Ohrenarzt. 9:151.

Warburg, M., 1963: Norrie's disease (atrofia bulborum hereditaria). Acta ophthal. 41:134.

Ward, P., Engel, E., and Nance, W., 1968: The larynx in the cri du chat (cat cry) syndrome. Trans. Amer. Acad. Ophthal. Otolaryng. 72:90.

Weibel, R., Stokes, J., Jr., Buynak, E., and Hilleman, M., 1969: Rubella vaccination in adult females. New Eng. J. Med. 280:682.

Wever, E., 1965: The degeneration processes in the ear of the shaker mouse. Ann. Otol. Rhinol. Laryng. 74:5.

Whalen, R., Huang, S., Peschel, E., and McIntosh, H., 1961: Hereditary nephropathy, deafness and renal foam cells. Amer. J. Med. 31:171.

Whiting, P., 1918: Inheritance of coat-color in cats. J. Exp. Zool. 25:539.

Wiegand, R., 1954: Dysostosis craniofacialis (Morbus Crouzon 1912) mit beitseitiger (häutiger) Gehörgangsatresie. Arch. Ohr. Nas-Kehlk-Heilk. 166:128.

Wildervanck, L., 1957: Deaf-mutism with Waardenburg-Klein syndrome in

children. Ned. T. Geneesk. 101:1120.

Wildervanck, L., 1962: Hereditary malformations of the ear in three generations. Acta oto-laryng. 54:553.

Wilson, T., and Kane, F., 1959: Congenital deafness in white cats. Acta oto-laryng. 50:269.

Windle, W., Becker, R., and Weil, A., 1944: Alterations in brain structure after asphyxiation at birth. J. Neouropath. Exp. Neurol. 3:224.

Windmiller, J., Whalley, P., and Fink, C., 1963: Cockayne's syndrome with chromosomal analysis. Amer. J. Dis. Child. 105:204.

Winter, L., Cram, B., and Banovetz, J., 1968: Hearing loss in hereditary renal disease. Arch. Otolaryng. 88:238.

Wolff, D., 1964: Malformations of the ear. Arch. Otolaryng. 79:288.

Wolff, D., and Maniglia, A., 1967: Microscopic observations of temporal bones from a stillborn. Anencephalic of seven months. Rev. panamer. Otorinolaring. Bronchoesofagol. 1:54.

Wright, J., and Etholm, B., 1973: Anomalies of the middle-ear muscles. J. Laryng. 87:281.

Wright, J., Jr., Taylor, C., and McKay, D., 1967: Variations in the course of the facial nerve as illustrated by tomography. Laryngoscope 77:717.

Zechner, G., and Altmann, P., 1968: The temporal bone in Hunter's syndrome (gargoylism). Arch. Ohr. Nas.-Kehlk-Heilk. 192:137.

Zellweger, H., 1965: Chromosomal aberrations and their significance for ophthalmo-otorhinolaryngology. Trans. Amer. Acad. Opthal. Otolaryng. 69:33.

Zellweger, H., Giaccai, L., and Firzli, S., 1952: Gargoylism and Marquio's disease. Amer. J. Dis. Child 84:421.

Ziprowski, L., and Adam, A., 1964: Recessive total albinism and congenital deaf-mutism. Arch. Derm. 89:151.

Ziprowski, L., Krakowski, A., Adam, A., Costeff, H., and Sade, J., 1962: Partial albinism and deaf-mutism due to a recessive sex-linked gene. Arch. Derm. 86:530.

Zonderman, B., 1959: The preschool nerve-deaf child. Laryngoscope 69:54.

5 Infections

A. BACTERIAL INFECTIONS

Bacterial infections of the ear usually occur in association with, or as a complication of, an upper respiratory infection. The symptoms vary according to the type of organism, the age of the patient, and certain anatomical features of the temporal bone (such as the extent of pneumatization and functional effectiveness of the eustachian tube). The most common infecting organisms, according to Stewart (1928) and Palva et al. (1964) are *Diplococcus pneumoniae, Haemophilus influenzae,* and beta-hemolytic streptococci. Viruses have been isolated from the middle ears of patients with viral pneumonia (Zippel, 1963); however, they are not common invaders.

1. DISORDERS OF THE TYMPANIC MEMBRANE

a. Myringitis

Acute myringitis. Acute myringitis usually occurs in association with infection of the middle ear or external auditory canal. It is characterized by thickening of the tympanic membrane due to hypervascularity, edema, and invasion with polymorphonuclear leucocytes (PMNs) and may be accompanied by serous and hemorrhagic blebs (Fig. 5.1). The accumulation of products of inflammation in the middle ear may cause bulging of the tympanic membrane. The infection may subside spontaneously or progress to the stage of focal necrosis, followed by perforation and suppurative otorrhea. Total necrosis of the tympanic membrane may occur in virulent hemolytic streptococcal infections; however, this complication is rare today because of the effectiveness of antibiotic drugs in controlling the growth of these organisms.

Bullous myringitis. This disorder is an inflammation of the tympanic membrane and adjacent skin of the external auditory canal occurring most commonly in association with influenza epidemics. It is characterized by blebs of serum and blood between the fibrous and dermal layers and causes only a minimal hearing loss.

Fig. 5.1: Acute serohemmorrhagic myringitis in a 67-year-old female with acute pneumococcal otitis media and meningitis. The tympanic membrane is thickened by collections of serum and blood between the fibrous and dermal layers. The mucous membrane of the middle ear and mastoid is thickened by hypervascularity, edema, and invasion with polymorphonuclear leucocytes (PMNs), and the spaces contain purulent exudate.

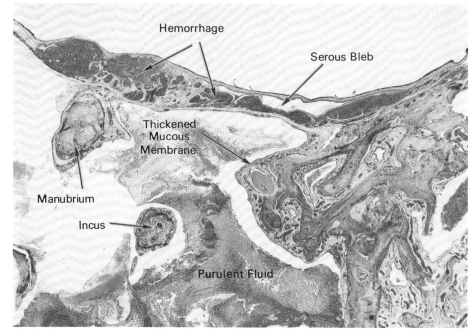

Fig. 5.2: Anterior marginal perforation. The mucocutaneous junction is located in the middle area about 3 mm from the tympanic annulus.

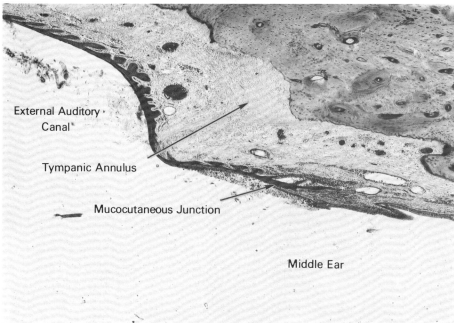

Fig. 5.3: Anterior central perforation. The rim of the tympanic membrane is thickened by fibrous tissue and a plaque of hyalin and the mucocutaneous junction is located on its medial surface.

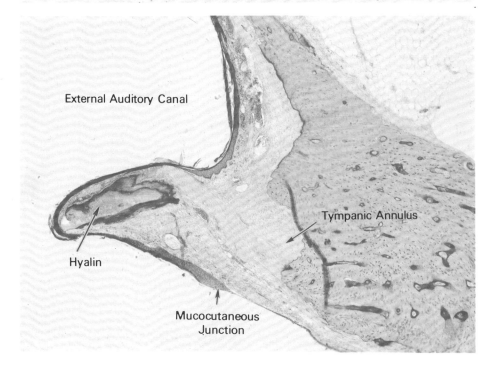

Fig. 5.4: Posterior central perforation. The tympanic membrane is thickened by fibrous tissue proliferation, and the mucucutaneous junction is located at the rim of the perforation.

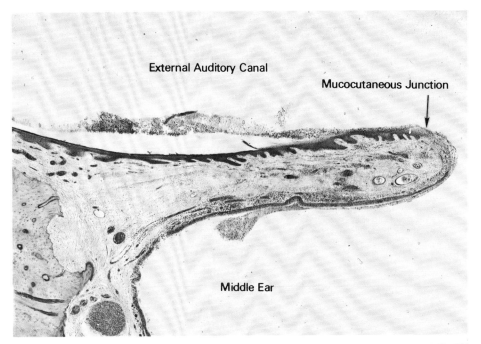

Fig. 5.5: Posterior marginal perforation. The mucocutaneous junction is located in the external auditory canal 5 mm lateral to the tympanic annulus.

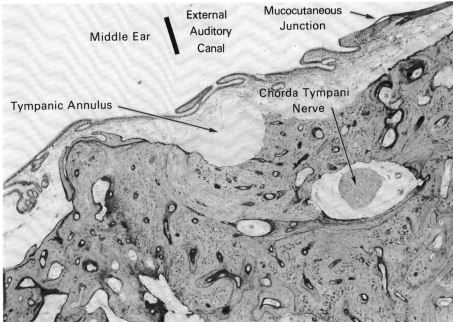

Fig. 5.6: Barrier membrane. A fibrous membrane bridges the external auditory canal and is associated with fibrous obliteration of the anteromedial part of the canal.

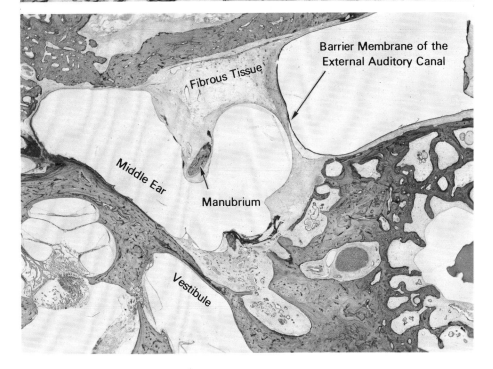

Hemorrhagic bullous myringitis may occur in association with meningo-encephalitis and is thought to be of viral etiology. These bullae frequently become invaded secondarily by bacteria, and the condition may be confused with acute otitis media.

Granular myringitis. This disorder is characterized by focal or diffuse replacement of the dermis of the tympanic membrane by a thin layer of granulation tissue. It may be associated with dermatitis of the external auditory canal. The fibrous layers of the tympanic membrane are intact, and hearing is not affected. Thorough removal of the granulation tissue is usually followed by healing, and recurrence is unusual.

b. Perforation

Most perforations of the tympanic membrane, whether caused by infection or trauma, heal spontaneously. Permanent perforations may occur when the area of destruction is large or when infection is recurrent or prolonged. A perforation of the pars tensa, regardless of size, is described as "central" when a rim of tympanic membrane remains at all borders, and "marginal" when some part of the defect extends to the tympanic annulus. Defects of Schrapnell's membrane are commonly termed "attic" perforations. The location of a perforation is of clinical significance in that epidermal invasion of the middle ear is more common with "marginal" than with "central" perforations of the pars tensa and is very common with perforations of Schrapnell's membrane.

With marginal perforations squamous epithelium frequently extends 1 to 4 mm into the middle ear (Figs. 5.2, 5.3) whereas with central perforations, the mucocutaneous junction usually is located at the rim of the perforation (Fig. 5.4). Squamous epithelium has a velvety appearance which aids the surgeon in determining the location of the mucocutaneous junction.

In exceptional cases the mucous membrane of the middle ear may extend through a perforation to replace squamous epithelium of the external auditory canal (Fig. 5.5). Ulceration of the external auditory canal may heal with proliferation of fibrous tissue and may be followed by the formation of a barrier membrane in the bony part of the canal (Fig. 5.6).

McArdle and Tonndorf (1968) have shown experimentally that hearing loss from a perforation is caused by the direct admittance of sound pressures into the middle ear. Hearing losses were determined to be greatest for low frequencies but, other than that, the location of the perforation could not be correlated with any particular type of audiometric pattern.

c. Replacement membrane

The thickness of a membrane which heals a perforation is determined by the degree of fibrous tissue proliferation incited during the healing process. The replacement membrane may have a dense intermediate layer of collagenous fibrous tissue or it may consist of only a thin layer of epidermis and mucous membrane. Thick and thin areas may occur in the same tympanic membrane and may be associated with plaques of hyalinized collagen (Fig. 5.7).

d. Retraction pocket

A retraction pocket consists of an invagination into the middle ear space of a replacement membrane and may occur either in the pars tensa or Schrapnell's membrane (Figs. 5.8, 5.9). A retraction pocket may be "fixed", that is, adherent to structures in the middle ear, or "mobile", that is, free to move in response to pressure differences acting upon the membrane.

e. Umbo blebs

Umbo blebs are benign asymptomatic glistening vesicles located in the center of the tympanic membrane. In Armstrong's experience (1955) the incidence was one in 364 examinations. These thin-walled blebs contain a thin lipoid fluid. They are asymptomatic and disappear spontaneously after several weeks. The etiology is unknown, and no treatment is indicated.

Fig. 5.7: Replacement membrane. A large part of the tympanic membrane posterior to the manubrium has been replaced by a thin membrane consisting principally of epidermis and mucous membrane. The anterior part shows fibrous thickening.

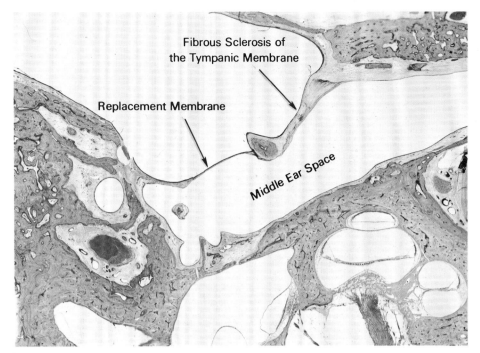

Fig. 5.8: Retraction pocket. There is a posterior marginal fixed retraction pocket and an anterior replacement membrane.

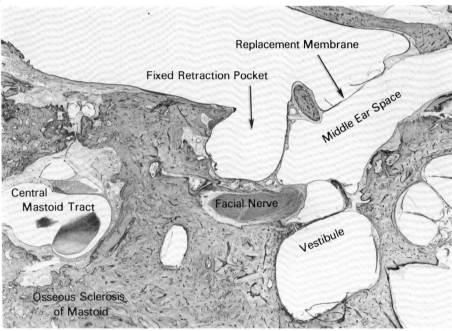

Fig. 5.9: Epitympanic (attic) retraction pocket. The epidermal lining is fixed to the head of the malleus and body of the incus.

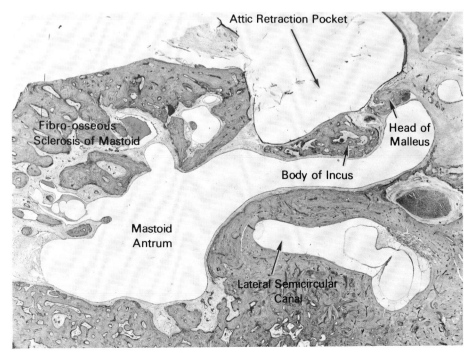

The middle ear, and adjacent pneumatized areas of the temporal bone, constitute an extension of the upper respiratory tract and are subject to bacterial invasion via the eustachian tube. Factors which determine the clinical manifestations of an infection are bacterial virulency, host response, and effectiveness of treatment. Mild infections may cause pain of short duration and hyperemia of the tympanic membrane, whereas severe suppurative and necrotizing infections cause prolonged pain, systemic reaction, and possible complications. The pathological changes include thickening of the mucous membrane from edema, vascular engorgement, and invasion with acute inflammatory cells (Fig. 5.10). Drainage through the eustachian tube is impaired because of inflammatory thickening of the mucous membrane and destruction of cilia. Purulent exudate may accumulate in the pneumatized spaces and distend and rupture the tympanic membrane, producing purulent otorrhea. Although most infections subside without significant permanent pathological or functional alterations, severe, persistent, or recurring infections usually result in irreversible pathological changes. Hůlka (1941) found that an acute attack of otitis media often causes a mild sensorineural hearing loss and that a permanent loss of hearing for high frequencies may persist after the infection has subsided. Presumably this is caused by the effect of bacterial exotoxins on the basal turn of the cochlea.

In severe and persisting infections the mucous membrane may become ulcerated, polypoid, or granulomatous. Prolonged infection may be associated with resorption of the ossicles and mastoid bone by demineralization and osteoclastic activity. The resorption of the mastoid trabeculae is frequently radiologically demonstrable and usually constitutes an indication for surgical intervention.

The local clinical manifestations of severe acute otitis media and mastoiditis are pain in the mastoid region, tenderness and swelling in the postauricular area, and edema of the posterosuperior wall of the external auditory canal. During the stage of rarefying osteitis the infectious process may break through the cortex of the mastoid to form subperiosteal accumulations of purulent exudate and granulation tissue. The infection may extend to the extradural regions of the posterior and middle cranial fossae, break through the mastoid tip into the neck (Bezold's abscess), or fistulize into the external auditory canal. Facial nerve palsy, thrombosis of the lateral sinus, labyrinthitis, and brain abscess are other complications of fulminating persistent acute otitis media and mastoiditis. Ordinarily, effective medical management and timely surgical intervention prevent the development of these complications.

Infections which occur in childhood frequently arrest the pneumatization process resulting in a small mastoid and minimal pneumatization of the temporal bone.

Tuberculosis. Tuberculosis of the middle ear and mastoid in adults usually has an insidious, painless onset and proceeds on a chronic course. Tuberculous involvement of the tympanic membrane leads to early perforation and aural discharge before there is sufficient accumulation of purulent exudate to cause pain. The onset of suppurative otitis media in a patient known to be suffering from pulmonary tuberculosis should lead the clinician to suspect a tubercular etiology. The presence of multiple perforations of the tympanic membrane or exuberant granulation tissue in the middle ear, particularly when occurring in a young child, is suggestive of tubercular infection.

Eschle (1883) identified the tubercle bacillus in an ear infection only one year after Koch's discovery of the organism. Some early investigators (Gradenigo, 1888; Bondy, 1909; Brieger, 1913) believed that the portal of entry was the eustachian tube, while others favored the idea that the infection was spread by the hematogenous route (Barnick, 1896; Preysing, 1898). In a clinical and histopathological study of temporal bones of eight cases, Proctor and Lindsay (1942) found strong evidence that the tubercle bacilli reached the ear

Fig. 5.10: Acute otitis media due to Haemophilus influenzae in a 7-month-old child. There is polypoid thickening of the mucous membrane and purulent exudate in the middle ear. The tympanic membrane is intact but thickened by vascular engorgement, edema, and invasion with acute inflammatory cells.

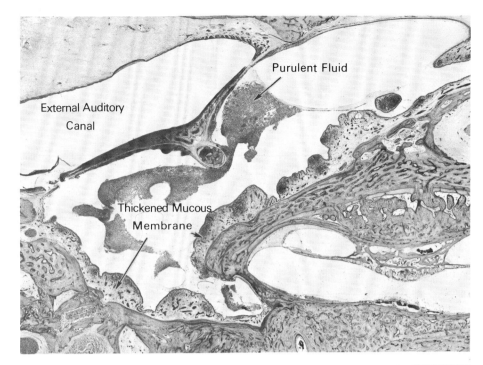

Fig. 5.11: Acute tuberculous otitis media and mastoiditis in a 57-year-old patient who died of miliary tuberculosis. The middle ear is filled with tuberculous granulation tissue. The tympanic membrane (inset) is intact but greatly thickened by tuberculous granulation tissue having the typical epithelioid cells, round cells, and multinucleated giant cells.

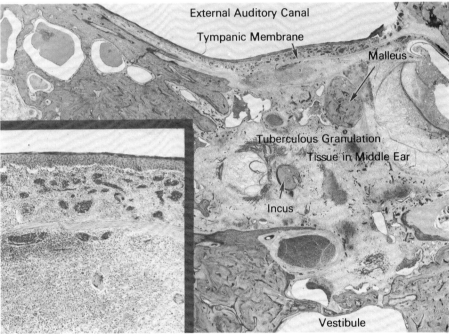

Fig. 5.12: Tuberculous otitis media in an adult showing obliteration of the middle ear by granulation tissue with large areas of necrosis and extensive ulceration of the mucous membrane.

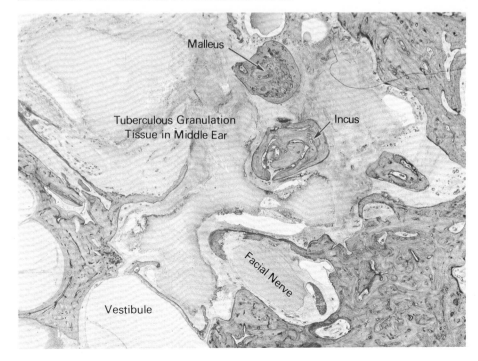

by the hematogenous route. Any caseous focus may be a source from which tubercle bacilli enter the blood stream to reach the temporal bone.

The incidence of tuberculous otitis media was very much higher during the early part of the century. Turner and Fraser, in a study reported in 1915, stated that 2.8 percent of all cases of suppurative otitis media were due to tuberculosis. Under the age of two years, 27 percent were tuberculous, while in infants under one year, the figure was 50 percent. Cox and Dwyer in 1929 found that 15 percent of cases of chronic aural discharge in children were tuberculous. These authors attributed the high incidence in children to the use of unsterilized milk.

Haslhofer (1969) found bilateral destruction of the temporal bones due to tuberculosis in an infant born of a mother with tuberculous salpingitis and endometritis. He believed the infection occurred either during the embryonal stage or during parturition, and that the organisms reached the temporal bones via the oral cavity and eustachian tube.

The infection begins with extensive edema and infiltration of the mucous membrane and tympanic membrane by round cells and giant cells (Fig. 5.11). As the infection progresses, numerous tubercles are formed consisting of epithelioid and lymphoid cells and containing characteristic giant cells of the Langhans type. Progression leads to caseation and ulceration (Fig. 5.12). The spaces not occupied by exuberant tuberculous granulation tissue become filled with purulent exudate, and this is followed by resorption of bone.

Many patients with tuberculous otitis media and mastoiditis are subjected to surgery without a correct etiological diagnosis having been made (Jeanes and Friedmann, 1960). An examination of the aural discharge for the presence of Mycobacterium tuberculosis should be made when otitis media does not respond readily to ordinary methods of treatment.

Diagnosis may be made from direct smears, cultures, or histological examination of granulation tissue removed from the middle ear or mastoid.

Previously untreated tuberculosis can nearly always be controlled by drugs alone. In the choice of drugs, laboratory testing of the susceptibility of the offending organisms to isoniazid, para-aminosalicylic acid (PAS), and streptomycin is of great importance. Isoniazid and PAS are commonly used for initial treatment. Streptomycin may be added for special problems, particularly in more severe infections. When the organism is resistant to isoniazid or PAS, one of the more toxic drugs (Cycloserine, Pyrazinanide, Viomycin, Kanamycin, Ethionamide) may be given (Tuberculosis, 1965). Chemoprophylaxis with isoniazid is effective in reducing morbidity from tuberculosis in high risk groups; thus, reactivation may be avoided, for example, in patients undergoing corticosteroid therapy or surgery, or in patients having leukemia or severe diabetes (Tuberculosis, 1967).

3. CHRONIC SUPPURATIVE OTITIS MEDIA AND MASTOIDITIS

Chronic suppurative otitis media and mastoiditis are characterized by perforation of the tympanic membrane and intermittent or constant purulent discharge associated with irreversible pathological changes in the middle ear, eustachian tube, and other pneumatized spaces of the temporal bone (Glorig and Gerwin, 1972). The mucous membrane throughout may be thickened by edema, submucosal fibrosis, and infiltration with chronic inflammatory cells (Fig. 5.13). Mucosal edema may proceed to formation of polyps (Figs. 5.14 to 5.17). In exceptional cases the polyps may become so large as to protrude from the meatus of the external auditory canal. Persistent suppuration may cause mucosal ulceration and the formation of granulation tissue. Ears with chronic suppurative disease have been found to exhibit an increased incidence of sensorineural hearing loss (Gardenghi, 1955; Bluvshtein, 1963; Paparella et al., 1970, 1972).

Chronic inflammation is commonly associated with rarefying osteitis of the ossicles, otic capsule, and mastoid bone (Fig. 5.18). Resorption of the otic capsule occurring with or without keratoma (cholesteatoma) may lead to

Fig. 5.13: Chronic suppurative otitis media in a 76-year-old patient. There is a large anterior marginal perforation, fibrous thickening of the mucous membrane, and partial resorption of the ossicles.

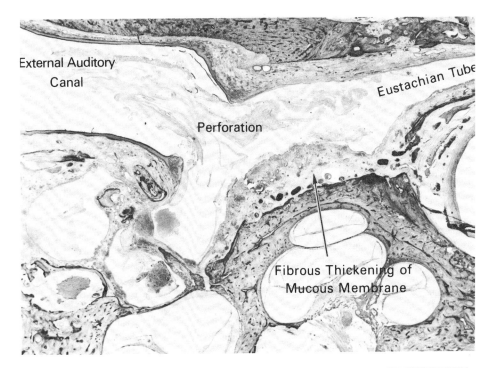

Fig. 5.14: Chronic suppurative otitis media in a 12-year-old boy. Edema, infiltration with inflammatory cells, and fibrous proliferation have resulted in polypoid hyperplasia of the mucous membrane.

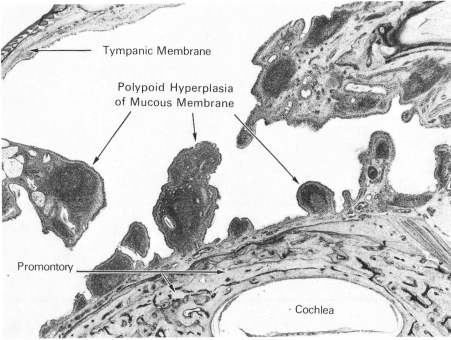

Fig. 5.15: Aural polyp arising from mucous membrane of the promontory in an 83-year-old female with chronic otorrhea. The tympanic membrane is missing, and the posterior mesotympanum is obliterated by fibrous tissue and cystic spaces.

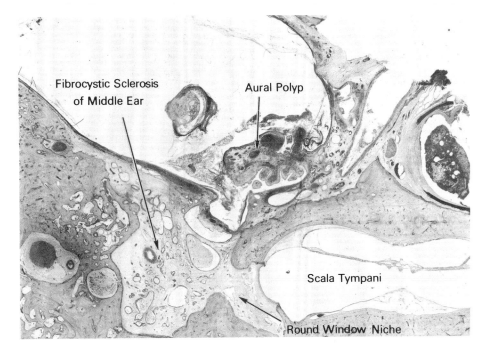

223   Infections

Fig. 5.16: Chronic suppurative otitis media and mastoiditis in a 48-year-old male. During childhood the ear was treated by the introduction of hot olive oil into the ear canal. The middle ear and mastoid are partially obliterated by polypoid granulomatous tissue containing lipoid droplets which presumably consist of olive oil. See also Fig. 5.17.

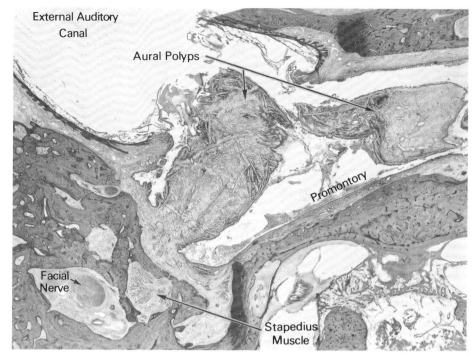

Fig. 5.17: Same case as Fig. 5.16. Higher magnification showing strata of lipoid droplets separated by plasma cells and lymphocytes. No lipophages, foreign body giant cells, or cholesterol clefts are present.

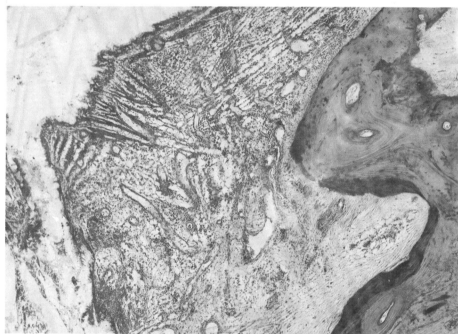

Fig. 5.18: Active rarefying osteitis adjacent to the incudal ligament associated with chronic suppurative otitis media and mastoiditis. Bone resorption is occurring by osteoclastic activity.

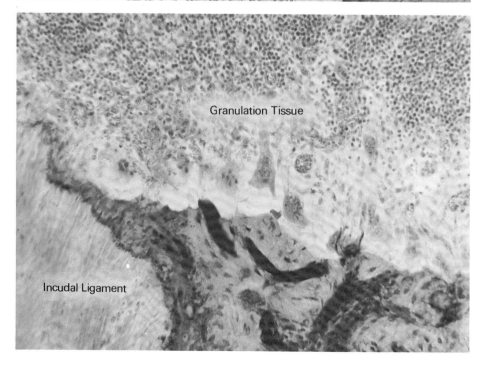

fistulization, invasion, and destruction of the inner ear (Figs. 5.19, 5.20).
Progressive osteitis is an indication for active medical and surgical therapy.

Chronic infection of the middle ear may lead to partial or complete obstruction of the eustachian tube. Fibrous and fibrocystic sclerosis may extend
into the osseous part of the tube to create narrowing of the lumen (Fig. 5.21).
Fibrosis, new bone growth, or deposition of hyalin may occlude the tympanic
orifice of the tube (Fig. 5.22).

4. KERATOMA (CHOLESTEATOMA)

Otologists are in general agreement about the pathogenesis and histopathology of keratoma (Harris, 1961; Harris and Weiss, 1962). Simply stated, it is
the accumulation of exfoliated keratin in the middle ear or other pneumatized areas of the temporal bone, arising from keratinizing squamous epithelium that has invaded these areas from the external auditory canal (Gray,
1964) and has commonly been misnamed cholesteatoma (Fig. 5.23). If the
epithelialized pocket is dry, the rate of exfoliation is slow and the keratin
mass may accumulate slowly for years without creating complications; however, in the presence of infection it may develop rapidly (Fig. 5.24). Keratoma
should not be confused with cholesterol granuloma, which is chronic gran-

Fig. 5.19: Active rarefying osteitis in the wall
of a radical mastoid cavity leading to a bony
fistula of the lateral semicircular canal.

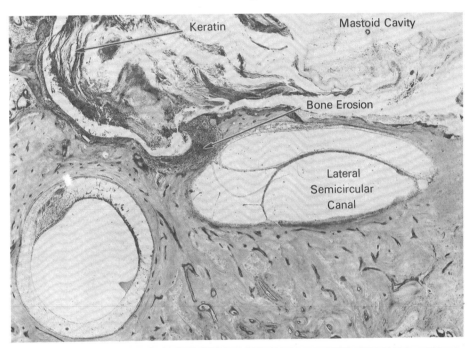

Fig. 5.20: Rarefying osteitis of the lateral semicircular canal associated with invasion of
squamous epithelium. Irregular resorption of
bone has created a small sequestrum. The endosteum is thickened by fibrous proliferation.

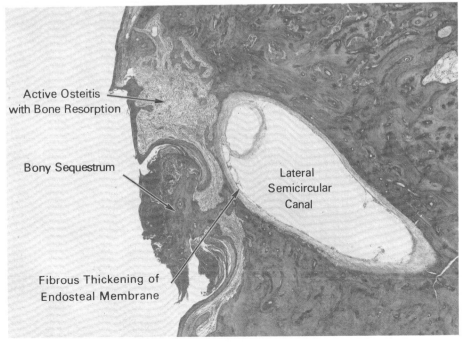

ulation tissue containing cholesterol crystals (Friedmann, 1959; Dota et al., 1963) (Fig. 5.25). The hypothesis that keratoma may develop by metaplasia of mucous membrane is untenable. Histological studies show that mucous membrane can change to pavement epithelium; however, there is no support for the concept that it can convert to keratinizing squamous epithelium.

Keratoma most commonly occurs in the epitympanum as a consequence of epidermal invasion through a perforation of Schrapnell's membrane. It may extend posteriorly into the antrum, periantral cells, and central mastoid tract, or inferiorly into the middle ear. Invasion through a posterosuperior marginal perforation of the pars tensa may lead to a keratoma of the posterior mesotympanum which may extend into the epitympanum and mastoid. Keratoma may be limited to the middle ear and, in rare cases, may be found behind an intact tympanic membrane. This occurs when epidermal ingrowth is followed by healing of a perforation of the tympanic membrane. When middle ear and mastoid keratoma occur behind an intact tympanic membrane without a prior history of otorrhea, the pathogenesis is more likely to be primary keratoma due to epithelial rests (Derlacki and Clemis, 1965; Derlacki et al., 1968).

Adults with keratoma usually have minimal pneumatization as the result

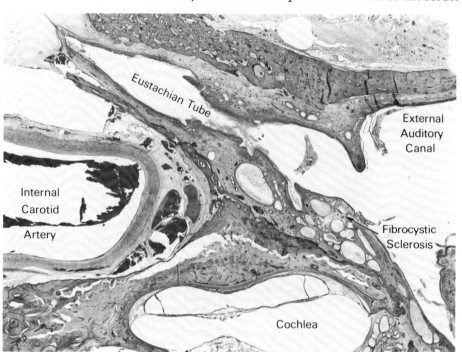

Fig. 5.21: The submucosal layer of the middle ear and osseous part of the eustachian tube is thickened by proliferation of fibrous tissue and epithelial-lined submucosal cystic spaces.

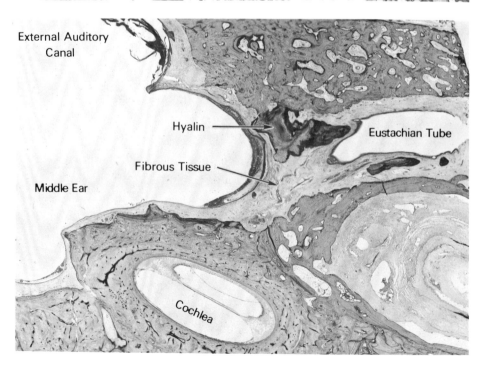

Fig. 5.22: The protympanum contains dense fibrous tissue with a deposit of hyalin which has blocked the orifice of the eustachian tube.

Fig. 5.23: Keratoma of the middle ear. Squamous epithelium has invaded the posterior mesotympanum through a small perforation of the tympanic membrane, and exfoliated keratin is retained within the pocket.

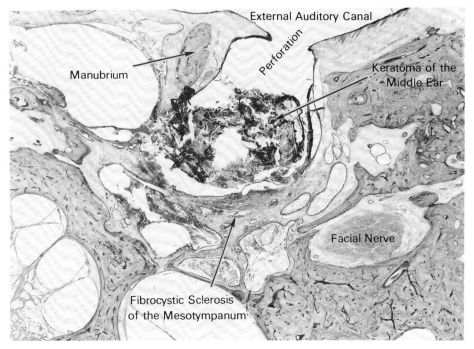

Fig. 5.24: This view shows finger-like extensions of squamous epithelium into the mesotympanum in the presence of chronic suppurative otitis media.

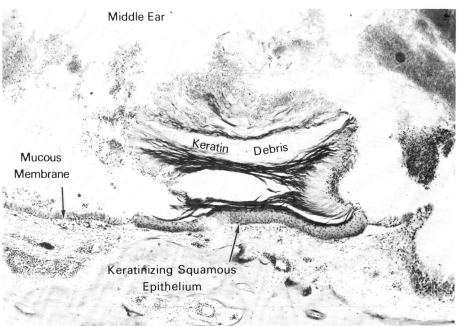

Fig. 5.25: Cholesterol granuloma. Chronic granulation tissue in the middle ear and mastoid frequently contains cholesterol crystals, demonstrated histologically as clefts. The condition should not be confused with keratoma.

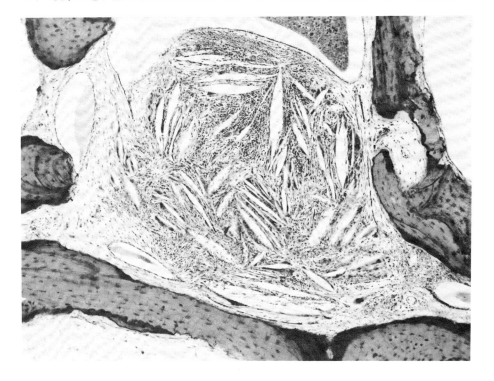

of childhood infections. Children with keratoma, on the other hand, frequently have extensively pneumatized temporal bones so that epidermal ingrowth may extend deeply into cell tracts.

The invading epidermis may form an incomplete surface lining of a space with its keratin debris spilling over into adjacent areas or it may completely line a space enveloping all structures within it.

It is well established that keratoma incites resorption of adjacent bone. The popular concept is that the bone gives way to the expanding mass through a process of pressure erosion. Sometimes, however, bone resorption occurs beneath an epidermal surface in the absence of a keratomatous mass. Abramson (1969; Abramson et al., 1971) believes that bone destruction may be due, in part, to the activity of collagenase and has presented evidence to show that the epidermis of keratomata, like skin elsewhere, is rich in collagenase. This tendency for keratoma to cause bone erosion may lead to destruction of ossicles, fistulization or invasion of the bony labyrinth, erosion of the fallopian canal, and extension into areas adjacent to the temporal bone. Keratomatous masses are often infected and when accompanied by bone erosion can lead to intracranial complications. For these reasons the identification of keratoma is considered by most otologists to be an indication for surgical intervention.

5. EPIDERMIZATION

Epidermization implies replacement of mucous membrane by keratinizing squamous epithelium without retention of keratin debris (Figs. 5.26, 5.27). The area of epidermization may involve part or all of the middle ear cavity and may include the antrum. It is often associated with resorption of the lateral epitympanic wall (scutum) or posterosuperior part of the bony tympanic annulus. Frequently a membrane bridges the tympanic orifice of the eustachian tube. The mastoid may communicate with the middle ear or it may be obliterated by fibro-osseous sclerosis. Epidermization may be associated with intermittent suppuration but does not in itself necessarily constitute an indication for surgical treatment.

6. SCLEROSIS

a. Fibrous sclerosis (adhesive otitis)

Fibrous sclerosis is the result of a healing reaction and is characterized by the proliferation of fibrous tissue in the middle ear and mastoid. The mucous membrane is thickened, and the partially pneumatized spaces contain dense strands of connective tissue which may impair ossicular movement (Fig. 5.28). This change may be associated with perforation or retraction of the tympanic membrane, resorption of ossicles, and deposits of hyalinized collagen (tympanosclerosis).

b. Fibrocystic sclerosis

Fibrocystic sclerosis implies partial or total obliteration of the middle ear and mastoid by fibrous tissue and cystic spaces. The cystic spaces develop as areas which have been isolated by fibrous tissue proliferation (Figs. 5.29 to 5.32). Hyperplasia of the mucous membrane may lead to numerous small cystic spaces within a fibrous matrix (Fig. 5.33). The cystic spaces are lined by nonsecreting flat or cuboidal epithelium and contain a thick protein-containing acidophilic fluid. The fluid may also contain exfoliated cells and cholesterol.

c. Fibro-osseous sclerosis

Fibro-osseous sclerosis is a healing reaction characterized by fibrous tissue proliferation and new bone growth. This reaction is extremely rare in the middle ear but is a common sequel to infection in the other pneumatized regions of the temporal bone. Osteoid tissue is deposited on existing bone by osteoblastic activity leading to the formation of lamellar new bone (Figs. 5.34, 5.35). The thickened bone trabeculae coalesce and progressively obliterate the intervening spaces. Central fibrous areas remain in the mastoid antrum and central mastoid tract even with the most advanced osseous sclerosis (Figs. 5.36, 5.37). Rarefying osteitis involving the trabeculae of the periantral cells or central mastoid tract may be associated with osseous sclerosis of the bordering areas. Should the central area subsequently become pneumatized, the radiological appearance can be that of an abnormal radiolucent area of the mastoid which may be misinterpreted as being bone erosion caused by keratoma (Fig. 5.38).

7. HYALINIZATION (TYMPANOSCLEROSIS)

The first description of this disorder appears in a publication of von Tröltsch in 1877. In 1955 Zöllner further elucidated the clinical nature of this condition and indicated its importance as an adverse factor in reconstructive middle ear surgery.

Chang (1969) and Sorensen and True (1971) have shown that hyalinization begins as fibroblastic invasion of the submucosal layers followed by thicken-

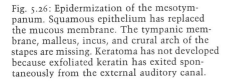

Fig. 5.26: Epidermization of the mesotympanum. Squamous epithelium has replaced the mucous membrane. The tympanic membrane, malleus, incus, and crural arch of the stapes are missing. Keratoma has not developed because exfoliated keratin has exited spontaneously from the external auditory canal.

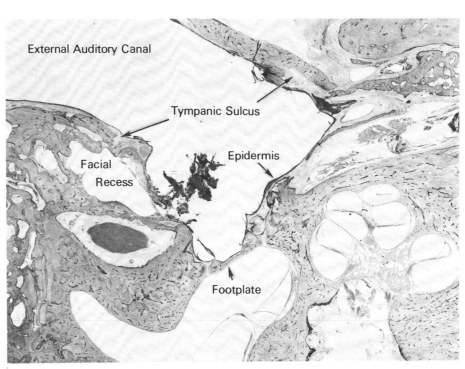

Fig. 5.27: Same specimen as Fig. 5.26 showing epidermization of the oval window niche. The footplate is fixed by a deposit of hyalin.

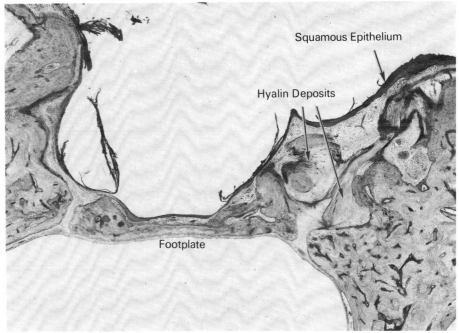

Fig. 5.28: Fibrous sclerosis of the posterior mesotympanum. The tympanic membrane is thickened and the middle ear contains interlacing strands of fibrous tissue causing partial fixation of the ossicles.

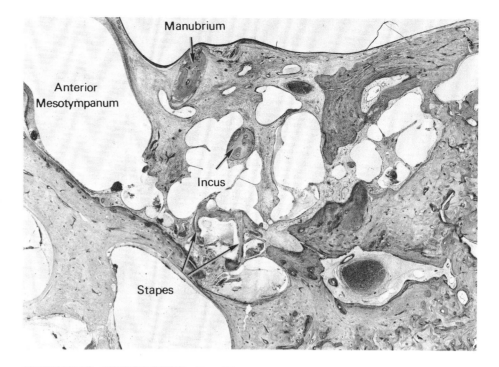

Fig. 5.29: Fibrocystic sclerosis of the middle ear. The tympanic cavity is partially obliterated by fibrous tissue and cystic spaces. The incus and crural arch of the stapes are missing.

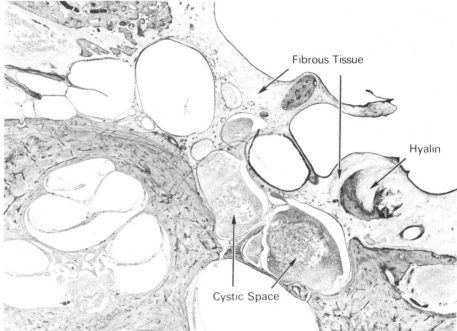

Fig. 5.30: Fibrocystic sclerosis of the posterior mesotympanum showing obliteration of the round window niche.

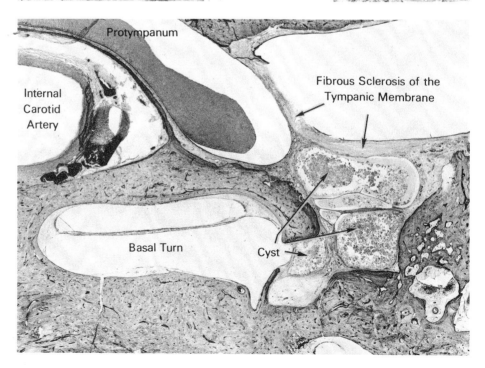

Fig. 5.31: Fibrocystic sclerosis of the mastoid. The intertrabecular spaces have been partially obliterated by fibrous tissue, leaving small central spaces lined by flat or cuboidal epithelium and containing acidophilic fluid.

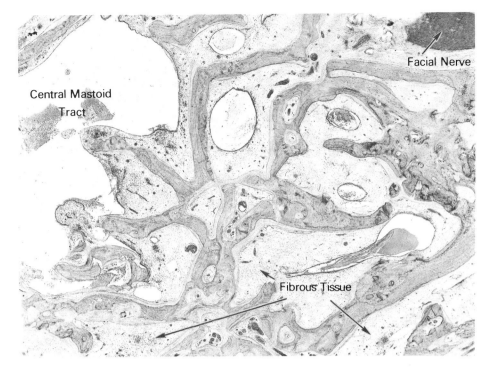

Fig. 5.32: Fibrocystic sclerosis of the central mastoid tract. Interlacing strands of fibrous tissue has resulted in loculated spaces containing granular acidophilic fluid with cellular debris and cholesterol crystals.

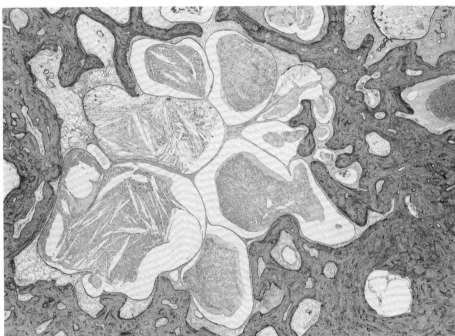

Fig. 5.33: Severe fibrocystic sclerosis with complete obliteration of the middle ear. The tympanic membrane and all ossicles, except the footplate of the stapes, have been destroyed.

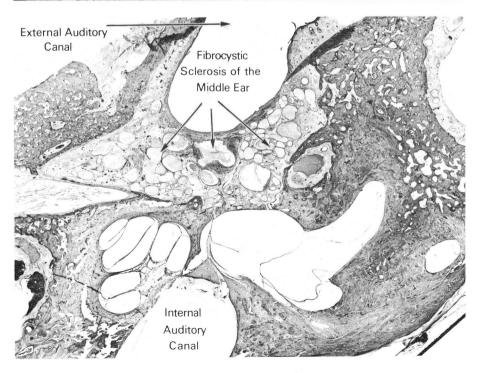

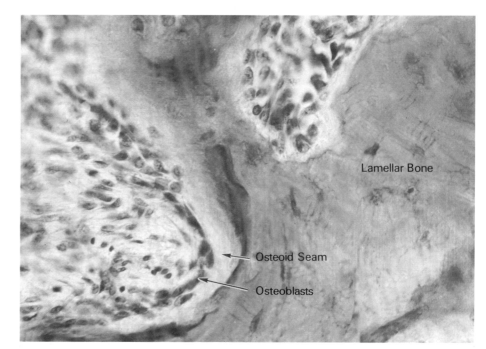

Fig. 5.34: Osseous sclerosis of the mastoid. Osteoid tissue is deposited on existing bone by osteoblastic activity.

Lamellar Bone

Osteoid Seam

Osteoblasts

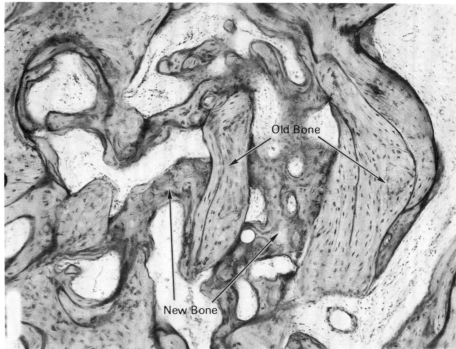

Fig. 5.35: Fibro-osseous sclerosis of the mastoid showing the intertrabecular spaces partially obliterated by new bone.

Old Bone

New Bone

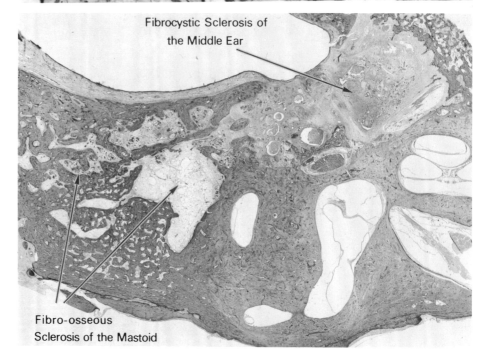

Fig. 5.36: Severe fibrocystic sclerosis of the middle ear and fibro-osseous sclerosis of the mastoid. The central mastoid tract is filled by a loosely structured fibrous tissue.

Fibrocystic Sclerosis of the Middle Ear

Fibro-osseous Sclerosis of the Mastoid

Fig. 5.37: Fibro-osseous obliteration of the mastoid. The obliterated central mastoid tract is identified by the central core of fibrous tissue.

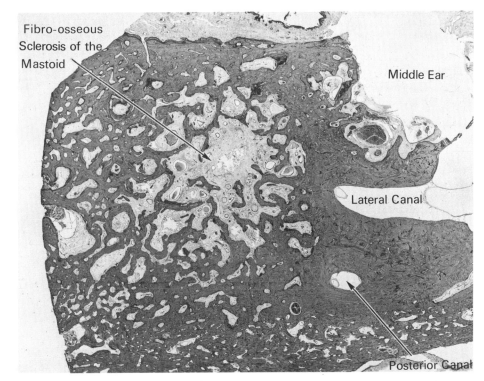

Fibro-osseous
Sclerosis of the
Mastoid

Middle Ear

Lateral Canal

Posterior Canal

Fig. 5.38: Osseous sclerosis surrounding enlarged pneumatized central mastoid tract. The radiologic appearance may be misinterpreted as keratoma of the mastoid. There is a large posterior retraction pocket.

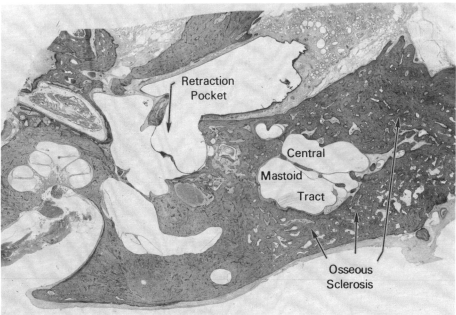

Retraction
Pocket

Central
Mastoid
Tract

Osseous
Sclerosis

ing and fusion of the collagenous fibers into a homogeneous mass and finally the deposition of scattered intracellular and extracellular calcium and phosphate crystals (Fig. 5.39). Although the pathogenesis is not clear, a prerequisite seems to be chronic otitis media followed by healing. Typically the ear with hyalinized collagen is free of suppuration. Inspection reveals whitish plaques in the tympanic membrane and nodular deposits in the submucosal layers of the middle ear (Igarashi et al., 1970) (Fig. 5.40). In severe cases much of the middle ear may be filled with this material. The underlying bone may appear normal but ossicles which are embedded in it lose their blood supply and become devitalized. The lacunae are empty although the bony framework remains. The overlying mucosa becomes very thin with diminished vascularity and may eventually disappear. In exceptional cases, particularly when reinfection occurs, masses of hyalinized collagen may extrude from the submucosa to become free masses in the middle ear (Fig. 5.41).

8. LESIONS OF THE OSSICLES

Rarefying osteitis of the ossicles is a common complication of chronic infections. The long process of the incus, crural arch of the stapes, body of the

Fig. 5.39: Hyalinized collagen (tympanosclerosis) of the tympanic cavity. Hyalin degeneration occurs as a healing reaction and is characterized by fibroblastic invasion of the submucosa followed by thickening and fusion of collagenous fibers into a homogeneous mass. No blood vessles and no viable cells are seen within the mass. The scattered small dark deposits presumably represent nuclear debris.

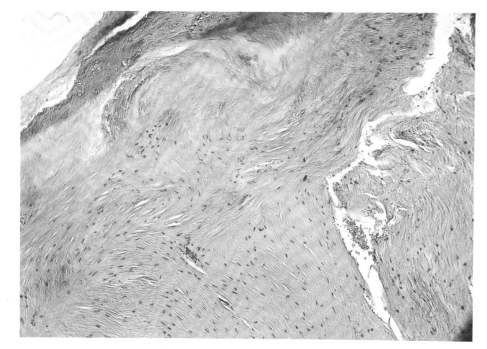

Fig. 5.40: Hyalin deposit in the tympanic membrane. These are often mistakenly termed calcium plaques.

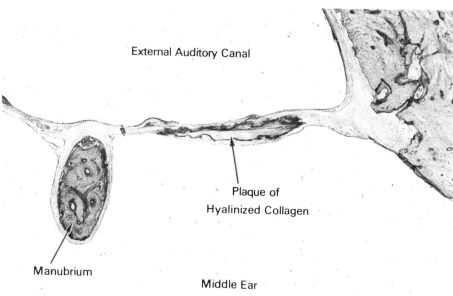

Fig. 5.41: Deposits of hyalin which extruded from the submucosa to lie free in the middle ear. The hyalin and ossicles were removed during reconstructive surgery of the middle ear.

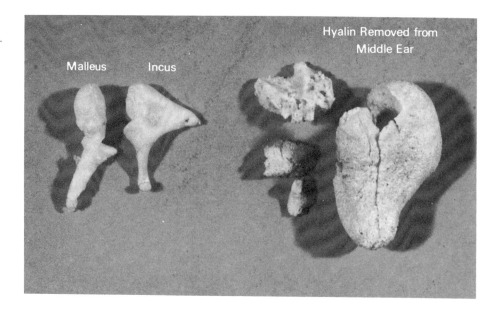

Fig. 5.42: Normal incus on the left. The other three incudes were removed during surgery and showed progressive stages of rarefying osteitis.

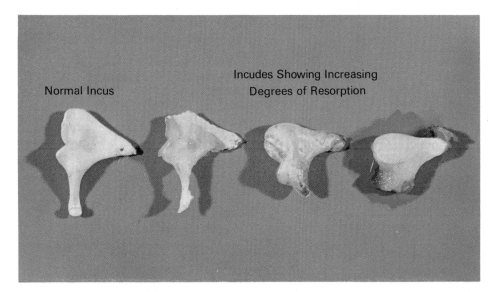

Fig. 5.43: Rarefying osteitis of the body of the incus. An irregular area of bone resorption contains dense fibrous tissue with scattered inflammatory cells and numerous vascular channels.

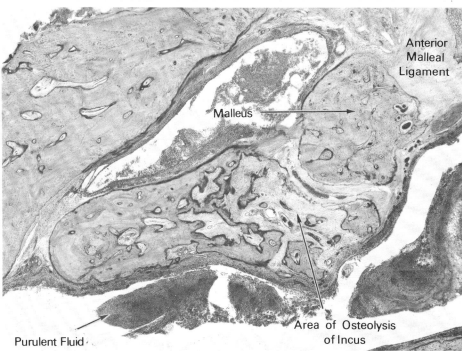

Fig. 5.44: Severe rarefying osteitis of the malleus and incus. The ossicles are partly replaced by and embedded in fibrous tissue, and the incus is ankylosed to the medial epitympanic wall.

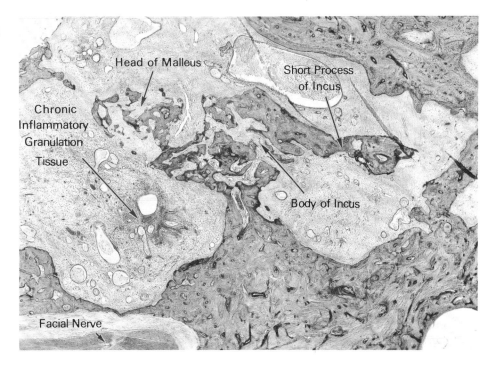

incus, and manubrium are involved in that order of frequency (Figs. 5.42, 5.43, 5.44).

Resorption of the lenticular process may result in a fibrous linkage between the long process of the incus and stapes and is characterized functionally by fluctuating conductive hearing loss. Acoustic transmission is improved when the fibrous band is placed under tension with forced inflation of the middle ear (Beickert, 1964).

Ossicular discontinuity in the presence of an intact tympanic membrane causes a large conductive hearing loss. An air-bone gap of 50 db or more is suggestive of this condition. When ossicular discontinuity is associated with a retracted replacement membrane which is adherent to the head of the stapes, the condition of "myringostapediopexy" is created which is compatible with excellent hearing (Fig. 5.45).

Many ingenious reconstructive procedures have been designed for the management of ossicular discontinuity (Harrison et al., 1959; Sheehy, 1965; Elbrønd, 1970). Operative procedures which attempt to recapture the acoustical advantages of the lever mechanism are termed Type II tympanoplasties (Wullstein, 1956a). When this is not possible, an attempt is made to establish sound transmission through a column of osseous or collagenous tissue, by a prosthesis, or by establishing the condition of myringostapediopexy (Juers, 1954).

The ossicles may be fixed by fibrous tissue, hyalinized collagen, and new bone growth (Hilding, 1965; Tos, 1970) (Figs. 5.46 to 5.50). The extent of ossicular resorption and fixation is an important determinant for the success of reconstructive middle ear surgery.

Fig. 5.45: A retracted posterior replacement membrane is in contact with the head of the stapes to produce "spontaneous myringostapediopexy," a condition which is compatible with good sound transmission.

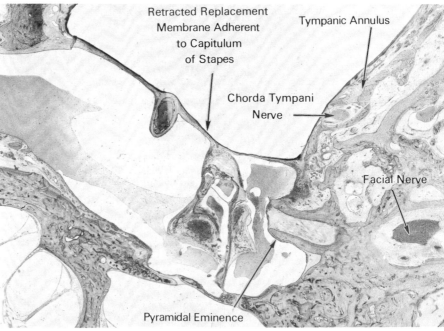

Fig. 5.46: Fixation of the incus to the lateral epitympanic wall by new bone growth. The epitympanic space, aditus, and antrum are obliterated by fibrocystic sclerosis.

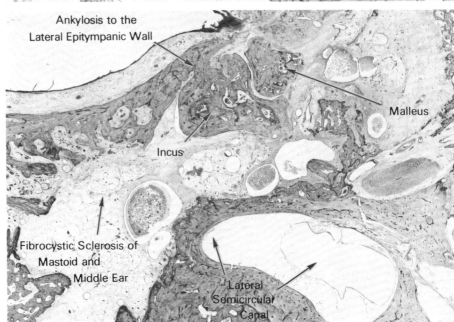

Fig. 5.47: Bony fixation of the head of the malleus to the anterior epitympanic wall by new bone growth.

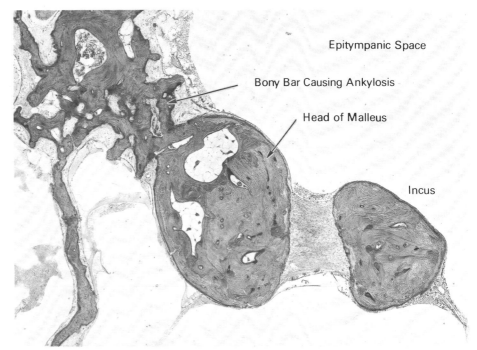

Epitympanic Space

Bony Bar Causing Ankylosis

Head of Malleus

Incus

Fig. 5.48: Fixation of the stapes by fibrous tissue and hyalin (tympanosclerosis). The head of the stapes has been resorbed.

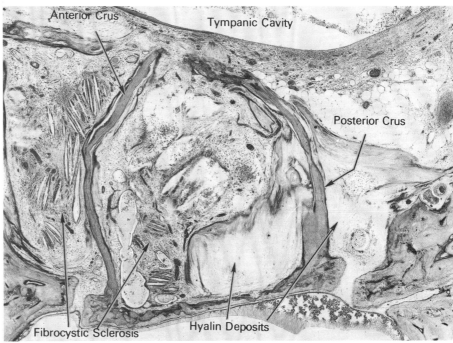

Anterior Crus

Tympanic Cavity

Posterior Crus

Fibrocystic Sclerosis

Hyalin Deposits

Fig. 5.49: The malleus and incus are fixed in the epitympanum by fibrous tissue and hyalin (tympanosclerosis). The ossicles show mild rarefying osteitis.

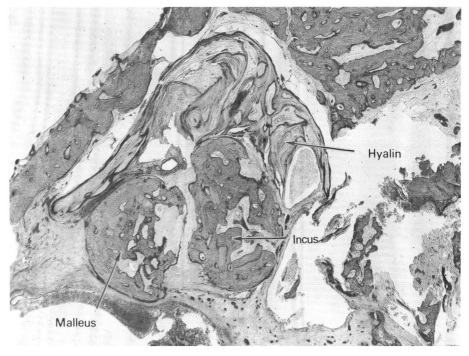

Hyalin

Incus

Malleus

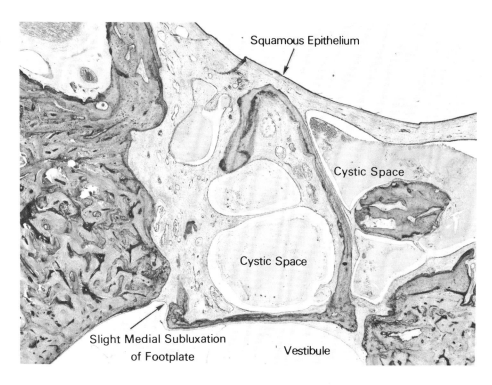

Fig. 5.50: Fibrous fixation of the stapes associated with fibrocystic sclerosis of the middle ear. The posterior crus has been partly resorbed.

9. PETROSITIS

Petrositis encompasses those infections which involve the perilabyrinthine and apical regions of the petrous bone. The pathways of pneumatization play an important role in the pathogenesis of acute petrositis and often provide routes of surgical approach to the apical region. Chronic petrositis occurring with chronic middle ear and mastoid infection is more often the result of direct extension from the peritubal area by progressive osteitis.

a. Acute petrositis

Acute petrositis is an acute inflammatory reaction in the pneumatized areas of the perilabyrinthine and apical regions. It is accompanied by all the changes in mucous membrane that characterize acute infection elsewhere in the temporal bone. Inflammatory reactions in this region assume special significance only when there is retention of the products of inflammation or when a prolonged acute infection leads to osteitis. The triad of symptoms consisting of (1) middle ear infection, (2) paralysis of the homolateral external rectus muscle (abducens nerve), and (3) pain in the homolateral orbit or behind the eye (trigeminal ganglionitis), constitutes Gradenigo's (1904) syndrome and is characteristic of infection of the petrous apex. The full triad may or may not be present depending upon the location and extent of inflammatory reaction. A lingering acute infection of the middle ear and mastoid which is associated with deep-seated pain should be regarded with concern.

b. Chronic petrositis

Chronic petrositis is a complication of chronic middle ear and mastoid suppuration. In addition to inflammatory changes and fibrosis in soft tissues, there is resorption of bone and new bone formation. It is possible for a low-grade infection of the petrous bone to persist for months or years without producing complications (Fig. 5.51).

Osteitis in the peritubal area may lead to inflammatory changes in the carotid canal (Fig. 5.52) and in rare instances can result in thrombosis and obliteration of the internal carotid artery (Fig. 5.53). Abscess formation may occur in either the peritubal area (Fig. 5.54) or the petrous apex area (Fig. 5.55).

The endochondral and endosteal layers of the otic capsule are quite resistant to destruction by infection, but, in exceptional cases, progressive rarefying osteitis may fistulize the otic capsule and destroy the labyrinth. If the

Fig. 5.51: Chronic low-grade petrositis showing bone resorption and new bone formation
involving the entire petrous apex. The semilunar ganglion is embedded in fibrotic granulation tissue.

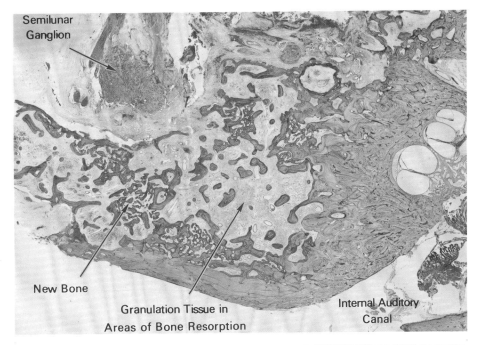

Fig. 5.52: Rarefying osteitis of the carotid
canal associated with chronic inflammation
and fibrosis of the pericarotid tissues in a 70-
year-old patient with chronic suppurative otitis media and mastoiditis and chronic lymphatic leukemia.

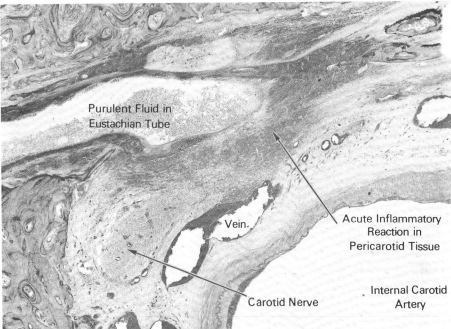

Fig. 5.53: Chronic petrositis in a 59-year-old
man showing destruction of the otic capsule
and obliteration of the carotid artery. There
are both resorption of bone and new bone
formation in the petrous apex.

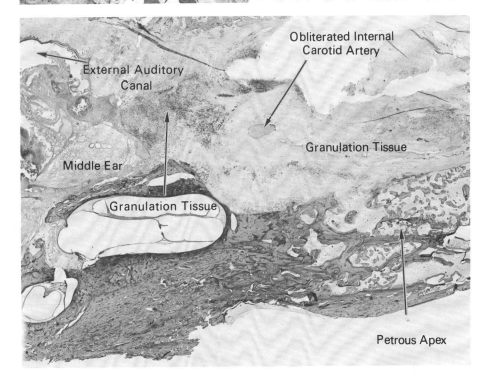

Fig. 5.54: Chronic petrositis showing an abscess in the peritubal area in a 76-year-old patient with chronic suppurative otitis media. The abscess extended into the retropharyngeal area and was associated with an extradural abscess.

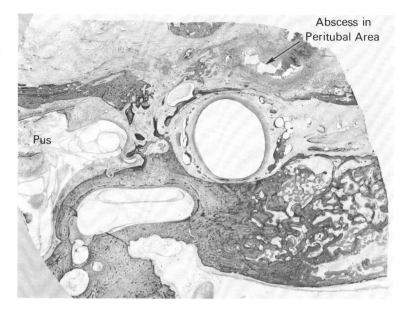

Fig. 5.55: Abscess of the petrous apex area of a 58-year-old man with chronic suppurative otitis media and mastoiditis. Death was due to meningitis.

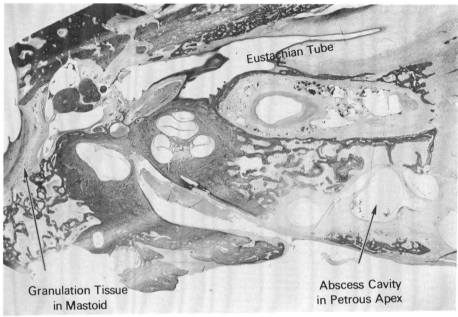

process is slow and associated with fibrosis, the labyrinth can be destroyed without causing intracranial complications.

Chronic petrositis may progress to involve contiguous structures and produce other serious complications, the most common of which are meningitis, extradural abscess, and brain abscess. Less common complications are destruction of the facial nerve, thrombosis of the lateral and petrosal sinuses, obliteration of the carotid artery, retropharyngeal abscess, and involvement of the abducens and trigeminal nerves, and nerves of the jugular foramen.

Brain abscess complicating petrositis is usually located in the temporal lobe. The mechanism by which microorganisms pass from the petrous bone to the brain substance without contaminating the meninges and subarachnoid spaces is not known. Retrograde phlebitis is the explanation most commonly offered, but proof of such process is lacking. The management of a temporal lobe abscess is usually considered a neurosurgical problem but arrest of the infection of the petrous bone during and after control of the brain abscess is the otologic surgeon's responsibility.

Petrositis may occur in the severe diabetic patient as a progression of infection from uncontrolled otitis externa, otitis media, and mastoiditis. It behaves as a low-grade osteomyelitis and may spread in the base of the skull from one petrous bone to the other. In spite of intensive medical therapy and surgery, the infection can be fatal (Chandler, 1968).

Petrositis demands prompt medical therapy and often requires surgical intervention. The apical region is most easily drained through tracts of pneumatization (Kopetzky and Armour, 1930–1931; Lempert, 1937; Lindsay, 1938). The approach of Ramadier (1933) through the bone between the cochlea and carotid artery may be feasible in some cases but is difficult and associated with some risk of injury to the carotid artery and cochlea.

10. LABYRINTHITIS

Many classifications have been proposed to encompass the various responses of the labyrinth to infection. The classification used here is derived from clinical and pathological observations and is based on the pathogenesis of labyrinthitis:

a. Acute toxic labyrinthitis
b. Acute suppurative labyrinthitis
c. Chronic labyrinthitis
d. Labyrinthine sclerosis

a. *Acute toxic labyrinthitis*

Acute toxic labyrinthitis, sometimes known as serous labyrinthitis, may be defined as an irritation of the labyrinth caused by otitic or meningitic infection without bacterial invasion of the inner ear. It is manifested by varying degrees of vertigo and hearing loss and is presumed to be caused by bacterial toxins or biochemical alterations. When occurring in mild form, recovery of function may be complete. In severe form the cytotoxic effects may be lethal to the sensory structures and result in partial or complete permanent loss of hearing and vestibular function. Acute toxic labyrinthitis may occur during the course of acute or chronic otitis media. Presumably the toxins enter the inner ear via the oval and round windows or through a pathologic bony labyrinthine fistula. Toxic labyrinthitis may also occur as a complication of meningitis, in which case the condition may be masked by the more severe meningeal symptoms. In the acute phase there is no clinical method for differentiating toxic from suppurative labyrinthitis. The diagnosis of toxic labyrinthitis can be made in retrospect if some auditory or vestibular function is preserved.

The principal pathological finding in mild acute toxic labyrinthitis is endolymphatic hydrops associated with a fine fibrillar or granular precipitate in the perilymphatic fluid (Figs. 5.56, 5.57). In more severe cases, the precipitate is also present in the endolymph.

In mild form no cytological changes are evident, whereas in severe form there is degeneration of the membranous labyrinth. Characteristically the changes are more severe in the auditory system than in the vestibular system.

b. *Acute suppurative labyrinthitis*

This condition is caused by bacterial invasion of the inner ear from contiguous areas of the temporal bone or meninges and, except when masked by coma, is manifested by severe vertigo and hearing loss.

Suppurative labyrinthitis of otitic origin may occur with either acute or chronic infections (Fig. 5.58). With acute infections the bacterial invasion is presumed to occur through the oval or round windows, whereas with chronic infection it may occur through either the windows or a pathologic fistula of the bony labyrinth. In 1904 Whitehead reported a 4 percent incidence of suppurative labyrinthitis in 691 patients requiring mastoidectomy and in 1914 Fraser reported a 1.4 percent incidence in patients with otitis media and mastoiditis. Fortunately, with the advent of antibiotics and improved surgical methods, suppurative labyrinthitis of otitic origin occurs only rarely.

Suppurative labyrinthitis of meningitic origin is the result of bacterial invasion from the subarachnoid space via either the cochlear aqueduct (Fig. 5.59) or internal auditory canal (Fig. 5.60).

A National Research Council survey (Shambaugh et al., 1933) revealed that meningitis was responsible for 20 percent of 5000 institutionalized deaf children. In a study of aural complications of meningococcic meningitis occurring during an epidemic in Russia in 1931, Zuckermann (1933) found a 3.8 percent incidence of total deafness in 230 children. Fraser and Dickie (1920) reported the incidence in different epidemics of meningococcic meningitis to range from 4 percent to 37.5 percent. In rare instances, it may also occur with pneumococcal infections; however, usually when pneumococcal meningitis has progressed to the stage of suppurative labyrinthitis, the patient does not survive.

In the first stage of suppurative labyrinthitis there is a collection of polymorphonuclear leucocytes (PMNs) in the perilymphatic space at the site of bacterial invasion. Presumably the leucocytes reach the area by diapedesis from adjacent labyrinthine vessels in response to a call for defensive action against the invading microorganisms. In the second stage, PMNs and a fine fibrillar precipitate accumulate throughout the perilymphatic system and eventually also in the endolymphatic spaces. Endolymphatic hydrops begins in the second stage and progresses into the third stage. The third stage is

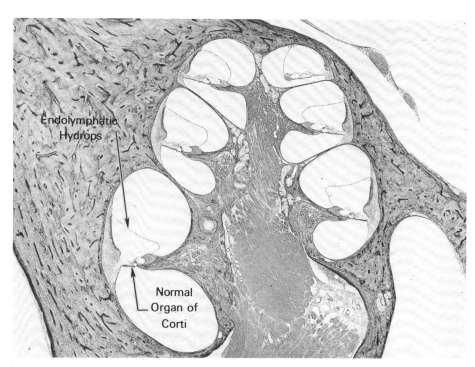

Fig. 5.56: Toxic labyrinthitis in the cat following surgical fistulization of the oval window. There is hydrops of the cochlear duct and saccule. The hair cell populations of the auditory and vestibular sense organs are normal.

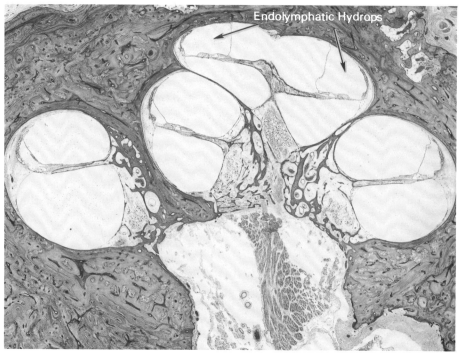

Fig. 5.57: Serous labyrinthitis in a patient with chronic suppurative otitis media and mastoiditis associated with a bony fistula of the lateral semicircular canal. There is moderate endolymphatic hydrops of the cochlear duct and saccule. The hair cell populations of the organ of Corti and vestibular sense organs are normal.

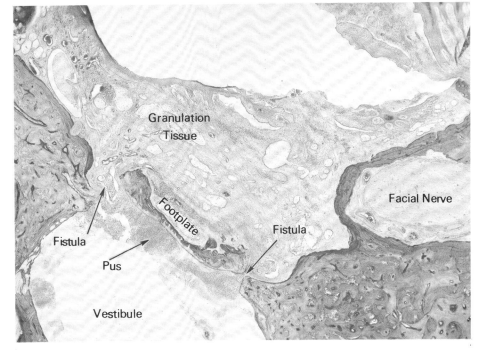

Fig. 5.58: Suppurative labyrinthitis of otitic origin. In this 57-year-old patient with chronic suppurative otitis media, the labyrinth is being invaded through the oval window following destruction of the annular ligament.

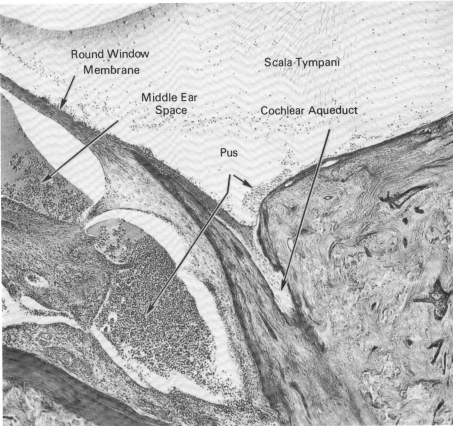

Fig. 5.59: Suppurative labyrinthitis associated with pneumococcal otitis media and meningitis in a 54-year-old woman. Polymorphonuclear leucocytes are seen in the cochlear aqueduct and scala tympani of the basal turn. Death occurred three days after the onset of meningeal symptoms.

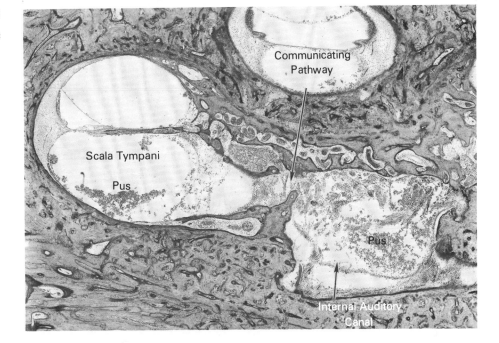

Fig. 5.60: Suppurative labyrinthitis associated with pneumococcal otitis media and meningitis. A communicating pathway between the internal auditory canal and scala tympani of the basal turn cointains numerous polymorphonuclear leucocytes.

characterized by necrosis of the membranous labyrinth. Infections of otitic origin often spread to the meninges during the second or third stage and constitute a serious threat to life. If the patient survives, the forth stage ensues and consists of healing with fibrosis and new bone formation (labyrinthine sclerosis). The end-result is profound loss of auditory and vestibular function.

The treatment of otitic suppurative labyrinthitis consists of intense antibiotic therapy and timely surgical intervention. With chronic infections, surgical exploration of the middle ear and mastoid may indicate a site of labyrinth invasion and provide a clear indication for labyrinthectomy. Many techniques for surgical drainage of the labyrinth have been proposed and all have a common objective, that being wide exposure of the canals, vestibule, and basal turn of the cochlea, without opening the subarachnoid space.

c. Chronic labyrinthitis

Chronic labyrinthitis varies in expression from a focal inflammatory reaction caused by a fistula of the bony labyrinth to diffuse destructive labyrinthitis. A fistula occurs most commonly in the lateral semicircular canal; however, the other semicircular canals and the cochlea may also be involved. Bone resorption is caused either by progressive rarefying osteitis or by keratomatous erosion, and frequently results in the characteristic fistula sign. Occasionally a fistula becomes so sensitive that sneezing, coughing, stooping, or head movement causes disequilibrium. Histological studies often show fibrous thickening of the endosteal membrane in the region of the fistula.

The development of a labyrinthine fistula in the presence of chronic infection is often an indication for surgical intervention. Granulation tissue, diseased bone, and ectopic squamous epithelium usually can be removed from the area of the fistula without opening the thickened endosteal lining. The fistula may then be covered with a bone graft.

Chronic diffuse labyrinthitis is caused by a slowly progressive osteitis of the bony labyrinth and invasion of the labyrinth by granulation tissue and fibrous tissue (Figs. 5.61, 5.62). Endolymphatic hydrops occurs and is followed by progressive degeneration of the auditory and vestibular sense organs. The patient may experience sudden or gradual loss of hearing and vestibular function.

In unusual cases squamous epithelium in the middle ear or mastoid can invade the labyrinth through a fistula and result in a keratoma of the inner ear.

Chronic labyrinthitis may become arrested at any stage, either spontaneously or because of effective medical or surgical therapy, and terminate in labyrinthine sclerosis. If not arrested it may progress and produce intracranial complications.

d. Labyrinthine sclerosis

Sclerosis of the labyrinth is the healed inactive state following labyrinthitis, whether of otitic or meningitic origin. Acute toxic labyrinthitis commonly terminates in endolymphatic hydrops with partial or complete degeneration of the labyrinth with little fibrous tissue proliferation. Suppurative labyrinthitis, on the other hand, often terminates with proliferation of fibrous and osseous tissue in the labyrinthine spaces. Sometimes there are cystic spaces containing acidophilic (protein-containing) fluid. The osseous spiral lamina, modiolus, and endosteal layer of the bony labyrinth may be partly resorbed and replaced by fibrous tissue and new bone (Figs. 5.63 to 5.66). Following meningococcal labyrinthitis, the proliferation of fibrous and osseous tissue is greatest in the basal turn near the cochlear aqueduct, suggesting that the infection may have reached the inner ear via this channel (Henneford and Lindsay, 1968).

Several theories have been advanced in regard to the pathogenesis of new bone in the labyrinth. It has been proposed that it arises from the endosteal lining (Baginsky, 1900; Turner and Fraser, 1928), by metaplasia of connective tissue (Wittmaack, 1926), and from granulation tissue (Georke, 1909; Zange,

Fig. 5.61: Chronic diffuse labyrinthitis in a 60-year-old patient with chronic suppurative otitis media and mastoiditis. The footplate of the stapes, part of the otic capsule, and the membranous labyrinth have been destroyed. The inner ear spaces and part of the internal auditory canal contain granulation tissue. There is a dense accumulation of polymorphonuclear leucocytes in the internal auditory canal surrounding the remaining nerve trunks. Death was caused by extradural abscess and purulent meningitis.

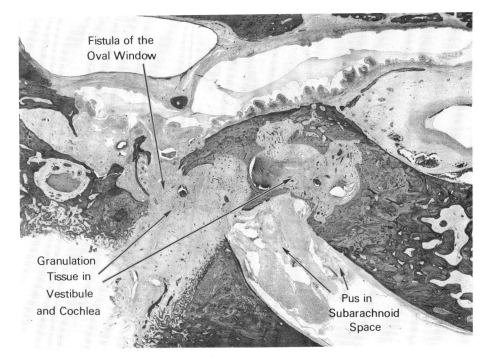

Fig. 5.62: This patient experienced chronic discharge from the right ear for many years and at the age of 67 developed chronic lymphatic leukemia. At the age of 68 she had a total hearing loss in this ear. At the age of 70 she experienced vertigo and progressive right facial paralysis. A radical mastoidectomy was performed, and the facial nerve was partially decompressed. She died of bronchopneumonia ten days later. There is resorption of much of the bony labyrinth, and the inner ear spaces are filled with granulation tissue. The facial nerve is degenerated.

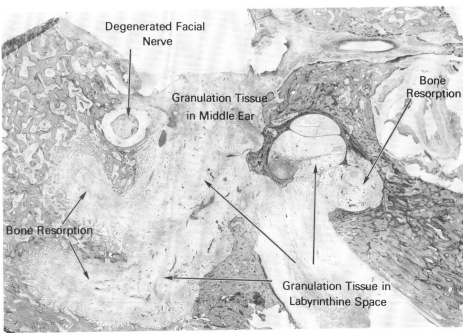

Fig. 5.63: Labyrinthine sclerosis. This patient experienced profound bilateral deafness from meningitis (probably meningococcic) at the age of three. Death occurred at the age of 46. Both ears show severe degeneration of the membranous labyrinths and fibro-osseous sclerosis of the apices of the cochleae.

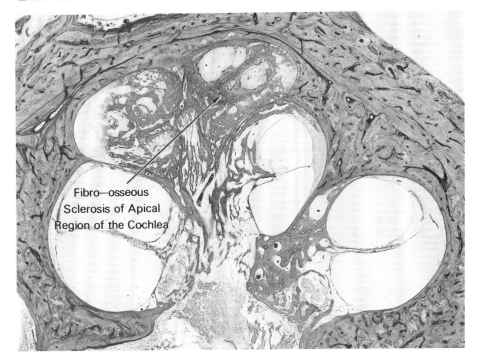

Fig. 5.64: Labyrinthine sclerosis. This patient could hear well until the age of two months when he developed a febrile illness, presumably a meningococcal meningitis, following which he was profoundly deaf. He died at the age of 84. Histological study of the right ear shows total degeneration of the membranous labyrinth, fibro-osseous sclerosis of the vestibule and basal half of the cochlea, and complete osseous sclerosis of the semicircular canals.

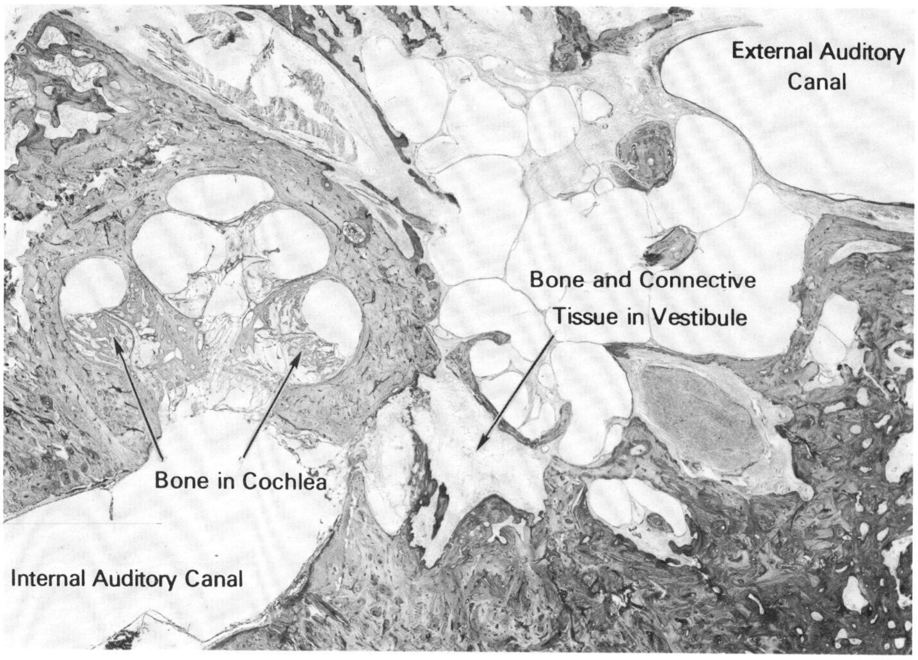

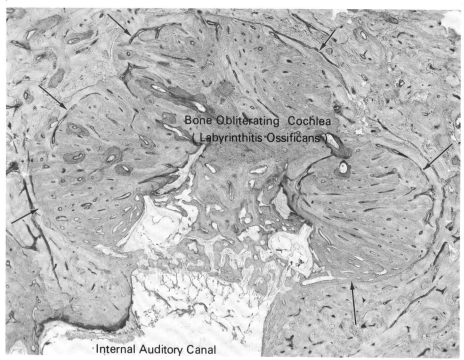

Fig. 5.65: Labyrinthine sclerosis. (Same patient as Fig. 5.64). There is total osseous sclerosis of the left cochlea. The labyrinthine spaces and most of the modiolus have been replaced by lamellar bone. The borders of the new bone can be readily distinguished (arrows) from the surrounding enchondral bone of the otic capsule.

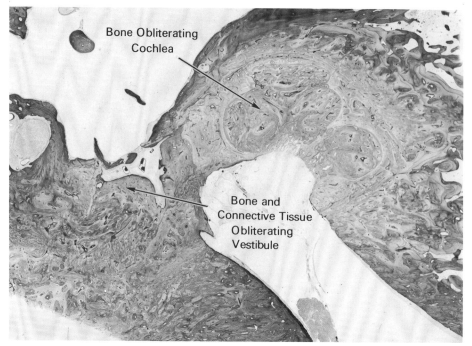

Fig. 5.66: Labyrinthine sclerosis. This patient experienced profound bilateral deafness in early childhood from meningitis, presumably due to meningococcal infection. She died at the age of 74. Histological study of the left ear shows total osseous sclerosis of the labyrinth.

1914; Preuss, 1922; Hagens, 1940). Paparella and Sugiura (1967) believe that the primordial cell responsible for labyrinthine fibrosis and ossification is the undifferentiated mesenchymal cell, which is a perivascular cell or adventitial cell located around capillaries. These undifferentiated mesenchymal cells are similar to tissue reticulum cells in the bloodstream, which are also multipotential primitive mononuclear cells. Presumably, the osteoblast may originate from the mesenchymal cell directly or from fibroblasts which have first differentiated from the mesenchymal cells.

11. OTITIC INTRACRANIAL COMPLICATIONS

Extension of infections beyond the confines of the temporal bones demands the earliest possible diagnosis for effective treatment. Mortality rates have diminished because of antimicrobial drugs and timely surgery; however, even today patients die of undiagnosed and inadequately treated complications of otitic infection.

a. Extradural abscess

Extradural abscess is the most common otitic intracranial complication and consists of a collection of purulent fluid between the dura mater and bone of the middle or posterior cranial fossae. There are no symptoms which are specific for extradural abscess. Headache and fever are common; however, most patients remain ambulatory. When the abscess communicates with the middle ear or mastoid because of resorption of intervening bone, there may be episodes of profuse otorrhea associated with temporary relief of headache. The dura may become covered by granulations and thickened. The squamous part of the temporal bone or the parietal bone may become perforated to produce a subperiosteal abscess on the lateral surface of the skull. Large abscesses may form in the middle cranial fossa and compress the temporal lobe; however, abscesses of the posterior cranial fossa are limited in size by the firm attachment of the dura at the internal auditory meatus, subarcuate fossa, and sigmoid sulcus. The extradural abscess may lead to thrombosis of the superior and inferior petrosal sinuses and the lateral sinus. If the dura is penetrated, the infection extends into the subarachnoid space where it may cause subdural abscess, meningitis, and possibly brain abscess.

Surgical exploration of a suspected extradural abscess should include the removal of parts of the tegmen and perisinus plate of bone and thorough exploration of the extradural region. The removal of mastoid cortex may release purulent fluid from a communicating extradural abscess. When headache and fever persist in spite of adequate medical management of acute or chronic suppurative otitis media and mastoiditis, extradural abscess should be suspected and surgical intervention should be considered.

b. Sinus thrombophlebitis

Dawes (1961) has found that lateral sinus thrombophlebitis is preceded by extradural abscess in over one-half of cases. An infected thrombus forms within the sinus and may in turn break down to form an intrasinus abscess which is excluded from the circulation by occlusive thrombi. Progression of the infection leads to thrombosis of the superior petrosal sinus and cavernous sinus anteriorly and the jugular bulb and vein inferiorly. The characteristic symptoms are recurring sudden rises in temperature associated with severe shivering and profuse sweating. This evidence of septicemia and pyemia may be accompanied by embolic abscesses in the lungs and other viscera, subcutaneous tissues, joint cavities, pleural cavity, and peritoneal cavity. Meningitis and brain abscess may appear at any time during the course of lateral sinus thrombophlebitis and may so dominate the clinical picture that the signs of thrombophlebitis may be obscured.

Early antibiotic therapy is usually adequate to control sinus thrombophlebitis complicating acute mastoiditis. When sinus thrombophlebitis occurs as a complication of mastoiditis, the mastoid should be explored after the initiation of intense medical therapy. The surgical management includes removal of the bony sinus plate and needling of the sinus to determine the nature of its contents. If indicated, the sinus wall is incised and the thrombus or abscess removed. When necessary, the internal jugular vein is ligated in the neck to prevent embolic spread of the infection.

c. Focal otitic encephalitis

Borries (1949) and Dawes (1953) regard this disorder as one which produces signs and symptoms of a brain abscess without intracerebral suppuration. It is frequently associated either with thrombotic lesions of the dural veins or with extradural abscess. Cerebral focal encephalitis is manifested by headache, drowsiness, disorientation, restlessness, convulsive seizures, and coma. Focal signs such as hemiplegia or aphasia may ensue. Cerebellar focal encephalitis is characterized by giddiness, vomiting, nystagmus, and ataxia. It may be impossible to differentiate focal otitic encephalitis from subdural abscess or brain abscess even with extensive diagnostic tests so that needle exploration of the brain through burr holes may be necessary.

Pathologically, the lesion consists of a focal area of brain edema and inflammation with scattered hemorrhages. Management consists of adequate antibiotic therapy and timely surgical intervention to control infection in the temporal bone and adjacent areas.

d. Otitic hydrocephalus

Otitic hydrocephalus occurs most frequently in children and adolescents as a complication of acute or chronic ear infection and is the result of sinus thrombosis which has impaired intracranial venous drainage. Dawes (1965) believes that impairment of the resorptive function of the arachnoid granulations in the superior sagittal sinus is a further cause for increased intracranial pressure.

The symptoms consist of nausea, vomiting, diplopia, and blurred vision. Severe papilledema may lead to optic atrophy and blindness. The cerebrospinal fluid pressure is greatly increased but is biochemically and bacteriologically normal. The electroencephalogram and skull films show no abnormality. Therapy consists of the elimination of otitic disease and measures aimed at reducing cerebrospinal fluid pressure. Dawes states that when bilateral sinus thrombosis has occurred, the otitic hydrocephalus is permanent. Optic atrophy invariably leaves only macular vision, and if the patient stoops, a convulsive seizure may be induced. Several types of operative procedures have been designed to shunt the cerebrospinal fluid into the venous system or other body cavities.

e. Subdural abscess and purulent pachymeningitis

Subdural abscess consists of a collection of purulent fluid between the dura mater and brain and usually is preceded by the clinical manifestations of otitic intracranial invasion. Symptoms include headache, drowsiness, paralyses, aphasia, convulsive seizures, nuchal rigidity, and coma. It occurs more commonly with chronic than with acute otitis media and usually is associated with infection in the extradural space or venous sinuses. The purulent infection may spread rapidly from the site of invasion or become loculated. A slowly developing infection may promote fibrous proliferation and formation of multiple localized abscesses sometimes associated with multiple small abscesses in adjacent brain tissue.

Subdural abscess requires intense antibiotic therapy and urgent surgical drainage. Burr holes should be made at appropriate locations and in sufficient number to insure the removal of purulent fluid and to provide access for tubes which can be used for irrigation with solutions containing antibiotic drugs.

f. Meningitis

Microorganisms may reach the meninges from the middle ear and mastoid via soft-tissue pathways, through areas of bone resorption, from infected venous sinuses and extradural spaces, and from an infected labyrinth. Among the organisms most commonly found are beta-hemolytic streptococci, *pneumococcus pneumoniae*, staphylococci, *Hemophilus influenzae*, bacillus *Proteus*, and *Pseudomonas aeruginosa*. The principal early clinical manifestations of meningitis are headache, fever, and nuchal rigidity. These symptoms are soon followed by restlessness, vomiting, photophobia, confusion, drowsiness, and coma. If there is a history suggestive of a probable other pre-existing intracranial infection, the sudden onset of meningitis suggests the possibility of rupture of a brain abscess into the subarachnoid space or ventricle.

Combinations of penicillin, streptomycin, sulfadiazine, sulfamethazine, chloromycetin, cephalosporins, and tetracylines are given in accordance with known sensitivities of offending microorganisms. The decision as to the need for otologic surgery and the appropriate time for that surgery is a matter of clinical judgment based on the history, clinical findings, type of microorganism, and response of the patient to medical therapy.

Survival rates for patients with otitic meningitis have ranged from 64 percent to 85 percent (Watson, 1948; McLay, 1954; Dawes, 1961).

Acute pneumococcal meningitis. Swartz and Dodge (1965), in a study of 207 cases of bacterial meningitis, found that 56 (27 percent) were caused by *Diplococcus pneumoniae.*

The incidence of pneumococcal meningitis is greatest at both extremes of the life span, with the greatest mortality in the group 50 to 90 years of age. Headache, lethargy or confusion, vomiting, irritability, and fever are consistent symptoms. Nuchal rigidity is present in about 80 percent of patients. Factors having an adverse effect on mortality are advanced age, coexisting illness, coma, delay in instituting therapy, and bacteremia. Otitis media is present in about 30 percent of cases. Throat cultures are of no value in establishing a bacteriologic diagnosis because pneumococci are isolated as frequently from the throats of patients with meningococcal as with pneumococcal meningitis. The number of leucocytes in the cerebrospinal fluid varies between 1,000 and 10,000 cells per cc; sugar concentration is usually 40 mg per 100 ml or less, and protein is elevated. *Diplococci pneumoniae* are readily identified on smear from cerebrospinal fluid.

Successful therapy depends upon an early bacterial diagnosis and prompt administration of intensive doses of penicillin. The recommended dose of penicillin is 1,000,000 to 2,000,000 units given intramuscularly or intravenously every two hours for adults and 16,000,000 units per sq. meter of body surface per day for children. It is doubtful that supplemental therapy with chemotherapeutic drugs (sulfadiazine, chloramphenicol) or the intrathecal injection of penicillin is helpful, and indeed may be harmful.

Prior to three decades ago, pneumococcal meningitis was frequently a fatal disease; however, antibiotic therapy has reduced the mortality rate to about 20 percent. Usually it is preceded by an upper respiratory infection in which the local and systemic reactions and the physical findings are more intense than those caused by viruses, and there is a higher incidence of associated infection of the middle ears and paranasal sinuses.

Increased intracranial pressure accompanying acute bacterial meningitis, from whatever causal microorganism, is a major cause of death.

Histological studies of the temporal bones of seven patients who died of pneumococcal meningitis show the middle ears and mastoids of six to have thick inflamed mucous membranes and small pools of exudate containing PMNs, and one to have large accumulations of pus throughout (Schuknecht and Montandon, 1970). The tympanic membranes were intact in six, and a small perforation was present in one. The tympanic membranes of two patients showed large serohemorrhagic blebs. One of the temporal bones showed a large petromastoid-subarcuate tract resulting in approximation of the lining membrane of the mastoid to the dura mater of the posterior cranial fossa (Fig. 5.67). The soft tissue throughout this tract, as well as the dura, was densely invaded by PMNs. (Voltolini [1868], in reporting the findings in a 27-year-old man who died of acute purulent meningitis, noted that pus extended through a petromastoid canal which was wider than usual.) Another temporal bone had large pacchionian bodies in the floor of the posterior cranial fossa extending into the mastoid cells (Fig. 5.68). The lining membrane of the cells, the pacchionian body, and the dura were densely invaded by inflammatory cells. In still another there was a congenital bony dehiscence of the posterior wall, placing the inflamed mucous membrane in contact with the dura.

The findings indicate that pneumococci spread rapidly throughout the upper respiratory tract and, when the dura is in juxtaposition to infected membranes, it is reasonable to assume that bacteria may take this route to reach the subarachnoid space. Other probable routes are the paranasal sinuses and blood stream.

Suppurative labyrinthitis was present in four of the seven cases. Inflam-

Fig. 5.67: This 68-year-old patient with acute pneumococcal meningitis was comatose on admission to the hospital and died 15 days later. In the right ear the petromastoid canal and subarcuate tract form a common pathway from the infected mastoid cells to the cranial cavity. Numerous polymorphonuclear leucocytes are seen within the tract.

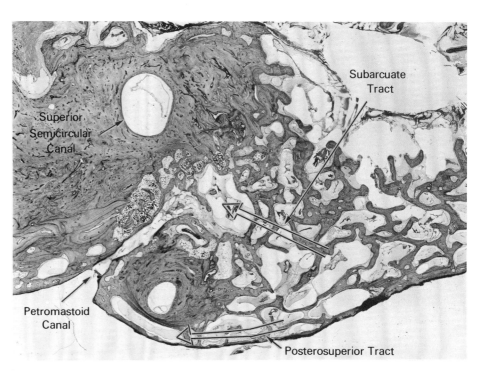

Fig. 5.68: This 81-year-old patient with acute pneumococcal meningitis was deeply comatose on admission to the hospital and died eight days later. Both ears show large infected pacchionian bodies extending from the dura of the posterior cranial fossa into the infected mastoid cells.

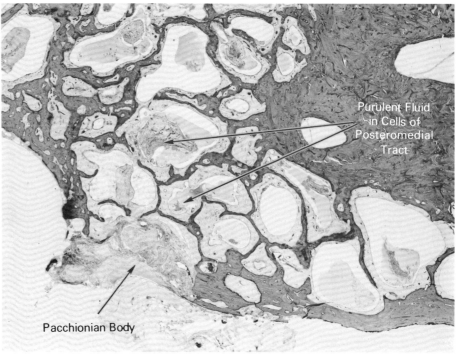

matory cells were found in patent cochlear aqueducts of two and in a communicating pathway between the internal auditory canal and scala tympani in another. These findings, coupled with the observation that most patients enter coma without previous labyrinthine symptoms, indicate that the suppurative labyrinthitis is of meningitic origin. Reversible hearing loss, as experienced by one of the seven patients who was recovering when he died of a perforated ileum, must be attributed to toxic labyrinthitis. Histological studies show a fine fibrillar precipitate in the perilymphatic spaces, without endolymphatic hydrops, in both ears of this patient.

It is doubtful that routine mastoidectomy for the drainage of pus is warranted for most patients with acute pneumococcal meningitis with associated otitis media. Rossberg (1960) performed simple mastoidectomies on five patients with pneumococcal meningitis and found only minimal inflammatory changes. If radiological studies show opacification of the pneumatized areas, it may be assumed that abundant purulent fluid is present and mastoidectomy should be considered.

g. Otitic brain abscess

Brain abscess may complicate chronic otitis media, mastoiditis, or petrositis and often is associated wth other intracranial complications. A brain abscess is most commonly located in either the temporal lobe or in the anterior part of the lateral lobe of the cerebellum. In rare instances an abscess occurs in a remote area of the brain presumably due to retrograde thrombophlebitis or to hematogenous bacterial metastasis. The most common offending microorganisms are Staphylococcus aureus, Staphylococcus albus, beta-hemolytic streptococci, and Pneumococcus pneumoniae. Other organisms occasionally involved are E. coli, bacillus Proteus, and Pseudomonas aeruginosa. The symptoms of brain abscess depend upon the rate of progression of the process and are due to increased intracranial pressure and to focal signs and symptoms related to dsyfunction of the affected part of the brain. The symptoms may be masked by the presence of other intracranial complications. The initial signs are headache, vomiting, and drowsiness, leading to stupor and coma. The temperature is often subnormal, and the pulse usually is slow. After two to three weeks, papilledema may be present. Cerebral focal signs consist of visual disturbances, aphasia, involvement of motor tracts, and ocular paralyses. Cerebellar signs consist of nystagmus, asynergia, and speech defects. In Pennybacker's series (1961) of 85 cases, the death rate was 36 percent prior to 1950 and 5.7 percent after 1950.

Immediate intense antibiotic therapy is imperative. Temporal lobe abscesses are generally managed by total surgical excision with otologic surgery delayed for some days or weeks until the patient's general condition has improved (Myers and Ballantine, 1965). Cerebellar abscesses appear to respond best to surgical drainage, which may be performed in conjunction with mastoid surgery.

12. SURGERY FOR SUPPURATIVE DISEASE OF THE TEMPORAL BONE

a. Simple mastoidectomy

The simple mastoidectomy is performed principally to establish drainage for acute infections of the middle ear and mastoid when these infections are not responding satisfactorily to medical therapy. Indications for the procedure are radiologic evidence of bone resorption, postauricular subperiosteal abscess, severe pain, high fever, or evidence of impending or existing complications. This operation is performed through a postauricular incision and consists of removing the lateral mastoid cortex and exenteration of the mastoid air cell system while preserving the posterior bony canal wall.

b. Modified radical mastoidectomy

The modified radical mastoidectomy is performed for chronic suppurative disease of the middle ear and mastoid and consists of removing the mastoid cortex, the posterior wall of the external auditory canal and the lateral wall of the epitympanic space. The mastoid air cell system is widely exenterated; however, the middle ear structures (tympanic membrane, ossicles, mucous membrane), or what remains of them, are meticulously preserved. The procedure was clearly described by Bondy (1910) and many otologic surgeons consider it the method of choice in selected cases (Baron, 1954).

c. Radical mastoidectomy

The classical radical mastoidectomy has been in routine use since the beginning of the century and consists of removal of the mastoid cortex, the posterior wall of the external auditory canal, and the lateral wall of the epitympanic space, followed by thorough exenteration of the air cell system and removal of the remaining parts of the malleus, incus, and tympanic membrane. Lempert (1938) advocated that the tensor tympani muscle and mucous membrane of the middle ear should also be removed. A frequent consequence of this procedure is a moderate to severe hearing loss.

d. Atticoantrotomy

The atticoantrotomy operation usually is performed by an approach through the external auditory canal for disease limited to the middle ear, epitympanum, and the mastoid antrum. It consists of partial removal of the posterosuperior part of the bony tympanic annulus and lateral wall of the epitympanum while preserving the pars tensa and ossicles. The most common pathological condition for which this procedure is performed is keratoma confined to the epitympanum and mastoid antrum. The cavity thus created is exteriorized to the external auditory canal.

e. Myringoplasty

Myringoplasty is a procedure in which a tissue graft is used to close a perforation of the tympanic membrane. Myringoplasty as first performed (Ely, 1880; Tangeman, 1883; Politzer, 1893) was generally unsuccessful; however, improvements in technique have led to a success rate of over 90 percent. The most commonly used tissue grafts are temporalis fascia, vein, split thickness skin, full thickness skin, ear lobe adipose tissue, and subcutaneous connective tissue.

f. Tympanoplasty

With the advent of antibiotics and the operation microscope, more emphasis has been placed on reconstructive procedures. Wullstein (1956b) and Zöllner (1955, 1957), after some years of experimentation and much clinical experience, presented the principles of tympanoplasty. Although several classifications have been suggested for these surgical procedures (Müsebeck, 1970), the one presented by Wullstein is used by most otologic surgeons (Lee and Schuknecht, 1971).

Type I tympanoplasty. Type I tympanoplasty is usually performed by an approach through the external auditory canal and consists of exploration of the middle ear, with possible removal of minor pathologies (retraction pockets, polypoid granulation tissue), inspection of the ossicular chain, and repair of the tympanic membrane with an autogenous tissue graft.

Type II tympanoplasty. Type II tympanoplasty implies a surgical operation for the removal of disease followed by a reconstructive procedure to reestablish the lever mechanism of the ossicular chain. It is usually performed through the external auditory canal and may include removal of the lateral epitympanic wall and posterior bony tympanic annulus as well as repair of a defect of the tympanic membrane. The most common ossicular reconstruction is the introduction of a bone or cartilage graft between the head of the stapes and long process of the incus for ears in which the lenticular process and tip of the long process of the incus are missing.

Type III tympanoplasty. Type III tympanoplasty is performed for ears in which the pathology precludes a re-establishment of a normal sound-conducting system. It implies removal of diseased tissue and preparation of the ear for either transposition of the tympanic membrane or introduction of a tissue graft to bridge the tympanic space while maintaining contact with the head of the stapes. The objectives are to create an aerated hypotympanum and mesotympanum which is ventilated by the eustachian tube, to provide a sound barrier to the round window, and to establish a mechanism by which sound energy is transmitted directly to the stapes. When mastoid exenteration is performed as part of the procedure, the term tympanomastoidectomy type III is applicable.

Type IV tympanoplasty. Type IV tympanoplasty is performed when there is extensive ossicular disease including absence of the crura of the stapes. In this procedure the tympanic membrane or tissue graft is positioned on the promontory, thus bridging the hypotympanic cavity and exteriorizing the oval window niche. Thus, sound energy passes directly to the footplate while the round window membrane is protected in an air-containing pocket ventilated by the eustachian tube. A thin split thickness skin graft may be placed in the oval window niche to prevent the formation of a fibrous tissue plug. When it is performed in combination with mastoid exenteration it is appropriately referred to as tympanomastoidectomy type IV.

Type V tympanoplasty. The type V tympanoplasty may be performed when a type III or IV tympanoplasty has succeeded in eliminating the disease process and in establishing an aerated hypotympanum but has failed to result in a hearing improvement because of fibrous or osseous fixation of the footplate. A second procedure is then performed to establish sound transmission by either creating a surgical fistula of the lateral canal or removing the footplate of the stapes (Gacek, 1973).

Tympanoplasty with autogenous or homologous bone (or cartilage) grafts. Autogenous or homologous grafts of bone (ossicles, cortical bone) or cartilage may be used in combination with various tympanoplasty procedures to improve sound transmission through the middle ear. For example, a better functional result might be achieved in a type IV tympanoplasty by placing a strut of reshaped incus on the footplate of the stapes, in which case the fascial graft would be positioned to contact the strut and bridge the mesotympanum, creating in effect a type III tympanoplasty. Farrior's (1966) classification would denote this particular procedure as a tympanoplasty type IV-IG, with IG meaning incus graft.

Homologous grafts of preserved tympanic membrane with attached malleus and incus have been attempted with variable success.

g. Mastoid obliteration

Mastoid obliteration implies the partial or complete obliteration of a surgically created mastoid cavity with free or pedicled autogenous tissue grafts or homologous tissue grafts (Guilford et al., 1958; Schiller, 1961; Thorburn, 1961; Palva, 1963; Schuknecht et al., 1966; Palva et al., 1968; Shea and Gardner, 1970). The method avoids a large radical mastoid cavity with its occasional attendant symptoms of discharge and crusting (Fig. 5.69). Many surgeons routinely obliterate the mastoid as part of the tympanomastoidectomy.

h. Intact canal wall tympanoplasty

Intact canal wall tympanoplasty consists of exenteration of the mastoid air cell system, combined with reconstruction of the middle ear, while preserving the external auditory canal (Myers and Schlosser, 1960; Palva, 1963; Jansen, 1963; Sheehy, 1965, 1970; Lapidot and Brandow, 1966; Smyth et al., 1967; Jako, 1967). Diseased areas are approached via both the external auditory canal and mastoid while preserving the intervening wall of the external auditory canal. The facial recess and posterior mesotympanum are exposed

Fig. 5.69: A modified radical mastoidectomy was performed on this ear when the patient was 59 years of age. The mastoid cells were widely exenterated; the lateral mastoid cortex and the posterior bony wall of the external auditory canal were removed. Granulation tissue was removed from the middle ear region; however, remnants of ossicles were left in place. Postoperatively she had a persistent mild chronic suppurative discharge and crusting in the middle ear and mastoid cavity. She died eight years later of subarachnoid hemorrhage. Histological studies show a large mastoid bowl bordered by sclerotic cortical bone and partly lined by squamous epithelium. In the midportion of the mastoid bowl there is a layer of highly cellular and vascular granulation tissue with areas of ulceration. The malleus and incus are partially resorbed and enveloped in fibrous tissue. Because discharge and crusting sometimes persist following radical mastoid surgery, otologic surgeons generally prefer surgical techniques which obviate the need to create an exteriorized mastoid cavity.

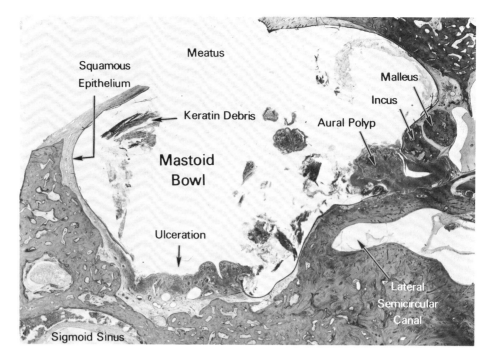

and entered posteriorly. By preserving the bony tympanic annulus it is sometimes possible to repair the tympanic membrane with tissue grafts and to bridge the middle ear space with tissue struts or prostheses and thereby establish an effective sound-conducting system.

i. Tympanotomy

Tympanotomy is a surgical procedure to expose the tympanic cavity in an ear with an intact tympanic membrane and to perform whatever further procedures are indicated. It consists of elevating a segment of the tympanic membrane in continuity with a collar of skin from the adjacent canal wall. A tympanotomy may be posterior, inferior, or anterior, depending upon the problem to be assessed. Exploratory tympanotomy is performed for diagnostic purposes; tympanotomy and biopsy are performed for histological diagnosis; tympanotomy and ossicular reconstruction are performed for ossicular disease resulting from infection or trauma; and tympanotomy and vestibular fluid tap are performed principally for the differential diagnosis of Ménière's disease and vestibular schwannoma.

j. Surgical procedures for complicated infections

Operative procedures performed for complicated infections, usually in association with radical mastoidectomy, include labyrinthectomy, petrosectomy, sequestrectomy, evacuation of extradural or subdural abscess, removal of infected thrombus of the sigmoid sinus, drainage of cerebellar abscess, and decompression of the facial nerve.

B. SEROMUCINOUS OTITIS MEDIA (OTIC SALPINGITIS)

Seromucinous otitis media is a disorder common to childhood but may occur at all ages. It is characterized by the accumulation of fluid of varying viscosity in the pneumatized spaces of the temporal bone. Although there is some disagreement regarding its pathogenesis, dysfunction of the eustachian tube appears to be an important factor. In young children the condition may go unnoticed for some months or years. The principal symptom is hearing loss, often of fluctuating character, due to alterations in the extent of ventilation of the middle ear.

Examination reveals intact tympanic membranes which may appear dull grey, pink, straw-colored, or near normal. A consistent finding is the chalky-white appearance of the manubrium. Pressure otoscopy reveals limitation of movement of the tympanic membrane. Fluid lines may be visible after forced inflation (Hantman, 1943). The fluid varies from serous to mucoid, the character being determined in great part by the activity of mucous-producing glands of the eustachian tube and middle ear (Sade, 1966).

The implication that eustachian tube dysfunction is the cause for seromucinous otitis media in children derives support from the investigations of Silverstein et al. (1966). Utilizing the eustachiometer they showed that nearly all the children tested who had seromucinous otitis media failed to demonstrate tubal opening during deglutition. The failure of the eustachian tube to open with the act of deglutition may be due to several factors: (1) an anatomically small eustachian tube; (2) extrinsic pressure on the cartilagenous part of the eustachian tube by enlarged glandular, lymphoid, or adipose tissue; (3) mucosal thickening due to allergic reaction or chronic inflammation; and (4) weakness of the tensor palati muscle. The mucoid content of the fluid probably is determined in part by hyperactivity of mucous-producing glands in the eustachian tube and middle ear, and in part by the degree to which tubal blockage interferes with movement of the mucous sheath through the eustachian tube. The fluid is more commonly mucinous in children and serous in adults. The presence of unilateral seromucinous otitis in an adult should raise the suspicion of carcinoma of the nasopharynx.

Idiopathic hemotympanum (blue ear drum) is a variant of seromucinous otitis media which apparently is associated with hemorrhage. The fluid is bluish or brownish in color and usually moderately viscid. Cholesterol granulomas have been found in the mastoids of some patients with this condition (Birrell, 1956; Friedmann, 1959; Paparella and Lim, 1967); however, it has not been demonstrated that these granulomas have a causal relationship to the disorder.

Clinical observation demonstrates that ears with seromucinous otitis media, particularly the mucoid type, are susceptible to bacterial infection which determines in great part the permanent pathological and functional alterations resulting from this disorder. Clinical observation demonstrates that prolonged seromucinous otitis media may lead to atrophy of the tympanic membrane and fibrous fixation or resorption of the ossicles. The pathological changes occurring with persistent seromucinous otitis media, having its onset in childhood and complicated by recurring infection, are similar to those associated with congenital cleft palate, and range from fibrocystic obliteration of the pneumatized spaces of the temporal bone to chronic suppurative otitis media and mastoiditis. On the other hand seromucinous otitis media in adults may persist for many years with no significant alterations in the middle ear or pneumatized spaces of the temporal bone (Fig. 5.70).

Fig. 5.70: Mastoid spaces in a 46-year-old male with seromucinous otitis media of undetermined cause of 19 years' duration. The subepithelial layer of the mucous membrane is thickened by fibrous tissue proliferation. The spaces are lined by a single layer of flat epithelial cells and contain an acidophilic fluid with degenerating exfoliated epithelial cells and scattered nuclear debris.

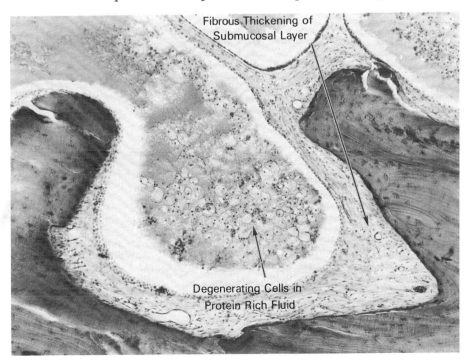

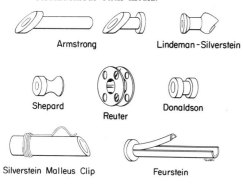

Fig. 5.71: Ventilating tubes which have been designed for aeration of the pneumatized spaces of the temporal bone for patients with seromucinous otitis media.

Armstrong

Lindeman-Silverstein

Shepard

Reuter

Donaldson

Silverstein Malleus Clip

Feurstein

The principal therapy for seromucinous otitis media is directed at re-establishing aeration of the temporal bone by eliminating the causes for tubal dysfunction. Thus allergic and infectious conditions are treated, and possibly lymphoid tissue is removed from the nasopharynx (Senturia et al., 1972).

Ventilating tubes. A popular method for establishing aeration of the temporal bone for patients with seromucinous otitis media is the use of the ventilation tube, first advocated by Armstrong (1957, 1962). Innovative otologists have designed these tubes in many forms (Lindeman and Silverstein, 1964; Silverstein, 1966; Armstrong, 1968) (Fig. 5.71). They are placed through the tympanic membrane and provide a by-pass by which the middle ear may be ventilated. Although most tubes remain patent and function for several months, some become blocked by dried exudate, epithelial debris and wax. They tend to be extruded spontaneously in three to six months, although some remain in place a year or more. Although a functional ventilating tube results in hearing improvement, there is no evidence that aeration by this method has any therapeutic effect on the malfunctioning eustachian tube (Kilby et al., 1972).

The following complications may follow the use of the ventilating tube: (1) permanent perforation of the tympanic membrane; (2) retracted replacement membrane at the site of the tube; and (3) keratoma of the middle ear. The author has observed the latter complication in two children and one adult (Figs. 5.72 to 5.76).

Silverstein (1970) has designed a more permanent tube which extends from the external auditory canal into the facial recess or aditus. The long-term effects of these permanent indwelling tubes are not presently known.

Fig. 5.72: This patient received radiation therapy for carcinoma of the nasopharynx at the age of 60 and died ten years later of unrelated causes. Fourteen months before death pressure-equalizing tubes (malleus-clip tubes) were introduced into both tympanic membranes because of seromucinous otitis media. This view shows the perforation in the anterior part of the left tympanic membrane at the site of the tube. The tympanic membrane at the anterior margin of the perforation is thickened and its luminal surface is lined by squamous epithelium. See Fig. 5.73.

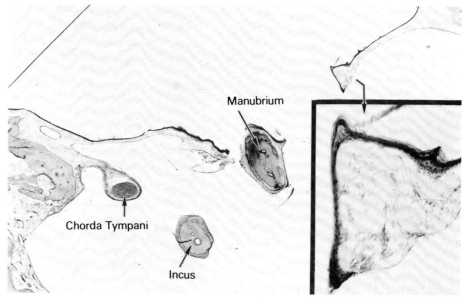

Fig. 5.73: Same ear as Fig. 5.72. This photograph shows the malleus-clip-tube in place.

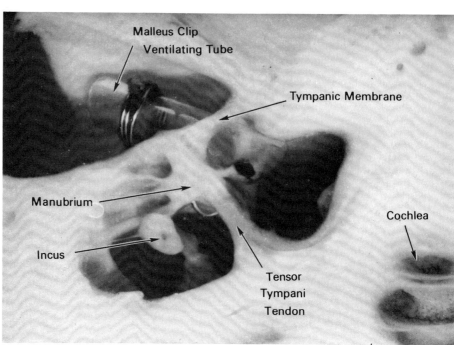

Fig. 5.74: Pressure-equalizing tube introduced two months before death in a 36-year-old male with seromucinous otitis media due to Wegener's granuloma. The lumen of the tube is blocked by dried exudate and squamous epithelium has invaded the middle ear. See Figs. 5.75 and 5.76.

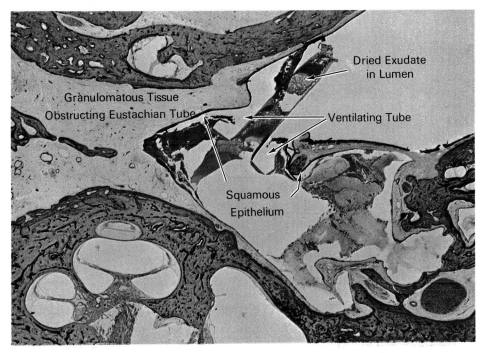

Fig. 5.75: Same ear as Fig. 5.74. The photograph shows the ventilating tube in place and blocked by a plug of exudate.

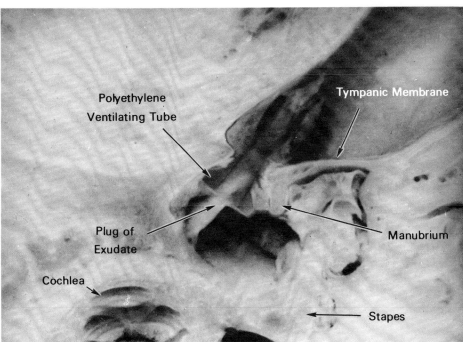

Fig. 5.76: Same ear as Figs. 5.74 and 5.75, showing squamous epithelium extending 3 to 4 mm into the middle ear.

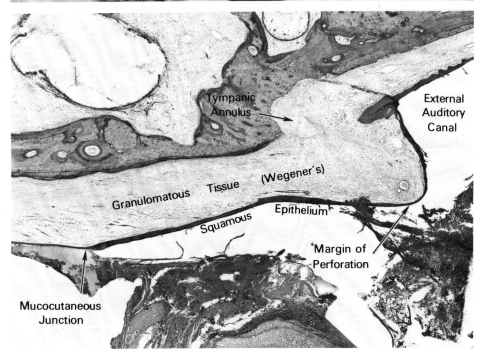

C. VIRAL INFECTIONS

1. HERPES ZOSTER OTICUS

It is now generally accepted that varicella (chicken pox) and herpes zoster are caused by the same DNA virus. Herpes zoster probably represents a reactivation of a latent varicella-zoster virus.

Tschiassny (1946) credits Tryde as providing the first description of herpes zoster with facial paralysis in 1872. In 1904 Körner coined the term "herpes zoster oticus" for cases having vesicular eruptions of the auricle, facial nerve palsy, and hearing loss. In 1907 Hunt provided a detailed description and classification for the disorder, and since then the terms "herpes zoster oticus" and "Ramsey Hunt syndrome" have become synonymous.

Frequently the first symptom is a deep, burning pain in the region of the ear. This is followed in one to four days by a vesicular eruption of the external auditory canal and concha, or less frequently of the face, neck, trunk, palate, and fauces (Johnson and Zonderman, 1948). Facial paralysis, hearing loss and vertigo may occur singly or in combination in varying degrees of severity, and may develop at any time after the initial symptom of pain and may precede evidence of vesiculation.

The various reports indicate that herpes zoster oticus is responsible for about 2 to 7 percent of all facial palsies (Taverner, 1955; Dalton, 1960; Matthews, 1961; Gregg, 1961; Cawthorne, 1952; Laumans, 1962; Jepsen, 1965; Peitersen and Andersen, 1967). The facial palsy may be partial or complete. The prognosis is poorest for complete palsy. About one-half of the patients with herpes zoster oticus retain some permanent facial motor disturbance and a few sustain permanent complete paralysis (Devriese, 1968).

Vestibular symptoms consist of disequilibrium varying from mild unsteadiness to severe vertigo with nausea and vomiting. Auditory symptoms consist of tinnitus and sensorineural hearing loss of varying degree. The loss usually is most severe for the high frequencies and may present the audiologic manifestations of either a sensory or neural lesion (Harbert and Young, 1967). Welsh and Welsh (1962) have found that recruitment, as tested by the alternate loudness balance test, is usually absent in patients with hearing loss due to herpes zoster oticus. Some recovery of hearing can be expected; with severe losses, however, recovery is rarely complete.

Pathological studies have failed to support Hunt's hypothesis that the facial paralysis is due to a herpetic geniculate ganglionitis. Denny-Brown et al. (1944), at autopsy, found degeneration of related motor and sensory roots, severe neuritis, unilateral segmental poliomyelitis, and localized leptomeningitis. The autopsy findings in patients with herpes zoster oticus with facial palsy (eight cases reviewed by Devriese, 1968) have consistently shown lymphocytic infiltration and degeneration of facial nerve fibers, but minimal changes in the geniculate ganglion.

Blackley et al. (1967) presented the findings in the temporal bone of a woman who died seven months after the onset of herpes zoster oticus. They found intense perivascular, perineural, and intraneural round cell aggregations in the facial nerve, auditory nerve, modiolus of the cochlea and mastoid process. Zajtchuk et al. (1972) reported the findings in a woman whose principal clinical manifestations were a vesicular eruption on the left auricle, severe vertigo, loss of taste on the left anterior two-thirds of the tongue, and absent left caloric response to ice water. The eruption and vertigo subsided in a few weeks, and she died two years later of Hodgkin's disease. Histological studies showed degeneration of the sensory and neural elements of the superior and lateral semicircular canals with fibrous tissue and new bone in the adjacent perilymphatic space of the lateral canal. Heilborn (1950) supports the hypothesis that herpes zoster oticus is a form of encephalomeningomyelitis in which the virus first gains virulence in the cerebrospinal fluid and then spreads from the meninges to the motor and sensory nerve roots.

The possibility that idiopathic facial palsy (Bell's palsy) is caused by the zoster virus seems to have been refuted by the studies of Aitken and Brian (1933) and Peitersen and Caunt (1970). These studies showed a low incidence of compliment fixation antibodies to zoster antigen in patients with acute nontraumatic peripheral facial palsies.

Most authors indicate that there is no satisfactory specific treatment for the viral infection of herpes zoster oticus. Decompression of the facial nerve has been advocated for selected cases (Crabtree, 1968); however, the usefulness of this procedure has not been clearly established. Steroid therapy has been endorsed by several authors (Gelfand, 1954; Sauer, 1955; Elliott, 1964; Harner et al., 1970) but, again, controlled studies have not been performed to determine the therapeutic value of these drugs.

2. VIRAL LABYRINTHITIS

The labyrinth may become involved in the course of specific viral infections such as measles, mumps, upper respiratory tract infection, and infectious mononucleosis. It is also probable that sudden deafness may be caused by viral infection without clinical evidence of systemic involvement.

a. Measles (Morbilli)

The incidence of measles as the suspected cause of sensorineural deafness in populations of deaf children has been studied by several investigators wi the following findings: Shambaugh et al. (1928), 6.7 percent; Yearsley (1934–1935), 9.3 percent; Goodman (1949), 4.4 percent; Simpson (1949), 5.0 percent; Bordley (1952), 6.4 percent; and Kinney (1953), 10.0 percent.

Usually the involvement is bilateral with moderate to severe permanent loss of auditory and vestibular function.

The pathological changes consist of severe degeneration of the organ of Corti, spiral ganglion and vestibular sense organs (Lewy and Hagens, 1937). Characteristically, the organ of Corti is shrunken and devoid of hair cells, or missing entirely. The atrophic change is most severe in the basal turn (Fig. 5.77). The stria vascularis is often atrophied (Nager, 1907) and the tectorial membrane is either missing, detached, or deformed into a round mass and often encapsulated with a layer of flattened cells (Lindsay and Hemenway, 1954). There may be a severe loss of cochlear neurons (Fig. 5.78). When the stria vascularis is severely atrophied Reissner's membrane is displaced toward the basilar membrane. The cristae and maculae show atrophied sensory epithelium (Fig. 5.79), which is consistent with the clinical demonstration of diminution or loss of caloric sensitivity.

Before antibiotics were available, otitis media was an occasional complication of measles but it is rarely seen today and is not a cause for profound bilateral deafness.

b. Mumps

Mumps is a common cause for unilateral but rarely for bilateral sensorineural hearing loss, and may vary from mild loss for high frequencies (Fig. 5.80) to profound deafness. Ears with an incomplete loss demonstrate audiometric findings consistent with a cochlear lesion. The incidence of vestibular involvement is small. Unilateral hearing loss from mumps labyrinthitis often goes undetected by patient or parents until school age.

The sex distribution is equal. There appears to be no relationsip between the severity of the clinical manifestations of the disease and the occurrence of deafness.

Sudden deafness occurring in apparently healthy children or adults may be due to a subclinical mumps infection. During a mumps epidemic a considerable number of healthy contact individuals will show positive serological tests (Wolff, 1953). Van Dishoeck and Bierman (1957) performed serological tests and viral cultures of the blood and stools on 66 patients with sudden

Fig. 5.77: Measles labyrinthitis. This patient experienced profound bilateral hearing loss while suffering from measles at the age of five. He died at the age of 72. The ears show identical changes. The organ of Corti is missing in the basal turn and consists of an epithelial mound without hair cells in the middle and apical turns. The stria vascularis is atrophied in the basal turn. There is atrophy of the cochlear neurons, most severe in the basal turn. The vestibular sensory and neural structures were also severely atrophied.

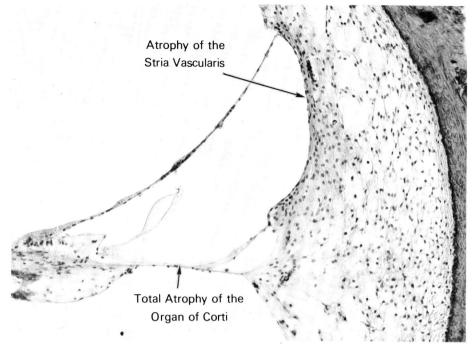

Atrophy of the
Stria Vascularis

Total Atrophy of the
Organ of Corti

Fig. 5.78: Measles labyrinthitis associated with encephalitis at the age of twelve. The auditory and vestibular sense organs are severely atrophied. An unusual feature is the complete loss of cochlear neurons. Not a single neuron can be found. The nerve fibers in Rosenthal's canal, seen most clearly near the apex, are presumed to be efferent fibers.

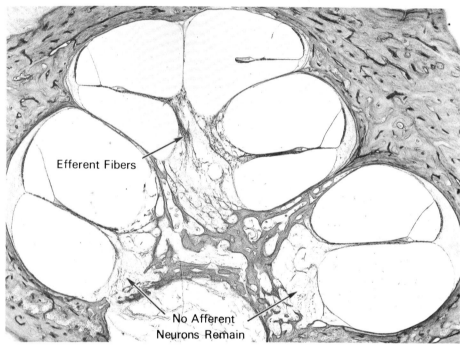

Efferent Fibers

No Afferent
Neurons Remain

Fig. 5.79: Measles labyrinthitis. The patient experienced profound hearing loss while suffering from measles at the age of four. At the age of forty audiometric tests revealed no responses and ice water caloric tests showed greatly reduced responses. She died at the age of 57. The auditory and vestibular sense organs are severely atrophied. This photomicrograph shows the changes in the crista of the posterior semicircular canal. Atrophy of the stroma has led to cystic spaces and an irregular distribution of fibrocytes. The sensory epithelium has an irregular contour and contains only a flattened distorted layer of supporting cells. The hair cells are missing.

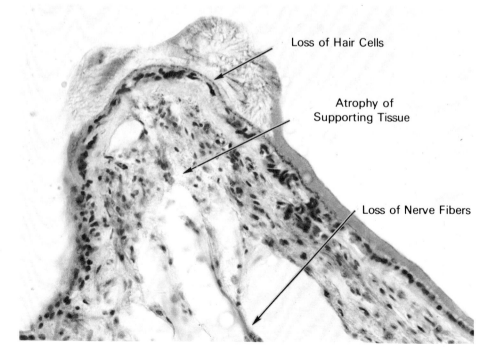

Loss of Hair Cells

Atrophy of
Supporting Tissue

Loss of Nerve Fibers

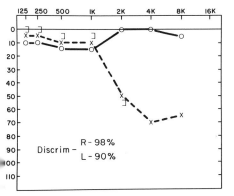

Fig. 5.80: Unilateral high-frequency sensorineural hearing loss resulting from mumps in early childhood.

deafness and found 14 to be positive for mumps. Saunders and Lippy (1959) studied the mumps antibody titers of 9 patients with sudden severe unilateral hearing loss and found that 4 had mumps and that 2 others probably had mumps. None of the patients had parotitis and each clearly recalled a previous childhood mumps infection.

Lindsay et al. (1960) examined the temporal bones of a six-year-old child who was profoundly deaf following mumps at the age of two. There was severe atrophy of the organ of Corti and stria vascularis and collapse of Reissner's membrane. In the basal and middle turns the tectorial membrane was detached from the limbus and appeared as an encapsulated homogeneous mass. There was moderate loss of cochlear neurons in the basal turn. The saccule, utricle, and semicircular canals appeared normal.

c. Upper respiratory tract illnesses

A large number of viruses of several morphologically different groups are known to cause illnesses of the upper respiratory tract (Mufson et al. 1966). Although most of these viruses are associated with benign disease, they are capable of an extremely virulent attack upon the central nervous system. It is not surprising that the inner ear may also be involved.

Lindsay (1959) found unilateral sudden deafness, tinnitus, and vertigo in four patients who had acute upper respiratory tract infections, with all experiencing partial recovery of hearing during the subsequent few months. Heller and Lindenberg (1955) reported five cases and Lieberman (1957) four cases who experienced sudden deafness with upper respiratory tract infections.

Beal et al. (1967) reported the pathological findings in the temporal bone of a patient who experienced sudden profound unilateral hearing loss while suffering from a "head cold." They found severe distortion and degeneration of the organ of Corti and stria vascularis with atrophy and encapsulation of the tectorial membrane.

Schuknecht et al. (1973) reported on the pathology of the inner ears of seven individuals with sudden deafness. At the time of onset two had "head colds," one had acute pharyngitis, and two had pneumonia. The principal pathological changes consisted of atrophy, in varying combinations and severity, of the organ of Corti, tectorial membrane, and stria vascularis. These changes were judged to be similar to those of sudden deafness due to known viral infections such as mumps and measles (Morbilli).

However, because there is still some doubt as to the pathogenesis of sudden deafness occurring in healthy individuals with or without upper respiratory tract illnesses, the pathology of these cases is described in Chapter 12, C: Sudden Deafness of Unknown Etiology.

d. Infectious mononucleosis

Infectious mononucleosis rarely involves the labyrinth; however, Gregg and Schaeffer (1964) reported the clinical findings in a 17-year-old male with infectious mononucleosis who developed sudden severe unilateral hearing loss and tinnitus. The patient also experienced unsteadiness and two episodes of severe vertigo. The profound unilateral hearing loss persisted after the patient had returned to good health. Bilateral severe loss of auditory and vestibular function may also occur (author's observation).

e. Cytomegalic inclusion disease

Cytomegalic inclusion disease occurs most commonly in infants as a result of intrauterine infection with a cytomegalovirus. The systemic form becomes clinically apparent soon after birth and is characterized by hemolytic anemia, purpura, jaundice, and hepatosplenomegaly. The brain may be involved and produce radiologically demonstrable cerebral calcifications. The focal form of the disease involves the salivary glands and constitutes an incidental finding at autopsy. The disorder may occur in adults with debilitating disease in both focal and systemic form (Ward et al., 1965).

Fig. 5.81: Cytomegalic inclusion disease. Inclusion-bearing cells (arrows) are seen on the endolymphatic side of Reissner's membrane in the region of the stria vascularis and in the spiral ligament. The infected cells are two to four times normal size, and each contains a deeply-staining central nuclear inclusion. A clear halo surrounds the inclusion and extends to the nuclear membrane. The arrangement of inclusions differs from cell to cell depending upon the stage of infection. (Courtesy of Myers and Stool)

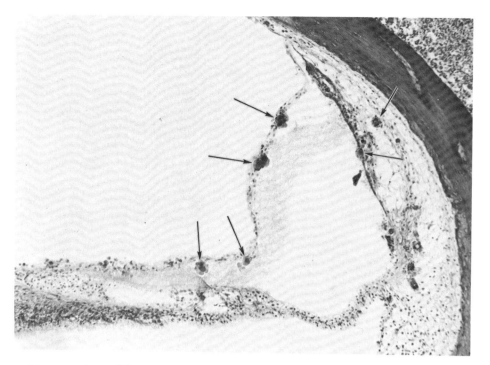

Myers and Stool (1968) and Davis (1969) studied the temporal bones of infants who died of the disease and found cytomegalic inclusions in the cochlea, saccule, utricle, and semicircular canals (Fig. 5.81).

f. Rubella

The clinical manifestations and pathology of Rubella deafness are described in Chapter 4C1, Maternal Rubella.

D. MYCOTIC DISEASES

The Mucorales are a group of ubiquitous fungi of low virulence which frequently occur as contaminants of laboratory cultures and are commonly found in refrigerators and incubators. Growth is rapid and is characterized by broad, branching, nonseptate hyphae known as rhizoids. Although commonly thought to be nonpathogenic, Gregory et al. in 1943 reported three diabetic patients with a rapidly fatal infection from this fungus. The fungus enters the nose and leads to sinusitis, orbital cellulitis, meningoencephalitis, and otitis media. The organisms have an affinity for arteries, penetrating the muscular walls and growing in their lumens where they incite thrombosis and infarction. The incidence of mucormycosis appears to be increasing, probably because these infections occur in chronically ill, frequently fatally debilitated patients who are now kept alive by modern medical therapy. The infection has been reported in patients with terminal malignancy, severe diabetes, and in those receiving chemotherapy and broad spectrum antibiotic therapy (Boyd, 1961; Robbins, 1962; New Eng. J. Med., 1968) (Fig. 5.82).

E. SYPHILITIC INFECTION

Syphilis, both congenital and acquired, can cause sensorineural hearing loss. The incidence of such loss among various forms of syphilis has been estimated as 18 percent for late congenital, 17 percent for early congenital, 25 percent for late latent, 29 percent for asymptomatic neurosyphilis, and 80 percent of symptomatic neurosyphilis (Tamari and Itkin, 1951). The histopathology of syphilitic infection is primarily twofold. Firstly, syphilis may cause a meningo-neuro-labyrinthitis as the predominant lesion in early (in-

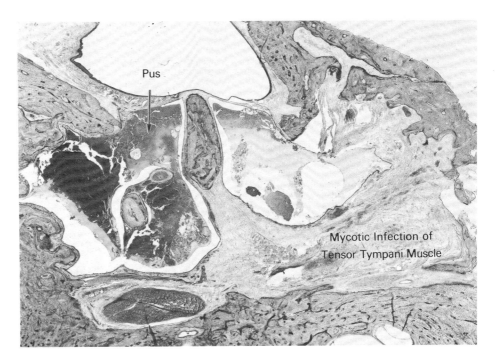

Fig. 5.82: Mucormycosis in a 38-year-old male with severe diabetes. The infection spread from the nasopharynx to both petrous apices and the middle ears. In spite of intensive therapy with amphotericin B, death was caused by rupture of the right internal carotid artery, nine weeks following onset of symptoms. The middle ears and mastoid are filled with acidophilic fluid, hemorrhages, collections of exfoliated epithelial cells and leucocytes. The mucosa and tensor tympani muscle are invaded by lymphocytes, large monocytes, and polymorphonuclear leucocytes. Similar changes are seen in the marrow spaces of the petrous apices associated with areas of bone destruction and new bone formation.

fantile) congenital syphilis and in the acute meningitides of secondary and tertiary syphilis (Goodhill, 1939). Secondly, syphilis may cause an osteitis of the temporal bone as the predominant lesion with secondary involvement of the membranous labyrinth in late (tardive) congenital, late latent and tertiary syphilis (Alexander, 1928; Mayer and Fraser, 1936; Goodhill, 1939). Pathologically, the lesions of congenital and acquired syphilis cannot be differentiated and similarly the hearing loss may be sudden or progressive, with or without vestibular involvement, in both congenital and acquired syphilis.

1. ACQUIRED SYPHILIS

Hearing loss may occur in the secondary and tertiary forms of acquired syphilis. Acute syphilitic labyrinthitis may occur in association with the acute lymphocytic meningitis of secondary syphilis. Goodhill (1939) described a case in which there was diffuse round cell infiltration in the membranous labyrinth in association with an overwhelming and fatal secondary syphilitic meningitis.

In late latent and tertiary syphilis the predominant lesion is a temporal bone osteitis with round cell infiltration (Goodhill, 1939) indistinguishable from that described by Mayer and Fraser (1936) in late congenital syphilis. Presumably neurosyphilis (meningovascular and taboparetic) may cause deafness by a meningo-neuro-labyrinthitis although temporal bones in such cases also show an extensive osteitis of the bony labyrinth (Goodhill, 1939).

Also in the tertiary stage of the disease gummatous lesions may involve the auricle, middle ear, mastoid and petrous bone. These lesions cause conductive and sensorineural hearing losses in varying combinations and in varying severity.

Because of the effectiveness of antibiotic therapy in the control of the disease, acquired syphilis is no longer an important cause of deafness.

2. CONGENITAL SYPHILIS

Congenital syphilis is caused by intrauterine infection as a consequence of acquired maternal syphilis. Even when the disease is detected and treatment is instituted early in life many patients eventually suffer from bilateral loss of auditory and vestibular function. Hearing loss is reported to occur in about 25 to 38 percent of patients with congenital syphilis (Dalsgaard-Neilson, 1938; Karmody and Schuknecht, 1966). The incidence is probably much higher than these figures indicate for the studies include young individuals with normal hearing, some of whom could be expected to develop deafness later in life.

Congenital syphilis exists in two forms, early (infantile) and late (tardive). Infantile congenital syphilis is often severe and fatal and the auditory and vestibular symptoms are overshadowed by multisystemic involvement. Goodhill (1939) has shown the otitic pathology in these cases to consist of severe degeneration of the organ of Corti and cochlear neurons with round cell infiltration, fibrinous deposits, and hemorrhage in the labyrinth.

Late or tardive congenital syphilis shows great variation in age of onset, progression, and severity. Onset in early childhood is often characterized by sudden, bilateral, severe deafness. Vestibular manifestations are uniformly present but often are poorly documented by the parents. Sometimes the disease presents a symptom complex similar to Ménière's disease with attacks of vertigo, nausea and vomiting associated with fluctuating hearing loss (Perlman and Leek, 1952). In the early stages of involvement, the hearing loss may be more severe for the low frequencies (Fig. 5.83). Onset may occur as late as the fifth decade (Rodger, 1940) in which case the hearing losses are often less severe.

Hutchinson, in 1863, provided the classical description of late congenital syphilis: "A form of deafness which occurs in these cases and which, as far as what little observation I have made on the subject goes, appears to be peculiar to them, is one in which the function fails without any external disease. It is usually symmetrical; not infrequently its stages are rapidly passed through and a patient who six months ago could hear almost perfectly becomes, without otorrhea and without any marked degree of pain, utterly deaf."

Hennebert's (1911) sign is frequently present in congenital syphilitics and consists of a positive fistula test without clinical evidence of middle ear disease. Tullio's sign occurs more often in association with congenital syphilis than any other disorder and consists of vertigo and nystagmus on stimulation with high intensity sound. An intact ossicular system seems to be an essential requirement for the Tullio phenomenon. It is readily elicited with a Bárány noise box (Perlman and Leek, 1952).

The pathophysiology of Hennebert's and Tullio's signs has generally been considered to be an inner ear fluid movement between the oval window and a bony fistula of a semicircular canal, thus resulting in movements of a cupula and stimulation of a crista. Perlman and Leek (1952) point out that Hennebert's sign is unlike the usual bony fistula response, as seen for example in association with chronic suppurative disease, in that the duration of the induced nystagmus is usually very brief, usually characterized by about three eye movements lasting about one second. Nadol (1973) has observed that Hennebert's sign may also exist in other diseases characterized by endolymphatic hydrops (e.g. Ménière's disease). He proposed that the phenomenon is

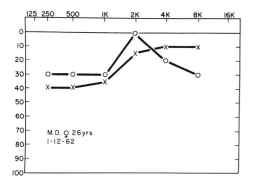

Fig. 5.83: Audiogram of a 26-year-old woman with congenital syphilis first diagnosed at the age of 6. At the age of 25 she first complained of fluctuating hearing loss and episodic vertigo. The fluctuating sensorineural hearing loss, worse for the low frequencies, simulates Ménière's disease.

Fig. 5.84: Osteitis of the bony labyrinth in a 43-year-old patient with congenital syphilis showing an area of bone resorption containing fibrous tissue with lymphocytes, plasma cells and multinucleated giant cells. See also Figs. 5.87, 5.88, and 5.89.

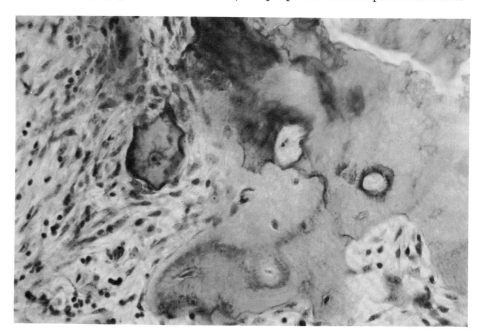

more probably caused by movements of the vestibular membranous labyrinth mediated by fibrous bands attached to the footplate of the stapes. He presented histopathological evidence to support this view.

Other sites commonly involved in congenital syphilis are (1) the nasal cartilaginous and bony framework (snuffles); (2) periostitis of the cranial bones (bossing of the skull); (3) periostitis of the tibia (sabre shins); (4) injury to odontogenous tissue (Hutchinson's teeth); (5) involvement of epiphyseal cartilages (reduction in stature); and (6) interstitial keratitis (cloudy cornea). Every tissue in the body may be affected to a greater or lesser degree. Only the most severe and untreated cases exhibit all of the classical manifestations.

Mononuclear leukocytic infiltration and obliterative endarteritis are common to all syphilitic lesions, whatever the organ affected. Mild reactions promote proliferation of fibrous tissue leading to an inflammatory fibrosis. Severe reactions result in gummatous lesions which are characterized by lymphocytic infiltration, vascular occlusion and central necrosis. The early histopathological changes of congenital infection parallel those of the secondary stage of acquired syphilis. Similarly the late pathological alterations of congenital syphilis are similar to those of the tertiary stage of the acquired disease.

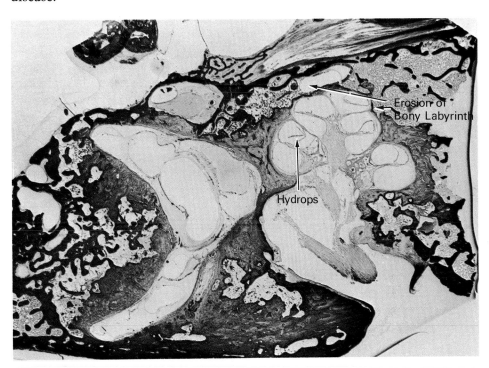

Fig. 5.85: This 70-year-old woman with congenital syphilis had been profoundly deaf for several decades. There is extensive erosion of all layers of the bony labyrinth. The areas of resorption are replaced by a highly cellular marrow-like tissue with areas of round cell infiltration. There is severe endolymphatic hydrops as well as degeneration of the membranous labyrinth. See Fig. 5.86.

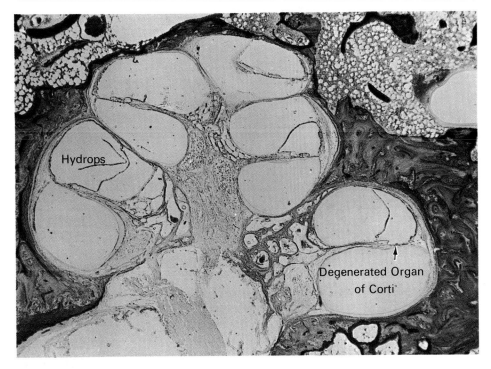

Fig. 5.86: Same patient as Fig. 5.85. High-power view shows patchy destruction of all layers of the bony labyrinth. The coalesced areas of bone destruction measure up to 2 mm in diameter, having irregular margins, and contain predominantly fatty marrow with areas of small round cell infiltration. No osteoclastic activity or new bone formation is seen. There is severe endolymphatic hydrops. The organ of Corti is missing in the basal 10 mm and severely degenerated in the remainder of the cochlea. The cochlear neurons are missing in the lower basal turn, and about 50 percent remain elsewhere. The sensory epithelia of the maculae are replaced by disorganized connective tissue, and the otolithic membranes are clumped into irregular masses.

The basic histological feature of bone involvement is an inflammatory rarefying osteitis featured by round cell infiltration, multinucleated giant cells and endarteritis leading to varying degrees of destruction of the bony labyrinth (Mayer and Fraser, 1936; Goodhill, 1939; Nager, 1955) (Fig. 5.84). The areas of resorption are first replaced by fibrous tissue heavily infiltrated with small round cells, and eventually by marrow tissue (Fig. 5.85).

The inner ear reaction is characterized by endolymphatic hydrops and progressive degeneration of the membranous labyrinth. Fibrous tissue proliferation may occur in areas adjacent to foci of bone resorption (Figs. 5.86 to 5.88).

Commonly the otitic involvement is nearly symmetrical both in terms of onset and rate of progression. It is of more than casual scientific interest that the only two diseases which are known to produce progressive endolymphatic hydrops, Ménière's disease and congenital syphilis, have similar clinical expressions, these being (1) severe episodic vertigo; (2) fluctuating hearing loss temporally related to the vertiginous attacks; (3) low-frequency hearing loss in the initial stages; and (4) flat audiometric patterns in later stages of the diseases. A reasonable assumption is that these symptoms are the result of over-accumulation of endolymph with the episodic feature caused by ruptures of the walls of the membranous labyrinth. Histological studies have provided evidence for these ruptures in both diseases. See Chapter 12A, Ménière's Disease.

There is progressive degeneration of the organ of Corti and cochlear neurons. The spiral ligament and basilar membrane undergo progressive atrophy which may lead to rupture of the cochlear duct (Nager, 1955). Similar changes involve the vestibular sense organs. Smith and Israel (1967) have reported finding spirochetes in the aqueous humor of the eye as well as in the cerebrospinal fluid, liver, lymph node, aorta, temporal artery, synovial fluid, frontal lobe cortex, and spinal cord in patients with congenital syphilis. Goldman and Girard (1967) also found intraocular treponemes in treated congenital syphilitics. Mack et al. (1969), utilizing the Krajian stain (Krajian, 1939), demonstrated spirochetes (presumably spirochaeta pallida) in the temporal bone of a patient with congenital syphilis (Fig. 5.89). Griffin and Silverstein (1969) searched for treponemes in fluid removed from the vestibules of the inner ears of patients with known congenital syphilis but were unable to demonstrate these organisms. Temporary improvement in hearing has been reported to follow the use of penicillin or ampicillin and steroid therapy (Hahn et al., 1962; Moore, 1963; Karmody and Schuknecht, 1966; Dawkins et al., 1968; Kerr et al., 1970 and 1973).

The continued presence of spirochetes in tissues despite courses of systemic penicillin is well known. Collart (1964) found spirochetes persisting in lymph nodes of patients who had received over 150 million units of penicillin therapy.

F. OTITIS EXTERNA

Infections of the external auditory canal are well-known problems to the otologist. Otitis externa may occur alone or in association with a broad spectrum of skin diseases and must be differentiated from otitis media and infections of adjacent structures, such as the parotid.

Furunculosis of the external auditory canal is a circumscribed erythematous pustular lesion surrounding a hair follicle and is usually due to staphylococci. Furunculosis may coexist with diffuse otitis externa.

Acute diffuse otitis externa is caused primarily by gram-negative bacilli, particularly *Pseudomonas aeruginosa*, and occurs mainly during hot, humid weather, and is often initiated by swimming (Senturia, 1945; Mitchell, 1955).

Otomycosis occurs primarily in tropical or subtropical climates and is caused by saprophytic fungi belonging to the classes *Aspergillacae, Mucoracae* dermatophytes, *Actinomycetaceae*, and yeast-like fungi. Wolf (1947) re-

Fig. 5.87: Same case as Figs. 5.84, 5.88, and 5.89. This patient with congenital syphilis developed bilateral interstitial keratitis at the age of 6 and bilateral hearing loss at the age of 18. In spite of intensive penicillin therapy, he became profoundly deaf. Death occurred at the age of 43. Examination shows severe endolymphatic hydrops with degeneration of the organ of Corti, stria vascularis, tectorial membrane, and cochlear neurons. The wall of the saccule is in contact with the footplate, and the utricle is distorted and displaced posteriorly. The vestibular sense organs are shrunken and show nearly total loss of hair cells. There is thickening of the dura mater lining the internal auditory canal.

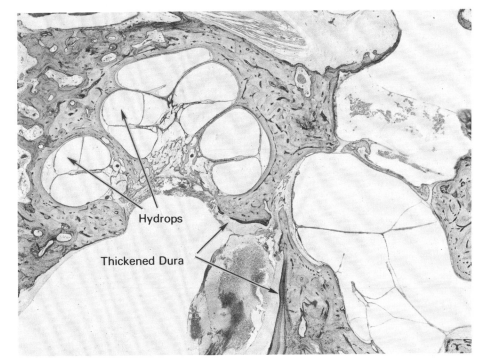

Fig. 5.88: Same specimen as in Figs. 5.84, 5.87, and 5.89, showing resorption of enchondral and endosteal bone and fibrous tissue proliferation in the posterior semicircular canal. Fistulization of the canals is responsible for Hennebert's and Tullio's signs, which are present in the early stages of congenital syphilitic infection of the temporal bone.

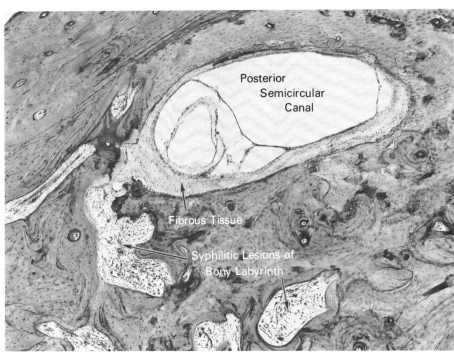

Fig. 5.89: Same specimen as Figs. 5.84, 5.87, and 5.88, showing a spirochete (arrow) at the margin of connective tissue in an area of bone resorption. Krajian stain. (Courtesy of Mack et al., 1969).

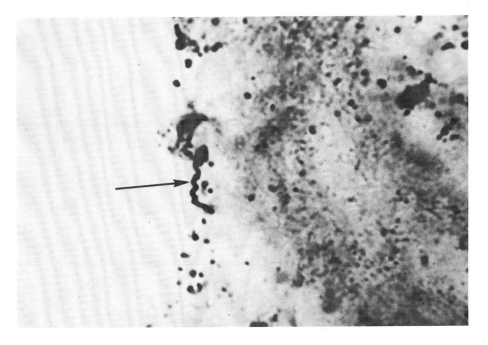

Fig. 5.90: At the age of 52 this patient complained of having had itching, discharging ears for many years. Examination revealed an exematoid dermatitis of the external auditory canals. She was treated with a variety of topical medicaments during the next twenty years but the condition was not completely controlled. She died at age 72. There is fibrous proliferation in the subepithelial layers, and the epithelium shows mild hyperkeratoses. The apocrine glands are severely atrophied.

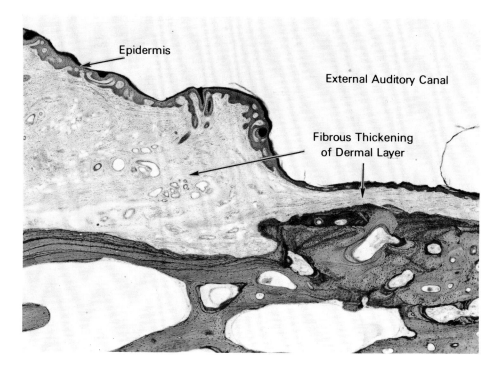

ported that at least 53 different species of fungi may cause otomycosis, with *Aspergillae* accounting for about 90 percent of the cases.

For a thorough review of this subject the reader is referred to the book *Diseases of the External Ear* by Senturia (1957).

Chronic diffuse otitis externa is characterized by pruritis and a persistent or recurring erythematous scaling or weeping dermatitis of one or both ears and sometimes associated with a seborrheic dermatitis of the scalp (Fig. 5.90). It is not primarily a bacterial infection, and the etiology is unknown. The disorder often involves the skin of the concha and tympanic membrane as well as the external auditory canal. Subcutaneous fibrous proliferation may result in narrowing of the lumen of the canal and, in rare cases the bony part of the canal may become completely obliterated by fibrous tissue. The surgical correction of chronic stenosing otitis externa, has been described by Paparella and Kurkjian (1966).

References

Abramson, M., 1969: Collagenolytic activity in middle ear cholesteatoma. Ann. Otol. Rhinol. Laryng. 78:112.

Abramson, M., and Gross, J., 1971: Further studies on a collagenase in middle ear cholesteatoma. Ann. Otol. Rhinol. Laryng. 80:177.

Aitken, R., and Brian, R., 1933: Facial palsy and infection with Zoster virus. Lancet 1:.19.

Alexander, G., 1928: New histopathological findings in the ear in lues and their importance in the general pathology of the ear. Laryngoscope 38:295.

Armstrong, B., 1955: External umbo blebs: non-inflammatory lipoid vesicles of the tympanic membrane. Laryngoscope 65:817.

Armstrong, B., 1957: Chronic secretory otitis media: diagnosis and treatment. Southern Med. J. 50:540.

Armstrong, B., 1962: Secretory otitis media —problems and pitfalls. J. Amer. Med. Assn. 179:505.

Armstrong, B., 1968: What your colleagues think of tympanostomy tubes. Laryngoscope 78:1303.

Baginsky, B., 1900: Zur Pathogenese der acuten Ertaubungen. Arch. Kinderheilk. 28:24.

Barnick, O., 1896: Klinische und pathologisch-anatomische Beiträge zur Tuberculose des mittleren und inneren Ohres. Arch. Ohren-heilk. 40:81.

Baron, S., 1954: Conservation of hearing the modified radical mastoidectomy. Laryngoscope 64:365.

Beal, D., Hemenway, W., and Lindsay, J., 1967: Inner ear pathology of sudden deafness. Arch. Otolaryng. 85:591.

Beickert, P., 1964: Alternation of hearing after tympanoplasty and stapedectomy. Arch. Otolaryng. 80:383.

Birrell, J., 1956: Black cellular cholesteatosis in childhood. J. Laryng. 70:260.

Blackley, B., Friedmann, I., and Wright, I., 1967: Herpes zoster auris associated with facial nerve palsy and auditory nerve symptoms. Acta oto-laryng. 63:533.

Bluvshtein, G., 1963: Audiologicheskaia Kharakteristika Khronicheskikh Gnoinykh Srednikh Otitiv. Vestn. Oto-Rino-Laring. 25:64.

Bondy, G., 1909: Zur Pathogenese der Mittelohrtuberkulose. Mschr. Ohrenheilk. 43:24.

Bondy, G., 1910: Totalaufmeisselung mit Erhaltung von Trommelfell und Gehörknöchelchen. Mschr. Ohrenheilk. 44:15.

Bordley, J., 1952: The problem of the preschool deaf child (diagnostic methods and the otologist's role in rehabilitation). Laryngoscope 62:514.

Borries, G., 1949: Otogenic non-purulent encephalitis. Acta oto-laryng. 37:483.

Boyd, W., 1961: A Textbook of Pathology, 7th ed. Lea and Febiger, Philadelphia, p. 327.

Brieger, O., 1913: Die Tuberkulose des Mittelohres. Verh. dtsch. otol. Ges. 22:31

Cawthorne, T., 1952: The role of surgery in the investigation and treatment of peripheral facial palsy. Lancet 1:1219.

Chandler, J., 1968: Malignant external otitis. Laryngoscope 78:1257.

Chang, I., 1969: Typmpanosclerosis. Acta oto-laryng. 68:62.

Collart, P., 1964: Persistence of treponema pallidum in late syphilis in rabbits and humans, notwithstanding treatment. Proc. Wld. Forum Syphilis and Other Treponematoses, p. 285. Public Health Service Publication 997, U.S. Government Printing Office, Washington, D.C.

Cox, G., and Dwyer, J., 1929: Tuberculosis of the middle ear. Arch. Otolaryng. 9:414.

Crabtree, J., 1968: Herpes zoster oticus. Laryngoscope 78:1853.

Dalsgaard-Neilson, E., 1938: Correlation between syphilitic interstitial keratitis and deafness. Acta Ophthal. 16:635.

Dalton, G., 1960: Bell's palsy: Some problems of prognosis and treatment. Brit. Med. J. 2:1765.

Davis, G., 1969: Cytomegalovirus in the inner ear: Case report and electron microscopic study. Ann. Otol. Rhinol. Laryng. 78:1179.

Dawes, J., 1953: Myringitis bullosa haemorrhagica its relationship to otogenic encephalitis and cranial nerve paralyses. J. Laryng. 67:313.

Dawes, J., 1961: Discussion on intracranial complications of otogenic origin. Proc. Roy. Soc. Med. 54:315.

Dawes, J., 1965: Complications of infections of the middle ear. In Diseases of the Ear, Nose, and Throat. Edited by W. Scott-Brown, J. Ballantyne, and J. Groves, Chap, 21. Butterworth & Co., London. Vol. 2, Chap. 21, pp. 478–554.

Dawkins, R., Sharp, M., and Morrison, A., 1968: Steroid treatment in congenital syphilitic deafness. J. Laryng. 82:1095.

Denny-Brown, D., Adams, R., and Fitzgerald, P., 1944: Pathologic features of herpes zoster. Arch. Neurol. Psychiat. 51:216.

Derlacki, E., and Clemis, J., 1965: Congenital cholesteatoma of the middle ear and mastoid. Ann. Otol. Rhinol. Laryng. 74:706.

Derlacki, E., Harrison, W., and Clemis, J., 1968: Congenital cholesteatoma of the middle ear and mastoid: a second report presenting seven additional cases. Laryngoscope 78:1050.

Devriese, P., 1968: Facial paralysis in cephalic herpes zoster. Ann. Otol. Rhinol. Laryng. 77:1101.

Dishoeck, H. van, and Bierman, Th., 1957: Sudden perceptive deafness and viral infection (report of the first one hundred patients). Ann. Otol. Rhinol. Laryng. 66:963.

Dota, T., Nakamura, K., Saheki, M., Sasaki, Y., 1963: Cholesterol granuloma: Experimental observations. Ann. Otol. Rhinol. Laryng. 72:346.

Elbrønd, O., 1970: Defects of the auditory ossicles in ears with intact tympanic membrane. Acta oto-laryng. Suppl. 264.

Elliott, F., 1964: Treatment of herpes zoster with high doses of Prednisone. Lancet 287:610.

Ely, E., 1880: Skin-grafting in chronic suppuration of the middle ear. Arch. Otol. 9:343.

Eschle, F., 1883: Tuberkelbacillen in dem Ausflusse bei Mittelohreiterungen von Phthisikerm. Dtsch. med. Wschr. 9:441.

Farrior, J., 1966: Principles of surgery in tympanoplasty and mastoidectomy. Laryngoscope 76:816.

Fraser, J., 1914: Acute suppurative otitis media, purulent labyrinthitis and leptomeningitis without rupture of the tympanic membrane. J. Laryng. 29:284.

Fraser, J., and Dickie, J., 1920: Meningitic neuro-labyrinthitis. Proc. Roy. Soc. Med. 13:23.

Friedmann, I., 1959: Epidermoid cholesteatoma and cholesterol granuloma: experimental and human. Ann. Otol. Rhinol. Laryng. 68:57.

Gacek, R., 1973: Results of modified type V tympanoplasty. Laryngoscope. 83:437.

Gardenghi, G., 1955: Contributo allo studio della funzione cocleare nell'otite media purulenta cronica. Boll. Mal. Orecch. 73:587.

Gelfand, M., 1954: Treatment of herpes zoster with Cortisone. J. Amer. Med. Assn. 154:911.

Georke, M., 1909: Die entzündlichen Erkrankungen des Labyrinthes. Arch. Ohr.-Nas.-KehlkHeilk. 80:1.

Glorig, A., and Gerwin, K., 1972: Otitis media. Proceedings of the National Conference, Callier Hearing and Speech Center, Dallas, Texas. C. C. Thomas, Springfield, Ill.

Goldman, J., and Girard, K., 1967: Intraocular treponemes in treated congenital syphilis. Arch. Ophthal. 78:47.

Goodhill, V., 1939: Syphilis of the ear: a histopathological study. Ann. Otol. Rhinol. Laryng. 48:676.

Goodman, A., 1949: Residual capacity to hear of pupils in schools for the deaf. J. Laryng. 63:551.

Gradenigo, G., 1888: Lupus des metteleren und inneren Ohres. Allg. wien. med. Ztg. 33:399.

Gradenigo, G., 1904: Sulla leptomeningite circoscritta e sulla paralisi dell'abducente di origine otitica. G. Accad. med. Torino 10:59.

Gray, J., 1964: The treatment of cholesteatoma in children. Proc. Roy. Soc. Med. 57:769.

Gregg, G., 1961: Some observations on Bell's palsy in Belfast during the period 1949-1958. Arch. phys. Med. 42:602.

Gregg, J., and Shaeffer, J., 1964: Unilateral inner ear deafness complicating infectious mononucleosis. S. Dakota J. Med. Pharm. 17:22.

Gregory, J., Golden, A., and Haymaker, W., 1943: Mucormycosis of central nervous system: report of three cases. Bull. Johns Hopkins Hosp. 73:405.

Griffin, W., Jr., and Silverstein, H., 1969: Inner ear fluids in certain human otologic disorders, Biochemical Mechanisms in Hearing and Deafness. Res. Otol. Int. Symp., p. 318, Edited by M. Paparella. C. C. Thomas, Springfield, Ill.

Guilford, F., Wright, W., and Draper, W., 1958: Controlled healing of mastoid and fenestration cavities. Trans. Amer. Acad. Ophthal. Otolaryng. 62:455.

Hagens, E., 1940: Pathology of the inner ear in a case of deafness from epidemic cerebrospinal meningitis. Ann. Otol. Rhinol. Laryng. 49:167.

Hahn, R., Rodin, P., and Haskins, H., 1962: Treatment of neural deafness with Prednisone. J. Chron. Dis. 15:395.

Hantman, I., 1943: Secretory otitis media. Arch. Otolaryng. 38:561.

Harbert, F., and Young, I., 1967: Audiologic findings in Ramsay Hunt syndrome. Arch. Otolaryng. 85:632.

Harner, S., Heiny, B., and Newell, R., 1970: Herpes zoster oticus. Arch. Otolaryng. 92:632.

Harris, I., 1961: Tympanosclerosis—a revived clinicopathologic entity. Laryngoscope 71:1488.

Harris, I., and Weiss, L., 1962: Tympanosclerosis: superficial and embedded forms. Trans. Amer. Acad. Ophthal. Otolaryng. 66:683.

Harrison, W., Shambaugh, G., Jr., Kaplan, J., and Derlacki, E., 1959: Prosthetics in the middle ear. Arch. Otolaryng. 69:661.

Haslhofer, L., 1969: Primäre kongenitale Mittelohrtuberkulose beim Säugling. Arch. klin. exp. Ohr.-Nas.-Kehlk.Heilk. 193:236.

Heilborn, F., 1950: Morphologische Studien zur Pathogenese des Zoster. Acta Anat. 10:363.

Heller, M., and Lindenberg, P., 1955: Sudden perceptive deafness: Report of five cases. Ann. Otol. Rhinol. Laryng. 64:931.

Henneford, G., and Lindsay, J., 1968: Deafmutism due to meningogenic labyrinthitis. Laryngoscope 78:251.

Hennebert, C., 1911: Un syndrome nouveau dans la labyrinthite hérédosyphilitique. Clinique, Brux 25:545; also Presse méd. 63:467.

Hilding, D., 1965: Postinflammatory fixation of the malleus. Arch. Otolaryng. 81:17.

Hůlka, J., 1941: Bone conduction changes in acute otitis media. Arch. Otolaryng. 33:333.

Hunt, J., 1907: On herpetic inflammations of the geniculate ganglion. A new syndrome and its complications. J. Nerv. Ment. Dis. 34:73.

Hutchinson, J., 1863: A Clinical Memoir on Certain Disease of the Eye and Ear Consequent on Inherited Syphilis. J. Churchill, London.

Igarashi, M., Konishi, S., Alford, B., and Guilford, F., 1970: The pathology of tympanosclerosis. Laryngoscope 80:233.

Jako, G., 1967: The posterior route to the middle ear: Posterior tympanotomy. Laryngoscope 77:306.

Jansen, C., 1963: Cartilage-tympanoplasty. Laryngoscope 73:1288.

Jeanes, A., and Friedmann, I., 1960: Tuberculosis of the middle ear. Tubercle, The Journal of the British Tuberculosis Association 41:109.

Jepsen, O., 1965: Topognosis (topographic diagnosis) of facial nerve lesions. Arch. Otolaryng. 81:446.

Johnson, L., and Zonderman, B., 1948: Herpes zoster oticus ("Ramsay Hunt syndrome"): Report of a case. Arch. Otolaryng. 48:1.

Juers, A., 1954: Preservation of hearing in surgery for chronic ear disease: a consideration of factors involved. Laryngoscope 64:235.

Karmody, C., and Schuknecht, H., 1966: Deafness in congenital syphilis. Arch. Otolaryng. 83:18.

Kerr, A., Smyth, G., and Landau, H., 1970: Congenital syphilitic labyrinthitis. Arch. Otolaryng. 91:474.

Kerr, A., Smyth, G., and Cinnamond, M., 1973: Congenital syphilitic deafness. J. Laryng. 87:1.

Kilby, D., Richards, S., and Hart, G., 1972: Grommets and glue ears: Two-year results. J. Laryng. 86:881.

Kinney, C., 1953: Hearing impairments in children. Laryngoscope 63:220.

Kopetzky, S., and Armour, R., 1930–1931: Suppuration of the petrous pyramid: Pathology, symptomatology and surgical treatment. Ann. Otol. Rhinol. Laryng. 39:996, 40:157.

Körner, O., 1904: Ueber den Herpes zoster oticus. Münch. med. Wschr. 1:6.

Krajian, A., 1939: The clinical application of a twenty-minute staining method for spirochaeta pallida in tissue sections. Amer. J. Syph. Gon. Ven. Dis. 23:617.

Lapidot, A., and Brandow, E., 1966: A method for preserving the posterior canal wall and bridge in the surgery for cholesteatoma: Preliminary report. Acta oto-laryng. 62:88.

Laumans, E., 1962: On the prognosis of peripheral facial paralysis of endotemporal origin. Thesis Amsterdam (H. J. Koersen en Zonen).

Lee, K., and Schuknecht, H., 1971: Results of tympanoplasty and mastoidectomy at the Massachusetts Eye and Ear Infirmary. Laryngoscope 81:529.

Lempert, J., 1937: Complete apicectomy (mastoidotympano-apicectomy): a new technique for the complete exenteration of the apical carotid portion of the petrous pyramid. Arch. Otolaryng. 25:144.

Lempert, J., 1938: Improvement of hearing in cases of otosclerosis: A new, one stage surgical technic. Arch. Otolaryng. 28:42.

Lewy, A., and Hagens, E., 1937: Report of the Chicago committee on otitic meningitis. Laryngoscope 47:761.

Lieberman, A., 1957: Unilateral deafness. Laryngoscope 67:1237.

Lindeman, R., and Silverstein, H., 1964: The "Arrow Tube". Arch. Otolaryng. 80:473.

Lindsay, J., 1938: Suppuration in the petrous pyramid. Ann. Otol. Rhinol. Laryng. 47:1.

Lindsay, J., 1959: Sudden deafness due to virus infection. Arch. Otolaryng. 69:13.

Lindsay, J., Davey, P., and Ward, P., 1960: Inner ear pathology in deafness due to mumps. Ann. Otol. Rhinol. Laryng. 69:918.

Lindsay, J., and Hemenway, W., 1954: Inner ear pathology due to measles. Ann. Otol. Rhinol. Laryng. 63:754.

Mack, L., Smith, J., Walter, E., and Montenegro, E., 1969: Spirochetes in the temporal bone in congenital syphilitic deafness despite penicillin therapy. Arch. Otolaryng. 90:11.

Matthews, W., 1961: Bell's palsy. Brit. Med. J. 2:215.

Mayer, O., and Fraser, J., 1936: Pathological changes in ear in late congenital syphilis. J. Laryng. 51:683 and 755.

McArdle, F., and Tonndorf, J., 1968: Perforations of the tympanic membrane and their effects upon middle-ear transmission. Arch. klin. exp. Ohren-, Nas.-KehlkHeilk. 192:145.

McLay, K., 1954: Otogenic meningitis. J. Laryng. 68:140.

Mitchell, R., 1955: Rapid microbiologic methodology in military medicine. Milit. Med. 166:85.

Moore, M., Jr., 1963: The epidemiology of syphilis. J. Amer. Med. Assn. 186:831.

Mufson, M., Webb, P., Kennedy, H., Gill, V., and Chanock, R., 1966: Etiology of upper respiratory tract illnesses among civilian adults. J. Amer. Med. Assn. 195:91.

Müsebeck, K., 1970: Zur Klassifikation der Tympanomastoidplastik. Relation zwischen Verlaufsform der chronischen Otitis media und sanierenden Operationstyp. Z. Laryng. Rhinol. 41:212.

Myers, D., and Schlosser, W., 1960: Anterior-posterior technique for the treatment of chronic otitis media and mastoiditis: Preliminary report. Laryngoscope 70:78.

Myers, E., and Ballantine, H., 1965: The management of otogenic brain abscess. Laryngoscope 75:273.

Myers, E., and Stool, S., 1968: Cytomegalic inclusion disease of the inner ear. Laryngoscope 78:1904.

Nadol, J., Jr., 1973: Personal commun.

Nager, F. von, 1907: Beitrage zur Histologie der erworbenen, Taubstummheit. Z. Ohrenheilk. 54:217.

Nager, F. von, 1955: Die Lues hereditaria tarda des Innerohreseine Folge chronischer Osteomyelitis des Felsenbeins. Pract. Oto-rhino-laryng. 17:1.

New England Journal of Medicine, 1968: Case records of the Massachusetts General Hospital 279:1220.

Palva, T., 1963: Surgery of chronic ear without cavity. Arch. Otolaryng. 77:570.

Palva, T., Friedmann, I., and Palva, A., 1964: Mastoiditis in children. J. Laryng. 78:977.

Palva, T., Palva, A., Salmivalli, O., and Salmivalli, A., 1968: Radical mastoidectomy with cavity obliteration. Arch. Otolaryng. 88:119.

Paparella, M., Brady, D., and Hoel, R., 1970: Sensorineural hearing loss in chronic otitis media and mastoiditis. Trans. Amer. Acad. Opthal. Otolaryng. 74:108.

Paparella, M., and Kurkjian, J., 1966: Surgical treatment for chronic stenosing external otitis (including finding of unusual canal tumor). Laryngoscope 76:232.

Paparella, M., and Lim, D., 1967: Pathogenesis and pathology of the "Idiopathic" blue ear drum. Arch. Otolaryng. 85:249.

Paparella, M., Oda, M., Hiraide, F., and Brady, D., 1972: Pathology of sensorineural hearing loss in otitis media. Ann. Otol. Rhinol. Laryng. 81:632.

Paparella, M., and Sugiura, S., 1967: The pathology of suppurative labyrinthitis. Ann. Otol. Rhinol. Laryng. 76:554.

Peitersen, E., and Andersen, P., 1967: Spontaneous course of 220 peripheral non-traumatic facial palsies. Acta oto-laryng. Suppl. 224:296.

Peitersen, E., and Caunt, A., 1970: The incidence of herpes zoster antibodies in patients with peripheral facial palsy. J. Laryng. 84:65.

Pennybacker, J., 1961: Discussion on intracranial complications of otogenic origin. Proc. Roy. Soc. Med. 54:309.

Perlman, H., and Leek, J., 1952: Late congenital syphilis of the ear. Laryngoscope 62:1175.

Politzer, A., 1893: Lehrbuch der Ohrenheilkunde, p. 376. Ferdinand Enke, Verlag, Stuttgart.

Preuss, L., 1922: Selbstheilung nach vollständiger Zerstörung des Labyrinthes. Z. Hals-Nas.-Ohrenheilk. 2:11.

Preysing, H., 1898: Multiple tuberkulöse Tumoren am Schädel und in beiden Trommelfellen. Z. Ohrenheilk. 32:369.

Proctor, B., and Lindsay, J., 1942: Tuberculosis of the ear. Arch. Otolaryng. 35:221.

Ramadier, J., 1933: Les osteites petreuses profondes (petrosites). Oto-Rhino-Laryng. Int. 17:816.

Robbins, S., 1962: Textbook of Pathology, 2nd Ed. W. B. Saunders, Philadelphia and London, chap. XII, p. 319.

Rodger, T., 1940: Syphilis as seen by the aural surgeon. J. Laryng. 55:168.

Rossberg, G., 1960: Pneumokokkenmeningitis und otitis media acuta. Arch. Ohrenheilk. 176:691.

Sade, J., 1966: Pathology and pathogenesis of serous otitis media. Arch. Otolaryng. 84:297.

Sauer, G., 1955: Herpes zoster: treatment of postherpetic neuralgia with Cortisone, Corticotropin and placebo. Arch. Derm. 71:488.

Saunders, W., and Lippy, W., 1959: Sudden deafness and Bell's palsy: a common cause. Ann. Otol. Rhinol. Laryng. 68:830.

Schiller, A., 1961: "Mastoid osteoplasty" using autogenous cancellous bone. J. Laryng. 75:647.

Schuknecht, H., Chasin, W., and Kurkjian, J., 1966: Stereoscopic Atlas of Mastoidotympanoplastic Surgery. C. V. Mosby Co., St. Louis, Mo.

Schuknecht, H., Kimura, R., and Naufal, P., 1973: The pathology of sudden deafness. Acta oto-laryng 76:75.

Schuknecht, H., and Montandon, P., 1970: Pathology of the ear in pneumococcal meningitis. Arch. Klin. exp. Ohr.-Nas.-Kehlk Heilk. 195:207.

Senturia, B., 1945: Etiology of external otitis. Laryngoscope 55:277.

Senturia, B., 1957: Diseases of the External Ear. C. C. Thomas, Springfield, Ill.

Senturia, B., Lim, D., Proud, G., Lupovich, P., and Bluestone, C., 1972: Symposium on Prophylaxis and Treatment of Middle Ear Effusions. Laryngoscope 82:1622.

Shambaugh, G., Hagens, E., Holderman, J.,

and Watkins, R., 1928: Statistical studies of children in public schools for the deaf. Arch. Otolaryng. 7:424.

Shambaugh, G., Wallner, L., Greene, L., and Shambaugh, G., Jr., 1933: Severe deafness in adults: a clinical study. Arch. Otolaryng. 18:430.

Shea, M., and Gardner, G., 1970: Mastoid obliteration using homograft bone. Arch. Otolaryng. 92:358.

Sheehy, J., 1965: Ossicular problems in tympanoplasty. Arch. Otolaryng. 81:115.

Sheehy, J., 1970: The intact canal wall technique in management of aural cholesteatoma. J. Laryng. 84:1.

Silverstein, H., 1966: Malleus clip tube for long-term equalization of middle ear pressure. Trans Amer. Acad. Ophthal. Otolaryng. 70:640.

Silverstein, H., 1970: Permanent middle ear aeration. Arch. Otolaryng. 91:313.

Silverstein, H., Miller, G., Jr., and Lindeman, R., 1966: Eustachian tube dysfunction as a cause for chronic secretory otitis in children (correction by pressure-equalization). Laryngoscope 76:259.

Simpson, R., 1949: The causes of perceptive deafness. Proc. Roy. Soc. Med. 42:536.

Smith, J., and Israel, C., 1967: Spirochetes in the aqueous humor in seronegative ocular syphilis: persistence after penicillin therapy. Arch. Ophthal. 77: 474.

Smyth, G., England, R., Gibson, R., Kerr, A., 1967: Posterior tympanotomy, its importance in combined approach tympanoplasty. J. Laryng. 81:69.

Sorensen, H., and True, O., 1971: Histology of tympanosclerosis. Acta oto-laryng. 73:18.

Stewart, J., 1928: Histopathology of mastoiditis. J. Laryng. 43:689.

Swartz, M., and Dodge, P., 1965: Bacterial meningitis: a review of selected aspects. New Eng. J. Med. 272:725, 777, 842, 898, 954, 1003.

Tamari, M., and Itkin, P., 1951: Penicillin and syphilis of the ear. Eye, Ear, Nose, Throat Monthly 30:252, 301, 358.

Tangeman, C., 1883: Reproduction of the membranae tympani by skin grafting. Arch. Otol. 12:228.

Taverner, D., 1955: Bell's palsy. Brain 78:209.

Thorburn, I., 1961: Experience with pedicled temporal muscle flaps in radical mastoid and tympanoplasty operations. J. Laryng. 75:885.

Tos, M., 1970: Bony fixation of the malleus and incus. Acta oto-laryng. 70:95.

Tröltsch, A. von, 1877: Lehrbuch der Ohrenheilkunde mit Einschluss der Anatomie des Ohres, 6th ed. Vogel, Leipzig. pp. 150–174.

Tschiassny, K., 1946: The site of the facial nerve lesion in cases of Ramsay Hunt's syndrome. Ann. Otol. Rhinol. Laryng. 55:152.

Tuberculosis, 1965: Chemotherapy of pulmonary tuberculosis in adults, the choice of drugs in relation to drug susceptibility. Amer. Thoracic Society, Committee on Therapy, Amer. Rev. of

Resp. Diseases 92: (No. 3), September.

Tuberculosis, 1967: Chemoprophylaxis for the prevention of tuberculosis. Report of Ad Hoc Committee on Chemoprophylaxis, National Tuberculosis Association, New York.

Turner, A., and Fraser, J., 1915: Tuberculosis of the middle-ear cleft in children: a clinical and pathological study. J. Laryng. 30:209.

Turner, A., and Fraser, J., 1928: A complication of middle ear suppuration: a clinical and pathological study. J. Laryng. 43:609.

Voltolini, R., 1868: Der Canalis petromastoideus im Schläfenbeine. Mscher. Ohrenheilk. 2:21.

Ward, P., Lindsay, J., and Warner, N., 1965: Cytomegalic inclusion disease affecting the temporal bone. Laryngoscope 75:628.

Watson, D., 1948: Progress in treatment of mastoid infection and some of its complications. President's Address. Proc. roy. Soc. Med. 41:155.

Welsh, L., and Welsh, J., 1962: Herpes zoster involving the head and neck. Laryngoscope 72:653.

Whitehead, A., 1904: Suppuration in the labyrinth. J. Laryng. 19:242.

Wittmaack, K., 1926: Die eitrige Labyrinthitis under ihre Folgezustände. Labyrinthitis Purulenta; Empyema sacculi endolymphatici. Henke u. Lubarsch, Hand. d. spez. path. Anat. u. Histol. Verlag von Julius Springer, Berlin.

Wolf, F., 1947: Relation of various fungi to otomycosis. Arch. Otolaryng. 46:361.

Wolff, H., 1953: Early diagnosis of mumps. Acta Leidensia 23:130.

Wullstein, H., 1956a: The restoration of the function of the middle ear in chronic otitis media. Ann. Otol. Rhinol. Laryng. 65:1020.

Wullstein, H., 1956b: Theory and practice of tympanoplasty. Laryngoscope 66:1076.

Yearsley, M., 1934–1935: An analysis of over four thousand cases of educational deafness studied during the past twenty-five years. Brit. J. Child. Dis. 31:177, 1934; 31:272 (Oct.-Dec.), 1934; 32:21 (Jan.-Mar.), 1935 32:107 (Apr.-June), 1935; 32:196 (July-Sept.), 1935; 32:264 (Oct-Dec.), 1935.

Zajtchuk, J., Matz, G., and Lindsay, J., 1972: Temporal bone pathology in herpes oticus. Ann. Otol. Rhinol. Laryng. 81:331.

Zange, J., 1914: Über umschriebene Entzündungen des Ohrlabyrinthes. Virchows Arch. Path. Anat. 216:500.

Zippel, R., 1963: Zür Pathogenese der akuten Mittelohrentzundung bei Virusgrippe. Z. Laryng. Rhinol. 42:823.

Zöllner, F., 1955: The principles of plastic surgery of the sound-conducting apparatus. J. Laryng. 69:637.

Zöllner, F., 1957: Hörverbessernde Operationen bei entzündlich bedingten Mittelohrveränderungen. Arch. Ohr.-Nas.-Kehlk-Heilk. 171:1.

Zuckermann, M., 1933: Aural complications of epidemic cerebrospinal meningitis. Vrach. delo 16:706.

6 Disorders of Intoxication

Because all biologically active substances exhibit some kinds of undesirable effects, the history of a new drug is frequently marked by early enthusiastic endorsements of its therapeutic value followed by later condemnations because of its adverse side reactions. Drugs interfere, in one way or another, with the chemical system which governs the homeostatic mechanisms of an organism. To be useful, drug-induced changes must do one of three things: (1) normalize pathological functions, (2) alleviate disease symptoms, or (3) combat infection. The obvious goal is to recognize the harmful effects of newly developed drugs by animal tests before any injury is done to human subjects. Unfortunately, present experimental methods have not been standardized, with the result that the final analyses cannot be considered dependable.

The following methods of study should be used when conducting animal experiments for the purpose of determining possible ototoxic effects of a new drug:

(1) Tests of auditory and vestibular function.
(2) Histological studies for both acute and permanent effects.
(3) Controls. These are essential to avoid the introduction of personal bias, misinterpretation of pre-existing pathology, aging effects, nutritional effects, habituation and learning factors, possible injuries from test procedures, artifacts of histological preparation, effects from the drug vehicle, etc.
(4) Quantitative estimations of cytological changes in the cochlear and vestibular systems.
(5) The study of brain tissues of experimental and control animals. Misinterpretations are frequent in the evaluation of changes in the central nervous system. A high degree of sophistication is required to differentiate pathological changes from preparation artifact and from postmortem autolysis.

The toxic properties of drugs may have a high order of organ specificity (Ballantyne, 1970). There are a number of drugs which affect the inner ear to create temporary or permanent alterations in auditory or vestibular function.

Drugs which are used extensively and manifest ototoxic side effects are the aminoglycoside antibiotics, quinine and related chemicals, and salicylates.

Other therapeutic agents with known ototoxic effects but not so commonly used are ethacrynic acid, thalidomide (toxic to embryo), nitrogen mustard, tetanus antitoxin, ascaridole (active principle in oil of chenapodium), and atoxyl.

A. AMINOGLYCOSIDE OTOTOXICITY

Very little of the aminoglycoside drugs is absorbed from the intestinal tract even after oral administration of large doses. They are readily absorbed from intramuscular and subcutaneous sites. In the blood the drugs are located mainly in the plasma and from there are distributed to all the extracellular fluids. Approximately 50 percent of the parenterally administered dose is excreted unchanged in the urine in 24 hours. In the presence of renal insufficiency, tubular resorption is minimal and the blood levels may remain high for many days.

Untoward responses to the drug consist of hypersensitivity reactions and toxic reactions. Among the hypersensitivity reactions are skin rashes, eosinophilia, fever, angioedema, exfoliative dermatitis, blood dyscrasias, and anaphalactic shock. These reactions are not dose-related.

Toxic reactions include degenerative changes in the inner ear, involving both the auditory and vestibular systems, neurotoxic effects of the optic and peripheral nerves and cerebral cortex, and renal toxicity characterized by albuminuria, cylindruria, and reduced urine output (Weinstein, 1965).

The studies of Jacoby and Gorini (1967) on the mode of action of streptomycin and its analogues on microorganisms suggest that these drugs not only inhibit protein synthesis, but also produce misreading of the genetic code. This concept is compatible with the delayed ototoxic effects demonstrated by dihydrostreptomycin and neomycin, for protein synthesis in the mature inner ear is a slow process (Koburg and Plester, 1962).

The intramuscular injection of tritium-labeled dihydrostreptomycin into guinea pigs has shown that the drug reaches all cells of the cochlea without any preferential localization (Balogh et al., 1970). The drug reaches the perilymph within 15 minutes, and the concentration is highest in both perilymph and endolymph in two hours. The drug almost disappears from these fluids in 24 hours.

Determination of the relative concentrations of streptomycin in the blood, spinal fluid, and perilymph has demonstrated an accumulation in the inner ear fluids with repeated injections of the drug (Vrabec et al., 1965). The same behavior has been demonstrated for neomycin and kanamycin (Meyer zum Gottesberge and Stupp, 1969). In a well-executed series of experiments, Stupp (1970) showed that the aminoglycoside antibiotics are concentrated in the perilymph and endolymph, accounting for the ototoxic behavior of these drugs. He also found that in therapeutic dosages only small amounts of penicillin reach the inner ear, while tetracycline and polymyxin E fail to enter the inner ear fluids.

1. STREPTOMYCIN

Streptomycin was isolated from cultures of a soil organism (streptomyces griseus) in 1944 (Schatz et al., 1944). It was the first antibacterial agent to be effective against tuberculosis. In the treatment of this disease it became apparent that streptomycin was toxic to the inner ear (Hinshaw and Feldman, 1945; Brown and Hinshaw, 1946; Farrington et al., 1947). It was found that parenterally administered streptomycin in doses of 2 to 3 gm per day usually resulted in loss of vestibular function in two to four weeks, and with higher daily doses or prolonged treatment, hearing loss also occurred.

Several animal experiments have been performed on different species, and these have shown that the drug affects mainly the vestibular endorgans

Fig. 6.1: Crista of the posterior canal showing loss of hair cells from the toxic effects of streptomycin sulfate. This 42-year-old patient, with impairment of cardiac and renal function, received 1 gm of streptomycin sulfate per day intramuscularly (in four equally divided doses of 0.025 gm) for ten days for a total of 10 gm. At the completion of therapy he was extremely ataxic, and ice water caloric tests failed to evoke a response in either ear. The ataxia improved but persisted to some extent until the time of his death four years later. He had no subjective change in hearing. Histological studies show a loss of 75 percent of the hair cells in all cristae and about 25 percent of the hair cells of the utricles of both ears. The saccules and cochleae appear normal.

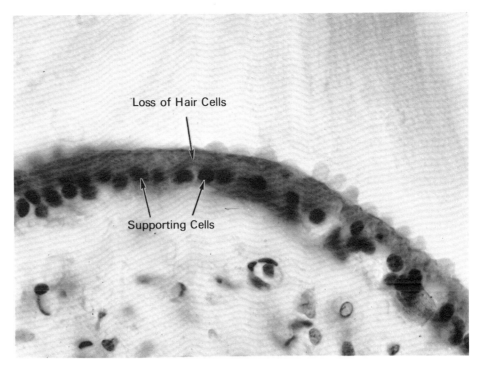

(Causse, 1949; Berg, 1951; McGee and Olszewski, 1962; Wersäll and Hawkins, 1962; Duvall and Wersäll, 1964). In cats, squirrel monkeys, and mice the vestibular lesions are confined primarily to the hair cells of the cristae with little or no damage to the maculae. The same change has been observed in the human inner ear (Fig. 6.1).

Numerous experimental studies on animals have shown that the loss of hair cells is most severe in the central part or summit of the crista and that the type I hair cells are more vulnerable to injury than the type II hair cells (Wersäll and Hawkins, 1962; Spoendlin, 1966; Lindeman, 1969; Kanda and Igarashi, 1969; Watanuki, 1971).

Based on the relatively selective toxic action of streptomycin on the vestibular endorgans, several investigators have utilized the parenteral administration of this drug for ablation of vestibular function in the treatment of disabling vertigo in patients with Ménière's disease. Fowler (1948) reported having treated four cases of bilateral Ménière's disease with 4 gm of streptomycin daily. He concluded that this treatment is indicated for any patient under the age of fifty years with bilateral Ménière's disease in whom conservative management has failed. Hamberger et al. (1949) reported treatment of four cases of Ménière's disease, two with bilateral disease, with 3 gm streptomycin daily. These patients were free from attacks of vertigo during the follow-up period, but they had undesirable ataxia for many months. Rüedi (1951) treated three cases with 2 to 3 gm daily, and Hanson (1951) treated five patients with 2 gm daily with similar results.

In 1957 Schuknecht reported treatment of eight cases, and in 1968 Singleton and Schuknecht reported their total experience with the treatment of 15 cases of Ménière's disease, of which nine had bilateral disease and six had unilateral disease. All were relieved of vertigo and none experienced hearing loss from the treatment. The first symptom of streptomycin ototoxicity reported by the patients was unsteadiness. This was generally followed by ataxia, anorexia, nausea, and occasional vomiting. Many patients developed spontaneous nystagmus during the course of treatment. The direction of the quick component was opposite to the ear showing the more rapid decreasing caloric response. It was not unusual for the spontaneous nystagmus to change direction during the course of treatment.

For unilateral Ménière's disease the streptomycin injections were discontinued on the first day the ice water caloric test failed to elicit a response in the diseased ear, and for bilateral disease when no response occurred in either ear. Several of the patients were given 3 gm of streptomycin daily, but this was found to cause too rapid an onset and progression of ototoxicity for deter-

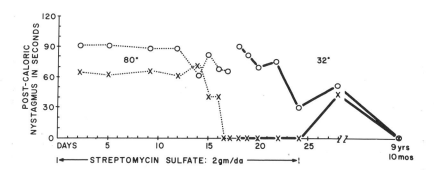

Fig. 6.2: Graph showing vestibular test results of a 32-year-old male who was treated with 2 gm of streptomycin sulfate per day for 24 days for the ablation of vestibular function because of bilateral Ménière's disease. For the first 17 days caloric tests were performed with 5 cc of water at 80°F, and thereafter with 5 cc of ice water. He first noticed disequilibrium on the eleventh day of treatment, following which ataxia increased and vestibular response decreased until the termination of treatment. He had no further vertiginous episodes and returned to a full work load in two and one-half months. Tests performed at the United States Naval Aerospace Medical Institute, United States Naval Aviation Medical Center, Pensacola, Florida, twelve years following treatment, revealed great diminution of canal and otolith function, immunity to motion sickness, and hearing unchanged from the pretreatment level. (Graybiel et al., 1965)

Fig. 6.3: Audiograms and cochlear chart of cat that received 200 mg/kg/day of streptomycin sulfate for 28 days. Post-treatment survival time was 15 months. Behavioral audiograms show a high-frequency hearing loss. Studies of cochlear pathology show a loss of hair cells and cochlear neurons in the basal 7 mm and in the 12–18 mm region. See also Figs. 6.4 and 6.5. (Courtesy of McGee and Olszewski)

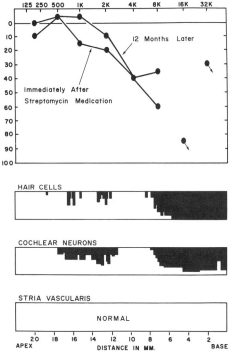

mining the appropriate time to discontinue therapy. The ideal dose appeared to be 2 gm daily, given intramuscularly in two equally divided doses. This resulted in a more gradual onset of ototoxicity. If no ototoxic effect was evident after ten days of treatment the dose was increased to 3 gm daily for one or more days, after which the 2 gm daily dose was resumed. Likewise, if the progression of ototoxicity was too rapid, the dose was decreased to 1 gm daily to assure a more careful control of the end point of therapy. The average total dose was 30 gm, and the average duration of treatment was 18 days (Fig. 6.2). In all cases ataxia was moderately severe upon termination of treatment and generally lasted a few months. The average duration of recovery for return to full activity was four months (range: one to nine months). After one or two years the patients experienced ataxia only when walking in the dark. In these 15 cases and in previously reported cases of Ménière's disease treated with streptomycin, there has been no hearing loss attributable to streptomycin. It seems quite clear, however, that the prolonged use of large dosages of streptomycin can lead to hearing loss (Lidén, 1953).

Graybiel et al. (1965, 1967) reported the results of extensive vestibular and auditory testing of four patients with Ménière's disease who had been treated by Schuknecht (1957). None had experienced a return of vertiginous symptoms over the follow-up period of 11 to 13 years. All exhibited great suppression of otolith and canal function and immunity from motion sickness. Hearing was not significantly different from pretreatment levels.

McGee and Olszewski (1962) gave streptomycin to cats in two equally divided doses varying from 25 mg/kg/day to 200 mg/kg/day. The smaller doses created changes only in vestibular function whereas the larger doses when given over long periods of time, produced high-frequency hearing losses as well. With 200 mg/kg/day postrotatory nystagmus disappeared on about the twelfth day of treatment. Ataxia developed simultaneously with the decrease of postrotatory nystagmus. Ataxia was severe for two or three weeks, after which there was gradual improvement; but even at the end of one year, gait had not returned to normal. All animals lost body weight while receiving the drug. The hearing loss and cochlear pathology of an animal which received 200 mg/kg/day for 28 days in a purposeful attempt to produce severe ototoxicity are shown in Fig. 6.3. Histological studies revealed the primary pathological change to be a loss of hair cells in the vestibular endorgans without changes in the supporting elements or the vestibular nerves. Estimates of the hair cell populations indicated that animals with total loss of postrotatory nystagmus had lost from 50 to 90 percent of the hair cells in the cristae but not more than 10 percent of the hair cells in the maculae of the utricle and saccule (Fig. 6.4). Changes in the cochlea varied from a loss of hair cells only to total loss of the organ of Corti (Fig. 6.5). The changes were always most severe in the basal turn. There was neural degeneration only in those areas where the supporting elements of the organ of Corti were damaged.

Schuknecht (1957) studied the effect of injecting streptomycin solution into the auditory bullae of cats. A concentration of 0.25 gm streptomycin sulfate in 0.5 cc of normal saline was slowly injected. Upon recovering from the anesthetic, the animals showed severe disequilibrium (nystagmus toward the opposite side, falling toward the same side, nausea, vomiting, and ataxia). Animals given 0.125 gm of streptomycin in 0.5 cc of normal saline solution

Fig. 6.4: Cristae of the horizontal canals of a normal animal (left) and an animal exhibiting loss of vestibular function caused by the intramuscular administration of 200 mg/kg/day for 28 days of streptomycin sulfate (right). In the treated ear the sensory epithelium is flattened and about 50 percent of the hair cells are missing. The remaining hair cells appear shrunken and have pyknotic nuclei. Posttreatment survival time was 15 months. See also Figs. 6.3 and 6.5.

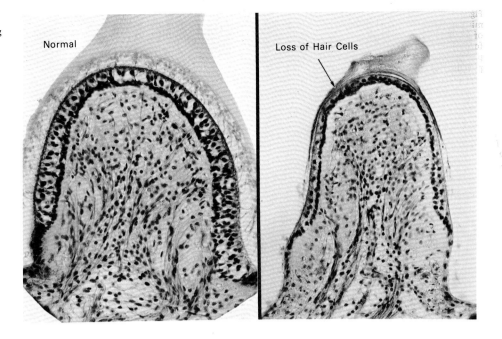

Fig. 6.5: Loss of second and third rows of external hair cells in the 13 mm region. See audiogram and cochlear chart of this cat in Fig. 6.3. (Streptomycin sulfate: 200 mg/kg/day for 28 days).

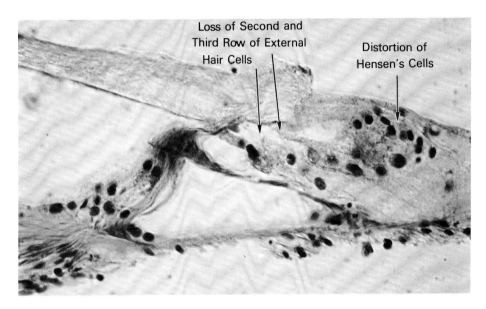

Fig. 6.6: The ablation of auditory and vestibular function can be achieved by the repeated intratympanic injection of a solution of streptomycin sulfate (0.125 gm/cc). This technique has been used to accomplish vestibular ablation for individuals with disabling Ménière's disease (Schuknecht, 1957).

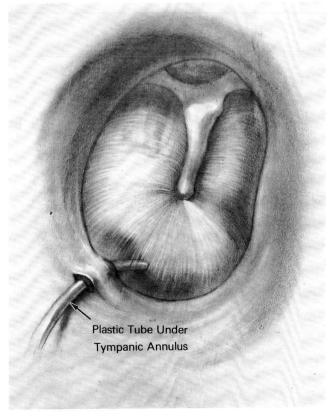

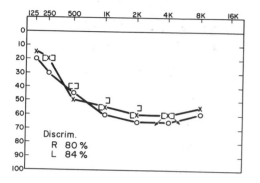

Fig. 6.7: Hearing loss due to intramuscular administration of dihydrostreptomycin. A dosage of 0.5 gm was given twice daily for 18 days for a total of 18 gm. Three months later the patient first noted bilateral hearing loss which progressed for three weeks after which there was no further change. Caloric responses were normal bilaterally. Good speech discrimination indicates minimal degeneration of cochlear neurons.

Fig. 6.8: Graph showing vestibular test results and pathological changes in a cat receiving 300 mg/kg/day of dihydrostreptomycin for 21 days. The tests for vestibular function consisted of placing the animal on a turntable with its head fixed in the axis of rotation and the horizontal canal in the plane of rotation. The table was rotated manually at the rate of one turn per second for ten seconds and then stopped abruptly. The duration of postrotatory nystagmus was timed by two independent observers after spinning the animal both to the right and to the left. The graphs showed that postrotatory nystagmus was lost between the 14th and 20th day in both ears and remained absent during the 14-month observation period. Control animals demonstrated that loss of reaction was not caused by habituation. Histological studies show loss of about half of the hair cells of the cristae and a slight loss of hair cells in the utricle (15-month survival time) See also Figs. 6.9 and 6.10. (Courtesy of McGee and Olszewski)

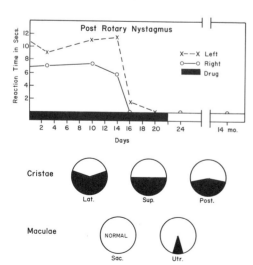

experienced less severe disequilibrium. Histological studies showed a severe loss of the hair cells in the cristae and maculae. There was also a loss of hair cells in the organ of Corti, most severe in the basal turn.

A control group of animals given intratympanic injections of saturated solution of sodium chloride exhibited no vestibular reaction. Because the osmotic and ionic concentration of the salt solution exceeded that of the streptomycin solution, the reaction to streptomycin was assumed to be a true chemical ototoxic effect.

Davis et al. (1958) subsequently used the method of intratympanic injection of streptomycin to achieve a selective loss of external hair cells in studies designed to locate the origin of bioelectric potentials of the inner ear.

Schuknecht (1957) also injected streptomycin solution (Squibb) via indwelling intratympanic tubes into the middle ears of patients with Ménière's disease in the hope of destroying vestibular function while preserving hearing (Fig. 6.6). With the injection of 0.5 cc in a strength of 0.125 gm/cc every six hours, disequilibrium became manifest on the third day and was fully developed by the sixth day.

Daily audiograms revealed that hearing loss occurred simultaneously with the onset of vestibular symptoms in all cases and proceeded to profound or total loss in the treated ear. An active spontaneous nystagmus toward the opposite side occurred coincidently with the sensation of disequilibrium; therefore, caloric testing was not feasible during treatment or for several weeks thereafter. Caloric tests performed two to three months following treatment showed total loss of response to ice water stimulation.

The finding that cats have a vestibular disturbance after one injection whereas human subjects required multiple injections may be related to the fact that the round window membrane of the cat is relatively much larger than that of the human being. On the other hand, when cats are given equivalent dosages based on body weight, they are less sensitive than human beings to parenterally administered streptomycin.

2. DIHYDROSTREPTOMYCIN

Dihydrostreptomycin, like neomycin, exhibits the peculiar feature that the ototoxic effects may be delayed for some weeks or months following administration of the drug (Fig. 6.7). Glorig (1951) reported that about one-third of a group of tuberculosis patients who received dihydrostreptomycin in doses of 2 to 7 gm weekly over a period of several weeks experienced the onset of hearing losses as long as five months after the medication had been discontinued.

Because clinical experience demonstrated that streptomycin had a greater toxic effect on the vestibular system and dihydrostreptomycin on the auditory system, the pharmaceutical companies prepared injectable preparations with half-doses of each with the expectation of preserving the therapeutic effects while minimizing the ototoxic effects. Dihydrostreptomycin also was prepared in combination with other antibiotics, particularly penicillin, to increase the antibacterial spectrum of the preparation. In 1959 Shambaugh et al. reported deafness of delayed onset in 32 patients receiving dihydrostreptomycin, mostly in combination with penicillin. Nine of the patients received dihydrostreptomycin in total doses of 4 gm or less. Subsequently, the United States Food and Drug Administration forbade the manufacture and sale of antibiotic preparations combining dihydrostreptomycin with other antibiotics.

Streptomycin is preferable to dihydrostreptomycin for routine clinical use because: (1) the ototoxic effect is more closely related to daily and total dosage which renders it more predictable; and (2) its toxic effect is mainly on the vestibular system and results in a mildly disabling dysfunction from which good compensatory recovery can be expected.

Experimenting on cats, McGee and Olszeweski (1962) gave dihydrostreptomycin in doses of 100 to 300 mg/kg/day for periods of time varying from 11 to 60 days. All of the animals receiving larger doses demonstrated severe disequilibrium and loss of postrotatory nystagmus. Several animals demonstrated hearing losses, and of these, two were delayed in onset. Histological studies showed loss of hair cells in all cristae and, in some animals, slight loss of hair cells in the utricle (Fig. 6.8). The hair cells losses in the organ of Corti of those animals developing hearing loss were most severe in the upper basal and middle turns (Figs. 6.9, 6.10). There was no loss of auditory or vestibular neurons. Detailed histological study of the brains revealed no changes in the lateral, superior, medial, or descending vestibular nuclei. In particular, there was no gliosis, loss of nerve cells, or other evidence of neuronal degeneration.

3. KANAMYCIN

Kanamycin, discovered by Umezawa et al. (1957), resembles neomycin in its structural formula. It is sometimes administered in spite of its known ototoxic effects when other antibiotics fail to produce the desired therapeutic result (Naunton and Ward, 1959). The drug is cleared from the blood stream by glomerular filtration, the half-life of blood levels being about four hours (Finland, 1958). In patients with impaired renal function very small doses can create high blood levels with an increase in the incidence of ototoxic effects.

Stupp et al. (1967) and others (Voldrich, 1965) have demonstrated high concentrations of kanamycin in the perilymphatic fluid with therapeutic dosage levels in the blood serum. Hawkins (1959), Ward and Fernandez (1961), and Matz et al. (1965) demonstrated in animal experiments the selective effect of the drug on the hair cells of the organ of Corti. Lindeman (1969) showed that kanamycin given to guinea pigs had its greatest effect on the external hair cells of the basal turn of the cochlea. In the vestibular system the greatest damage was to the sensory cells on the crests of the cristae and striola of the utricle, with minimal effect on the striola of the saccule. The type I hair cells were more sensitive than the type II hair cells. Ishii et al. (1968) studied the effect of kanamycin on three lysosomal enzymes in guinea pigs. They found that the drug caused a decrease in enzymatic activity in the hair cells and cochlear neurons prior to cell death. The first damage was to external hair cells in the basal turn with progressive damage in an apical direction. The first cochlear neurons to be involved were in the apex with progressive damage in a basal direction.

The histological findings in two human subjects experiencing hearing loss from kanamycin were reported by Benitez et al. (1962) and demonstrated a loss of hair cells in the organ of Corti, most severe in the basal turn (Figs. 6.11,

Fig. 6.9: Audiograms and chart of cochlear pathology of the same animal as Figs. 6.8 and 6.10. The cat was given 300 mg/kg/day of dihydrostreptomycin for 21 days. Audiograms were obtained by the avoidance conditioning technique by which the cat was trained to avoid shock by moving forward in a rotating cage in response to auditory stimuli. Beginning after two months the animal exhibited a progressive hearing loss for the frequency range 500 to 800 Hz. After a survival time of 15 months, histological studies show a loss of hair cells in the organ of Corti, most severe in the 10 to 20 mm region. The cochlear neurons, stria vascularis, and other structures of the cochlea appear normal. (Courtesy of McGee and Olszewski)

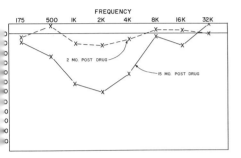
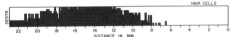

Fig. 6.10: Total loss of hair cells of the organ of Corti in the 14 mm region of the cochlea following the administration of 300 mg/kg/day of dihydrostreptomycin for 21 days. Same cat as in Figs. 6.8 and 6.9.

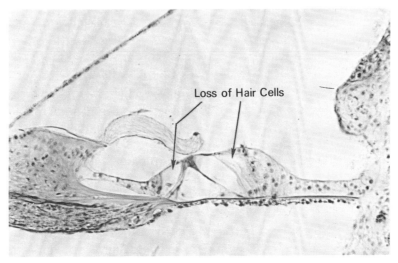

Fig. 6.11: Audiogram of a 27-year-old female with severe renal failure who received an initial dose of 1 gm of kanamycin followed by 0.25 gm every other day for a total of 3 gm over a period of 18 days. Tinnitus and high-frequency hearing loss developed on the 18th day, following which there was no further change on repeated testing. She died two weeks after completion of therapy. Histological studies show a severe loss of hair cells in the basal 15 mm of both cochleae (see also Fig. 6.12). The population of cochlear neurons was normal and the vestibular sense organs appeared normal.

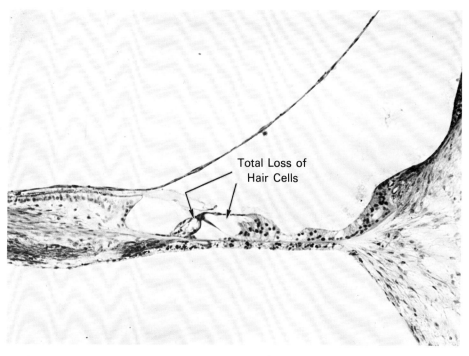

Fig. 6.12: Kanamycin ototoxicity (see Fig. 6.11). Organ of Corti showing a total loss of hair cells in the 8 mm region of the right cochlea.

Fig. 6.13: This 49-year-old female with renal failure was treated with kanamycin in a daily dosage of 1.5 gm for a period of eight days to a total dosage of 12 gm. On the eighth day she developed bilateral hearing loss, and the drug was discontinued; however, the hearing loss progressed to profound deafness during the ensuing three days. She died three months later. Histological studies of the cochleae reveal a near total loss of internal and external hair cells except in the apical 3 or 4 mm. The population of cochlear neurons is normal. See Fig. 6.14.

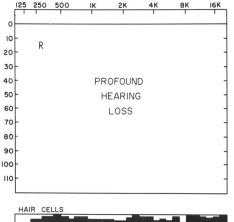

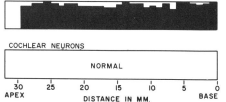

6.12). Similar observations were made by Igarashi and Yoshinobu (1963) (Figs. 6.13, 6.14). The drug is often given orally to suppress intestinal flora in preparation of patients for intestinal surgery.

The drug has been used extensively in the treatment of gram-negative bacillary infections in infants and children in doses of 15 mg/kg/day for short courses of therapy (six to ten days) without eliciting an ototoxic effect (Yow, 1966; Eichenwald, 1966; Sanders et al., 1967). However, other antibiotics to which patients have not become sensitized and to which infecting agents are sensitive should be employed when possible in place of kanamycin. When it is used, the dose should be reduced in older individuals and those with renal insufficiency, audiometric tests should be made at frequent intervals, and the state of renal function should be known at all times. The daily parenteral dose should not be greater than 15 mg/kg, and the total quantity administered should not exceed 40 gm.

4. NEOMYCIN

The severe ototoxic effects of neomycin make this an unpopular antibiotic; however, it is used occasionally as a life-saving measure in severe bacterial infections when bacteriologic studies indicate a specific sensitivity of the organism to the drug, to suppress intestinal flora preoperatively, and to

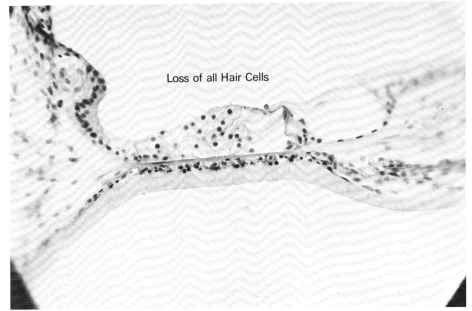

Loss of all Hair Cells

Fig. 6.14: Organ of Corti of the upper basal turn showing total loss of hair cells as a result of kanamycin ototoxicity. All other structures of the cochlear duct appear normal. See Fig. 6.13.

Fig. 6.15: Audiogram and cochlear chart of the right ear of an 87-year-old woman who experienced profound bilateral hearing loss after 18 daily irrigations of an infected wound with a solution containing neomycin in a concentration of 1 gm per 1000 cc. See Fig. 6.16.

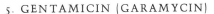

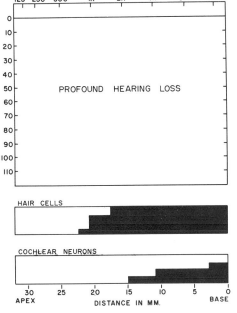

reduce arterial ammonia concentration in patients with hepatic encephalopathy. Profound loss of hearing after intravenous or intramuscular administration was reported shortly after the drug was introduced (Waisbren and Spink, 1950).

When taken orally, about 3 percent is absorbed and excreted by the kidney (Waksman, 1958). Even when taken by this route the drug can cause hearing loss after extended use (Last and Sherlock, 1960; Halpern and Heller, 1961; Gibson, 1967; Berk and Chalmers, 1970). Neomycin may also cause hearing loss when used in colonic irrigation (Fields, 1964), wound irrigation (Kelly et al., 1969), and following intrapleural instillation (Myerson et al., 1970) (Figs. 6.15, 6.16).

Lindsay et al. (1960) reported the findings in a patient who received 18 gm of the drug in 19 days and suffered profound bilateral sensorineural deafness. Histological examination showed the primary effect to be severe loss of internal hair cells and, to a lesser extent, of external hair cells of the organ of Corti.

In studies on guinea pigs, Kohonen (1965) found that neomycin, as well as kanamycin, first damages the external hair cells of the basal turn, followed by progressive damage to external hair cells in an apical direction, and then by damage to internal hair cells, most severe in the apex and progressing in a basal direction.

The audiograms of three patients who exhibited severe hearing loss from the intramuscular administration of neomycin for infection of the urinary tract are shown in Fig. 6.17. The ototoxic manifestations of neomycin may occur immediately after administration or after a delay of several weeks and frequently is progressive. The hearing loss is characterized by a severe decrease in speech discrimination. The toxic effect on the vestibular system is less severe. Neomycin should be used only with the full understanding of physician and patient that profound deafness is a possible complication of parenteral therapy and to a lesser extent of oral therapy and irrigation procedures.

5. GENTAMICIN (GARAMYCIN)

Gentamicin is an effective antibiotic drug against Pseudomonas, Proteus, Staphylococcus aureus, E. coli, and certain other enteric gram-negative bacilli. It is excreted almost exclusively by the kidneys as a glomerular filtrate (Weinstein et al., 1963) and, like the other aminoglycosides, is nephrotoxic.

Gentamicin is an important therapeutic agent in the treatment of Pseudomonas infections and other infections with gram-negative organisms. It has been used successfully, for example, to treat Pseudomonas cellulitis of the

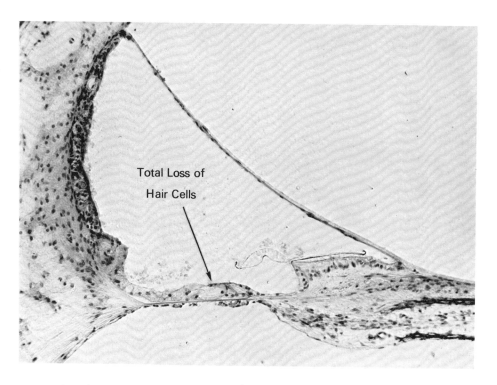

Fig. 6.16: Same case as Fig. 6.15. This photomicrograph shows the organ of Corti in the 10 mm region. There is a total loss of hair cells and partial loss of supporting cells. This region of the cochlea showed a 40 percent loss of cochlear neurons.

Total Loss of
Hair Cells

external auditory canal in diabetic patients. The daily dosage of drug is carefully regulated on the basis of daily determinations of plasma levels of the drug, renal and hepatic function, and auditory and vestibular tests.

Gentamicin was found by Black et al. (1963) to damage vestibular function in the rat, cat, and dog. Lundquist and Wersäll (1967) found the drug to be more toxic than kanamycin and streptomycin when given in the same doses to guinea pigs. The changes were more severe in the vestibular hair cells and consisted of ballooning of the cell surface and degeneration of mitochondria, leading to complete degeneration first of the type I and then of the type II hair cells. A striking early change is the fusion of stereocilia (Wersäll et al., 1971).

Webster et al. (1970) demonstrated in an experiment on cats that gentamicin has a greater effect on the vestibular endorgans than on the organ of Corti.

6. VIOMYCIN

Viomycin, like streptomycin, has been used extensively for the treatment of tuberculosis (Amberson, 1952). It exhibits no cross resistance with streptomycin and is used most often in those patients who have previously received streptomycin and require further treatment. Daly and Cohen (1965) compared the ototoxic effects on 75 patients receiving viomycin and 61 receiving streptomycin in doses of 1 gm per day and found viomycin to exhibit slightly greater ototoxicity, its toxic effects involving mainly the vestibular system.

B. QUININE AND CHLOROQUINE OTOTOXICITY

The toxic effects of quinine on hearing have been known since the inception of this drug and its extensive use as an antimalarial agent. Apparently the effect may be temporary but can be permanent when given in large doses or to sensitive individuals, although documentation of this point is vague.

The developing embryo appears to be exceedingly sensitive to quinine. The etiologic role of quinine as a cause of deafness for the newborn was proposed by Taylor in 1934. Schuknecht's experience with this problem (unpublished data) concerns the children of parents who were medical missionaries in Ethiopia. While living in Canada, the mother gave birth to two children

Fig. 6.17: Audiograms of three patients who experienced hearing loss from intramuscular administration of neomycin. Severe loss of speech discrimination suggests that atrophy of the organ of Corti was accompanied by neural degeneration.
A: This patient received a total of 13.5 gm over an eight-day period. She first noticed bilateral deafness and unsteadiness two months following administration of the drug. The hearing loss progressed for several weeks. The audiogram was made five months after treatment. Caloric response was diminished in the left ear only.

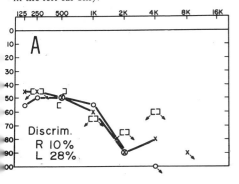

B: This patient received 32.25 gm in 45 days and noticed a progressive bilateral hearing loss beginning one month after cessation of treatment. Caloric response was diminished in the left ear only.

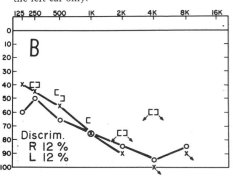

C: This patient received a total dose of 4 gm in eight days. He developed a diffuse erythematous rash and bilateral symmetrical hearing loss four days after completion of therapy. The hearing loss progressed for several months. Caloric tests revealed a decreased response in the right ear.

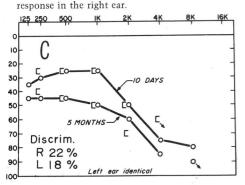

with normal hearing; then in Ethiopia she acquired malaria and was treated for several years intermittently with quinine, atabrine, and other antimalarial drugs. During this time she gave birth to three children all of whom were found to be profoundly deaf from the time of birth.

Forbes (1943) reports the case of a mother receiving quinine at hourly intervals during the 24 hours immediately preceding the birth of a male child. This child developed amblyopia and a bilateral symmetrical hearing loss of about 30 to 40 db, worse for the high frequencies. He also examined a patient, age 21, who had been given massive doses of quinine when 8½ years of age and, after that, experienced a loss of hearing and of vision. The audiograms showed a bilateral sensorineural hearing loss of 20 to 30 db for frequencies up to 2000 Hz and an abrupt severe high-frequency hearing loss for frequencies above that level.

One of the best animals studies is reported by Rüedi et al. (1951, 1952) in which adult guinea pigs were given quinine in doses of 50 to 100 mg/kg/day for periods varying from 95 to 522 days. None of the animals exhibited disequilibrium; however, hearing, as tested by the pinna reflex, was lost in some animals and greatly diminished in others. Histological examination revealed normal peripheral vestibular sense organs; however, there were advanced degenerative changes in the organs of Corti, cochlear neurons, and striae vasculares in all ears. In most animals the injury was most severe in the basal portions of the cochleae. The changes varied from a loss of external hair cells (Fig. 6.18) to total destruction of the organ of Corti. In those ears with involvement of the supporting structures of the organ of Corti there was a loss of cochlear neurons. A pathological change not seen in streptomycin toxicity was atrophy of the striae vasculares. This consisted of a decrease in cellular tissue and the formation of large vacuolated spaces in the strial tissue (Fig. 6.19). Histological studies of the brain stems showed the vestibular and cochlear nuclei to be normal.

Chloroquine is a synthetic drug having a molecular structure similar to that of quinine. It is also used chiefly for its antimalarial properties and like quinine may cause fetal injury (Med. Letter, 1965). Prolonged use of the drug in the treatment of arthritis and other chronic diseases may lead to retinopathy and ototoxicity (Dewar and Mann, 1954; Scherbel et al., 1958).

Hart and Naunton (1964) describe the findings in children of a mother who had been taking chloroquine intermittently in excess of the recommended dosage for over six years. Although she experienced no toxic symptoms herself, evidence of toxicity of the drug was seen in her offspring. She took the drug during four pregnancies which resulted in one miscarriage and three children with congenital defects. The damage included dorsal column disease in two, mental retardation in one, and deafness and vestibular disorders in all three. One of the children had neonatal convulsions and hemiatrophy of the body. Three other pregnancies, during which she did not take the drug, resulted in normal healthy children.

C. SALICYLATE OTOTOXICITY

Salicylates are used in large quantities, particularly in the form of aspirin (acetylsalicylic acid) as a therapeutic agent in the treatment of arthritis, rheumatic fever, and other connective tissue disorders. The drug relieves pain and has a general salutary effect on these disorders. In high therapeutic dosages, it produces hearing loss, tinnitus, and occasionally vertigo. Because these symptoms are reversible, they are often used by rheumatologists to establish the optimum dosage of the medication.

Jager and Alway (1946) reported tinnitus and a moderate reduction in hearing in 34 of 38 patients being treated with large doses of salicylates for acute rheumatic fever and other diseases. They demonstrated reversibility of the

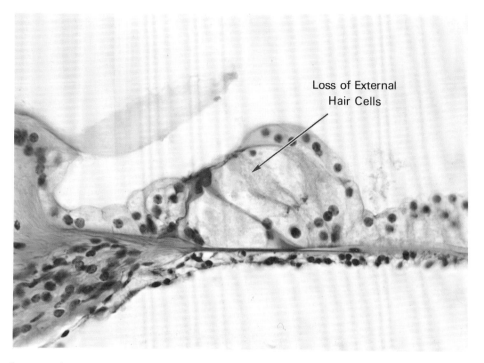

Fig. 6.18: Loss of external hair cells in the guinea pig cochlea caused by the oral administration of ototoxic doses of quinine (0.1 gm/day for 182 days). (Courtesy of Rüedi et al., 1951)

Loss of External Hair Cells

Fig. 6.19: Degeneration and cystic formation of the stria vascularis of the guinea pig following the oral administration of ototoxic doses of quinine (0.1 gm/day for 248 days). (Courtesy of Rüedi)

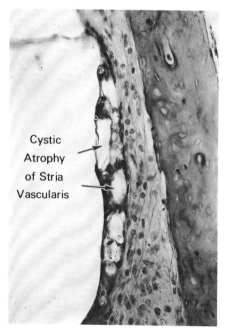

Cystic Atrophy of Stria Vascularis

hearing loss upon discontinuance of the drug. Graham and Parker (1948), in a study of 58 patients, showed that deafness and tinnitus occurred when the plasma concentration of salicylates approached 35 mg percent. Waltner (1955) described bilateral severe sensorineural hearing loss and loudness recruitment in a 28-year-old patient who had ingested 200 aspirin tablets (300 mg each) in six days. The hearing loss was completely reversed within seven days. Studies by McCabe and Dey (1965) on aspirin toxicity in five patients with normal hearing showed the audiometric patterns to be consistent with toxicity of the cochlea rather than the central nervous system.

Myers and Bernstein (1965) and Myers et al. (1965) studied patients at the Massachusetts Eye and Ear Infirmary by giving increasing doses of acetylsalicylic acid until high-pitched tinnitus and subjective hearing loss were noted. About 6 to 8 gm per day were required to achieve this effect. Audiometric tests were performed before, during, and after the treatment and plasma salicylate levels were determined during these periods. (Fig. 6.20).

When salicylates were withdrawn from another group of patients who had hearing losses from taking large doses for long periods of time, there was rapid disappearance of tinnitus and improvement in hearing within 72 hours (Fig. 6.21).

Bernstein and Weiss (1967) also showed that vestibular function is depressed by salicylate toxicity. Caloric responses, recorded electronystagmographically, showed depression of both the slow phase velocity and the duration of nystagmus.

Myers and Bernstein (1965) also studied the effect of salicylate toxicity on ten behaviorally trained squirrel monkeys (Saimiri). After obtaining baseline audiograms, the animals were given one subcutaneous injection of sodium salicylate. The LD 50 dosage for small animals for sodium salicylate is 650/mg/kg. The squirrel monkeys were given doses varying from 500–600 mg/kg. Twenty-four hours after injection the average hearing loss for these animals was 30 db and the average plasma salicylate level was 36 mg percent. The hearing returned to normal in two to three days, and microscopic studies failed to show any abnormality in the sensory epithelia, cochlear neurons, or striae vasculares.

Silverstein et al. (1967) studied the effect of a single intraperitoneal infusion of salicylate (350 mg/kg) upon the electrical activity of the cochlea and inner ear fluids of the cat. After four hours the voltage amplitudes of the neural responses had decreased 70 to 75 percent and cochlear microphonics had decreased 50 to 60 percent of the original values, the thresholds of the responses at the same time were elevated 20 to 25 db. Salicylate level in the perilymph averaged 28 mg/100 ml, while malic acid dehydrogenase activity decreased 50 percent. Sodium, potassium, and total protein concentration of the endolymph and perilymph were unchanged. These authors postulated that salicylate intoxication interferes with enzymatic activity in either (or both) the hair cells and cochlear neurons.

Other studies suggest that salicylates may uncouple oxydative phosphorylation in association with the entire respiratory chain (Lutwak-Mann, 1942). Salicylates also appear to inhibit certain transaminases and puridine nucleotide-linked dehydrogenases (Smith, 1963; Westernhagen, 1967). Ishii et al. (1967) injected tritium-labeled salicylate into guinea pigs and showed that the drug is rapidly absorbed and promptly reaches the cochlea where it diffuses to all parts of the cochlear duct without exhibiting an affinity for any specific cell type.

D. ETHACRYNIC ACID OTOTOXICITY

Ethacrynic acid is a relatively new and valuable diuretic, the renal effect of which is to promote the excretion of large volumes of iso-osmotic urine. In 1966 Schneider and Becker reported temporary hearing loss following the administration of ethacrynic acid, and since then many other reports have alluded to the transient ototoxicity of this drug (Meriwether et al., 1971).

Mathog and Klein (1969) observed permanent hearing losses in three uremic patients after administration of ethacrynic acid and small amounts of aminoglycoside antibiotics. Matz et al. (1969) reported a case of ototoxicity to ethacrynic acid twenty minutes after the infusion of a single dose of the drug. The patient had poor renal and hepatic function and died ten days later. Histological studies revealed bilateral loss of external hair cells, most severe in the basal turn. This patient also received 18 gm of neomycin orally in seven days which could possibly have been responsible for the deafness and hair cell loss.

Quick and Duvall (1970) administered ethacrynic acid intravenously to guinea pigs and found the pinna reflex to be lost suddenly six minutes following injection. Electron microscopic studies showed degenerative changes in the intermediate cell layer of the stria vascularis. Mathog et al. (1970) administered the drug to cats and demonstrated an immediate decrease in cochlear microphonic response. Animals which received a single large dose (30 mg/kg of body weight) or multiple doses and were permitted to survive for several days showed a loss of external hair cells, most severe in the basal turn.

Kohonen et al. (1970) in animal experiments elicited an immediate decrease in microphonic cochlear responses following the intravenous injection of the drug but could not find permanent functional or morphological alterations. Silverstein and Yules (1971) also demonstrated, in an experiment on cats, that the intravenous injection of ethacrynic acid caused a prompt and prolonged decrease in cochlear microphonic responses. There was marked swelling of the cells of the striae vasculares, however, the electrolyte and protein concentrations of the endolymph were not significantly altered. They postulated that ethacrynic acid probably has a direct effect on the hair cells of the organ of Corti.

Ernstson (1972) administered ethacrynic acid intraperitoneally to guinea pigs in doses of 2, 4, and 8 mg/kg of body weight in separate tests. Behavioral audiograms revealed hearing losses worse for the high frequencies, which reverted to normal within 24 hours.

E. THALIDOMIDE OTOTOXICITY

The story of the tranquilizing drug, thalidomide, is a tragic chapter in the development of drug therapy. The drug is alleged to be responsible for birth

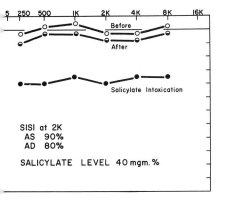

Fig. 6.20: Audiometric thresholds in a 20-year-old patient before the administration of salicylates, during salicylate intoxication, and 24 hours after discontinuing the administration of salicylates. The audiometric thresholds of the two ears were symmetrical; however, only the right is shown. At the height of intoxication the serum salicylate level was 40 mg percent and the threshold elevation was 40 db for all frequencies tested. The short increment sensitivity index (SISI test) was positive indicating a toxic effect on the sense organ.) (Courtesy of Myers and Bernstein)

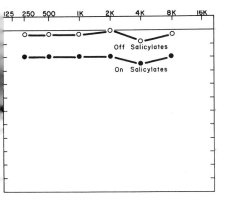

Fig. 6.21: Audiometric thresholds of a 40-year-old female who had been taking 20 aspirin tablets daily for two years. Audiometric thresholds were symmetrical in the two ears; only the right is shown. The hearing returned to normal two weeks after discontinuing the drug. (Courtesy of Myers and Bernstein)

deformities in 5,000 to 6,000 babies, some 4,000 of them in West Germany alone. The trial against the German pharmaceutical company, Chemie Grünenthal, ended on December 18, 1969, with a financial settlement of $27,000,000, plus interest, to the parents of 2,000 surviving children (approximately $19,000 per child) and $1,100,000 to some 800 adults who suffered nervous disorders from taking the drug. The company also met court costs of $1,600,000.

Thalidomide was an over-the-counter prescription-free drug in Germany from late 1957 until 1961. It was a popular tranquilizer without noticeable side effects and was used extensively by women in the early months of pregnancy. The drug was never released in the United States but was used for investigational purposes for a short time and is presumed to be responsible for some of the 17 cases of phocomelia occurring in this country.

The suspicion that thalidomide might be responsible for congenital anomalies when ingested by pregnant women was first reported by Lenz and Knapp (1962). In addition to ectromelia (hypoplasia or aplasia of one or more limbs), the drug causes malformations of the intestinal and urinary tracts, the heart, and the ears. In 1963 Miehlke and Partsch reported the finding in 13 patients with deformities of the ears and paralyses of the facial and abducens nerves. The critical period when thalidomide ingestion by the mother may cause anomalies is generally between the 37th and 50th day after the last menstruation.

In Sweden the use of the drug for three years resulted in the birth of at least 150 abnormal children. In 1964, d'Avignon and Barr reported the otoneurological findings in 100 of these children who were surviving at that time. They described a syndrome consisting of paralysis of the soft palate and oculomotor muscles in addition to hearing loss and paralyses of the facial and abducens nerves. All degrees of malformation of the auricles, external auditory canals, and middle ears have been described. The hearing losses may vary from moderate impairment to total deafness. Vestibular dysfunction may range from mild hypoactivity to total absence of response to caloric testing. Jorgensen et al. (1964), in temporal bone studies of an infant born of a mother who took thalidomide during the first month of pregnancy, found total absence of the bony labyrinth on one side. The cochlear, vestibular, and facial nerves were also totally missing (Fig. 6.22).

Livingstone (1965) reported his findings in the ears of children suffering thalidomide anomalies. In the fourteen thalidomide cases examined, surgery was performed on both ears in five cases and on one ear in six cases. Three were found unsuitable for surgery. Among the anomalies observed at the time of surgery were persistent branchial cyst or sinus, atresia of the ex-

Fig. 6.22: Michel type aplasia (total absence of the bony and membranous labyrinth) in an infant born of a mother who ingested thalidomide during the first month of pregnancy. (Courtesy of Jorgensen et al., 1964)

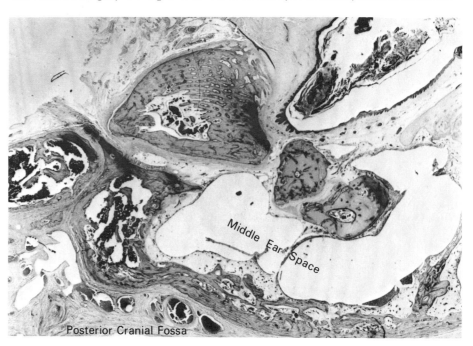

Fig. 6.23: Audiometric thresholds showing hearing loss from intra-arterial nitrogen mustard (methyl-bis (2) chloroethyl, 1, 2-c amine hydrochloride) therapy in a 30-year-old female with Hodgkin's disease. Prior to treatment her hearing was subjectively normal. She received nitrogen mustard in a total dose of 32 mg/kg over a time span of 20 minutes. She remained fully conscious during and after the procedure but immediately after the completion of treatment she experienced vertigo, severe tinnitus, and diminished hearing. She died one year later, and histological studies show a diffuse shrunken appearance of the organ of Corti and vestibular sense organs. The populations of hair cells and nerve fibers appear to be normal. This shrunken appearance is presumably due to the toxic effect of nitrogen mustard; however, the change cannot be clearly differentiated from compression artifact.

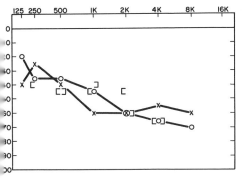

Fig. 6.24: Behavioral audiometric thresholds of the cat two weeks following the administration of 1.0 mg/kg of nitrogen mustard delivered into the carotid artery. (Courtesy of Cummings, 1968)

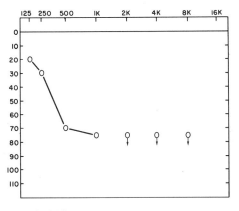

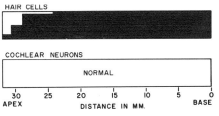

Fig. 6.25: Organ of Corti of the cat showing loss of external hair cells following the intra-carotid administration of nitrogen mustard in a dose of 1.0 mg/kg. (Courtesy of Cummings, 1968)

ternal auditory canal, middle ear filled with sticky mucous-like material, persistent cartilaginous styloid process, fused ossicular mass, and discontinuity of the incudostapedial joint. Livingstone felt that 75 percent of the children with bilateral atresia were suitable for surgery and that in 75 percent of those operated upon it was possible to improve hearing. (See also Chapter 4C4, Drugs.)

F. NITROGEN MUSTARD OTOTOXICITY

The toxic side effects of anticancer drugs necessitate dosages which are generally too small to be curative. Total-body perfusion requires the removal of marrow from the sternum and iliac crests immediately prior to treatment to counteract the severe depression of hematopoiesis. Drugs are then perfused via catheters which have been passed into the thoracic aorta and inferior vena cava by way of the common femoral artery and vein. When perfusion has been completed, the marrow is returned to the patient by intravenous infusion. Because total-body perfusion often results in a severe general toxic reaction, sometimes with fatal hematologic depression, various techniques for regional perfusion are performed.

Chemotherapeutic anticancer agents fall into three general classes, the alkylating agents, the antimetabolites, and the antibiotics. Nitrogen mustard, an alkylating agent when given by the technique of total-body perfusion, has ototoxic properties. Histological study of the cochleae of an individual who experienced a moderately severe bilateral sensorineural hearing loss from nitrogen mustard revealed shrinkage of the organ of Corti without loss of hair cells (Schuknecht, 1964) (Fig. 6.23).

In an experiment on cats which were behaviorally trained for auditory testing Cummings (1968) produced severe hearing losses by carotid perfusion with nitrogen mustard (Fig. 6.24). Histological studies revealed severe loss of internal and external hair cells throughout the basal and middle turns of the cochleae (Fig. 6.25).

G. TETANUS ANTITOXIN OTOTOXICITY

The neurological complications following the prophylactic or therapeutic use of sera may be classified into meningeal, cerebral, spinal, radicular, and peripheral nerve types. Tetanus antitoxin of horse origin is the most common cause of serum sickness and neurological complications. Deafness oc-

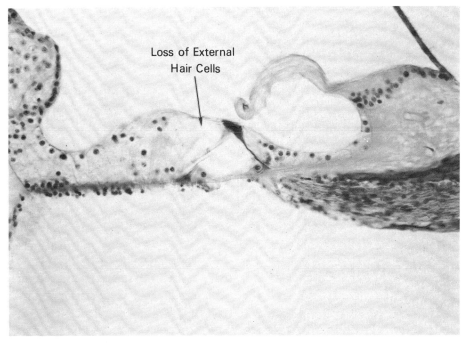

Loss of External Hair Cells

curring in patients being treated for clinical tetanus has been reported by Amberg and Hewitt (1935) and by Cutter (1936). McCready (1938) reported the first case of deafness following the prophylactic use of tetanus antitoxin. Further cases have been reported by Taylor (1942), Berger and Sachs (1953), and by Pantazopoulos (1965). In all cases the hearing loss developed several days after injection of tetanus antitoxin and was associated with severe serum sickness. The hearing losses were profound and permanent.

References

Amberg, E., and Hewitt, R., 1935: Tetanus, tetanus antitoxin or phenobarbital deafness. J. Amer. Med. Assn. 105:585.

Amberson, J., 1952: A summary of the second viomycin conference. Trans. XI Conference on the Chemotherapy of Tuberculosis, 286.

Ballantyne, J., 1970: Iatrogenic deafness. J. Laryng. 84:967.

Balogh, K., Hiraide, F., and Ishii, D., 1970: Distribution of radioactive dihydrostreptomycin in the cochlea: An autoradiographic study. Ann. Otol. Rhinol. Laryng. 79:641.

Benitez, J., Schuknecht, H., and Brandenburg, J., 1962: Pathologic changes in human ear after kanamycin. Arch. Otolaryng. 75:192.

Berg, K., 1951: The toxic effect of streptomycin on the vestibular and cochlear apparatus. Acta oto-laryng. Suppl. 97:1.

Berger, M., and Sachs, A., 1953: Perceptive deafness associated with prophylactic use of tetanus antitoxin. Arch. Otolaryng. 57:501.

Berk, D., and Chalmers, T., 1970: Deafness complicating antibiotic therapy of hepatic encephalopathy. Ann. Int. Med. 73:393.

Bernstein, J., and Weiss, A., 1967: Further observations on salicylate ototoxicity. J. Laryng. Otol. 81:915.

Black, J., Calesnick, B., Williams, D., and Weinstein, M., 1963: Pharmacology of gentamicin: A new broad-spectrum antibiotic. Antimicrob. Agents Chemother., p. 138.

Brown, H., and Hinshaw, H., 1946: Toxic reaction of streptomycin on the eighth nerve apparatus. Proc. Staff Meeting, Mayo Clinic 21:347.

Causse, R., 1949: Action toxique vestibulaire et cochleaire de la strepomycine au point de vue experimental. Ann. d'Otolaryng. 66:518.

Cummings, C., 1968: Experimental observations on the ototoxicity of nitrogen mustard. Laryngoscope 78:530.

Cutter, R., 1936: Auditory nerve involvement after T.A.T.: First reported cases. J. Amer. Med. Assn. 106:1006.

Daly, J., and Cohen, N., 1965: Viomycin ototoxicity in man: A cupulometric study. Ann. Otol. Rhinol. Laryng. 74:521.

d'Avignon, M., and Barr, B., 1964: Ear abnormalities and cranial nerve palsies in thalidomide children. Arch. Otolaryng. 80:136.

Davis, H., Deatherage, B., Rosenblut, B., Fernandez, C., Kimura, R., and Smith, C., 1958: Modification of cochlear potentials produced by streptomycin poisoning and by extensive venous obstruction. Laryngosope 68:596.

Dewar, W., and Mann, H., 1954: Chloroquine in lupus erythematosis. Lancet 1:780.

Duvall, A., and Wersäll, J., 1964: Site of action of streptomycin upon inner ear sensory cells. Acta oto-laryng. 57:581.

Eichenwald, H., 1966: Some observations on dosage and toxicity of kanamycin in premature and full-term infants. Ann. N.Y. Acad. Sci. 132:984.

Ernstson, S., 1972: Ethacrynic acid-induced hearing loss in guinea pigs. Acta oto-laryng. 73:476.

Farrington, R., Hull-Smith, H., Bunn, P., and McDermott, W., 1947: Streptomycin toxicity. Reactions to highly purified drug on long-continued administration to human subjects. J. Amer. Med. Assn. 134:679.

Fields, R., 1964: Neomycin ototoxicity: Report of a case due to rectal and colonic irrigations. Arch. Otolaryng. 79:67.

Finland, M., 1958: Summary of the monograph on the basic and clinical research of the new antibiotic, kanamycin. Ann. N.Y. Acad. Sci. 76:391.

Forbes, S., 1943: Quinine in relation to nerve deafness. Ann. Otol. Rhinol. Laryng. 52:109.

Fowler, E., Jr., 1948: Streptomycin treatment of vertigo. Trans. Amer. Acad. Ophthal. Otolaryng. 52:239.

Gibson, W., Jr., 1967: Deafness due to orally administered neomycin. Arch. Otolaryng. 86:163.

Glorig, A., 1951: The effect of dihydrostreptomycin hydrochloride and sulfate on the auditory mechanism. Ann. Otol. Rhinol. Laryng. 60:327.

Graham, J., and Parker, W., 1948: The toxic manifestations of sodium salicylate therapy. Quart. J. Med. 17:153.

Graybiel, A., Schuknecht, H., Fregly, A., Miller, E., and McLeod, M., 1965: Practical and theoretical implications based on long-term follow-up of Ménière's patients treated with streptomycin sulfate. NASA Order R-93, Naval Aerospace Med. Inst. 948:23.

Graybiel, A., Schuknecht, H., Fregly, A., Miller, E., and McLeod, M., 1967: Streptomycin in Ménière's disease. Arch. Otolaryng. 85:156.

Halpern, E., and Heller, M., 1961: Ototoxicity of orally administered neomycin: Report of a case. Arch. Otolaryng. 73:675.

Hamberger, C., Hyden, H., and Koch, H., 1949: Streptomycin bei der Ménièreschen Krankheit. Arch. Ohr. Nas.-Kehlk Heilk. 155:667.

Hanson, H., 1951: The treatment of endolymphatic hydrops (Ménière's disease) with streptomycin. Ann. Otol. Rhinol. Laryng. 60:676.

Hart, C., and Naunton, R., 1964: The ototoxicity of chloroquine phosphate. Arch. Otolaryng. 80:407.

Hawkins, J., Jr., 1959: The ototoxicity of kanamycin. Ann. Otol. Rhinol. Laryng. 68:698.

Hinshaw, H., and Feldman, W., 1945: Streptomycin in treatment of clinical tuberculosis: A preliminary report. Proc. Staff Meet. Mayo Clinic 20:313.

Igarashi, M., and Yoshinobu, T., 1963: Kanamycin deafness: A human temporal bone report. Otolaryng. Clin. (Kyoto) 56:301.

Ishii, T., Bernstein, J., and Balogh, K., 1967: Distribution of tritium-labeled salicylate in the cochlea: An autoradiographical study. Ann. Otol. Rhinol. Laryng. 76:368.

Ishii, T., Ishii, D., and Balogh, K., Jr., 1968: Lysosomal enzymes in the inner ears of kanamycin-treated guinea pigs. Acta oto-laryng. 65:449.

Jacoby, G., and Gorini, L., 1967: The effect of streptomycin and other aminoglycoside antibiotics on protein synthesis, In: Antibiotics I. Mechanism of Action. Edited by D. Gottlieb and P. Shaw. Springer-Verlag, New York, p. 726.

Jager, B., and Alway, R., 1946: The treatment of acute rheumatic fever with large doses of sodium salicylate. Amer. J. Med. Sci. 211:273.

Jorgensen, M., Kristensen, H., and Buch, N., 1964: Thalidomide-induced aplasia of the inner ear. J. Laryng. Otol. 78:1095.

Kanda, T., and Igarashi, M., 1969: Ultrastructural changes in vestibular sensory endorgans after viomycin sulfate intoxication. Acta oto-laryng. 68:474.

Kelly, D., Nilo, E., Berggren, R., 1969: Deafness after topical neomycin wound irrigation. New Eng. J. Med. 280:1338.

Koburg, E., and Plester, D., 1962: Zur Grösse des Eiweisstoffwechsels der Gewebe der Cochlea: Autoradiographische Untersuchungen an Meerschweinchen nach Gabe von H-3-Leucin und H-3-Lysin. Acta oto-laryng. 54:319.

Kohonen, A., 1965: Effect of some ototoxic drugs upon the pattern and innervation of cochlear sensory cells in the guinea pig. Acta oto-laryng. Suppl. 208:1.

Kohonen, A., Jauhiainen, T., and Tarkkanen, J., 1970: Experimental deafness caused by ethacrynic acid. Acta oto-laryng. 70:187.

Last, P., and Sherlock, S., 1960: Systemic absorption of orally administered neomycin in liver disease. New Eng. J. Med. 262:385.

Lenz, W., and Knapp, R., 1962: Die thalidomidembryopathie. Dtsch. med.

Wschr. 87:1232.

Lidén, G., 1953: Loss of hearing following treatment with dihydrostreptomycin or streptomycin. Acta oto-laryng. 43:551.

Lindeman, H., 1969: Regional differences in sensitivity of the vestibular sensory epithelia to ototoxic antibiotics. Acta oto-laryng. 67:177.

Lindsay, J., Proctor, L., and Work, W., 1960: Histopathologic inner ear changes in deafness due to neomycin in a human. Laryngoscope 70:382.

Livingstone, G., 1965: Congenital ear abnormalities due to thalidomide. Proc. Roy. Soc. Med. 58:493.

Lundquist, P., and Wersäll, J., 1967: The ototoxic effect of gentamicin: An electron microscopical study, in Gentamicin, First International Symposium, Paris, p. 26.

Lutwak-Mann, C., 1942: The effect of salicylates and chincophen on enzymes and metabolic processes. Biochem. J. 36:706.

Mathog, R., and Klein, W., Jr., 1969: Ototoxicity of ethacrynic acid and aminoglycoside antibiotics in uremia. New Eng. J. Med. 280:1223.

Mathog, R., Thomas, W., and Hudson, W., 1970: Ototoxicity of new and potent diuretics. A preliminary study. Arch. Otolaryng. 92:7.

Matz, G., Beal, D., and Krames, L., 1969: Ototoxicity of ethacrynic acid: Demonstrated in a human temporal bone. Arch. Otolaryng. 90:152.

Matz, G., Wallace, T., and Ward, P., 1965: The ototoxicity of kanamycin: A comparative histopathological study. Laryngoscope 75:1690.

McCabe, P., and Dey, F., 1965: The effect of aspirin upon auditory sensitivity. Ann. Otol. Rhinol. Laryng. 74:312.

McCready, P., 1938: Inner ear deafness from tetanus antitoxin injection. Ann. Otol. Rhinol. Laryng. 47:247.

McGee, T., and Olszewski, J., 1962: Streptomycin sulfate and dihydrostreptomycin toxicity. Arch. Otolaryng. 75:295.

Medical Letter. Drug Therapy, 1965: Chloraquine (aralen) and fetal injury. 7:9.

Meriwether, W., Mangi, R., and Serpick, A., 1971: Deafness following standard intravenous dose of ethacrynic acid. J. Amer. Med. Assn. 216:795.

Meyer zum Gottesberge, A., and Stupp, H., 1969: Streptomycinspiegel in der Perilymphe des Menschen. Acta oto-laryng. 67:171.

Miehlke, A., and Partsch, C., 1963: Ohrmissbildung, facialis-und Abducenlähmung als Syndrom der Thalidomideschädigung. Arch. Ohr. Nas.-Kehlk Heilk. 181:154.

Myers, E., and Bernstein, J., 1965: Salicylate ototoxicity: A clinical and experimental study. Arch. Otolaryng. 82:483.

Myers, E., Bernstein, J., and Fostiropolous, G., 1965: Salicylate ototoxicity. A clinical study. New Eng. J. Med. 273:587.

Myerson, M., Knight, H., Gambarini, A., and Curran, T., 1970: Intrapleural neomycin causing ototoxicity. Ann. thorac. Surg. 9:483.

Naunton, R., and Ward, P., 1959: The ototoxicity of kanamycin sulfate in the presence of compromised renal function. Arch. Otolaryng. 69:398.

Pantazopoulos, P., 1965: Perceptive deafness following prophylactic use of tetanus antitoxin. Laryngoscope 75:1832.

Quick, C., and Duvall, A., 1970: Early changes in the cochlear duct from ethacrynic acid: An electronmicroscopic evaluation. Laryngoscope 80:954.

Ruben, R., Toriyama, M., Dische, M., Bransilver, B., and Daly, J., 1969: External and middle ear malformations associated with mandibulo-facial dysostosis and renal abnormalities: a case report. Ann. Otol. Rhinol. Laryng. 78:605.

Rüedi, L., 1951: Therapeutic and toxic effects of streptomycin in otology. Laryngoscope 61:613.

Rüedi, L., Furrer, W., Graf, K., Lüthy, F., Nager, G., and Tschirren, B., 1951: Weitere Befunde über die Toxischen Wirkungen von Streptomycin und Chinin am Gehörorgan des Meerschweinchens. Bull. schweiz. Akad. med. Wiss. 7:276.

Rüedi, L., Furrer, W., Lüthy, F., Nager, G., and Tschirren, B., 1952: Further observations concerning the toxic effects of streptomycin and quinine on the auditory organ of guinea pigs. Laryngoscope 62:333.

Sanders, O., Eliot, D., Cramblett, H., 1967: Retrospective study for possible kanamycin ototoxicity among neonatal infants. J. Pediat. 70:960.

Schatz, A., Bugie, E., and Waksman, S., 1944: Streptomycin, a substance exhibiting antibiotic activity against gram-positive and gram-negative bacteria. Proc. Soc. Exp. Biol. 57:244.

Scherbel, A., Harrison, J., and Atdjian, M., 1958: Further observations on the use of 4-aminoquinaline compounds in patients with rheumatoid arthritis or related diseases. Cleveland Clin. Quart. 25:95.

Schneider, W., and Becker, E., 1966: Acute transient hearing loss after ethacrynic acid therapy. Arch. Int. Med. 117:715.

Schuknecht, H., 1957: Ablation therapy in the management of Ménière's disease. Acta oto-laryng. Suppl. 132:1.

Schuknecht, H., 1964: The pathology of several disorders of the inner ear which cause vertigo. Southern Med. J. 57:1161.

Schwartz, G., David, D., Riggio, R., Stengel, K., and Rubin, A., 1970: Ototoxicity induced by furosemide. New Eng. J. Med. 282:1413.

Shambaugh, G., Jr., Derlacki, E., Harrison, W., House, H., House, W., Hildyard, V., Schuknecht, H., and Shea, J., 1959: Dihydrostreptomycin deafness. J. Amer. Med. Assn. 170:1657.

Silverstein, H., Bernstein, J., and Davies, D., 1967: Salicylate ototoxicity. A biochemical and electrophysiological study. Ann. Otol. Rhinol. Laryng. 76:118.

Silverstein, H., and Yules, R., 1971: The effect of diuretics on cochlear potentials and inner ear fluids. Laryngoscope 81:873.

Singleton, E., and Schuknecht, H., 1968: Streptomycin sulfate in the management of Ménière's disease. Otol. Clin. North Amer., p. 531.

Smith, M., 1963: Salicylates and intermediary metabolism. In Salicylates. J. & A. Churchill, Ltd., London, p. 47.

Spoendlin, H., 1966: Zur ototoxizität des streptomyzins. Pract. oto-rhino-laryng. 28:305.

Stupp, H., 1970: Untersuchung der Antibiotikaspiegel in den Innenohrflussigkeiten und ihre Bedeutung für die Spezifische Ototoxizität der Aminoglykosidantibiotika. Acta oto-laryng. Suppl. 262.

Stupp, H., Rauch, S., Sous, H., Brun, J., and Lagler, F., 1967: Kanamycin dosage and levels in ear and other organs. Arch. Otolaryng. 86:515.

Taylor, H., 1934: Prenatal medication as a possible etiologic factor of deafness in the newborn. Arch. Otolaryng. 20:790.

Taylor, H., 1942: Neurological complications of serum sickness with special reference to the ear. Laryngoscope 52:923.

Umezawa, H., Veda, M., Maeda, K., Yagashita, K., Kondo, S., Okami, Y., Utiara, K., Osato, Y., Nitta, K., and Takeuchi, T., 1957: Production and isolation of a new antibiotic, kanamycin. J. Antibiot., Tokyo, 10:181.

Voldrich, L., 1965: The kinetics of streptomycin, kanamycin and neomycin in the inner ear. Acta oto-laryng. 60:243.

Vrabec, D., Cody, D., and Ulrich, J., 1965: A study of the relative concentrations of antibiotics in the blood, spinal fluid, and perilymph in animals. Ann. Otol. Rhinol. Laryng. 74:688.

Waisbren, B., and Spink, W., 1950: A clinical appraisal of neomycin. Ann. intern. Med. 33:1099.

Waksman, S., 1958: Neomycin: Its Nature and Practical Applications. Edited by S. A. Waksman, Upjohn of England, Crawley, Sussex, England, 400 pp.

Waltner, J., 1955: The effects of salicylate on the inner ear. Ann. Otol. Rhinol. Laryng. 64:617.

Ward, P., and Fernandez, C., 1961: The ototoxicity of kanamycin in guinea pigs. Ann. Otol. Rhinol. Laryng. 70:132.

Watanuki, K., 1971: Pathology of the vestibular sensory epithelia in streptomycin and kanamycin ototoxicosis. Jap. J. Otol. (Tokyo) 74:52.

Webster, J., McGee, T., Carroll, R., Benitez, J., and Williams, M., 1970: Ototoxicity of gentamicin: Histopathologic and functional results in the cat. Trans. Amer. Acad. Ophthal. Otolaryng. 74:1155.

Weinstein, L., 1965: Streptomycin, Chap. 58 in The Pharmacological Basis of Therapeutics, Edited by I. Goodman and A. Gilman, MacMillan, New York, p. 1230.

Weinstein, M., Luedemann, G., Oden, E., and Wagman, G., 1963: Gentamicin: A new broad-spectrum antibiotic complex. Antimicrobiol. Agents chemother., p. 1.

Wersäll, J., Björkroth, B., Flock, Å., and Lundquist, P-G., 1971: Sensory hair fusion in vestibular sensory cells after gentamicin exposure. Arch. Klin. exp. Ohr. Nase.-KehlkHeilk. 200:1.

Wersäll, J., and Hawkins, J., Jr., 1962: The vestibular sensory epithelia in the cat labyrinth and their reactions in chronic streptomycin intoxication. Acta oto-laryng. 54:1.

Westernhagen, B. von, 1968: Histochemische Untersuchungen zur Wirkung der Salicylsäure auf das Innenohr. Arch. klin. exp. Ohr. Nas-KehlkHeilk. 190:86.

Yow M., 1966: Panel discussion: Kanamycin in pediatric practice with special reference to observations on ototoxicity. Ann. N.Y. Acad. Sci. 132:1037.

7 Trauma

A. DIRECT TRAUMA TO THE TEMPORAL BONE

Disturbances in cochlear and vestibular function comprise the largest group of objectively demonstrable, late complications subsequent to head injury. In a study of 551 patients with head injury of which 80 percent had skull fractures, Alexander and Scholl (1938) found that 15 percent demonstrated signs of cerebral injury and 33 percent had hearing losses probably attributable to the injury.

1. FRACTURE OF THE TEMPORAL BONE

a. Longitudinal fracture

Typically a longitudinal fracture of the temporal bone is a linear break through the floor of the middle cranial fossa which passes parallel and adjacent to the anterior margin of the petrous pyramid. It extends from the region of the gasserian ganglion medially and to the middle ear and mastoid air cells laterally. On roentgenograms there is frequently a linear fracture in the squamous portion of the temporal bone, and the air cell system of the middle ear and mastoid are rendered opaque by blood or cerebrospinal fluid. About 80 percent of temporal bone fractures are of the longitudinal type (Fischer and Wolfsen, 1943).

The experiments of Proctor and his associates (1956), as well as Gurdjian and Lissner (1946), have shown that longitudinal fractures occur more commonly from blows to the parietal and temporal regions of the skull than from blows to the occipital or frontal regions. Characteristically, the fracture line traverses the annulus tympanicus, creating a laceration of the tympanic membrane and bleeding from the external auditory canal. A step-like deformity is sometiimes seen in the external auditory canal. Facial weakness or paralysis occurs in less than 25 percent of cases and usually is temporary (Ulrich, 1926). Cerebrospinal otorrhea is common and usually subsides in a few days as the fracture heals. Among the middle ear lesions which have been demonstrated histologically are dislocation of the incudomalleal and incudostapedial joints

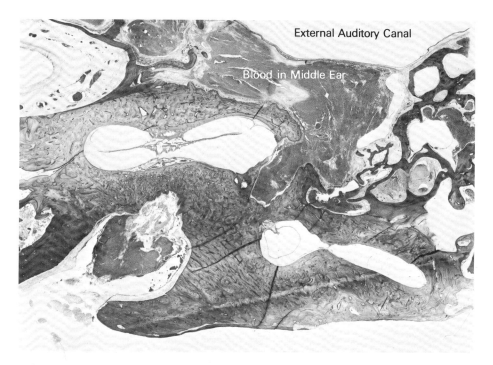

Fig. 7.1: Massive hemotympanum with intact tympanic membrane associated with longitudinal fracture of the temporal bone in an individual suffering a fatal head injury.

External Auditory Canal

Blood in Middle Ear

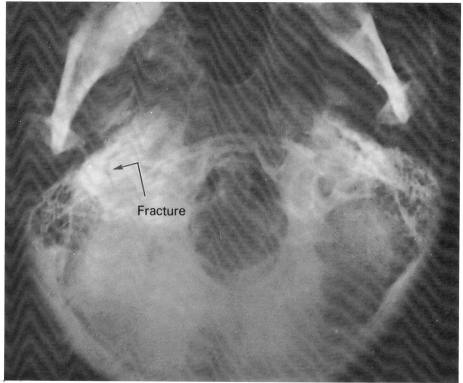

Fig. 7.2: Roentgenogram showing a transverse fracture of the temporal bone in an individual with a nonfatal head injury.

Fracture

and rupture of the annular ligament with luxation of the stapes (Kelemen, 1944).

Laceration of the tympanic membrane, ossicular injuries, and hemotympanum cause a conductive hearing loss (Fig. 7.1).

Lacerations of the tympanic membrane usually heal spontaneously; but, when ossicles have been dislocated, there is frequently a severe conductive hearing loss which is permanent unless corrected by reconstructive middle ear surgery.

Many ears in which a longitudinal temporal bone fracture has occurred show a sensorineural hearing loss which exhibits all the characteristics of inner ear concussion (Schuknecht and Davison, 1956). It can vary from a loss for high frequencies, centering on 4000 Hz, to severe involvement of a wide range of frequencies (Nassulphis, 1946; Schuknecht, 1950). Some improvement in bone conduction thresholds can be expected during the first three weeks following injury as the cochlea recovers from that component of the hearing loss which is attributable to temporary threshold shift (TTS).

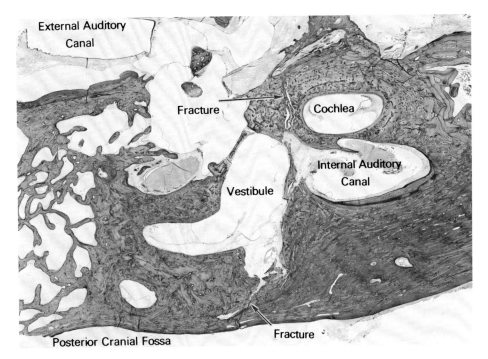

Fig. 7.3: Transverse fracture of the temporal bone in a 21-year-old man which occurred four months before death from unrelated causes. The fracture extends through the fallopian canal, vestibule, lateral and posterior semicircular canals, basal turn of the cochlea, and vestibular aqueduct. The fracture line is well healed with new bone and connective tissue. See Fig. 7.4.

b. Transverse fracture

A transverse fracture of the temporal bone occurs perpendicular to the long axis of the petrous pyramid and is most likely to result from blows to the occiput (Gurdjian and Lissner, 1946) (Fig. 7.2). In about 50 percent of cases the fracture can be demonstrated radiologically in either the submentovertical or Stenvers' position of the skull (Grove, 1939). Also, in about 50 percent of cases the facial nerve is lacerated and the resultant palsy may be permanent unless timely surgical repair is instituted. Bleeding from the ear is uncommon although hemotympanum is a frequent finding. The tympanic membrane is at first dark blue, later becoming light blue and then rose red before complete resolution occurs in two to four weeks (Rutin, 1937). Cerebrospinal fluid may continue to fill the middle ear after the blood is absorbed. In such cases the fluid may drain through the eustachian tube into the nasopharynx (Ecker, 1947).

The transverse fracture passes through the vestibule of the inner ear, causing extensive destruction of the membranous labyrinth and usually complete loss of cochlear and vestibular function (Stenger, 1909) (Figs. 7.3 to 7.5). Severe vertigo exists for several days and is accompanied by nausea and vomiting. It gradually subsides over a period of two to three weeks, although unsteadiness and a tendency to sway to the side of the involved ear when walking may persist for months. A mild spontaneous nystagmus with the quick component to the opposite side may also persist for many months or years, and may persist indefinitely. This is best demonstrated by electronystagmography with the eyes closed. Some cases of incomplete loss of auditory and vestibular function following transverse fracture of the temporal bone have been reported (Nager, 1949; Hofmann, 1925; Gordon, 1954). In such cases there may have been an isolated or incomplete fracture of the labyrinthine capsule. Isolated fractures of the cochlea and internal auditory canal have been described in autopsy specimens (Schlittler, 1936).

c. Delayed meningitis following fracture

Meningitis may occur as a late complication of a temporal bone fracture. The infection usually develops some months or even years later in association with an upper respiratory illness. Applebaum (1960) reported 91 cases of meningitis complicating injuries to the head. Skull fractures were identified in 48, rhinorrhea or otorrhea in 15, and bleeding from the ears or nose in 13. *Diplococcus pneumoniae* was the etiologic agent in 47, and the onset of meningitis ranged from several hours to years after injury. Three patients had

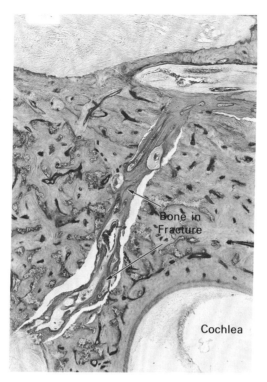

Fig. 7.4: Same case as Fig. 7.3. The fracture of the bony labyrinth is firmly healed by fibrous tissue and bone. The new bone derives from the periosteal and endosteal layers of the bony labyrinth.

repeated bouts of meningitis. New bone and fibrous tissue are generated from the endosteal and periosteal layers of the bony labyrinth and normally grow into the fissure to seal the defect within three or four weeks (Fig. 7.6). The enchondral layer of the bony labyrinth generates very little, if any, fibrous tissue or new bone (Perlman, 1939). This may account for an occasional persistent cerebrospinal fluid fistula following fracture. Other determinants of the development of a fistula are the width of the fissure and ingrowth of epithelium from the mucous membrane (Klestadt, 1913; Manasse, 1924; Hofmann, 1925). A more common site for a persisting cerebrospinal fluid fistula is in the tegmen of the middle ear or mastoid.

Patients having had temporal bone fractures should be kept under close surveillance for several years so that prompt treatment may be instituted should meningitis occur. Management requires identification of the site of the fistula and an otological or neurosurgical procedure to close the defect. The diagnosis, pathology, and management of patients with temporal bone fracture have been treated in depth by Kley (1968).

d. Cholesteatoma following fracture

Cholesteatoma of the mastoid may occur as a delayed complication of longitudinal fracture of the temporal bone. The condition develops as the result of ingrowth of squamous epithelium into a fissure in the bony wall of the external auditory canal. Cholesteatomas developing under these conditions in well-pneumatized temporal bones may be exceedingly extensive and difficult to remove surgically.

2. OSSICULAR INJURIES

Trauma to the ossicles may occur with or without temporal bone fracture. Hough (1969) found the most common injuries to be subluxation of the incus with separation of the incudostapedial joint, luxation of the incus with an intact stapes, fracture of the crura, and fracture of the malleus. Surgical treatment consists of a variety of techniques, including the use of autogenous bone graft, repositioning of dislocated ossicles, transplantation of the body of the incus to the head of the stapes, transplant of homograft incus or malleus, and partial or total ossiculectomy and introduction of prosthetic material. Ossicular injuries can often be demonstrated radiographically (Wright et al., 1969).

Fee (1968) has demonstrated perilymph fistulas of the oval window in patients having head injury without evidence of skull fracture. The symptoms consisted of persistent disequilibrium and fluctuating hearing loss for weeks or months following the head trauma. Surgical exploration revealed fracture dislocations of the footplates which were successfully treated by autogenous tissue grafts.

3. LABYRINTHINE CONCUSSION FROM HEAD BLOW

It is a matter of common clinical experience that deafness and disequilibrium may follow a blow to the head when there is no radiological or other

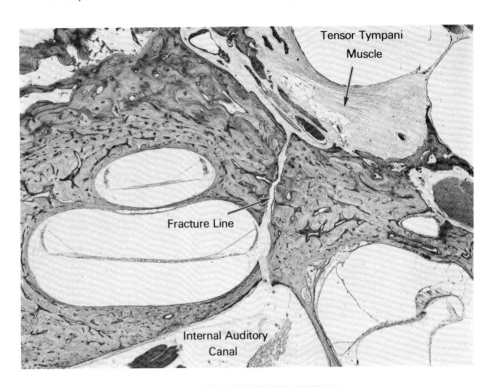

Fig. 7.5: Transverse fracture of the temporal bone in a 79-year-old individual incurred fifty years before death. The fissure contains fibrous tissue. There is no evidence of bony healing.

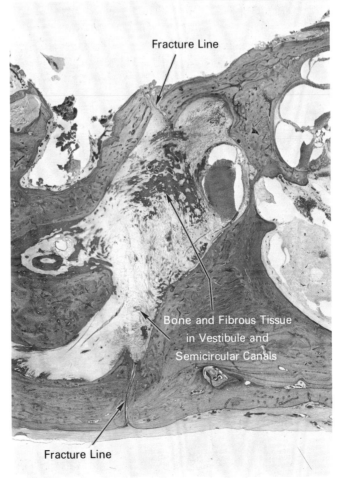

Fig. 7.6: This patient died of otitic meningitis at the age of 25, nine months following transverse fracture of the temporal bone. The membranous labyrinth is completely degenerated, and the vestibule and semicircular canals contain bone and connective tissue. There is no evidence of a fistulous tract through the labyrinth. Presumably meningeal infection occurred through an unhealed fracture elsewhere in the temporal bone.

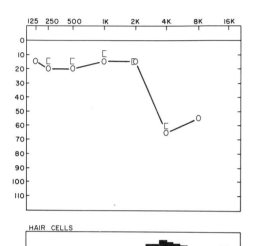

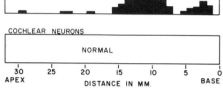

Fig. 7.7: At the age of 53 this individual sustained a severe head injury followed by unconsciousness. Subsequent audiometric studies showed a high-frequency sensorineural hearing loss characteristic of stimulation injury. The hearing loss was most severe for 4000 Hz and was associated with a loss of external hair cells in the 7 to 15 mm region. See Fig. 7.8.

Fig. 7.8: Same individual as Fig. 7.7. There is a loss of external hair cells in the 10 mm region of the cochlea. The inset shows normal hair cells in the 20 mm region.

evidence of a labyrinthine fracture. Probably in most cases these symptoms are caused by combined injury to the central nervous system and to the labyrinth. The extent to which each is involved depends in large part on the nature of the head blow. For example, a blow to the vertex by a large blunt object, resulting in depressed skull fracture, would be expected to create brain injury, whereas a sharp blow to the temporal or mastoid area by a smaller object, without fracture, would be more likely to create inner ear concussion injury.

Petechial hemorrhages into the brain and brain stem and areas of necrosis with traumatic cyst formation are well-known sequellae of a severe head blow and may occasionally be responsible for some of the auditory and vestibular symptoms following head blow (Oppenheim, 1902; Kirikae et al., 1969). There seems to be ample evidence to show, however, that the principal mechanism involved is concussion injury to the inner ear structures.

a. Auditory concussion

This type of deafness has also been termed inner ear concussion, commotio labyrinthi, and otitis interna vasomotoria by various authors. To produce labyrinthine concussion, a head injury ordinarily must be severe enough to cause loss of consciousness. A relatively moderate blow, however, can create a permanent sensorineural hearing loss, particularly when delivered to the occiput (Hofmann, 1925; Klingenberg, 1929; Wittmaack, 1932; Koch, 1933; Voss, 1936; Escher, 1948). In 1892, Schwartze, being aware that the hearing losses are often partially reversible (temporary threshold shift), suggested the cause to be transient hyperemia of the membranous labyrinth. Linck (1921) and Stenger (1909) delivered head blows to rats and Brunner (1940) to guinea pigs, and all demonstrated inner ear hemorrhages which they believed to be responsible for the hearing loss. In a well-executed experiment Wittmaack (1932) found degeneration of hair cells and cochlear neurons in the middle turns of the cochleae of cats subjected to head blows and reasoned that a traveling pressure wave resembling an acoustic stimulus injured these structures directly. Rüedi and Furrer (1946) produced temporary high-frequency hearing losses in two human volunteers to whom mallet blows were delivered to the mastoid cortex through a postauricular incision under local anesthesia.

Igarashi et al. (1964) reported the temporal bone findings in a patient with well-documented head injury. A high-frequency hearing loss was found to correlate with injury to the organ of Corti in the midbasal turn. The histological changes were like those known to result from high-intensity acoustic stimulation (Figs. 7.7, 7.8).

Some investigators (Hellmann, 1922; Manasse, 1924; Alexander, 1928;

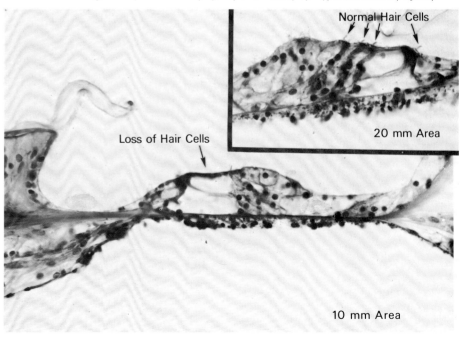

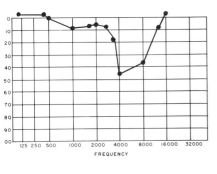

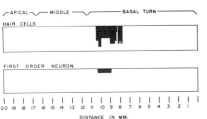

B

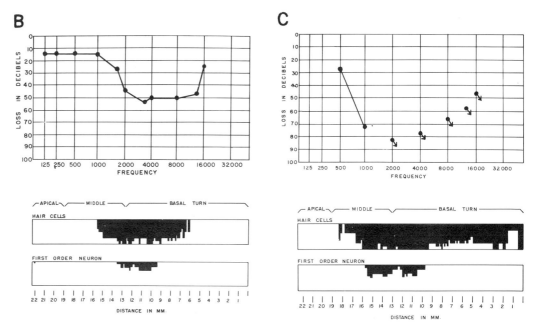

C

Fig. 7.9: Audiograms and cochlear charts of three animals sustaining experimental blows to the head. Frequencies are plotted on the abscissa of the audiogram in accordance with the anatomical frequency scale and distance along the cochlear duct is indicated in mm. The injuries are most severe in the 8 to 14 mm regions and are morphologically identical to injuries resulting from airborne stimuli.

Fischer and Wolfsen, 1943; Nager, 1949) found severe degeneration with fibrous tissue and bone in the inner ear, and others (Theodore, 1910; Wittmaack, 1932; Nassulphis, 1946) demonstrated degenerative changes in the organ of Corti and cochlear neurons, most severe in the basal turn. These reports are not provided with sufficient histological or functional test data to permit an assessment of the mechanism of injury.

In 1951, Schuknecht et al. recorded the hearing losses and pathological changes in nine cats subjected to head blows (Fig. 7.9). The postconcussion behavioral audiograms of these animals revealed hearing losses which were most severe for the high tones. Three animals exhibited losses confined to the 3000 to 8000 Hz range of hearing. All animals showed some recovery of hearing during the first two weeks following injury (Fig. 7.10).

In all cochleae the most severe changes were located in the middle part of the basal turn which serves 4000 to 8000 Hz. The slightest observable change in the organ of Corti was a derangement in cytoarchitecture in which the external hair cells appear to be shortened and widened and contained pyknotic nuclei. More severe injuries consisted of loss of internal hair cells, flattening of the organ of Corti, and finally complete disappearance of the organ of Corti (Fig. 7.11). Degeneration of cochlear neurons occurred in the same regions of the cochleae as the organ of Corti lesions, but were less severe.

These pathological changes are like those reported by Lurie et al. (1944), Perlman (1948), Lindquist (1949), and others for intense airborne sound stimuli.

Presumably a blow to the head creates a pressure wave in the skull which is transmitted through bone to the cochlea just as a pressure wave in air is carried by the conducting mechanism, and the injury must be attributed to intense acoustic stimulation. Another possible mechanism is that the sudden acceleration or deceleration of the head creates a relative movement of the footplate due to the inertia of the tympanic membrane and ossicles.

b. Vestibular concussion

The mechanism of injury to the vestibular system from a blow to the head cannot be defined as clearly as for the auditory system. Windle et al. (1944) have demonstrated degenerative changes in the lateral vestibular nuclei from experimental head blows. Certainly contusions and petechial hemorrhages into the vestibular nuclei and injury to the cerebellum can be expected to produce disequilibrium.

The most common type of postconcussion disequilibrium is generally known as positional vertigo of the benign paroxysmal type (Bárány, 1921; Dix and Hallpike, 1952) and more recently termed cupulolithiasis (Schuk-

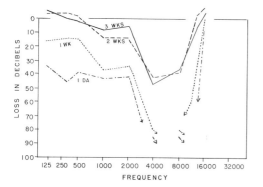

Fig. 7.10: Behavioral audiograms made on a cat following an experimental blow to the head. Serial audiograms show improvement in thresholds during a two-week period following injury, after which the thresholds remained stable until the animal was sacrificed three months later.

Fig. 7.11: Organ of Corti in the 10 mm region of the cochlea of a cat who sustained a severe high-frequency hearing loss following a blow to the head (see behavioral audiogram C in Fig. 7.9). There is a total loss of hair cells, external Deiters' cells, Hensen's cells, and the Claudius cells. The pillar cells, internal hair cells, internal Deiters' cells and cochlear neurons appear normal.

necht, 1969). Blows to the occipital and temporal regions are most likely to produce this symptom. It may persist for weeks or months following an injury but is usually self-limiting (Cawthorne, 1954; Gordon, 1954; Schuknecht and Davison, 1956).

The principal complaint of the patient is the occurrence of sudden attacks of vertigo precipitated by certain head positions. The sensation of vertigo is always of short duration (five to ten seconds) but may be very severe and sometimes is associated with nausea. The attack can be elicited by placing the patient in the supine head hanging position with the head turned to one side. The attack is provoked when the injured ear is in the undermost position. For further details regarding method of examination, clinical features and pathology, see Chapter 12B, Cupulolithiasis.

Injury to the utricular otolithic membrane may provide a mechanism for this type of vertigo (Schuknecht, 1962). A head blow conceivably could induce sufficiently intense utricular stimulation to cause disruption of the otolithic membrane and detachment of otoconia. These free otoconia might then settle into the ampulla of the posterior semicircular canal, which is the most dependent part of the labyrinth, and with changes in head position, cause

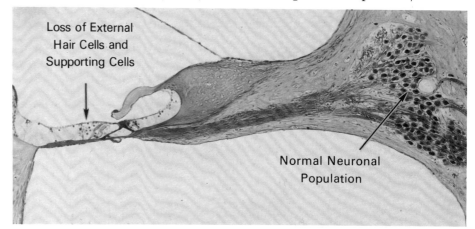

displacement of the cupula of this canal. Several investigators have demonstrated in experimental animals that intense gravitational stresses cause disruption of the otolithic membranes (Wittmaack, 1909; Hasegawa, 1931; de Kleyn and Versteegh, 1933; Parker et al., 1968).

Barber (1964) found this type of positional vertigo in 47 percent of 47 patients with longitudinal fracture of the temporal bone and in 20.8 percent of 77 individuals with head injuries of comparable severity but without skull fracture.

Whiplash injury. Toglia et al. (1970) found vestibular abnormalities to be as common following whiplash injuries as after direct head trauma. About one-half of 116 patients demonstrated objective evidence of either caloric abnormality or nystagmus. They emphasize the importance of utilizing electronystagmography to detect small degrees of vestibular disturbance. They also stated that about 50 percent of their patients with whiplash injury experienced hearing loss or tinnitus, or both, but provided no documentation for this comment. Several authors (Denny-Brown, 1945; Russell, 1954; Toglia et al., 1970) state that the vertiginous symptoms usually subside within a few months following injury. Gotten (1956) states that 95 percent of the whiplash patients become symptom-free following litigation, but this might be due to its self-limiting course.

4. PENETRATING WOUNDS

a. Trauma via the external auditory canal

Trauma to the tympanic membrane and ossicles may be incurred by an object which traverses the external auditory canal. Hair pins, tooth-picks and cotton applicators are frequently used to scratch or clean the ear canal and are a common cause for such injuries.

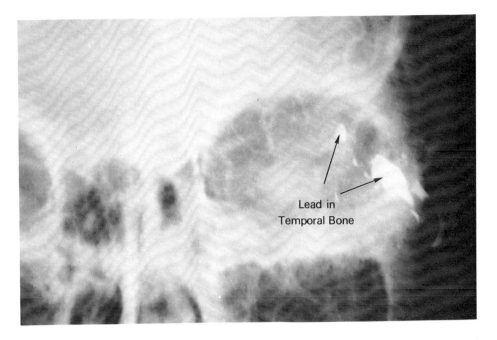

Fig. 7.12: This individual was shot in the temporal bone in 1920 at the age of 28 while fighting with the British forces in Ireland. After healing, the wound was asymptomatic except for a conductive hearing loss. He died in Boston, Mass. in 1964, 44 years later at the age of 72 of cerebrovascular hemorrhage. The roentgenograms, taken at the time of his terminal admission to the hospital, show a large metallic deposit in the temporal bone. See Fig. 7.13.

In addition to tears in the tympanic membrane, the ossicles may be dislocated and foreign material may be introduced into the middle ear. Any patient experiencing vertigo from such an injury must be suspected of having a subluxated or fractured stapes. Puncture wounds or small tears of the tympanic membrane heal spontaneously; however, more severe injuries should be treated by immediate exploration and surgical repair (Silverstein, 1973). Infolded flaps of tympanic membrane and disarticulated ossicles may be repositioned. A subluxated or fractured stapes associated with an oval window fistula may be replaced by an autogenous tissue graft and the continuity of the sound transmission system re-established immediately or subsequently by reconstructive techniques (Arragg and Paparella, 1964).

b. Gunshot wounds

Gunshot wounds to the temporal bone create all degrees and combinations of injuries including tears of the major vessels, facial nerve injury, tears of the dura, and destruction of the structures of the middle and inner ear. Surgical exploration and repair should be instituted as soon as practicable. Although there is ample evidence that lead from bullets may lie dormant in bone for many years (Hempstead, 1932; Martin, 1940; Mosher, 1942; Kerr, 1967), thorough debridement and removal of foreign material is indicated (Figs. 7.12, 7.13).

Fig. 7.13: Same individual as Fig. 7.12. The metallic deposit, shown to be lead by electron microprobe analysis, caused no significant tissue reaction during the 44 years of its existence in the temporal bone.

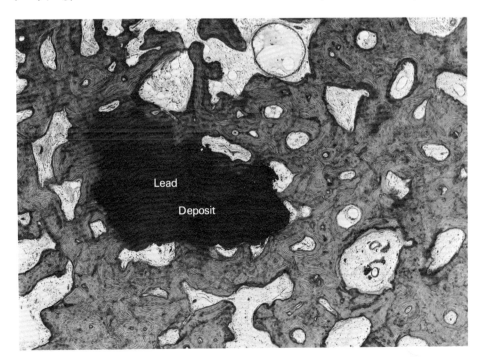

B. SURGICAL TRAUMA

1. SURGICAL FISTULIZATION OF THE LABYRINTH

Probably the most common injury to the inner ear during mastoid surgery is inadvertent opening of the lateral semicircular canal. The canal is vulnerable because of its prominent position in the floor of the mastoid antrum. The creation of a small bony fistula without tearing of the membranous semicircular canal may be tolerated without incident; however, when the membranous canal is injured, the usual result is a profound hearing loss and moderate to severe loss of vestibular function (Altmann, 1946) (Fig. 7.14).

Fig. 7.14: This ear, which had previously been subjected to a radical mastoidectomy, shows a surgical fistula of the lateral semicircular canal which is presumed to be iatrogenic. The canal is filled with dense fibrous tissue, and the auditory and vestibular sense organs are severely degenerated.

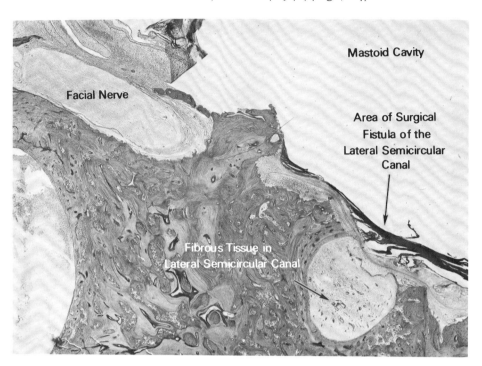

2. DISLOCATION OF THE STAPES AND INCUS

Accidental luxation or fracture of the stapes associated with fistulization of the oval window may occur during mastoid and middle ear surgery and was more common prior to the development of surgical microscopes. A study of the histopatholgy of the temporal bones of such cases indicates that the extent of the inner ear damage depends upon the size of the fistula created in the oval window and the amount of associated trauma to the structures of the vestibule (Kohonen, 1970) (Figs. 7.15 to 7.17). With modern surgical techniques the injury occurs less frequently, but should it occur and be recognized, it is sometimes possible to avoid subsequent hearing loss by repositioning the footplate or closing the fistula with an autogenous tissue graft.

Altmann and Waltner (1945) found multiple fractures in the footplate of a patient who died of unrelated causes five days following surgery and ascribed the injury to curetting in the oval window niche. There was moderate bleeding into the vestibule and mild labyrinthitis.

Luxation of the incus is usually caused by inadvertent dislocation of the short process. This process is located in the floor of the aditus ad antrum where it is vulnerable to the surgeon's instruments (Ballantyne, 1970). The injury results in ossicular discontinuity and a conductive hearing loss. The loss is moderately severe when associated with a perforation of the tympanic membrane and very severe when the tympanic membrane is intact.

3. SURGICALLY INDUCED STIMULATION DEAFNESS (ACOUSTIC TRAUMA)

Stimulation deafness may be induced during manipulative procedures in the external and middle ear. High-frequency hearing losses may result from

Fig. 7.15: A left modified radical mastoidectomy was performed on this woman at the age of 46. She had no vertigo following surgery, and her postoperative pure tone air conduction thresholds in this ear were in the 20 to 30 db range. She died 14 years later. There is subluxation of the posterior margin of the footplate into the vestibule. The oval window fistula is healed with fibrous tissue. The sensory and neural structures of the auditory and vestibular systems appear normal.

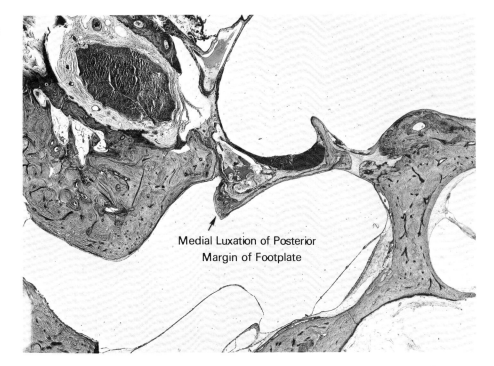

Medial Luxation of Posterior
Margin of Footplate

Fig. 7.16: A radical mastoidectomy was performed on this ear when the patient was 50 years of age. It is not known whether she had vestibular symptoms following surgery; however, audiometric tests two years later revealed profound hearing loss in this ear. She died 26 years after surgery. Histological studies show fibrous replacement of the anterior one-third of the footplate and fragments of the crura embedded in connective tissue. These changes are presumed to be of iatrogenic origin. There is severe endolymphatic hydrops and degeneration of the organ of Corti and cochlear neurons. The vestibular sense organs and nerves appear normal.

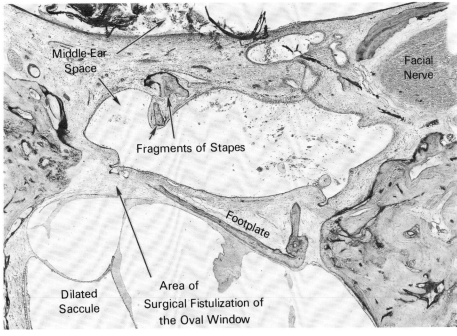

Middle Ear
Space

Facial
Nerve

Fragments of Stapes

Footplate

Dilated
Saccule

Area of
Surgical Fistulization of
the Oval Window

Fig. 7.17: A radical mastoidectomy was performed on this ear when the patient was 41 years of age. He experienced severe vertigo for some days following surgery and permanent profound deafness in this ear. He died at the age of 55. Histological study shows the stapes deeply displaced into the vestibule with the anterior margin of the footplate in contact with the saccular wall. There is moderate endolymphatic hydrops of the utricle and saccule; however, the vestibular sense organs appear normal. The organ of Corti has near total loss of hair cells and 90 percent loss of cochlear neurons but no cochlear hydrops is present.

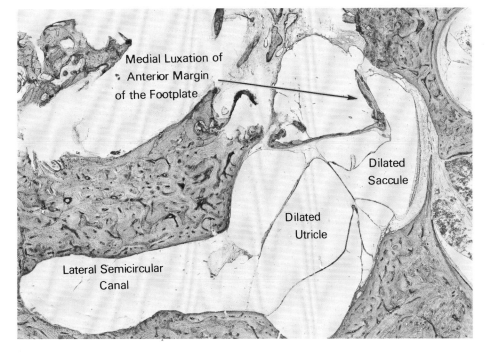

Medial Luxation of
Anterior Margin
of the Footplate

Dilated
Saccule

Dilated
Utricle

Lateral Semicircular
Canal

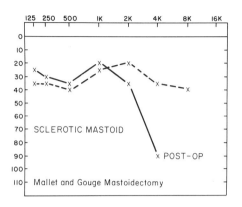

Fig. 7.18: High-frequency hearing loss following the use of a mallet and gouge to exenterate a small sclerotic mastoid (author's case, 1949). The mechanism of injury is presumed to be acoustic trauma.

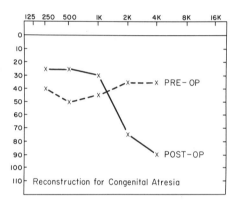

Fig. 7.19: High-frequency hearing loss following surgical reconstruction for the correction of congenital aural atresia. It seems probable that the hearing loss was induced by contact of the bone-cutting burr with the incus during removal of bony atresia plate.

the use of the mallet and gouge during exenteration of a sclerotic mastoid (Fig. 7.18) or from contact of the burr on the intact ossicular chain (Fig. 7.19). In an experiment on cats, Paparella (1962) placed 4.0 mm sharp cutting burrs (six grooves) rotating at 15,000 to 18,000 rpm, as commonly used in otologic surgery, on the body of the incus for periods of time varying from 5 to 20 seconds for the different animals. On behavioral audiograms these animals exhibited severe high-frequency hearing losses. Histological studies showed cochlear injuries characteristic of acoustic trauma. Paparella also demonstrated that a 0.5 mm cutting burr rotating at 4000 to 5000 rpm, as commonly used in surgery for otosclerosis, failed to produce hearing losses or inner ear injury when applied to the ossicles. In another experiment Paparella (1961) found that direct stimulation of the ossicular chain with a vibrator (cavitron instrument, frequency 25,000 vibrations per second, probe tip excursion —.001 inch) produced severe cochlear injuries (Fig. 7.20).

Singleton and Schuknecht (1959) studied the pathological changes and reparative processes consequent to experimentally induced stapes fractures in cats. They found that inward subluxation of the footplate of the stapes caused injury to the organ of Corti in the upper basal turn in some animals. The histopathological changes at the site of the injury were similar to those resulting from head blows or air-conducted blast injuries (Fig. 7.21). Schuknecht and Tonndorf (1960) postulated that some of the high-frequency hearing losses which follow surgical removal of the stapes for otosclerosis may be the result of surgically induced stimulation injury.

4. UTRICULAR INJURY

Otologic surgeons have learned that manipulations within the vestibule, such as attempts to remove depressed fragments of footplate, are frequently followed by vertigo which may be immediate and prolonged. It seems probable, on an anatomical basis, that the structure most commonly injured is the utricle, for it frequently lies in a vulnerable position medial to the superior part of the oval window. Tears of the utricular wall would undoubtedly cause severe and probably permanent vestibular dysfunction as well as hearing loss. Contact injuries to the utricular macula may incite not only immediate disequilibrium but also paroxysmal positional vertigo due to dislodged otoconia (see Chapter 12B, Cupulolithiasis).

Surgical destruction of the saccule in animals produces mild temporary disequilibrium (Igarashi, 1965). Although the effects of saccular injuries in the human ear are not known, it seems probable that functional changes are less severe than those following utricular injuries.

C. NOISE DEAFNESS

The temporary loss of hearing from exposure to high-intensity noise (steady state, intermittent, impact) is known as the temporary threshold shift (TTS). One of the most informative experimental studies of temporary deafness in human subjects following exposure to loud tones and noise was performed by Davis et al. (1950). They exposed ten volunteers to pure tone stimuli at intensities of 110 to 130 db for periods of 1 to 64 minutes and consistently produced temporary high-tone hearing losses.

Much study has been given to the etiology and cytological alterations occurring in both temporary and permanent stimulation deafness. Siebenmann and Yoshii (1908) provided one of the first good descriptions of the histological changes observed by light microscopy in experimentally induced noise deafness. The earliest changes occurred in the external hair cells and consisted of loss of sensory hairs followed by deformation, swelling, and disintegration of the cell body. With progressive severity of the injury, there was involvement of the pillar cells, Deiters' cells, and Hensen's cells. Finally, the internal hair cells became affected and eventually the cochlear neurons atrophied.

Fig. 7.20: Injuries of the organs of Corti caused by contact of a vibrating probe (25,000 vibrations per second) to the ossicular chain of the cat. *Above:* Application of the probe to the malleus for 20 seconds has resulted in avulsion of the organ of Corti from the basilar membrane (48 hours post injury). *Middle:* Loss of external hair cells in the upper basal turn following application of the probe to the handle of the malleus for 20 seconds (9 weeks post injury). *Below:* Total degeneration of the organ of Corti in the basal and middle turns following application of probe to the incudostapedial joint for 10 seconds (8 weeks post injury). (Courtesy of Paparella)

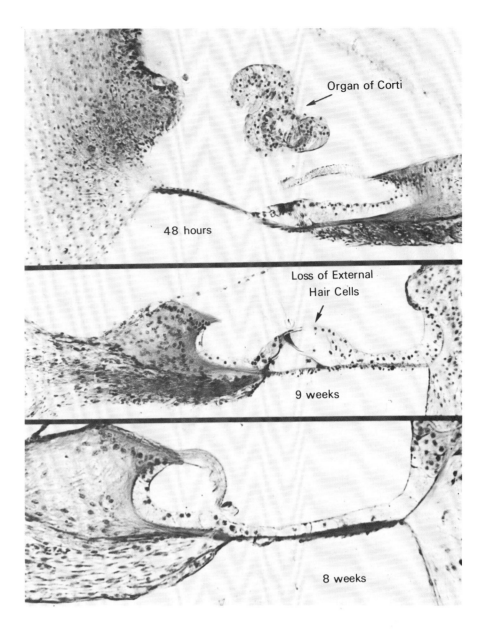

Fig. 7.21: Loss of hair cells in the midregion of the basal turn following intentional fracture of the footplate in the cat.

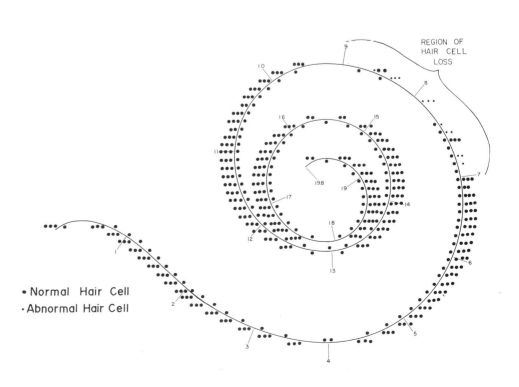

Merkle (1954) and Neubert and Wuestenfeld (1955), utilizing the surface preparation technique, demonstrated swelling of the hair cell nuclei in direct relationship to the intensity and duration of noise exposure. Mizukoshi et al. (1957) and Beck (1959a, 1959b), utilizing the surface preparation technique with histochemical methods, showed a decrease in ribonucleic acid in the hair cells, the magnitude of which was directly related to stimulus intensity. Misrahy et al. (1958) found that the endolymphatic oxygen tension first increases after noise exposure and then decreases rapidly and markedly. The original levels of oxygen tension are restored only after prolonged recovery times and are directly related to the duration and intensity of the noise exposure. Vosteen (1958) showed that the respiratory enzyme, succinicdehydrogenase, decreases first in the nerve endings and then in the external hair cells following prolonged exposures to sound pressure levels of 80 to 85 db (re. 002 dynes/cm²). The effect was considerably less when the stimulus was interrupted periodically. Zorzoli and Oriani (1958) reported that after exposure at levels of 50 db for one-half hour, the glycogen content of the hair cells diminished, and suggested that the energy consumed during sound exposure is obtained from glucose metabolism.

Electron microscopic studies of sound-injured guinea pig ears by Spoendlin (1958, 1971) showed the early alterations to be distortion of external hair cells, buckling of sensory hairs, swelling of the dendrites to the internal hair cells, and increase in the density of efferent nerve endings for the external hair cells (Fig. 7.22). The swelling of dendrites appeared to be reversible; however, the buckling of sensory hairs of the internal hair cells was permanent. More intense stimulation resulted in disintegration of hair cells and rupture of dendrites.

In a study utilizing scanning and transmission electron microscopy, Lim and Melnick (1971) found high-intensity noise exposure to produce a progression of changes in the organ of Corti consisting of blebs on the surface of the hair cells, vesiculation and vacuolization of the smooth endoplasmic reticulum, accumulation of lysosomal granules in the subcuticular region, deformation of cuticular plates, and eventual cell rupture and lysis (Figs. 7.23 and 7.24).

Fig. 7.22: Electron micrograph showing external hair cell area of the guinea pig immediately after exposure to one hour of noise at 130 db. There is swelling and buckling of the hair cells and shifting of nuclei from a basal to a subapical location. The mitochondria and endoplasmic reticulum become randomly distributed throughout the cells. The efferent nerve endings are more densely packed with synaptic vesicles, and there is a denser ground substance between the vesicles. (Courtesy of Spoendlin)

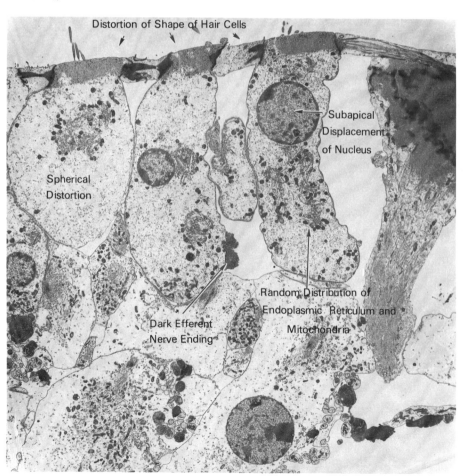

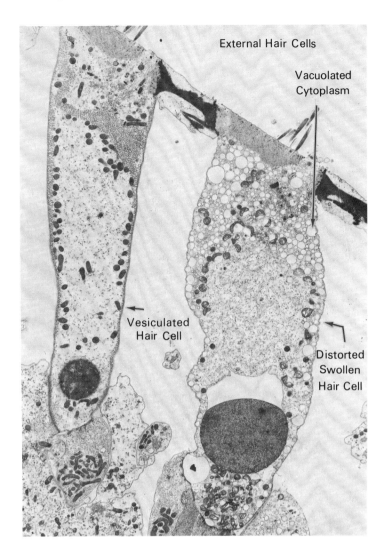

Fig. 7.23: Transmission electron microscopic view showing vesiculation and vacuolization of the endoplasmic reticulum in the external hair cells of the second turn of a guinea pig exposed to a noise band of 300 to 600 Hz at an intensity of 117 db for 4 hours. The animal was killed 10 days following exposure. (Courtesy of Lim)

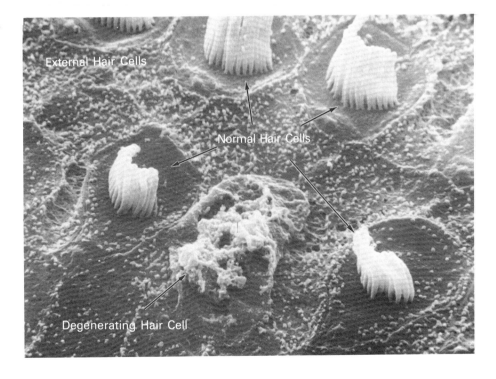

Fig. 7.24: Scanning electron micrograph showing a degenerating external hair cell of a guinea pig after 14 hours' exposure to a 1 to 2 K Hz noise band at an intensity of 117 db. (Courtesy of Lim)

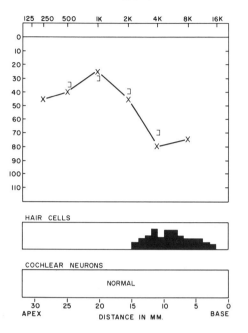

Fig. 7.25: Audiogram and cochlear chart of a man who worked for several years as a boiler-maker and steam fitter in a shipyard where he was exposed to high-intensity noise. He died at the age of 47. The severe loss of hearing for 4000 to 8000 Hz is correlated with a loss of external hair cells in the 2 to 15 mm region of the cochlea. See Fig. 7.24.

Thus it appears that moderate intensities of acoustic stimulation incite metabolic activity leading to exhaustion of enzymes and glycogen stores, diminished oxygen tension, decreased energy output, and reversible alterations in organelles of the sensory cells and nerve endings. The functional manifestation is auditory fatigue or temporary threshold shift. More intense stimulation results in irreversible morphological alterations and permanent hearing loss.

The remarkable tendency for stimulation injuries to involve the 8 to 10 mm region of the cochlea with hearing losses centering around 4000 Hz is well known and the object of much conjecture. Two schools of thought appear to exist specifically with regard to the cause of the 4000 Hz dip: (1) the mechanistic view which holds that strong destructive forces develop in this particular region of the cochlea [e.g. the "dual eddy" theory of Rüedi and Furrer (1946) and the "jet" theory of Hilding (1953)]; and (2) the locus-minoris-resistentiae view which maintains that this region is especially vulnerable to injury [e.g. insufficient blood supply at the juncture of the main cochlear artery and the cochlear ramus artery as suggested by Crowe et al. (1934)].

Based on observations from cochlear models, Schuknecht and Tonndorf (1960) presented a concept which falls into the mechanistic viewpoint. Experiments on cochlear models using transient signals showed that the closer the stress is concentrated to the basal end of the cochlea, the shorter is the time constant of the applied signal. Since the sensitivity falls off for signals with very short time constants, a region of optimal stress develops close to, but not directly at, the basal end of the cochlea.

The functional and pathological changes characteristic of noise deafness in human subjects are shown in Figs. 7.25 to 7.28.

Cochlear injury produced by intense sinusoidal sound (pure tones) has been the subject of numerous investigations (Upton, 1929; Davis et al., 1935; Wever and Smith, 1944; Lurie et al., 1944; Smith, 1947; Covell and Eldridge, 1951; Stockwell et al., 1969). Several studies showed a systematic relationship between the frequency of the stimulating tone and the location of injury in the cochlea. The experiment of Stockwell et al. (1969) on guinea pigs provides the best information on this subject. They found that lower frequencies produced proportionally greater damage to external hair cell rows than did

Fig. 7.26: Same ear as Fig. 7.23. Photomicrographs showing organ of Corti with loss of external hair cells in the 10 mm region (above) and normal organ of Corti in the 20 mm region.

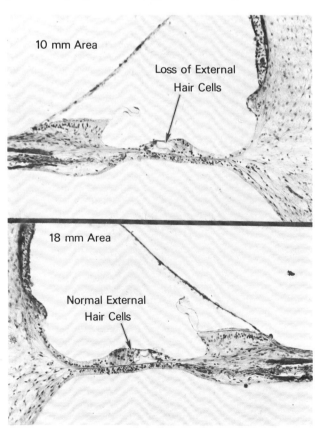

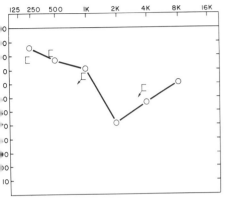

Fig. 7.27: Audiogram of a 71-year-old man who had been exposed to high-intensity noise in a sawmill for many years. See Fig. 7.28. (Courtesy of Bredberg)

Fig. 7.28: For history see legend, Fig. 7.27. The surface preparation of the cochlea shows loss of hair cells and radial nerve fibers in the 10.5 to 14 mm regions. (Courtesy of Bredberg)

higher frequencies. Hair cell injury caused by exposures to 150 db was severe over wide areas, extending from the supposed sites of maximum stimulation toward the basal end of the cochlea. Lesions produced by a 4000 Hz tone appeared near the stimulation maximum for that frequency, whereas lesions caused by lower frequencies tended to appear progressively nearer the base with respect to stimulation maxima. Multiple peaks of injury were commonly observed in their animals. Taylor and Williams (1966) found that shoulder weapons produce a hearing loss for high frequencies (Fig. 7.29). This effect of small arms noise on hearing was confirmed by Keim (1969) (Fig. 7.30). Both authors observed, furthermore, that the right ear is protected by the "head shadow" effect during the firing of arms from the right shoulder.

Severe impact noise can cause severe sensorineural hearing loss. In one such case of unilateral severe deafness, Schuknecht (1972a) observed a large tear in the round window membrane on surgical exploration.

In recent years, there has been an increasing awareness of the need for damage-risk criteria (the maximum levels and durations of sound of different spectra to which the ear can be safely exposed). Noises generated in industry, in the military services, and even in the home (e.g. amplified music) can lead to permanent hearing impairment. Damage-risk criteria have been formulated by the NAS-NRC Committee on Hearing, Bio-acoustics and Bio-mechanics for steady-state and impact noise (Kryter, 1965, 1970; Kryter et al., 1966; Ward, 1968). An example of a damage-risk contour is shown in Figure 7.31.

Most industrial noises can be classified as either impact noise (drop hammers, punch presses, paper shredders, etc.) or as steady noise (diesel engines, lathes, etc.). The acoustic energy in noise is seldom distributed uniformly among the component frequencies; thus piston engines, pit fur-

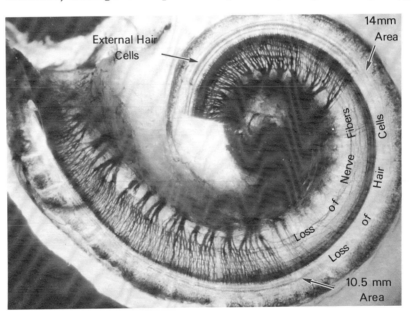

Fig. 7.29: Median audiometric thresholds for the left ears of 32 hunters (ages 40–49) and 9 matched controls (non-hunters). (Courtesy of Taylor)

Fig. 7.30: Average audiometric thresholds (ASA-1951 calibration) of 14 individuals before and 10 weeks after exposure to rifle shooting in the course of military training. All were right-handed and placed the weapon on the right shoulder. In this position the right ear is somewhat protected by the head shadow. (Courtesy of Keim)

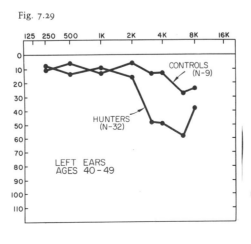

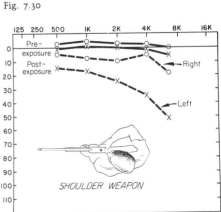

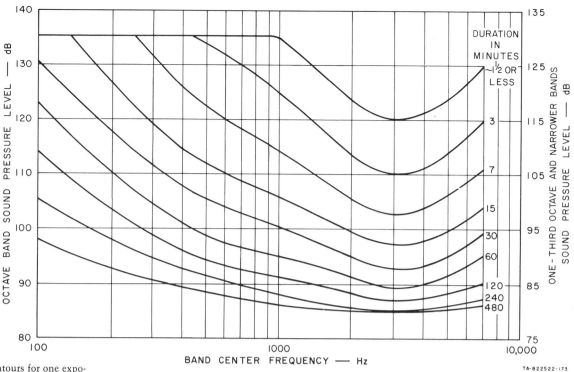

Fig. 7.31: Damage-risk contours for one exposure per day to full octave (left-hand ordinate) and one-third octave narrower (right-hand ordinate) bands of noise. This graph can be applied to the individual band levels present in the broad band noise. It is predicted that daily exposures to these levels for five years or longer will cause hearing losses equal to or greater than 10 db at 1000 Hz, 15 db at 2000 Hz, and 30 db at 3000 Hz in about 50 percent of individuals. (Courtesy of Kryter)

naces, etc., produce mainly low frequencies, and pneumatic peen hammers, high-speed cut-off saws, etc., produce predominantly middle and high frequencies. The measurements of noise levels, therefore, must include octave band levels as well as overall levels. Steady noises can be measured with a sound level meter and octave band analyzer; however, special equipment is required for the measurement of impact noises. The effects of continuous noise exposure differ from those of exposures interrupted by periods of reduced noise levels; therefore, an analysis of occupational noise should include a study of its distribution, timed throughout a representative work day, as well as the total exposure during a work life. Any assessment for the need of hearing conservation must consider both the noise levels and exposure times. Early noise-induced hearing losses are usually confined to the frequencies around 4000 Hz, and as the exposure lengthens, the losses spread to lower frequencies. Because the most important frequencies to be protected against are in the range of 500 to 2000 Hz, it follows that the 300 to 600 and 600 to 1200 Hz bands deserve particular attention.

In the *Guide for Conservation of Hearing in Noise* (1969), the Committee for the Conservation of Hearing of the American Academy of Ophthalmology and Otolaryngology has recommended that noise exposure controls and tests of hearing are advisable if individuals are to be exposed regularly to steady noise which has levels of 90 db or greater as measured on the A scale of the sound level meter. The A scale performs by introducing the electrical equivalent of the noise through a broad-band filter that has frequency characteristics similar to the human ear. The Committee also recommended that a hearing conservation program should be considered whenever persons have (1) difficulty communicating by speech while they are in the noise, (2) tinnitus after several hours of noise exposure, or (3) temporary threshold shift after noise exposure. An occupational hearing conservation program includes an attempt at environmental control through reduction of noise produced by the source, isolation by sound proofing, and revision of operational procedures. The use of ear plugs or ear muffs is particularly important when noise cannot be controlled by environmental changes. Both pre-employment hearing tests and subsequent periodic tests should be part of a conservation program. Some individuals appear to be highly susceptible to noise-induced hearing loss, and until a valid test is developed to identify these individuals, periodic hearing tests must be used to identify them.

D. OTITIC BAROTRAUMA (AEROTITIS)

Otitic barotrauma (aerotitis) is a traumatic inflammatory disorder of the middle ear resulting from sudden severe negative pressure in the pneumatized spaces of the temporal bone. It occurs most commonly during descent from altitudes or during ascent from underwater diving. It is caused by failure of the eustachian tube to open sufficiently to permit the equalization of middle ear pressures.

During ascent to altitude, the middle ear pressure slowly increases and the tympanic membrane bulges laterally until the pressure is great enough to force open the eustachian tube at which time the individual detects a distinct "click" in the ear. On the average, successive expulsions of air through the eustachian tube occur every 435 feet of ascent, regardless of the speed at which the ascent is made (Armstrong and Heim, 1937). After eustachian tube closure has taken place, there is a small residual intratympanic positive pressure of about 3.6 mm of mercury.

During descent from altitude, the eustachian tube behaves in an entirely different manner, for a normal tube does not open passively and air does not enter the tympanic cavity without the intervention of muscular activity.

The difference between the extra- and intratympanic pressures depends not only upon the altitude lost in terms of distance but also upon the level at which this change takes place. A loss of height from 30,000 to 20,000 feet creates an atmospheric pressure difference of 126.6 mm of mercury, whereas a loss of height from 12,000 feet to 2,000 feet creates a pressure differential of 223.4 mm of mercury.

The failure to equalize tympanic pressures on descent may be caused by (1) poor function of the eustachian tube as a result of congenital, anatomical, or chronic pathological conditions, (2) acute pathological changes in the eustachian tube such as edema associated with upper respiratory infection, and (3) incidental conditions, such as sleeping during descent.

Dickson and King (1954) found the incidence of otitic barotrauma in individuals flying in jet engine fighter aircraft to be three times greater than that for individuals employed on piston-engine aircraft. For those training in jet fighters the incidence was six and one-half times greater.

Intense negative pressure results in medial displacement and stretching of the tympanic membrane, hyperemia, and edema and ecchymosis of the mucous membrane of the middle ear, followed by transudation of fluid which may become sanguinous in severe cases. With sudden and intense pressure changes the pars tensa may rupture. King (1966) reported a case in which the incus was dislocated as the result of otitic barotrauma. Pain may be excruciating in the acute phase but gradually subsides over a period of hours after which the only remaining symptom is moderate conductive hearing loss. As eustachian tube function is re-established and pressures are equalized, the pathological changes spontaneously resolve over a period of two to three weeks. The condition rarely occurs in pressurized aircraft; however, individuals with marginal tubal function or those who fly with head colds are more apt to experience otitic barotrauma. The incidence of its occurrence may be reduced in susceptible individuals by the use of nasal shrinking agents, and repeated gentle autoinflation by the Valsalva maneuver is also helpful.

Mackay (1963) found that an air crewman who constantly experienced severe ear pain when reaching altitude had a polyp in the middle ear behaving as a ball valve to prevent the normal escape of air from the eustachian tube. Removal of the polyp gave complete relief.

Sensorineural hearing loss has been reported in association with otitic barotrauma due to altitude change (Simpson, 1942; Scott-Brown et al., 1965) but is more common with underwater diving.

Middle ear changes, such as serous otitis and perforated tympanic membrane, resulting from the pressure changes associated with diving have been well documented (Sims, 1961; Bayliss, 1968). In a study of sports and recreational divers, Lundgren (1965) found that 26 percent experienced vertigo during scuba diving or when diving by breath holding. Seventy-three percent of the group related the onset of their vertigo to ascent or surfacing, while the remaining 27 percent experienced vertigo on descent or while on the bottom. MacFie (1964) found permanent unilateral sensorineural hearing loss in three patients following diving. A fourth patient who maintained normal hearing but suffered vertigo had a hypoactive caloric response in one ear. Three of the four patients were also found to have middle ear barotrauma. Stucker and Echols (1969) reported five cases, Eichel and Landes (1970) two cases, Soss (1971) three cases, and Freeman and Edmonds (1972) five cases of sensorineural hearing loss associated with diving.

Simmons (1968), in a report of fifteen cases of sudden sensorineural hearing loss, described two which were associated with skin diving. One of them related the hearing loss to the Valsalva maneuver, and his hearing did not return to normal until three weeks later. The other noted the onset 14 hours after diving and regained his hearing in one week.

Eichel and Landes (1970) suspect a relationship to forceful overinflation which is frequently performed by divers to avert barotrauma. Stucker and Echols (1969) postulate that gas bubbles might be released as small emboli to occlude the endarteries of the inner ear, and Simmons (1968) suspects a rupture of Reissner's membrane due to pressure changes. Recent observations suggest that many of these cases of sensorineural hearing loss occurring in association with deep water diving are the result of traumatic fistulization of the round or oval window. Pullen (1972, 1973), Freeman (1972), and Schuknecht (1972a) have performed emergency surgery in such cases and observed round window ruptures. Hearing in these ears was improved following closure with autogenous tissue.

The forced inflation of air into the external auditory canal as a diagnostic or therapeutic maneuver can result in sudden death. Air may be forced into the cranial cavity through bony and dural defects (Åhrén and Thulin, 1965) or into the venous system resulting in air embolus (Fairman et al., 1968). In a study on guinea pigs Goldstein and Mundie (1971) demonstrated that pressures of 400 to 475 mm of mercury applied to the external auditory canal not only cause rupture of the tympanic membrane but force air into the cranial cavity with immediate death.

E. RUPTURES OF THE LABYRINTHINE WINDOWS

Previously in this chapter it has been pointed out that fistulae of the oval window can occur as the result of a head injury without evidence of skull fracture (Fee, 1968), and that fistulae of the oval or round windows may result from impact noise (Schuknecht, 1972a) and from deep water diving (Pullen, 1972, 1973; Schuknecht, 1972b).

In 1971, Goodhill performed middle ear surgical explorations on three individuals who experienced sudden deafness in association with physical exertion and found fistulae of both oval and round windows in two and of the oval window only in one. Goodhill et al. (1973) subsequently reported on eighteen additional cases. Of the total twenty-one cases, fistulae of one or both windows were found in fifteen. In ten of the fifteen, there was a definite history of exertion or trauma prior to onset. The oval window alone was ruptured in nine, the round window alone in one, and both windows were ruptured in five ears. Most of the patients suffered from vertigo and showed vestibular dysfunction on testing.

It should be understood that Goodhill et al. (1973) did not actually see the fistulae but assumed their presence on the basis of observing clear fluid in the windows. To obtain a clear and total view of the round window membrane, it is usually necessary to remove the lateral margins of the round window niche which normally hides the membrane from view.

There are several important considerations relative to the identification of labyrinthine fistulae: (1) observation of fluid is presumptive evidence only for a fistula, as tissue fluid may ooze from even slight mucosal trauma; (2) exposure of the round window membrane by drilling away the bony margins of the round window niche can result in a traumatic tear of the membrane; (3) the round window niche frequently is partly bridged by a sheath of mucous membrane which may be difficult to differentiate from the round window membrane on visual inspection.

It is quite obvious that ruptures of the labyrinthine windows are the cause for some cases of sudden deafness but certainly not all of them. To this time, there has been insufficient experience upon which to develop sound indications for surgical exploration of ears with sudden deafness. It seems reasonable, however, to perform surgical exploration on those cases which exhibit a clear history of onset with exertion, barometric change, head injury, or impact noise.

F. IRRADIATION INJURY

X-ray irradiation is frequently used either alone or in combination with surgery for the treatment of malignant disease of the head and neck. It is the therapy of choice for some lesions and is the only treatment for others. In the application of x-ray irradiation to any disease, its effect on adjacent normal tissues is an integral part of the therapy relative to morbidity and mortality. Its effect on tissue depends upon the amount absorbed rather than on the quantity delivered. The character of the response is determined by the intensity of the irradiation and the size of the area exposed. Although all tissue will be damaged by x-ray irradiation in the dosage ranges commonly used in therapy, some tissues are regarded as being radio-resistant (bone and nervous tissue) and others as being radio-sensitive (lymphocytes). The use of fractionated dosages is designed to achieve its maximum effect in the inhibition of mitoses. The effects of irradiation may be discussed in terms of early and late reactions.

1. EARLY IRRADIATION REACTIONS

The first effect of irradiation on tissues is the splitting of molecules into radicals and ions, thus upsetting the chemical balance of the cells. Winther (1969a, 1969b, 1970a, 1970b) studied the immediate effect of single doses of x-ray on the sensory cells of the inner ear of the guinea pig. Single dose exposures to 2000r and 4000r created no changes; however, degenerative changes resulted from exposures to 6000r and 7000r. Many of the animals exhibited disequilibrium without nystagmus beginning one hour after exposure to 7000r. It was not determined whether the disequilibrium was due to injury to the labyrinth or to other parts of the central nervous system. Degenerative changes were seen as early as three hours after irradiation and were well developed at six hours. Sites of predilection were the external hair cells of the basal turns and the peripheral zones of the maculae and cristae. The type II hair cells appeared to be more sensitive to injury than the type I hair cells. In an animal experiment Kelemen (1963) demonstrated that high doses may result in hemorrhages and aseptic labyrinthitis.

A basic reaction to irradiation given at therapeutic levels is a vasculitis consisting of an inflammatory reaction in the endothelium of the blood vessels which leads at first to vasodilatation and later to obliteration of the vascular lumen.

The inflammatory changes in the skin of the auricle and external auditory canal and in the mucous membrane of the middle ear have been studied clinically (Borsanyi et al., 1961) and experimentally in animals (Nýlen et al., 1960;

Berg and Lindgren, 1961); however, the inner ear reactions to fractionated therapeutic dosages of irradiation have not been clearly documented.

2. LATE IRRADIATION REACTIONS

The late reactions of the temporal bone to irradiation consist of atrophy of the membranous labyrinth and osteoradionecrosis. Irradiation atrophy of the membranous labyrinth is an infrequent late complication consisting of a progressive hearing loss beginning soon after treatment and often progressing to profound deafness. The degenerative changes are particularly prominent in the spiral and annular ligaments. Severe atrophy of the spiral ligament may result in distortion and rupture of the cochlear duct leading to degeneration of the organ of Corti (Figs. 7.32, 7.33). Atrophy of the annular ligament may be severe and could conceivably lead to fistulization of the oval window (Figs. 7.34, 7.35).

Osteoradionecrosis may become clinically evident many years following x-ray treatment. Frey (1954) showed that single doses of 5000r given to one focus of bone causes immediate massive local necrosis. Even fractionated doses given at sufficiently high intensity to a small field result in bone necrosis, which develops insidiously. Histological changes in bone architecture following exposure to x-ray irradiation are (1) death of osteocytes resulting in empty lacunae; (2) disturbance of the normal dynamic changes of the tissue with a preponderance of osteolysis; (3) infiltration by a fibrillar connective tissue around spicules of dead or hypoactive bone; (4) decrease or total absence of new bone formation; and (5) loss of marrow substance. The reaction is one of bone necrosis with compensatory reparative fibrosis. The result is a tissue which is not only prone to injury and to spontaneous fracture but is highly susceptible to infection. Block (1952) described the development of irradiation osteitis in the mastoids of a patient 15 years after x-ray therapy for syringobulbia. Gyorkey and Pollock (1960) found absorption of the long process of the incus seven years after irradiation for a malignancy of the posterior cranial fossa. Schuknecht and Karmody (1966) reported osteoradionecrosis of the temporal bone in two patients 13 years and 4 years after therapy for malignancies which existed in adjacent areas.

Osteoradionecrosis of the temporal bone may constitute a life-threatening complication of irradiation therapy. Death of bone leads to sequestration and is usually followed by infection and a fetid discharge from the ear canal. Areas of bone resorption contain fibrous tissue, bone sequestrae, granulation tissue, and collections of pus (Figs. 7.36, 7.37). Squamous epithelium may invade the mastoid through fistulae of the external auditory canal (Fig. 7.38). Necrosis of the tegmen of the middle ear or mastoid leads to fistulization into the middle cranial fossa and intracranial infection (Fig. 7.39).

When cancercidal doses of irradiation are administered to bone in the treatment of malignant neoplasms, there will be an effect on normal bone. The temporal bone seems particularly susceptible to irradiation necrosis. It is readily infected from the external auditory canal and eustachian tube, and this in turn may lead to extension of infection to the cranial cavity. With current radiotherapeutic methods this complication may become less frequent, but it remains an important consideration in the management of patients with malignant disease in this area.

Fig. 7.32: At the age of 63 a radical mastoid-ectomy was performed for the partial removal of a glomus body tumor, and this was followed by the administration of 4000r (200 kv) of radiation therapy. At the time of treatment the patient exhibited a 50 to 60 db conductive hearing loss in this ear but no subsequent auditory tests were made. She died 10 years later at the age of 73 of cerebral hemorrhage. Histological study reveals severe atrophy of the spiral ligament throughout the cochlea, most severe on the medial side where the ligament is separated from the cochlear wall and displaced internally. There are hair cells in the middle and apical turns, but in some areas the organ of Corti is severely distorted because of atrophy of the spiral ligament. There is severe degeneration of the cochlear neurons in the basal turn. The stroma of the maculae and cristae show moderate loss of cellularity and replacement with cystic spaces, although the sensory epithelium appears normal. These atrophic changes are assumed to be caused by the irradiation treatments as the opposite ear shows only mild atrophy of the spiral ligament in the middle and apical turns. See also Figs. 7.34, 7.36.

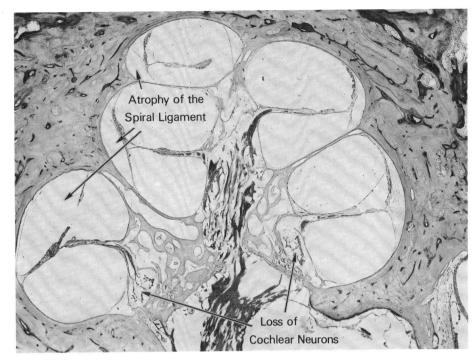

Fig. 7.33: At the age of 67 this patient received 5200r of x-ray treatment for carcinoma of the left parotid. The therapy was given in fractionated doses over a 12-day period. During an examination nine years later at the age of 76 he complained of hearing loss in the left ear. At the age of 77 he had a fetid discharge from the ear canal and areas of osteoradionecrosis of the temporal bone. He died of broncho-pneumonia at the age of 80, 13 years after irradiation therapy. Histological study reveals severe atrophy of the basilar membrane, spiral ligament and stria vascularis throughout the cochlea. The cochlear duct is ruptured in the middle turn. The organ of Corti is atrophied and shows a severe diffuse loss of hair cells. There is partial degeneration of both divisions of the vestibular nerve; however, the vestibular sense organs appear normal. Although no audiometric studies were done he had no complaints referable to his right ear. See also Figs. 7.35, 7.37, 7.38.

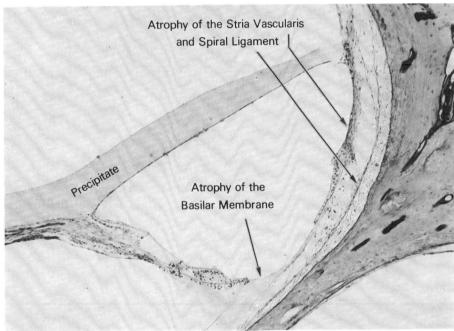

Fig. 7.34: For history see legend, Fig. 7.32. There is severe atrophy of the annular ligament ten years following 4000r x-ray therapy.

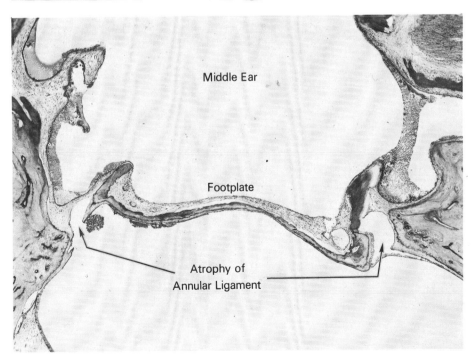

Fig. 7.35: For history see legend, Fig. 7.33. There is moderate atrophy of the annular ligament 13 years following 5200r of x-ray treatment.

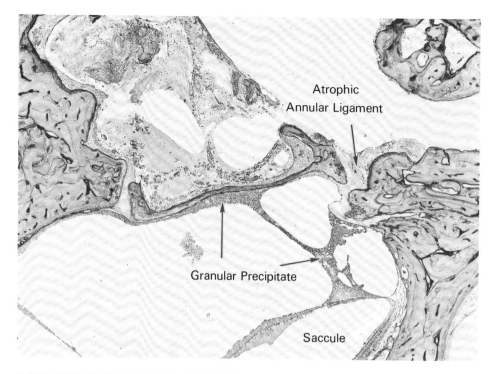

Fig. 7.36: For history see legend, Fig. 7.32. Ten years following the administration of 4000r to the temporal bone there is extensive resorption of the bony labyrinth. In the region of the semicircular canals, the osteolytic process extends to the endosteum; however, no fistulization has occurred. The mastoid bone is partly replaced by fibrous tissue. Glomus body tumor is present in the anterior part of the mastoid and infralabyrinthine areas. All structures of the membranous labyrinth show severe atrophic changes.

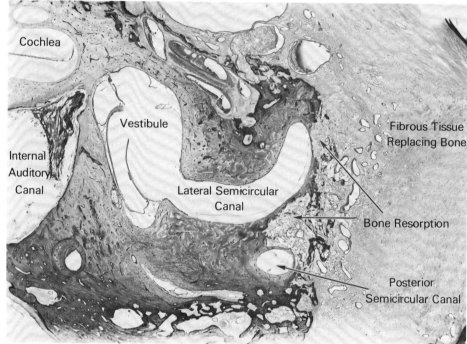

Fig. 7.37: For history see legend, Fig. 7.33. Thirteen years after the administration of 5200r there is severe osteoradionecrosis and infection of the temporal bone. In the mastoid there are numerous sequestrae surrounded by fibrous tissue. An abscess is seen in the area of the central mastoid tract. There is partial resorption of the bony labyrinth around the semicircular canals.

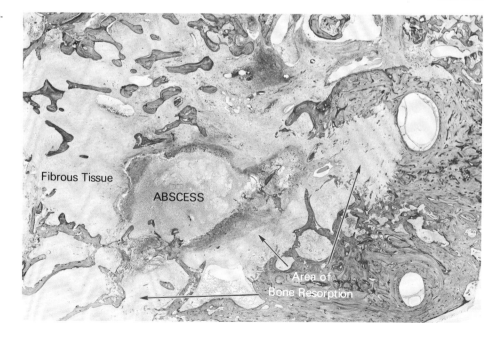

Fig. 7.38: For history see legend, Fig. 7.33. There is extensive destruction of the mastoid with deep invasion of squamous epithelium from the external auditory canal. There is an area of resorption of the posterior wall of the mastoid and thickening of the dura of the posterior cranial fossa.

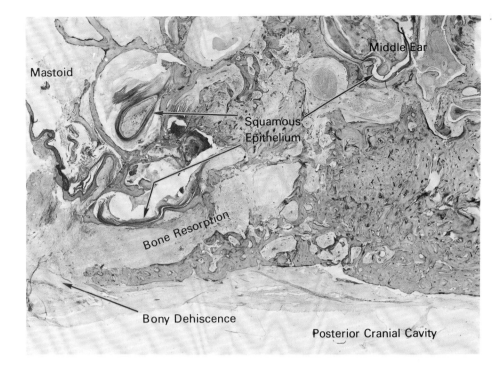

Fig. 7.39: At the age of 56 this individual received 6700r (200 kv) to the posterior wall of the right maxillary sinus for adenoid cystic carcinoma. Coincident with the therapy he noted tinnitus and hearing loss in the right ear. He died four years later of meningitis complicating osteoradionecrosis of the maxilla and temporal bone. Autopsy showed a fistulous tract in the tegmen tympani. Histological study shows the fistula to be located anterolateral to the geniculate ganglion. Its margins consist of devitalized spicules of bone embedded in fibrous tissue. There is resorption of bone in the anterior parts of the petrous, tympanic, and squamous portions of the temporal bone. Purulent fluid is seen throughout the middle ear and mastoid. The mastoid contains fibrous tissue and granulation tissue.

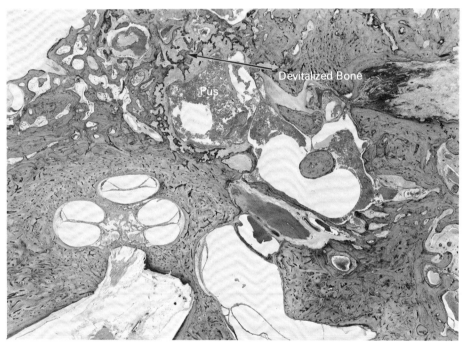

References

Åhrén, C., and Thulin, C.-A., 1965: Lethal intracranial complications following inflation in the external auditory canal in treatment of serous otitis media and due to defects in the petrous bone. Acta otolaryng. 60:407.

Alexander, A., and Scholl, R., 1938: Beschwerden und Störungen im Hör- und Gleichgewichtsorgan bei der Nachuntersuchung Schädelverletzter. Mschr. Ohrenheilk. 72:1021.

Alexander, G., 1928: Die Schussverletzungen des Ohres. Hdb. Neurol. Ohres. 2:449.

Altmann, F., 1946: Healing of fistulas of the human labyrinth: Histopathologic studies. Arch. Otolaryng. 43:409.

Altmann, F., and Waltner, J., 1945: Slight operative injuries of the stapes: Histopathologic study of a case. Arch. Otolaryng. 42:42.

Applebaum, E., 1960: Meningitis following trauma to the head and face. J. Amer. Med. Assn. 173:1818.

Armstrong, H., and Heim, J., 1937: Effect of flight on middle ear. J. Amer. Med. Assn. 109:417.

Arragg, F., and Paparella, M., 1964: Traumatic fracture of the stapes. Laryngoscope 74:1329.

Ballantyne, J., 1970: Iatrogenic deafness. J. Laryng. 84:967.

Bárány, R., 1921: Diagnose von Krankheitserscheinungen im Bereiche des Otolithenapparates. Acta oto-laryng. 2:434.

Barber, H., 1964: Positional nystagmus, especially after head injury. Laryngoscope 74:891.

Bayliss, G., 1968: Aural barotrauma in naval divers. Arch. Otolaryng. 88:141.

Beck, C., 1959a: Läsionen der Meerschwenchencochlea durch Kälteeinwirkung. Arch. Ohr. Nas.-KehlkHeilk. 174:169.

Beck, C., 1959b: Die Antwort des Cortischen Organs auf transkapsuläre Ultraschallapplikation (Experimentelle Untersuchungen am Meerschweinchen). Arch. Ohr. Nas.-KehlkHeilk. 174:173.

Berg, N., and Lindgren, M., 1961: Dose factors and morphology of delayed radiation lesions of the internal and middle ears in rabbits. Acta Radiol. 56:305.

Block, E., 1952: Rontgenschädigung des Schläfenbeines. Z. Hals-Nas.- Ohrenheilk. 3:45.

Borsanyi, S., Blanchard, C., and Thorne, B., 1961: The effects of ionizing radiation on the ear. Ann. Otol. Rhinol. Laryng. 70:255.

Brunner, H., 1940: Disturbances of the function of the ear after concussion of the brain. Laryngoscope 50:921.

Cawthorne, T., 1954: Positional nystagmus. Ann. Otol. Rhinol. Laryng. 63:481.

Committee on Conservation of Hearing of the American Academy of Ophthalmology and Otolaryngology, 1969: Guide for conservation of hearing in noise. Trans. Amer. Acad. Ophthal. Otolaryng. Suppl.

Covell, W., and Eldredge, D., 1951: Injury to animal ears by intense sound. Report from Aero Medical Laboratory, Research Division, U.S. Air Force, Wright-Patterson Air Force Base, Dayton, Ohio (No. 6561–July).

Crowe, S., Guild, S., and Polvogt, L., 1934: Observations on pathology of high-tone deafness. Bull. Johns Hopkins Hosp. 54:315.

Davis, H., Derbyshire, A., Kemp, E., Lurie, M., and Upton, M., 1935: Functional and histological changes in the cochlea of the guinea pig resulting from prolonged stimulation. J. Gen. Psychol. 12:251.

Davis, H., Morgan, C., Hawkins, J., Jr., Galambos, R., and Smith, F., 1950: Temporary deafness following exposure to loud tones and noise. Acta oto-laryng. Suppl. 88.

Denny-Brown, C., 1945: Disability arising from closed head injury. J. Amer. Med. Assn. 127:429.

Dickson, E., and King, P., 1954: Report 881, Flying Personnel Research Committee, Air Ministry, London.

Dix, M., and Hallpike, C., 1952: The pathology, symptomatology and diagnosis of certain common disorders of the vestibular system. Ann. Otol. Rhinol. Laryng. 61:987.

Ecker, A., 1947: Cerebrospinal rhinorrhea by way of the eustachian tube. J. Neurosurg. 4:177.

Eichel, B., and Landes, B., 1970: Sensorineural hearing loss caused by skin diving. Arch. Otolaryng. 92:128.

Escher, F., 1948: Die Otologische Beurteilung des Schädeltraumatikers. Pract. oto-rhino-laryng. Suppl. 1, vol. 10.

Fairman, H., Brown, N., and Hallpike, C., 1968: Air embolism as a complication of inflation of the tympanum through the external auditory meatus. Acta otolaryng. 66:65.

Fee, G., 1968: Traumatic perilymphatic fistulas. Arch. Otolaryng. 88:477.

Fischer, J., and Wolfsen, L., 1943: The Inner Ear. Grune and Stratton, New York.

Freeman, P., 1972: Personal communication.

Freeman, P., and Edmonds, C., 1972: Inner ear barotrauma. Arch. Otolaryng. 95:556.

Frey, J., 1954: Über die Kombinationsbehandlung von Rontgenspätschäden der Haut mit Kurzwellen und Vitamin E. Strahlentherapie 95:440.

Goldstein, A., and Mundie, J., 1971: Rupture of the tympanic membrane followed by sudden death. Arch. Otolaryng. 93:140.

Goodhill, V., 1971: Sudden deafness and round window rupture. Laryngoscope 81:1462.

Goodhill, V., Harris, I., Brockman, S., Hantz, O., 1973: Sudden deafness and labyrinthine window ruptures: audiovestibular observations. Ann. Otol. Rhinol. Laryng. 82:2.

Gordon, N., 1954: Post-traumatic vertigo, with special reference to positional nystagmus. Lancet 1:1216.

Gotten, N., 1956: Survey of 100 cases of whiplash injury after settlement of litigation. J. Amer. Med. Assn. 162:865.

Grove, W. E., 1939: Skull fractures involving the ear: a clinical study of 211 cases. Laryngoscope 49:678.

Gurdjian, E., and Lissner, H., 1946: Deformations of the skull in head injury studied by "stresscoat" technique, quantitative determinations. Surg. Gynec. Obstet. 83:219.

Gyorkey, J., and Pollock, F., 1960: Radiation necrosis of the ossicles. Arch. Otolaryng. 71:793.

Hasegawa, T., 1931: Die Veränderung der labyrinthären Reflexe bei zentrifugiertem Meerschweinchen. Pflügers Arch. ges. Physiol. 229:205.

Hellmann, K., 1922: Zur pathologishen Anatomie der Taubheit nach Kopfschuss. Z. Hals-Nas.-Ohrenheilk. 1:358.

Hempstead, B., 1932: Bullets in the ear. J. Amer. Med. Assn. 98:2281.

Hilding, A., 1953: Studies on the otic labyrinth; anatomic explanation for hearing dip at 4,096 characteristic of acoustic trauma and presbycusis. Ann. Otol. Rhinol. Laryng. 62:950.

Hofmann, L., 1925: Fracturen der Schläfenbein pyramide. Zbl. Hals-Nas.-Ohrenheilk. 7:539.

Hough, J., 1969: Restoration of hearing loss after head trauma. Ann. Otol. Rhinol. Laryng. 78:210.

Igarashi, M., 1965: Histopathological findings after experimental saccular destruction in the squirrel monkey. Laryngoscope 75:1048.

Igarashi, M., Schuknecht, H., and Myers, E., 1964: Cochlear pathology in humans with stimulation deafness. J. Laryng. 78:115.

Keim, R., 1969: Sensorineural hearing loss associated with firearms. Arch. Otolaryng. 90:581.

Kelemen, G., 1944: Fractures of the temporal bone. Arch. Otolaryng. 40:333.

Kelemen, G., 1963: Radiation and ear: Experimental studies. Acta oto-laryng.

Suppl. 184.

Kerr, A., 1967: Gunshot injury of the temporal bone: A histological report. J. Irish Med. Assn. 60:446.

King, P., 1966: Otitic barotrauma. Proc. Roy. Soc. Med. 59:543.

Kirikae, I., Eguchi, K., Okamoto, M., and Nakamura, K., 1969: Histopathological changes in the auditory pathway in cases of fatal head injury. Acta oto-laryng. 67:341.

Klestadt, A., 1913: Spätmeningitis nach Labyrinthfractur. Z. Ohrenheilk. 69:229.

Kley, W., 1968: Die Unfallchirurgie der Schädelbasis und der pneumatischen Räume. Arch. Klin. exp. Ohr. Nas.-KehlkHeilk. 191:1.

Kleyn, A. de, and Versteegh, C., 1933: Labyrinthreflex nach Abschleuderung der Otolithen Membrane bei Meerschweinchen. Pflüger Arch. ges Physiol. 232:454.

Klingenberg, A., 1929: Die Isolierte Schneckenfracture bei Schädelbasisbruchen. Z. Hals-Nas.-Ohrenheilk 22:452.

Koch, J., 1933: Studien über Veränderungen des Gehörorgans, inbesondere Störungen der Innenohrfunction nach Schädelunfallen mit und ohne Verletzung des Schläfenbeins. Arch. f. Ohrenh. 137:105.

Kohonen, A., 1970: Surgical luxation of the footplate of the stapes. Arch. Otolaryng. 91:242.

Kryter, K., 1965: Hazardous exposure to intermittent and steady-state noise, Report of working Group 46. Committee on Hearing, Bioacoustics and Biomechanics, Office of Naval Research, Washington, D.C.

Kryter, K., 1970: The Effects of Noise on Man. Academic Press, New York.

Kryter, K., Ward, W., Miller, J., and Eldredge, D., 1966: Hazardous exposure to intermittent and steady-state noise. J. Acoust. Soc. Amer. 39:451.

Lim, D., and Melnick, W., 1971: Acoustic damage of the cochlea: A scanning and transmission electron microscopic observation. Arch. Otolaryng. 94:294.

Linck, A., 1921: Beitrag zur klinik und Pathologie der Schädelbasisfrakturen. Z. Ohrenheilk. 81:265.

Lindquist, S., 1949: Stimulation deafness: A study of temporary and permanent hearing losses resulting from exposure to noise and blast impulses. Thesis. Department of Psychology, University of Chicago.

Lundgren, C., 1965: Alternobaric vertigo: a diving hazard. Brit. Med. J. 2:500.

Lurie, M., Davis, H., and Hawkins, J., Jr., 1944: Acoustic trauma of the organ of Corti in guinea pigs. Laryngoscope 54:375.

MacFie, D., 1964: ENT problems of diving. Med. J. Canada 20:845.

Mackay, R., 1963: Eustachian obstruction due to middle ear polyp. Arch. Otolaryng. 77:474.

Manasse, P., 1924: Schädelbasisfracture. Beitr. Anat. Physiol. Path. Therap. Ohr. 21:230.

Martin, R., 1940: Recent experiences with operation on the facial nerve. Arch. Otolaryng. 32:1071.

Merkle, U., 1954: Eine Methode zur morphologischen Erfassung der Ansprechgebiete in der Cochlea des Meerschweinchens. Z. Anat. EntwGesch. 117:504.

Misrahy, G., Shinabarger, W., and Arnold, I., 1958: Changes in cochlear endolymphatic oxygen availability action potential, and microphonics during and following asphyxia, hypoxia, and exposure to sounds. J. Acoust. Soc. Amer. 30:712.

Mizukoshi, O., Konishi, T., and Nakamura, F., 1957: Physico-chemical process in hair cells of the organ of Corti. Ann. Otol. Rhinol. Laryng. 66:106.

Mosher, W., 1942: Foreign bodies of external canal, middle ear and mastoid and their complications. Arch. Otolaryng. 36:679.

Nager, F., 1949: Zur Histologie der isolierten Schneckenfraktur. Pract. oto-rhino-laryng. 11:134.

Nassulphis, P., 1946: Die Schädigung des Innenohres und Seiner Nerven nach Schädeltrauma. Mschr. Ohrenheilk. 79:68 and 222.

Neubert, K., and Wuestenfeld, E., 1955: Nachweis der zellulaeren Ansprechgebiete im Innenohr. Naturwissenschaften 42:350.

Nylén, C., Engfeldt, B., and Larsson, B., 1960: The effect of local irradiation of the labyrinth in the rat with ionizing particles. Acta oto-laryng. Suppl. 158:217.

Oppenheim, H., 1902: Lehrbuch d. Nervenkrank. S. Karger, Berlin.

Paparella, M., 1961: A high-frequency microvibrator: Bioacoustical effects. Arch. Otolaryng. 74:220.

Paparella, M., 1962: Acoustic trauma from the bone cutting burr. Laryngoscope 72:116.

Parker, D., Covell, W., and Gierke, H. von., 1968: Exploration of vestibular damage in guinea pigs following mechanical stimulation. Acta oto-laryng. Suppl. 239.

Perlman, H., 1939: Process of healing in injuries to capsule of labyrinth. Arch. Otolaryng. 29:287.

Perlman, H., 1948: Minimal shock pulse trauma to the cochlea: Acute and chronic. Laryngoscope 58:466.

Proctor, B., Gurdjian, E., and Webster, J., 1956: The ear in head trauma. Laryngoscope 66:16

Pullen, F., II, 1972: Round window membrane rupture: a cause of sudden deafness. Trans. Amer. Acad. Ophth. Otol. 76:1444.

Pullen, F., II, 1973: Personal communication.

Rüedi, L., and Furrer, W., 1946: Das akustische Trauma. Pract. Oto-rhino-laryng. 8:177.

Russell, W., 1954: Studies on head injury. Brit. med. Bull. 10:65.

Rutin, E., 1937: Zur Klinik der Schläfenbeinbruche. Mschr. Ohrenheilk 71:179.

Schlittler, E., 1936: Labyrinthzersplitterung-isolierte Vestibularfraktur-Spätmeningitis nach 16 Jahren. Acta oto-laryng. 24:213.

Schuknecht, H., 1950: A clinical study of auditory damage following blows to the head. Ann. Otol. Rhinol. Laryng. 59:331.

Schuknecht, H., 1962: Positional vertigo: clinical and experimental observations. Trans. Amer. Acad. Ophthal. Otolaryng. 66:319.

Schuknecht, H., 1969: Cupulolithiasis.. Arch. Otolaryng. 90:765.

Schuknecht, H., 1972a: Unpublished data.

Schuknecht, H., 1972b: Unpublished data.

Schuknecht, H., and Davison, R., 1956: Deafness and vertigo from head injury. Arch. Otolaryng. 63:513.

Schuknecht, H., and Karmody, C., 1966: Radionecrosis of the temporal bone. Laryngoscope 76:1416.

Schuknecht, H., Neff, W., and Perlman, H., 1951: An experimental study of auditory damage following blows to the head. Ann. Otol. Rhinol. Laryng. 60:273.

Schuknecht, H., and Tonndorf, J., 1960: Acoustic trauma of the cochlea from ear surgery. Laryngoscope 70:479.

Schwartze, H., 1892: Handbuch der Ohrenheilkunde. F. C. W. Vogel, Leipzig.

Scott-Brown, W., Ballantyne, J., and Groves, J., 1965: Diseases of the Ear, Nose and Throat. Vol. II. Appleton-Century-Crofts, New York.

Siebenmann, F., Yoshii, U., 1908: Demonstration von experimentellen akustischen Schädigungen des Gehörorganes. Verh. dtsch. Ges. Otolog. 17:114.

Silverstein, H., 1973: Penetrating wounds of the tympanic membrane and ossicular chain. Trans. Am. Acad. Ophth. and Otolar. 77:ORL, 125.

Simmons, F., 1968: Theory of membrane breaks in sudden hearing loss. Arch. Otolaryng. 88:41.

Simpson, J., 1942: Discussion on effects of flying on nose and ear. Proc. Roy. Soc. Med. 35:245.

Sims, R., 1961: Otitis barotrauma in divers. Med. J. Austr. 2:1040.

Singleton, G., and Schuknecht, H., 1959: Experimental fracture of the stapes in cats. Ann. Otol. Rhinol. Laryng. 68:1069.

Smith, K., 1947: The problem of stimulation deafness. II. Histological changes in the cochlea as a function of tonal frequency. J. Exp. Psychol. 37:304.

Soss, S., 1971: Sensorineural hearing loss with diving. Arch. Otolaryng. 93:501.

Spoendlin, H., 1958: Submikroskopische Veränderungen am Corti'schen Organ des Meerschweinchens nach akustischer Belastung. Pract. oto-rhino-laryng. 20:197.

Spoendlin, H., 1971: Primary structural changes in the organ of Corti after acoustic overstimulation. Acta oto-laryng. 71:166.

Stenger, P., 1909: Beitrag zur Kenntnis der nach Kopfverletzungen auftretenden Veränderungen im Inneren Ohr. Arch. Ohrenheilk. 79:43.

Stockwell, C., Ades, H., and Engström, H., 1969: Patterns of hair cell damage after intense auditory stimulation. Ann. Otol. Rhinol. Laryng. 78:1144.

Stucker, F., and Echols, W., 1969: Clinical trends. Vol. 8.

Taylor, G., and Williams, E., 1966: Acoustic trauma in the sports hunter. Laryngoscope 76:863.

Theodore, E., 1910: Beitrag zur Pathologie der Labyrinthershutterung. Z. Ohrenheilk. 61:299.

Toglia, J., Rosenberg, P., and Ronis, M., 1970: Post traumatic dizziness: vestibular, audiologic and medicolegal aspects. Arch. Otolaryng. 92:485.

Ulrich, K., 1926: Verletzungen des Gehörsorgans bei Schädelbasisfrakturen. Acta oto-laryng. Suppl. 6.

Upton, M., 1929: Functional disturbances of hearing in guinea pigs after long exposure to an intense tone. J. Gen. Psychol. 2:397.

Voss, O., 1936: Die Chirurgie der Schädelbasisfrakturen. Ambrosius Barth, Leipzig.

Vosteen, K., 1958: Die Erschoepfung der Phonoreceptoren nach funktioneller Belastung. Arch. Nas.-KehlkHeilk. 172:489.

Ward, W., 1968: Proposed damage-risk criterion for impulse noise (gunfire). Report NAS-NRC Committee on Hearing, Bioacoustics and Biomechanics, no. 57, Office of Naval Research, Washington, D.C.

Wever, E., and Smith, K., 1944: The problem of stimulation deafness. I. Cochlear impairment as a function of tonal frequency. J. Exp. Psychol. 34:239.

Windle, W., Groat, R., and Fox, C., 1944: Experimental structural alterations in the brain during and after concussion. Surg. Gynec. Obstet. 79:561.

Winther, F., 1969a: Early degenerative

changes in the inner ear sensory cells of the guinea pig following local x-ray irradiation. Acta oto-laryng. 67:262.

Winther, F., 1969b: X-ray irradiation of inner ear of the guinea pig. Acta oto-laryng. 68:514.

Winther, F., 1970a: X-ray irradiation of the inner ear of the guinea pig: An electron microscopic study of the degenerating outer hair cells of the organ of Corti. Acta oto-laryng. 69:61.

Winther, F., 1970b: X-ray irradiation of the inner ear of the guinea pig: An electron microscopic study of the degenerating vestibular sensory cell. Acta oto-laryng. 69:307.

Wittmaack, K., 1909: Über die Veränderungen im Innen Ohr nach Rotationen. Verh. Dtsch. ges. Otol. 18:150.

Wittmaack, K., 1932: Über die traumatische Labyrinthdegenration. Arch. Ohr. Nas.-KehlkHeilk. 131:59.

Wright, J., Taylor, C., and Bizal, J., 1969: Tomography and the vulnerable incus. Ann. Otol. Rhinol. Laryng. 78:263.

Zorzoli, G., and Oriani, A., 1958: Recherches histochemiques sur les cellules ciliees de l'organe de Corti soumises a des stimulations acoustiques. Rev. Laryng. 79:213.

8 Disorders of Circulation

A. HEMORRHAGE

1. HEMORRHAGE INTO THE MIDDLE EAR

There are a variety of diseases and injuries which produce hemorrhage into the middle ear. It is particularly common with bleeding disorders such as leukemia, thrombocytopenic purpura, and hemophilia.

Fracture of the temporal bone is commonly associated with hemorrhage into the middle ear. With longitudinal fractures the tympanic membrane is frequently torn and there is bleeding from the ear. With transverse fractures the tympanic membrane frequently remains intact, resulting in hemotympanum manifested by the characteristic bluish discoloration of the tympanic membrane.

Bleeding into the middle ear may occasionally follow middle ear surgery, such as stapedectomy or exploratory tympanotomy, resulting in a postoperative hemotympanum. Ordinarily this complication does not adversely affect the results of surgery, as the blood is resorbed spontaneously or drains from the eustachian tube in ten to fifteen days.

Hemotympanum may follow the introduction of tight anterior and posterior nasal packing for epistaxis. Continuous bleeding forces blood up the eustachian tube and into the middle ear space. Again resolution is complete in ten to fifteen days.

Idiopathic hemotympanum is a poorly understood disorder that is considered to be a variant of seromucinous otitis media which is discussed in Chapter 6. It is characterized by the insidious development of a bluish fluid in the pneumatized spaces of the temporal bone. The bluish, brownish, or yellowish discoloration of the fluid is presumably caused by hemolyzed blood. Exploratory mastoidectomy has frequently revealed one or more discrete granulomas in the mastoid cells. Characteristically, these granulomas contain numerous cholesterol clefts and are highly vascularized. It is presumed that the bleeding is from these granulomas; however, it is not known whether these granulomas have a causal relationship or are a consequence of the seromucinous otitis media. Surgical removal of the granulomas has been reported to have successfully eliminated the condition in some ears but not in others (Paparella and Lim, 1967).

Spontaneous hemorrhage into the inner ear occurs mainly as a complication of bleeding diseases or of diseases which are characterized by hemorrhages in their terminal stages, the most common being leukemia. Hemorrhage associated with varying degrees of degenerative change have been found in the inner ears of leukemic patients by Steinbrugge (1886), Schwabach (1897), Finlaysin (1898), Kock (1905), Alexander (1906), Nishio (1926) and Paparella et al. (1973). In 1928, Fraser reported on four patients with leukemia who developed unilateral hearing losses. The temporal bones of two patients, one who died fourteen days after the hearing loss and the other seven days after the hearing loss showed "degeneration of the ganglion cells but no evidence of hemorrhage". Druss (1945) found otologic complications in 25 of 148 patients with leukemia. The changes consisted of acute otitis media, leukemic infiltration of the middle and inner ear structures, and hemorrhage into the middle and inner ears. Hallpike and Harrison (1950) found an extensive cellular infiltrate, possibly due to hemorrhage, in the inner ears of a leukemic patient who experienced a sudden vertiginous episode ten days prior to death.

Schuknecht et al. (1965) reported the findings in the temporal bones of an 11-year-old girl with leukemia who experienced sudden profound hearing loss in her right ear six days prior to death. There was a massive hemorrhage in the perilymphatic spaces of the inner ear; however, no blood was found in the cochlear duct and there were no morphological changes in the organ of Corti or spiral ganglion except those characteristic of postmortem autolysis (Fig. 8.1). The invasion of blood into the perilymphatic space appears to render the auditory sense organ nonfunctional, possibly because of alterations in chemistry.

Histological study of the temporal bone of a 69-year-old patient with Wegener's granulomatosis, who experienced a severe prolonged vertiginous episode six weeks before death, demonstrates an organizing blood clot in the vestibular labyrinth (Fig. 8.2). Neither history nor histological study indicated involvement of the cochlea.

It seems doubtful that spontaneous hemorrhage is a common cause for sudden deafness in healthy individuals. In none of our seven temporal bones from healthy individuals with sudden deafness is there evidence of blood or fibrosis which would indicate that hemorrhage had occurred into the inner ear. [see discussions on Viral labyrinthitis (Chapter 5C2), Sudden deafness of vascular etiology (this chapter), and Sudden Deafness (Chapter 12C)].

It is apparent that inner ear hemorrhage can result from a head blow without fracture of the bony labyrinth. Schuknecht et al. (1951) demonstrated hemorrhages in the perilymphatic spaces of five of nine cats receiving experimental head blows. Blood was found in the endolymphatic space (cochlear duct) of one animal. In none of these animals was there evidence of fracture of the temporal bone. By plotting the location of the blood in cochlear reconstructions it was demonstrated that blood had collected in adjacent parts of the three cochlear turns (Fig. 8.3). The location of the blood was not spatially correlated with areas of injury to the organ of Corti or cochlear neurons (Fig. 8.4). It appears that the red blood corpuscles were free to respond to gravitational forces and settled to adjacent parts of the cochlear turns where they were fixed during histological preparation of the ear. The animals were killed at times varying from three days to five months following head blows, and it was found that the white blood cells disappeared from hemorrhages that were older than three weeks. Even after five months there was no evidence of fibrous tissue proliferation (Fig. 8.5). Although red blood corpuscles normally have a life expectancy of about 120 days in the vascular system, they apparently persist for extended periods of time in the perilymphatic fluid. It would seem probable, however, that massive hemorrhages might interfere with the inner ear fluid physiology or biochemistry and incite de-

Fig. 8.1: This 11-year-old girl with acute leukemia experienced sudden hearing loss in the right ear six days before death. Examination showed a fine horizontal nystagmus to the left and total loss of hearing in the right ear (left masked with Bárány noise apparatus). Histological study of the right ear shows a massive collection of blood in the perilymphatic spaces and smaller hemorrhages in the endolymphatic spaces of the posterior semicircular canal and saccule. Reissner's membrane is intact. The hair cells of the organ of Corti and vestibular sense organs, as well as the cochlear and vestibular nerves, appear normal.

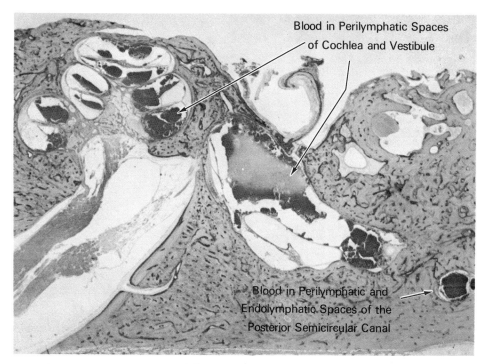

Blood in Perilymphatic Spaces of Cochlea and Vestibule

Blood in Perilymphatic and Endolymphatic Spaces of the Posterior Semicircular Canal

Fig. 8.2: At the age of 69 this woman with Wegener's granulomatosis, while standing motionless in her home, experienced a sudden severe attack of vertigo and fell to the floor. She did not lose consciousness but remained severely vertiginous for several hours and finally summoned neighbors by shouting. The disequilibrium subsided gradually over a three-week period and she died six weeks after the attack. Histological studies show collections of red blood cells in the perilymphatic spaces of the vestibule and semicircular canals. Within and surrounding the areas of hemorrhage is a network of loose fibrous tissue containing numerous pigment-laden macrophages and a few capillaries. There is severe degeneration of the cristae of the superior and lateral semicircular canals. The maculae of the utricle and saccule have normal hair cell populations.

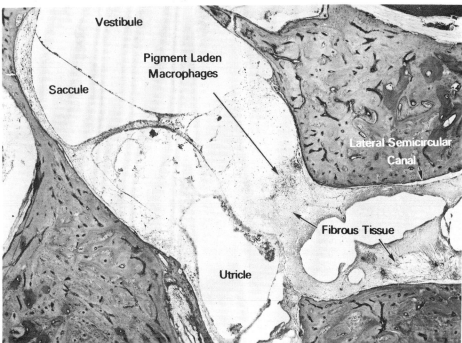

Vestibule

Pigment Laden Macrophages

Saccule

Lateral Semicircular Canal

Fibrous Tissue

Utricle

generative change in the sensory and neural structures. Likewise, bleeding from important nutrient vessels would probably result in associated ischemia of structures in the inner ear with resulting degeneration and fibrosis. The introduction of moderate amounts of blood into the inner ear at the time of surgery during stapedectomy, for example, does not appear to cause damage to the inner ear (Linthicum and Sheehy, 1969).

3. SUBARACHNOID HEMORRHAGE

Acute subarachnoid hemorrhage causes severe head pain which usually overshadows all other symptoms; however, some patients complain of vertigo. It has not been determined if this is a true vestibular disorder and, if so, if it is caused by central or peripheral involvement of the vestibular system.

It is known that cochlear aqueduct is larger and more often patent in the newborn infant. Voss (1926) studied 30 temporal bones from infants who died from birth trauma and found blood in the scala tympani of the basal turns in every case. Smutneva (1951), in a study of 15 newborns who died as the result

Fig. 8.3: Graphic reconstruction to show the location of red blood cells in the cochlea of a cat six weeks following an experimental blow to the head. Presumably, following the intra-cochlear hemorrhage, the red blood corpuscles were free to respond to gravitational forces and settled to the dependent parts of each cochlear turn where they were fixed by intra-vital perfusion.

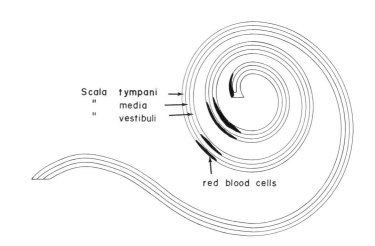

Scala tympani →
" media →
" vestibuli →

red blood cells

Fig. 8.4: Red blood cell mass in the scala tympani of the middle turn of the cochlea of a cat three weeks following an experimental blow to the head. The sensory and neural structures in the area of the blood mass appear normal.

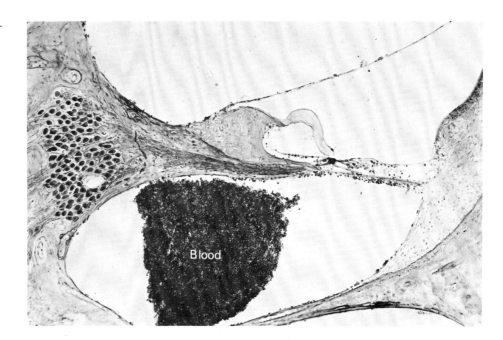

Blood

Fig. 8.5: Blood in the scala tympani of the basal turn of a cat five months following an experimental blow to the head. The severe inner ear concussion resulted in immediate profound hearing loss as determined by behavioral testing. The degenerative changes in the sensory and neural structures and the tear of Reissner's membrane are characteristic of severe stimulation injury.

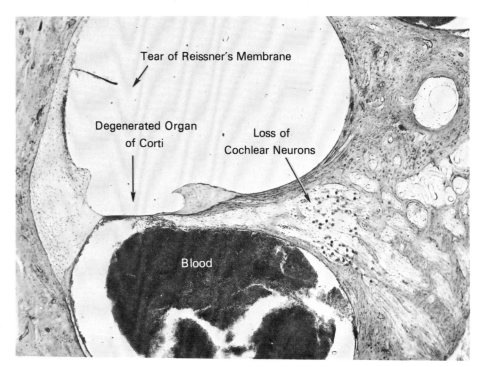

Tear of Reissner's Membrane

Degenerated Organ of Corti

Loss of Cochlear Neurons

Blood

Fig. 8.6: Spontaneous subarachnoid hemorrhage. This 44-year-old man, in apparent good health, suddenly experienced head pain and vertigo, lapsed into coma, and died 16 days later. Each ear showed extravascular blood in the internal auditory canal, cochlear aqueduct and scala tympani. The cochlear aqueduct of the right ear measured 266 microns in diameter at the isthmus.

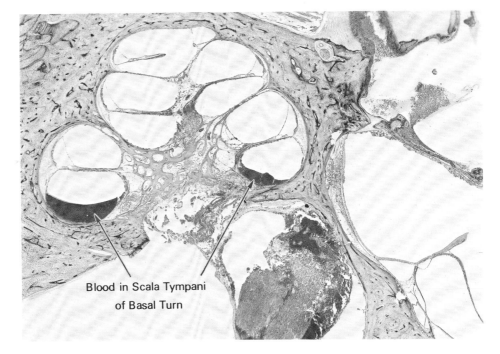

Blood in Scala Tympani
of Basal Turn

Fig. 8.7: Spontaneous subarachnoid hemorrhage. This 67-year-old woman developed severe headache, vomiting, vertigo, lapsed into coma, and died seven days later. The right ear, which was removed for study shows extravascular blood in Rosenthal's canal, the modiolar spaces, and the osseous spiral lamina. No blood is seen in the inner ear. The cochlear aqueduct measured 134 microns in diameter at the isthmus.

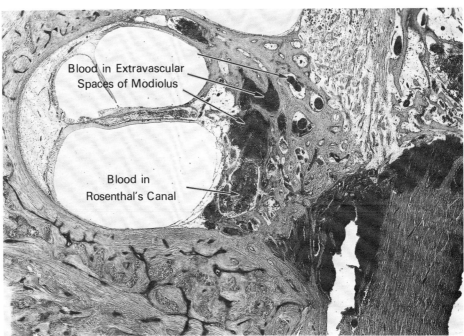

Blood in Extravascular
Spaces of Modiolus

Blood in
Rosenthal's Canal

Fig. 8.8: This 53-year-old woman died two days after spontaneous subarachnoid hemorrhage. Both temporal bones show massive hemorrhages in the internal auditory canals with extravascular blood extending into the spaces of the modioli and the subepithelial layers of the vestibular sense organs. This view shows extravascular blood extending into the subepithelial stroma of the saccular macula. The cochlear aqueduct of the ear, shown in this view, measured 164 microns in diameter at the isthmus.

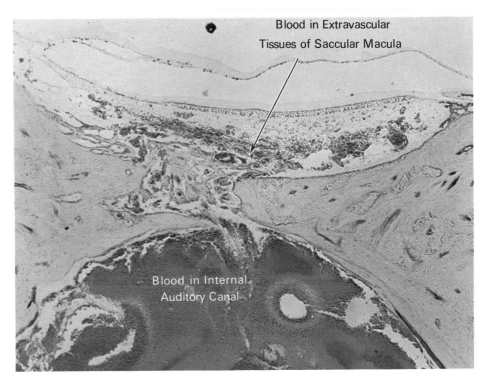

Blood in Extravascular
Tissues of Saccular Macula

Blood in Internal
Auditory Canal

of intracranial hemorrhage, found all to have blood in the internal auditory canals and cochleae. Blood is commonly found in the scala tympani of the basal turn following skull fracture (Ulrich, 1926), after intracranial surgery (Crowe, 1930), and after subarachnoid hemorrhage (Perlman and Lindsay, 1939).

Holden and Schuknecht (1968) studied the blood distribution pattern in twelve ears from patients who had suffered spontaneous subarachnoid hemorrhage and found that blood had entered the inner ears of six, all of which had patent cochlear aqueducts (Fig. 8.6). Blood was found in the internal auditory canals in all ears and had entered Rosenthal's canals in seven. It was also found in the osseous spiral lamina in three, all of which possessed small cochlear aqueducts, suggesting that circulation between the cerebrospinal fluid and perilymph occurred through the internal auditory canals and modioli in these ears (Fig. 8.7). Each of these ears with blood in the osseous spiral lamina had an eosinophilic precipitate in the scala tympani, suggesting that blood serum may have entered that area from the modiolus, possibly through the pores of the inferior shelf of the osseous spiral lamina (Schuknecht and El Seifi, 1963). Blood was found around the trunks of the vestibular nerves as far as the subepithelial layers of the saccular macula (Fig. 8.8) and the crista of the posterior semicircular canal. It was located within the perineural spaces of the fallopian canal as far as the descending part of the facial nerve (Fig. 8.9). There was no evidence that the subarachnoid hemorrhage had damaged the sensory or neural elements of the inner ears.

The findings of this study suggest that there is a free interchange between cerebrospinal fluid and perilymph. When the cochlear aqueduct is sufficiently large, the fluid interchange is through this channel; however, when the cochlear aqueduct is small, the interchange is primarily via the internal auditory canal and the fluid spaces of the modiolus. Particulate matter such as red blood corpuscles, on the other hand, can reach the inner ear via the cochlear aqueduct but not via the internal auditory canal.

B. VASCULAR STASIS OR OCCLUSION

1. SUDDEN DEAFNESS OF VASCULAR ETIOLOGY

Sudden deafness, when produced by vascular lesions, usually occurs in association with known systemic vascular disease. For example, massive inner ear hemorrhage has been identified as a cause for sudden deafness in leukemia (Schuknecht et al., 1965). Sudden deafness may also occur in Buerger's disease (thromboangiitis obliterans) (Kirikae et al., 1962), macroglobulinemia (Ruben et al., 1969; Schuknecht, unpublished observation), disorders characterized by hyperviscosity of the blood serum (Solomon and Fahey, 1963; Wilkinson et al., 1966), fat emboli, and hypercoagulation (Jaffe, 1970). Sudden deafness has been observed to follow a surgical procedure, such as a laparotomy, which is suggestive but not certain, of an embolic phenomenon.

The role, if any, of vascular lesions in the etiology of sudden deafness occurring in healthy individuals remains unknown. Lindsay and Zuidema (1950) studied the clinical features of 16 cases of sudden deafness and found that four were associated with systemic diseases and twelve were unexplainable. They concluded that the high incidence of the disorder in healthy adults under the age of 30 argues against a vascular etiology.

2. OCCLUSION OF THE ANTERIOR VESTIBULAR ARTERY

In 1956 Lindsay and Hemenway described a symptom complex observed in patients in the latter decades of life which they suspected was caused by occlusion of a vessel that supplies the vestibular labyrinth. The disorder was manifested by the sudden onset of severe vertigo without deafness or signs of

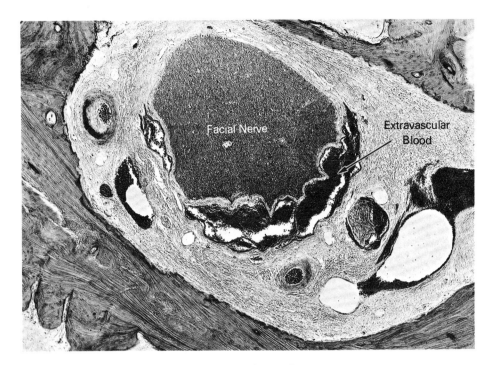

Fig. 8.9: Same patient as Fig. 8.8. Extravascular blood is found in the perineural region of the facial nerve as far distally as the middle of its vertical segment.

central nervous system disease and was followed by gradual recovery during the subsequent weeks. The clinical picture was consistent with that known to result from sudden destruction of one vestibular labyrinth. A further manifestation of the syndrome was the development of positional vertigo several weeks following the original attack and persisting for weeks or years. The pathological findings of the temporal bones from a patient with this syndrome showed severe degeneration of the utricular macula, the cristae of the lateral and superior semicircular canals, and the superior division of the vestibular nerve, all of which are supplied by the anterior vestibular artery (Fig. 8.10). Schuknecht (1962, 1969) suggested that ischemic necrosis of the utricular macula results in a release of otoconia which settle upon the cupula of the posterior semicircular canal to cause the positional vertigo (Chapter 12B, Cupulolithiasis). (See also Fig. 8.11.)

3. LATERAL MEDULLARY SYNDROME (WALLENBERG'S SYNDROME)

The lateral medullary syndrome is due to occlusion by embolism or thrombosis of either the vertebral or posterior inferior cerebellar artery, more commonly the former (Fisher et al., 1961). The symptoms may develop gradually or suddenly and consist of headache, pain in the side of the face, vertigo, vomiting, diplopia, dysphagia, and dysphonia, without loss of consciousness. Typical findings include (1) ipsilateral analgesia of the face due to injury to the descending spinal tract of the trigeminal nerve; (2) ipsilateral ptosis, enophthalmos, and miosis from a lesion of the reticular formation which contains sympathetic fibers from the hypothalamus to the spinal cord; (3) contralateral analgesia and thermanesthesia of the trunk and extremities from involvement of the crossed spinothalamic fibers; (4) ipsilateral paralysis of the soft palate, pharynx, and larynx due to involvement of the nucleus ambiguus and emerging fibers of the IXth and Xth cranial nerves; and (5) variable involvement of the VIth, VIIth, and VIIIth cranial nerves (Hiller, 1952; Grinker and Sahs, 1966).

Hallpike (1965) performed vestibular tests on eight subjects with this syndrome. All had severe vertigo at the time of onset, and tests demonstrated that all had directional preponderance to the side opposite the lesion. Serial sections of the brain stems showed that the lesions involved the descending vestibular nuclei and the caudal parts of the medial vestibular nuclei. These nuclei, according to Brodal et al. (1962) and Gacek (1969), receive their afferent fibers from the utricle. It was proposed by Carmichael et al. (1965), therefore, that the lesions involved the utricular tonus elements and thus

Fig. 8.10: At the age of 65 this woman experienced sudden onset of severe vertigo associated with vomiting. The vertigo gradually subsided over a period of one month following which she had vertiginous episodes on assuming the supine position with the head turned to the right. The vertigo was readily demonstrated by positional testing. Caloric response was absent in the right ear. The positional vertigo continued until her death thirteen years later. Histological study of the right ear shows degeneration of the superior division of the vestibular nerve, the utricular macula, and the cristae of the superior and lateral semicircular canals. It is presumed that this patient suffered occlusion of the right anterior vestibular artery. The left ear appears normal. (Courtesy of Lindsay and Hemenway)

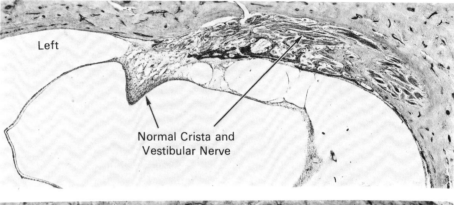

Fig. 8.11: At the age of 73 this individual experienced a severe attack of vertigo associated with nausea and vomiting. Six months later she complained of recurring vertiginous episodes, and examination revealed nystagmus and vertigo in the supine, right-ear-down position. There was latency of six seconds and duration of ten seconds. She died at the age of 87, and histological studies of the right ear show severe degeneration of the superior division of the vestibular nerve and the sense organs supplied by it (utricle, superior and lateral canals). There is a small basophilic deposit on the cupula of the right posterior semicircular canal. The left inner ear appears normal.

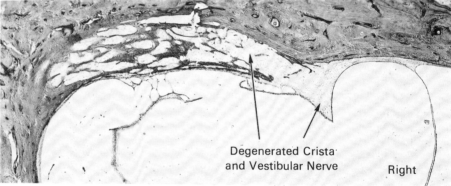

created a deviation of the eyes toward the side of the lesion. Thus, under the conditions of testing with eyes in the straight-ahead position, the eyes are subjected to the directional distortion which facilitates contralateral nystagmus, thereby explaining directional preponderance.

All patients had normal hearing, indicating that the bulk of the lesion was situated below the level of entry into the brain stem of the cochlear nerve.

4. OCCLUSION OF THE ANTERIOR INFERIOR CEREBELLAR ARTERY

The onset of this syndrome is sudden, with or without premonitory symptoms and usually is not accompanied by loss of consciousness. Vertigo is the first and most important symptom and often is associated with nausea and vomiting. The other principal symptoms are facial paralysis, hearing loss, sensory disturbances, and cerebellar asynergia, all of which appear in a few hours. The vertigo and hearing loss are caused by degenerative changes in the auditory and vestibular nuclei in the brain stem and to ischemic necrosis of the membranous labyrinth.

Ipsilateral loss of pain and temperature sensation on the face, as well as corneal hypesthesia are caused by interruption of the spinal tract and nucleus of the trigeminal nerve. Partial loss of pain and temperature sensation on the contralateral side of the body is due to partial involvement in varying degrees of the inferior and middle cerebellar peduncles (Adams, 1943).

The clinical course is one of gradual improvement over a variable period. The disorder by itself is rarely fatal, but the hypertensive and arteriosclerotic vascular disease, which is the usual pathologic basis for the vascular occlusion of the artery, often leads to other serious and often fatal complications.

5. VERTEBROBASILAR ISCHEMIA

Vertigo is a common symptom of vertebrobasilar ischemia or infarction (Weiss, 1968). Although the initial episode may have no associated visual, sensory, or somatic motor disturbances, they usually occur within a few days of onset (Barber and Dionne, 1971). Therefore, when repeated vertiginous episodes occur without the development of additional neurological findings, the diagnosis of ischemic vertebrobasilar disease is less probable.

Fields (1966) has suggested that the reason the vestibular nuclei are particularly vulnerable to ischemia is that they are situated far laterally in the pons and are supplied by long thin vessels devoid of branching. The most common cause for decreased blood flow is atherosclerosis of the vertebral or basilar arteries; however, mechanical compression of these vessels by cervical spondylosis with hyperextension or extreme rotation of the neck may be responsible in some cases. The diagnosis can sometimes be confirmed by arteriography. Transient vertigo may occur with momentary drops in blood pressure in the vertebrobasilar system such as with orthostatic hypotension, Stokes-Adams attacks, and the subclavian steal syndrome; however, in these cases the vertigo is overshadowed by the more severe signs of brain stem ischemia.

Stenosis or occlusion of the subclavian or innominate arteries proximal to the origin of the vertebral artery may result in the thyrocervical steal syndrome and basilar ischemia. Normally, the blood pressure in the vertebral artery is greater at its origin and lesser at the origin of the basilar artery, resulting in a cephalad flow of blood. When the blood pressure is reduced because of stenosis or occlusion of the subclavian or innominate arteries, the blood flow may be reversed, which in effect siphons blood from the basilar junction and deprives the basilar artery of effective blood supply. The usual underlying pathology is atherosclerotic occlusive vascular disease of the subclavian or innominate arteries, although arteritis, dissecting aneurysm, or syphilis may give rise to the condition. The most common symptom is vertigo (Trevino, 1970), although it is rarely an isolated finding. Other symptoms are diplopia, blurred vision, transient hemianopsia, headaches, syncope, speech difficulties, and hemiparesis. A constant finding in the syndrome is a difference in blood pressure and pulses between the two upper extremities.

6. DISORDERS OF THE MAJOR VESSELS

a. Carotid artery

Stallings and McCabe (1969) and Conley and Hildyard (1969) have described congenital aneurysms of the internal carotid artery. The surgical significance of these lesions is obvious, for incision or laceration of such a mass by the unsuspecting surgeon could lead to serious neurological complications or death. The true nature of this pulsatile mass can best be determined by carotid arteriogram.

Atherosclerosis of the internal carotid artery is a common finding in the temporal bones of individuals past the age of fifty. The incidence is directly

Fig. 8.12: Severe atherosclerosis of the internal carotid artery in a woman who died of cerebral hemorrhage at the age of 70. The lesion is characterized by lipoid deposition, fibrous proliferation, and calcification of the arterial wall.

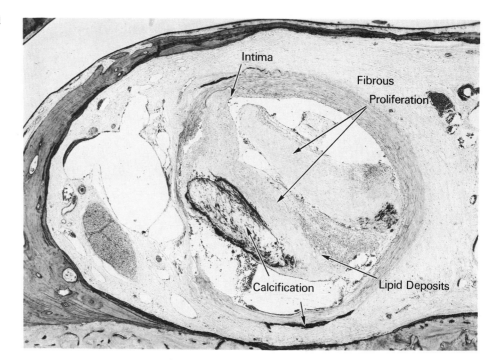

Fig. 8.13: Atrophy of the wall of the internal carotid artery in a woman who experienced a myocardial infarct at the age of 60 and at the age of 67 developed angina and heart failure. She died of a second myocardial infarct at the age of 72. The arterial wall is not atrophied in those regions where it is separated from bone by a layer of soft tissue. See Fig. 8.14.

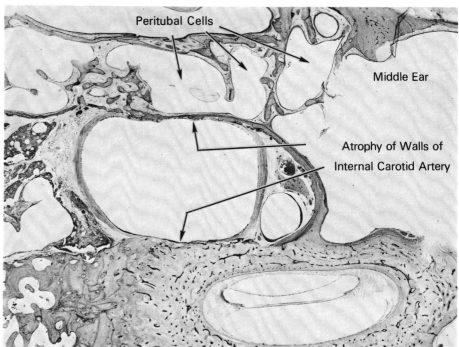

Fig. 8.14: Higher-power view of the internal carotid artery shown in Fig. 8.13. On the medial and lateral sides, the arterial wall consists only of a layer of endothelium lying directly on the bone of the carotid canal.

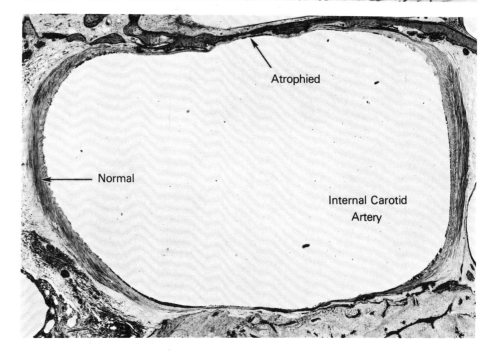

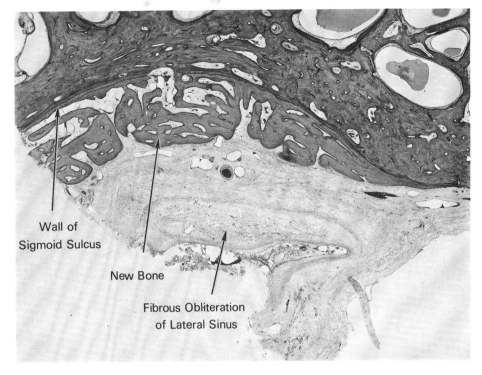

Wall of
Sigmoid Sulcus

New Bone

Fibrous Obliteration
of Lateral Sinus

related to age, as would be expected. Atherosclerosis is the most common alteration of arteriosclerosis and consists of intimal lipidosis and fibrosis. As lipid accumulates in the intima there is fibrous tissue proliferation near the inner surface. The fibrous layer often shows hyalinization and as it grows may form a thick plaque which bulges into the lumen of the artery. Calcification is often a conspicuous part of the atheromatous process and tends to occur in fibrous tissue at the margins of lipid accumulations (Radpour et al., 1962) (Fig. 8.12). Atherosclerosis of the internal carotid artery in its severest form may cause cerebral ischemia; however, it produces no specific otological manifestations.

Atrophy of the walls of the internal carotid artery would seem to have equal, if not more serious, implications for the otologic surgeon. This condition does not appear to be related to atherosclerosis. It is characterized by progressive thinning of the medial layer of the arterial wall. As the wall stretches, it comes to lie against the bony wall of the carotid canal. Finally the arterial wall may consist of only a thin endothelial layer lying directly on the bone of the carotid canal. Possibly the atrophic change is caused by the pulsating contact of the artery against the bony wall, because it does not occur in those regions where the arterial wall is separated from bone by soft tissue (Figs. 8.13, 8.14).

b. Lateral venous sinus

The principal disorders of the lateral venous sinus and jugular bulb are phlebitis, thrombosis, and abscess formation in association with infections of the middle ear and mastoid. These disorders are described in Chapter 11. Ligation of the internal jugular vein results in fibrous occlusion of the sinus (Fig. 8.15).

References

Adams, R., 1943: Occlusion of the anterior inferior cerebellar artery. Arch. Neurol. Psychiat. 49:765.

Alexander, G., 1906: Ueber lymphomatose Ohrenkrankungen. Z. Heilkunde. 7:331.

Barber, H., and Dionne, J., 1971: Vestibular findings in vertebro-basilar ischemia. Ann. Otol. Rhinol. Laryng. 80:805.

Brodal, A., Pomeiano, O., and Walberg, F., 1962: The Vestibular Nuclei and Their Connections, Anatomy and Functional Correlations. William Ramsay Henderson Trust, Oliver and Boyd, Publishers, Edinburgh, and London.

Carmichael, E., Dix, M., and Hallpike, C., 1965: Observations upon the neurological mechanism of directional preponderance of caloric nystagmus resulting from vascular lesions of the brain-stem. Brain 88:51.

Conley, J., and Hildyard, V., 1969: Aneurysm of the internal carotid artery presenting in the middle ear. Arch. Otolaryng. 90:35.

Crowe, S., 1930: Pathologic changes in meningitis of the internal ear. Arch. Otolaryng. 11:537.

Druss, J., 1945: Aural manifestations of leukemia. Arch. Otolaryng. 42:267.

Fields, W., 1966: Vertigo related to alteration in arterial blood flow. In The Vestibular System and Its Diseases, Edited by R. Wolfson, University of Pennsylvania Press, Philadelphia, Pa., pp. 472.

Finlaysin, J., 1898: The diagnosis during life of retinal and labyrinthine hemorrhages in a case of splenic leukemia. Brit. Med. J. 2:1925.

Fisher, C., Karnes, W., and Kubik, C., 1961: Lateral medullary infarction—the pattern of vascular occlusion. J. Neuropath. Exp. Neurol. 20:323.

Fraser, J., 1928: Affections of the labyrinth and eighth nerve in leukemia. Ann. Otol. Rhinol. Laryng. 37:361.

Gacek, R., 1969: The course and central termination of first order neurons supplying vestibular endorgans in the cat. Acta oto-laryng. Suppl. 254.

Grinker, R., and Sahs, A., 1966: Neurology, 11th ed. Charles C. Thomas, Springfield, Ill., pp. 904.

Hallpike, C., 1965: Clinical otoneurology and its contributions to theory and practice. Proc. Roy. Soc. Med. 58:185.

Hallpike, C., and Harrison, M., 1950: Clinical and pathological observations on a case of leukaemia with deafness and vertigo. J. Laryng. 64:427.

Hiller, F., 1952: "The tegmental pons syndrome," extract from The vascular syndromes of basilar and vertebral arteries and their branches. J. Nerv. Ment. Dis. 116:988.

Holden, H., and Schuknecht, H., 1968: Distribution pattern of blood in the inner ear following spontaneous subarachnoid haemorrhage. J. Laryng. 82:321.

Jaffe, B., 1970: Sudden deafness—a local manifestation of sytemic disorders: Fat emboli, hypercoagulation and infections. Laryngoscope 80:788.

Kirikae, I., Nomura, Y., Shitara, T., and Kobayashi, T., 1962: Sudden deafness due to Buerger's disease. Arch. Otolaryng. 75:502.

Kock, A., 1905: Ein Fall von Leukämischen Blutungen im innerin Ohre, mit besonderer Berücksichtigung der pathologischanatomischen Untersuchung der Schäfenbeine. Z. Ohrenheilk. 50:412.

Lindsay, J., and Hemenway, W., 1956: Postural vertigo due to unilateral sudden partial loss of vestibular function. Ann. Otol. Rhinol. Laryng. 65:692.

Lindsay, J., and Zuidema, J., 1950: Inner ear deafness of sudden onset. Laryngoscope 60:238.

Linthicum, F., and Sheehy, J., 1969: Blood in the vestibule at stapedectomy: human case report with histological findings. Ann. Otol. Rhinol. Laryng. 78:425.

Nishio, S., 1926: Ueber leukämische Veränderungen im Felsenbein. Z. Hals.-Nas.-Ohrenheilk. 16:541.

Paparella, M., Berlinger, N., Oda, M., and El Fiky, F., 1973: Otological manifestations of leukemia. Laryngoscope 83:1510.

Paparella, M., and Lim, D., 1967: Pathogenesis and pathology of the "idiopathic" blue ear drum. Arch. Otolaryng. 85:249.

Perlman, H., and Lindsay, J., 1939: Relation of the internal ear spaces to the meninges. Arch. Otolaryng. 29:12.

Radpour, S., Wolff, D., and Polisar, I., 1962: Atheromatous changes in the human internal carotid artery. Arch. Otolaryng. 76:261.

Ruben, R., Distenfeld, A., Berg, P., and Carr, R., 1969: Sudden sequential deafness as the presenting symptom of macroglobulinemia. J. Amer. Med. Assn. 209:1364.

Schuknecht, H., 1962: Positional vertigo: clinical and experimental observations. Trans. Amer. Acad. Ophthal. Otolaryng. 66:319.

Schuknecht, H., 1969: Cupulolithiasis. Arch. Otolaryng. 90:765.

Schuknecht, H., and El Seifi, A., 1963: Experimental observations on the fluid physiology of the inner ear. Ann. Otol. Rhinol. Laryng. 72:687.

Schuknecht, H., Igarashi, M., and Chasin, W., 1965: Inner ear hemorrhage in leukemia. Laryngoscope 75:662.

Schuknecht, H., Neff, W., and Perlman, H., 1951: An experimental study of auditory damage following blows to the head. Ann. Otol. Rhinol. Laryng. 60:273.

Schwabach, D., 1897: Ueber Erkrankungen des Gehörorgans bei Leukämie. Z. Ohrenheilk. 31:103.

Smutneva, A., 1951: Morfologicheski Izmenenilia Vukhe Novorozhdennykh Pri Vnutricherepnykh Krovoizluaniiakh (Morphological auricular changes associated with intracranial haemorrhage in neonates). Vestn. Oto-rino-laryng. 13:24.

Solomon, A., and Fahey, J., 1963: Plasmapheresis therapy in macroglobulinemia. Ann. Intern. Med. 58:789.

Stallings, J., and McCabe, B., 1969: Congenital middle ear aneurysm of internal carotid. Arch. Otolaryng. 90:39.

Steinbrugge, H., 1886: Labyrintherkrankung in einem Falle von Leukämie. Z. Ohrenheilk. 16:238.

Trevino, R., 1970: Thyrocervical steal syndrome. Arch. Otolaryng. 92:177.

Ulrich, K., 1926: Verletzungen des Gehörorgans bei Schädelbasis fracturen, Acta Oto-laryng. Suppl. 6.

Voss, O., 1926: Klinische und pathologisch-anatomische Folgeerscheinungen geburtstraumatischer Schädigungen des Felsenbeines. Mschr. Kinderheilk. 34:568.

Weiss, A., 1968: Neurological aspects of the differential diagnosis of vertigo. Ann. Otol. Rhinol. Laryng. 77:216.

Wilkinson, P., Davidson, W., and Sommaripa, A., 1966: Turnover of 131 I-labelled autologous macroglobulin in Waldenström's macroglobulinemia. Ann. Intern. Med. 65:308.

9 Disorders of Innervation

A. DEGENERATION OF THE COCHLEAR NEURONS

Degeneration of the cochlear neurons may occur as a primary or secondary condition.

1. PRIMARY DEGENERATION OF THE COCHLEAR NEURONS

A loss in population of cochlear neurons in the absence of any other cochlear pathology may occur as a normal consequence of aging (Fig. 9.1). The severity of neuronal loss is probably controlled principally by genetic factors. Moderate losses of neurons to the basal turn of the cochlea appear to have little effect on thresholds or on speech discrimination. Loss of neurons in the middle and apical turns, on the other hand, causes a loss of speech discrimination (Otte, 1968). Primary neural degeneration may be recognized by a distinctive pattern of auditory dysfunction. It is characterized by a loss of speech discrimination which is relatively more severe than the threshold elevations for pure tones (see Chapter 10J, Presbycusis).

2. SECONDARY DEGENERATION OF THE COCHLEAR NEURONS

Secondary neural degeneration implies a loss of cochlear neurons caused by factors extraneous to the neurons themselves. It is characteristic of the cochlear neurons to degenerate as a result of injury to either their axonal or dendritic fibers.

Experimental studies have shown that cutting the axons (central fibers) results in total degeneration of the neurons with no effect on the organ of Corti (Neff, 1947; Wever and Neff, 1947; Schuknecht and Woellner, 1953). Furthermore, injury to the dendritic (peripheral) fibers in their course within the osseous spiral lamina also results in neuronal degeneration (Hind and Schuknecht, 1954).

In experimentally induced lesions of the organ of Corti it is common to find the loss in hair cell population to greatly exceed the loss of cochlear neurons. It is actually possible for all the hair cells in a region of the cochlea to disap-

Fig. 9.1: Primary neural degeneration in a 67-year-old man who complained of hearing loss for two years. Autopsy was performed 11 hours after death. Histological preservation is excellent. About 30 percent of the neurons remain in the basal halves and about 60 percent in the middle and apical turns of both cochleae. All structures of the cochlear ducts appear normal throughout.

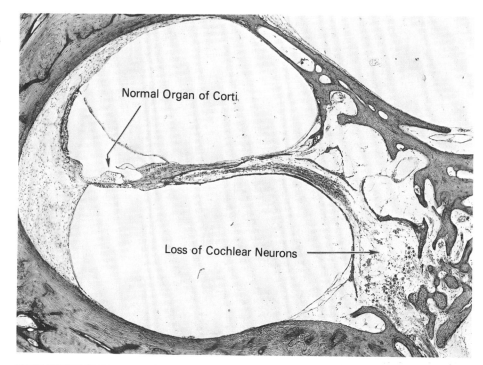

Fig. 9.2: Abnormal cochlear neurons in a cat with profound concussion deafness. The animal was sacrificed five months following a blow to the head (Schuknecht et al., 1951). Histological study shows the organ of Corti to be missing throughout most of the cochlea, there being only an epithelial mound in the apical turn. In this view from the basal turn, about 30 percent of the cochlear neurons remains. Each neuron has a normal-appearing axon but the dendrite is missing. The cell bodies are swollen, the cytoplasm is clear, and the nuclei are displaced toward the axonal poles of the cells. These pathological changes represent secondary neural degeneration following injury to the dendritic nerve endings in the organ of Corti.

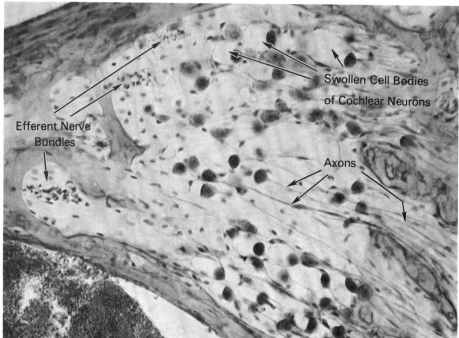

pear while the cochlear neuronal population remains normal. The extent of loss of cochlear neurons appears to parallel closely the magnitude of injury suffered by the supporting cells of the organ of Corti, particularly the pillar cells. If the pillars are erect and Deiters' cells are present, there often is little or no loss of cochlear neurons. When there is shortening of the height of the pillar arch or partial collapse of the internal or external pillars, there is usually a loss in the number of neurons in that area. A total loss of pillar cells is usually associated with severe loss of neurons; however, following experimental injuries to the cochlea as well as in pathological conditions in which the organ of Corti is entirely missing, it is common to find a few neurons remaining. These neurons appear to have survived a sublethal injury and persist in an altered morphological state. The nucleus is somewhat pyknotic and displaced toward the axonal side of the cell. The peripheral fiber (dendrite) is missing, and a large vacuole is present at the dendritic pole of the cell (Fig. 9.2). These observations apply to acquired lesions only and do not hold true for developmental defects. In the Scheibe type of aplasia, for example, the population of cochlear neurons may be normal although the organ of Corti may be grossly abnormal or missing (see Chapter 4E, Morphological Patterns of Aplasia).

Secondary neural degeneration can be expected to occur in any acquired peripheral cochlear disorder in which the atrophic changes in the organ of Corti are severe enough to involve the supporting elements. The hearing losses, however, are predominantly a reflection of the extent of injury to the sense organ because the loss of cochlear neurons is less severe than the loss of sensory cells both in terms of density and spatial distribution. The loss of cochlear neurons, therefore, would be expected to cause little or no additional functional deficit.

The magnitude of secondary cochlear neuronal degeneration becomes an important consideration, however, for those investigators who are attempting to develop electronic devices to substitute for cochlear function. Electrical stimulation of the cochlear neurons in profoundly deaf individuals has been attempted with limited success (Djourno et al., 1957; Doyle et al., 1964; Simmons, 1966; Michelson, 1971; House and Urban, 1973). The problem of developing a device which can perform the cochlear task of stimulus coding appears to be a formidable one. Be that as it may, for any such device to be capable of functioning successfully, it will be necessary for the ear to possess a certain minimum number of cochlear neurons.

Kerr and Schuknecht (1968) evaluated the cochlear neuronal population in human ears having profound sensorineural hearing losses caused by various etiologies. Of the series of 41 ears from 29 profoundly deaf patients there were 10 ears which had more than two-thirds of the cochlear neurons remaining, 3 with one-third to two-thirds remaining, and 28 with less than one-third remaining. The patterns of degenerative change in the cochlear neurons were consistent for some etiologies and inconsistent for others. It was found that the neuronal population was good in ears profoundly deaf from some types of congenital deafness, temporal bone fractures, and toxic drugs (Fig. 9.3). A greatly decreased population of cochlear neurons was found in profound deafness due to bacterial labyrinthitis and congenital syphilis (Fig. 9.4). When profound deafness was due to viral labyrinthitis, vascular occlusion, or otosclerosis, the extent of degeneration of the ganglion was variable. The precise number of neurons required for socially adequate hearing for speech has not been determined; however, Otte's (1968) study suggests that useful speech reception can exist when two-thirds or more of the cochlear neurons are present in the speech frequency area of the cochlea. Ten of the 41 profoundly deaf ears which were studied by Kerr and Schuknecht (1968) met this criterion.

B. DISORDERS OF THE VESTIBULAR NERVE

1. VESTIBULAR NEURITIS

The literature presents such a confusing picture of this vestibular disorder that the establishment of clinical entities remains rather vague. Vestibular neuritis seems the most appropriate term until such time as more definite pathological entities evolve. Vestibular neuritis implies a unilateral disorder of the vestibular system without involvement of the auditory mechanism, brain stem, or other cranial nerves. It may express itself in an acute form, typified by a single vertiginous episode, or in a chronic form in which vertigo of a milder but more persistent type recurs over a period of months or years.

a) Acute vestibular neuritis

The acute form of vestibular neuritis is characterized by a single severe attack of prolonged vertigo. It has been variously referred to as epidemic vertigo (Charters, 1957; Pedersen, 1961), neurolabyrinthitis epidemica (Meulengracht, 1950), acute labyrinthitis (Burrowes, 1952a, 1952b), vestibular paralysis (Hart, 1965), and vestibular neuronitis (Coats, 1969). The onset is sudden and almost always is severe enough to cause nausea and vomiting. Onset may

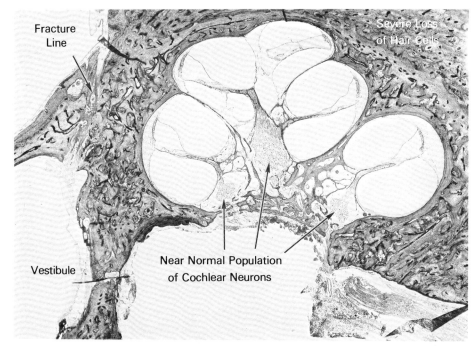

Fig. 9.3: Preservation of cochlear neurons in a profoundly deaf ear of a 21-year-old man following transverse fracture of the temporal bone. Four months after this injury he died from another accident.

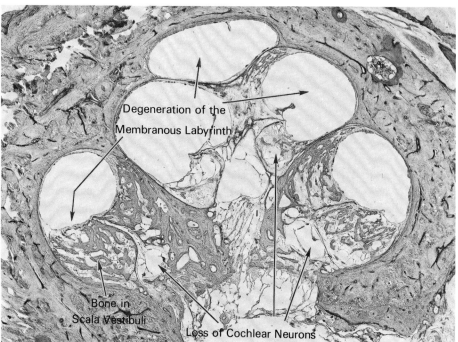

Fig. 9.4: Secondary neural degeneration in the cochlea of an 84-year-old man who was profoundly deaf from meningitis (presumably meningococcal) since early childhood. There is total degeneration of the membranous labyrinth, and the scalae contain fibrous tissue and bone. Only a few abnormal cochlear neurons remain.

occur during the night. Examination reveals spontaneous nystagmus, and caloric tests, performed after the nystagmus has subsided, show decreased vestibular response in the ear opposite to the direction of the spontaneous nystagmus (Coats, 1969). As with any acute unilateral vestibular paralysis, the vertigo subsides gradually over a period of days or weeks as compensation occurs. The severity and duration of symptoms is presumably dependent upon the number of vestibular neurons involved in the attack. It is a benign self-limiting disorder. Treatment is symptomatic.

Coats (1969), after studying a large group of patients with vestibular symptoms, evolved the following criteria for diagnosis of the disorder: (1) a unilateral peripheral vestibular deficit in the absence of a hearing loss; (2) occurrence predominantly in middle age (30 to 40 years); (3) a single episode of prolonged severe vertigo; (4) decreased vestibular response in the ear opposite to the direction of spontaneous nystagmus; and (5) complete subsidence of disequilibrium in six months. Two of Coats' patients who were tested with the body-sway galvanic test showed decreased galvanic responses on the side of the lesion which he interpreted as indicating a neural location for the lesion. There was no sex predominance in his patients. A preceding respiratory infection commonly occurred in the cases studied by

Coats (1969) as well as by Charters (1957) and Hart (1965).

Many authors report the disease to be most common in the spring and early summer months. It is frequently reported as involving several members of the same family or individuals in close contact with each other. Walford (1952) described an epidemic which occurred in an artist's colony where it became known locally as "the staggers". Because of its occasional epidemic nature many authors have suggested a viral etiology (Burrowes, 1952a, 1952b; Mackiewicz, 1963; Williams, 1963); however, laboratory attempts to establish a viral etiology have generally been unsuccessful (Pedersen, 1959; Walford, 1952; Merifield, 1965). Hart (1965) emphasizes the similarity in behavior of epidemic vertigo and herpes zoster infections, pointing out that both occasionally occur in epidemics and that both are almost always unilateral.

The site of involvement within the vestibular system has not been determined by pathological studies. Presumably the infrequent occurrence of associated hearing loss eliminates the possibility of labyrinthitis with involvement of the sense organs. On the basis of electronystagmographic studies, Pfaltz (1955) places the lesion in the vestibular nerves, somewhere between the end-organ and nucleus. Hart (1965) believes the site of the lesion to be in the vestibular nerve or labyrinth and the factors which mitigate against involvement of the vestibular nuclei to the lack of other brain stem involvement and the occurrence of rapid and relatively complete compensation. Marshall (1955) failed to find pathological changes in the inner ear of a patient who died eight weeks after experiencing an attack of acute vertigo.

Acute vestibular neuritis can usually be differentiated from the initial attack of Ménière's disease because the latter is of shorter duration. Other disorders to be considered in the differential diagnosis are multiple sclerosis, herpes zoster oticus, vestibular schwannoma, and occlusion of either the anterior or the posterior inferior cerebellar arteries. Occlusion of the anterior vestibular artery (Lindsay and Hemenway, 1956) may pesent symptoms identical to acute vestibular neuritis but occurs in an older age group, does not follow an upper respiratory infection, does not occur in epidemics, and usually is followed by persisting positional vertigo (see Chapter 12B, Cupulolithiasis). Acute diabetic neuropathy involving the vestibular nerve may also produce symptoms identical to that of acute vestibular neuritis. Differentiation is made on the basis of elevated blood sugar levels or abnormal glucose tolerance tests. Often these diabetic patients exhibit other cranial nerve or peripheral neuropathies (Naufal and Schuknecht, 1972).

b) Chronic vestibular neuritis

This disorder is characterized by recurring episodes of vertigo without signs of involvement of the auditory system, other cranial nerves, or the brain stem. Nylén (1924) first described the condition, but it was Hallpike (1949) and later Dix and Hallpike (1952) who gave better descriptions and termed it vestibular neuronitis. The main criteria they presented were "sudden and severe transient seizures accompanied by sensations of blackout." On the other hand, they described cases in which there were no severe paroxysms and the disequilibrium was a form of "feeling top heavy" or "off balance" particularly when walking or standing.

The attacks are usually less severe and of shorter duration than those of acute vestibular neuritis but may recur over a period of years (Harrison, 1962). The disorder is relatively uncommon, its incidence being one-tenth that of Ménière's disease (Stahle, 1966). Dix and Hallpike (1952), Pfaltz (1955), and Kattum and Mündnich (1957) found a preceding or accompanying infection of the upper respiratory system in a high percentage of patients. Most of their patients were middle aged.

Some patients, but not all, demonstrate a decreased vestibular response in one or both ears or directional preponderance. With the more severe attacks there is spontaneous nystagmus away from the ear exhibiting decreased caloric response (Stahle, 1966). It is a benign self-limiting disease. Therapy is symptomatic and required only for the most severe attacks.

Hilding et al. (1968) performed electron microscopic studies of vestibular nerves removed surgically from a 42-year-old woman with episodic vertigo and found nerve swelling and myelin degeneration believed to be a pathological change rather than preparation artifact. Morgenstein and Seung (1971) described severe degeneration of the sensory and neural structures of both the auditory and vestibular system in a patient with recurring vertigo. The patient had a profound hearing loss of unknown etiology in the involved ear since childhood. The diagnosis of vestibular neuronitis as made by the authors is subject to question. Weiss (1968) has pointed out that the clinical manifestations, etiology, and underlying pathology of the conditions, here termed acute and chronic vestibular neuritis, have not been clearly elucidated. Hallpike (1962) points out that in the last forty years many publications have appeared describing vertiginous syndromes which pursue a benign course without evidence of cochlear involvement. Some occur in epidemics in association with neurological abnormalities such as oculomotor weakness or cerebral disturbances (Barré and Reys, 1921; Dalsgaard-Nielsen, 1953).

The differential diagnosis must include Ménière's disease, cupulolithiasis, vestibular schwannoma and other lesions of the cerebellopontine angle, cerebellar space-occupying lesions, and multiple sclerosis. Usually these diseases present other characteristic symptoms and findings which facilitate differentiation from chronic vestibular neuritis.

2. DIABETIC VESTIBULAR NEUROPATHY

Neuropathies involving the central, peripheral, and autonomic nervous systems are common in diabetes mellitus. The pathogenesis for the pathological changes in the nervous system is assumed to be related to the associated vascular disease; however, a direct metabolic effect has not been completely excluded. Spratt and Hardin (1957) found the incidence of polyneuritis in diabetics to be 14 percent.

The most common cranial neuropathy involves the nerves of ocular movement. In five cases of cranial nerve paralysis in diabetes reported by Root (1933), the IIIrd nerve was involved in two, the VIth nerve in two, and both IVth nerves in one. Joslin et al. (1959) observed a case which developed bilateral IVth nerve palsy followed by recovery after adequate treatment. Dreyfus et al. (1957) reported the postmortem findings in a diabetic patient with oculomotor palsy and interpreted the morphological changes in the nerve and midbrain to be consistent with occlusion of an artery supplying the area.

Severe prolonged episodes of vertigo resembling acute vestibular neuritis may occur as an unusual manifestation of cranial neuropathies in diabetes mellitus. Naufal and Schuknecht (1972) presented the findings in a diabetic patient who exhibited recurring palsies of the IIIrd, VIIth, and vestibular division of the VIIIth cranial nerves. The episodes of vertigo occurred at ages 67, 69, and 85. The attacks were of acute onset, associated with nausea, aggravated by head movement, and required bed rest for several days. Disequilibrium of mild degree was present for some months following each attack but recovery was complete. Histological studies of the temporal bone of this patient showed a loss of vestibular neurons, most severe in the superior division of the nerve in both ears (Figs. 9.5, 9.6). The underlying pathology is presumed to be related to the microangiopathies which occur in diabetes mellitus. It has been demonstrated that the small arterioles, capillaries, and venules of nerves, skin, skeletal muscle, myocardium, kidney, retina, and placenta suffer narrowing of their lumens because of hypertrophy and proliferation of the intimal endothelium and by the deposition of polysaccharides and lipids.

Subsidence of symptoms of vestibular neuropathy apparently is the result of physiological compensation rather than of regeneration of the injured neurons. Recovery of function from diabetic neuropathy involving the cranial motor nerves, on the other hand, is by nerve regeneration.

Fig. 9.5: Vestibular neuropathy in an 86-year-woman with diabetes mellitus. She experienced palsies of cranial nerve III (oculomotor) at the ages of 54, 58, 79, and 81, cranial nerve VII (facial) at the ages of 56, 80, and 81, and cranial nerve VIII (vestibular division) at the ages of 67, 69, and 85. There is a loss of 55 percent of the neurons of the superior divisions of Scarpa's ganglia in both ears (Naufal and Schuknecht, 1972).

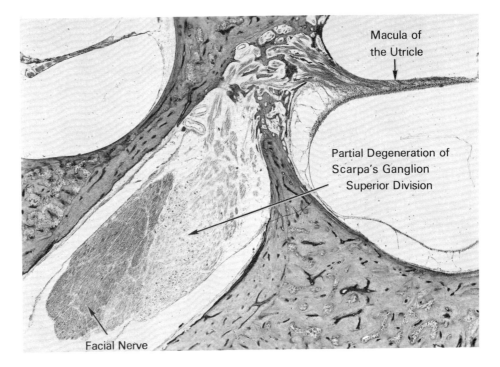

Fig. 9.6: Diabetic vestibular neuropathy. Same case as Fig. 9.5. There is a loss of 12 percent of the neurons in the inferior division of Scarpa's ganglion in the right ear (shown here) and 29 percent in the left ear.

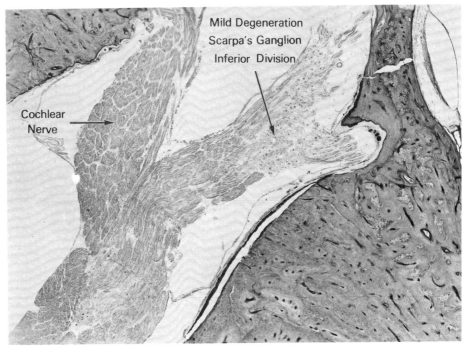

C. FACIAL NERVE PALSY

1. IDIOPATHIC FACIAL PALSY (BELL'S PALSY)

Sir Charles Bell (1833) first discovered that the facial musculature is innervated by a cranial nerve separate from the trigeminal nerve. In 1893 Gowers noted that exposure to cold sometimes precedes the onset of facial palsy and ascribed it to neuritis of the facial nerve. Peripheral facial palsy of undetermined etiology is now referred to as Bell's palsy, and little has been added regarding its etiology or pathology since Gowers' report. A common concept, although not universally accepted, is that Bell's palsy is due to a primary ischemia, possibly a vasospasm resulting in venous stasis and edema of the nerve. This idea implies that because of the unyielding nature of the walls of the fallopian canal, the swelling results in compression and ischemia with temporary or permanent injury to the axons. Ballance and Duel (1932), Kettel (1959), Jongkees (1961a), Miehlke (1960), Cawthorne (1965), and many others have reported finding swelling in the mastoid segment of the nerve

Fig. 9.7: At the age of 77 this woman developed a complete left facial paralysis diagnosed as Bell's palsy. There was nearly complete recovery of facial movement, but at the time of her death 10 years later at the age of 87, she still exhibited a mild facial droop on the left side. Histological study shows partial loss of the motor fibers beginning in the internal auditory canal and becoming progressively more severe to the distal part of the mastoid segment. The neurons of the geniculate ganglion, the chorda tympani nerve, and the greater superficial petrosal nerve appear normal. The fiber bundles appear uniform and parallel except in the superior part of the mastoid segment where they seem to intertwine to some extent.

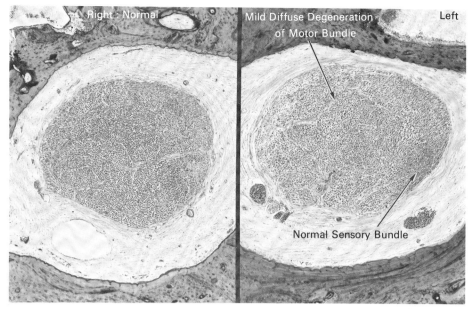

when performing exploratory and decompression operations for Bell's palsy.

The pathology of Bell's palsy remains largely unknown; however, the autopsy reports of Minkowski (1891), Dejerine and Theohari (1897), and André-Thomas (1907) describe gross degenerative changes in the nerve trunk in subjects who had Bell's palsy. Following recovery from Bell's palsy the facial nerve may appear entirely normal on histological study (author's observation, unpublished). Examination of the temporal bones of an individual with incomplete recovery showed partial loss of motor nerve fibers and a normal sensory bundle (Fig. 9.7). Alexander (1901–1902) found perivascular round cell infiltration in the endoneurium and Kettel (1947) described nerve degeneration and fibrosis after prolonged intervals following Bell's palsy. Fowler (1963) studied the temporal bone findings in a patient with Boeck's sarcoid who developed Bell's palsy, and found engorged vessels surrounding the nerve in its entire intratemporal course as well as degenerative changes in the nerve trunk. Sade et al. (1965) performed biopsies of the nerve sheath epineurium in four patients with Bell's palsy and found no evidence of edema, inflammatory changes, or vascular abnormalities and suggested that Bell's palsy might be due to a lower motor neuron paralysis of nuclear origin and possibly of viral etiology. Reports by Saunders and Lippy (1959) and Saunders (1963) suggest that at least some cases of unilateral Bell's palsy are due to viral disease. Blatt and Freeman (1966) suggest that Bell's palsy is a primary inflammatory neuropathy of the chorda tympani nerve with retrograde extension of the process to the main trunk of the facial nerve. Collier (1951, 1954) and Dalton (1960) pointed out that, while Bell's palsy is probably a condition of multiple etiologies, some cases are caused by vasospasm on exposure to cold and others, which occur in epidemics or are associated with poliomyelitis or herpes zoster, are of viral etiolgy (see Chapter 5C1, Herpes zoster oticus).

The high incidence of Bell's palsy in diabetics has been clearly established (Wechsler, 1963). Diabetes mellitus is a more common disorder than ordinarily supposed, occurring in about 15 percent of the general population (Sharp et al., 1964). Korczyn (1971) studied 130 patients with Bell's palsy and found evidence of diabetes in 88 for an incidence of 66 percent. Of this group, 18 were known diabetics, 8 were found to have fasting blood glucose levels above 130 mg per 100 ml, and 62 had abnormal glucose tolerance tests. He pointed out that the incidence of diabetes in the general population is about 12 to 14 percent and that Bell's palsy may be the first manifestation of diabetes. He suggests a glucose tolerance test should be performed on every patient presenting this neurological finding. Utilizing similar diagnostic criteria, Adour and Bell (1971), on the other hand, found the incidence of diabetes in patients with Bell's palsy to be 10 percent, the same as that in the general population.

Presumably the pathogenesis of the facial palsy in these cases is ischemia of an area of the facial nerve caused by the microangiopathy associated with diabetes. The frequent history of onset following exposure to cold would be explained by vasospasm occurring in small vessels with already narrowed lumens.

It seems probable that some cases of Bell's palsy are due to a Varicella-Zoster virus infection of the nerve. Tomita et al. (1972) determined the complement fixing antibody titers of this virus in 80 cases of peripheral facial nerve palsy. Significant increases in titer were found in 81 percent of 22 patients with the Ramsey-Hunt syndrome (herpes zoster oticus) and in 25 percent of 44 patients who had been diagnosed as having idiopathic (Bell's) palsy.

Nystagmus has been found to occur in association with idiopathic facial palsy. Philipszoon (1962) found that 10 of 12 patients studied exhibited either spontaneous or positional nystagmus. More recently, Robert and Pfaltz (1970), in a study of 29 patients with facial palsy, found spontaneous nystagmus to the opposite side of the lesion in 50 percent, decreased vestibular response on the side of the lesion in 70 percent, and directional preponderance of galvanic response toward the unimpaired side in 70 percent. A possible explanation for this phenomenon might be found in the close anatomical relationship of the facial nerve and superior division of the vestibular nerve in the internal auditory canal (Fig. 9.5).

Facial diplegia (bilateral Bell's palsy) may occur with polyneuritis (Landry-Guillain syndrome) (Patrick, 1916), infectious mononucleosis (Creaturo, 1950), and influenza (Barkas, 1895). Schuring and Saunders (1964) described a patient with facial diplegia associated with a rash and submandibular lymphadenopathy, malaise, headache, and aphthous stomatitis which was presumed to be on a viral basis.

The incidence of complete recovery of function in idiopathic unilateral facial palsy, with or without treatment, appears to be about 70 to 80 percent, with about 15 percent retaining some permanent weakness or synkinesia and less than 5 percent sustaining severe or total paralysis. Dalton (1960), in a study of 86 patients, found that complete recovery occurred in 59 percent of those who complained of pain with the paralysis and in 74 percent of those without pain.

More controlled studies are needed to determine whether medical therapy is helpful in the management of Bell's palsy. Adour et al. (1972) are of the opinion that prednisone administered orally results in fuller recovery of motor function and less severe complications. The usefulness of vasodilators and antibiotics seems doubtful.

The physiological extent of nerve involvement can be assessed by nerve excitability tests and electromyography, and a relatively accurate determination can be made of the location of the lesion along the course of the nerve by the Schirmer test for lacrimation, the stapedial reflex test, electrogustometry and submaxillary gland secretion studies (Alford et al., 1973). The value of testing nerve response to electrical stimulation as a guide for determining surgical intervention has not been clearly ascertained. Giancarlo and Mattucci (1970) observed a greater incidence of recovery among 19 patients having surgical decompression of the facial nerve than in 8 patients who refused surgery.

Kettel (1963) suggested the following guidelines for surgical intervention: (1) Decompression of the nerve should be performed as an emergency procedure if the palsy is accompanied by severe pain from the beginning; (2) It should be performed if, in the presence of complete palsy, electromyographic studies show complete block of conduction, and if fibrillations are present; (3) Surgery should be performed if spontaneous recovery has ceased before complete restitution of movement has occurred; (4) Surgery is indicated for recurring facial palsy; and (5) When there has been complete palsy of long duration but without atrophy of muscles, the atrophic segment of the nerve should be resected and a nerve graft inserted.

Based on observations made at the time of surgery, Fisch and Esslen (1972) believe that in idiopathic palsy the nerve is frequently more involved proximal to the geniculate ganglion rather than toward the stylomastoid foramen. They recommend total decompression of the nerve throughout its intratemporal course, including the segment in the internal auditory canal.

A recent report by Mechelse et al. (1971) suggests that surgical decompression when performed in the second or third week following the onset of facial paralysis does not influence the natural course of the disease. Patients with presumed bad prognoses, as determined by clinical and electromyographic criteria, were divided into control and surgical groups. No difference was observed in facial recovery after follow-up periods of one year. Adour and Swanson (1971) also found that early or late facial nerve decompression is not of benefit in patients with Bell's palsy who show evidence of impending or actual denervation as based on nerve excitability testing.

2. TRAUMATIC FACIAL PALSY

Traumatic facial palsy may be due to accidental direct trauma or to surgical injury. Regardless of cause, a distinction should be made between immediate palsy where the nerve may have been transected or torn and delayed palsy where the continuity of the nerve trunk has been preserved.

For immediate palsies associated with fracture of the temporal bone, most authors advocate surgery as soon as the patient's general condition permits (Kley, 1961; von Schulthess, 1961). For palsies which are delayed or develop slowly, Jongkees (1961b) and Kettel (1963) advocate a conservative approach. Greiner et al. (1960) have pointed out that surgical exploration sometimes reveals a macroscopically normal nerve trunk. A patient having complete peripheral facial palsy following a transverse fracture of the temporal bone was found on surgical exploration to have a normal appearing facial nerve from the internal auditory canal to the stylomastoid foramen (author's observation). No recovery occurred during the subsequent 3 years. The nature and site of injury for some cases of facial palsy following temporal bone fracture remains obscure.

Surgical injuries to the facial nerve in its intratemporal course may occur at any level. Total facial palsy observed immediately after surgery demands prompt surgical exploration and repair. A postoperative palsy which is delayed in onset has a much better prognosis than a palsy which occurs immediately after surgery; however, if after six weeks of observation there are no signs of spontaneous recovery, facial nerve exploration should be considered (Kettel, 1963).

The method of repair of facial nerve injuries has been described in detail by Pulec (1969) and Guilford (1970). The principal techniques which are employed to facilitate return of function are simple decompression, end-to-end anastomosis, and nerve grafting. Accurate approximation of cut nerve surfaces is most important for successful nerve grafting. Extremely long segments of the nerve may be encouraged to regenerate through grafts. Dott (1963) and Drake (1963) have been successful in restoring some degree of facial motor activity with grafts extending from the nerve trunk at the brain stem, following an extratemporal course, to the distal segment at the posterior border of the parotid gland.

3. MELKERSSON-ROSENTHAL SYNDROME

The simultaneous occurrence of facial paralysis and swelling of the face has been known for over a century, but it was Melkersson in 1928 who postulated the relationship between the two conditions. Rosenthal (1931) added a third component, that being a fissured tongue (lingua plicata). Swelling of the lips, either unilateral or bilateral, is a typical feature of the syndrome. The edema of the lip may be preceded by or occur simultaneously with unilateral or bilateral facial palsy. Onset occurs at any age with the peak incidence being at the age of twenty. The palatal and buccal mucosa may also exhibit swelling and plication. Histologically the lesion of the lip shows dilated lymphatic vessels, scattered inflammatory cells, and occasionally giant cells (Saberman and Tenta, 1966). The etiology is obscure. The histological appearance is suggestive of a possible relationship to sarcoidosis. A more popular hypothesis is that the disorder is due to a dysfunction of the autonomic nervous system.

4. OTHER LESIONS OF THE FACIAL NERVE

The facial nerve may be involved in a large number of neoplastic, inflammatory, and granulomatous disorders. Schwannoma is the most common primary neoplasm of the facial nerve (see Chapter 11A8, Facial nerve neoplasms).

Metastatic neoplasms of the temporal bone may involve the nerve anywhere along its course from the internal auditory meatus to the stylomastoid foramen. The nerve trunk may be destroyed by direct invasion (Fig. 9.8) or by compression (Fig. 9.9).

Both acute and chronic inflammatory disease may involve the facial nerve. Facial paralysis associated with acute otitis media is caused by extension of the inflammatory process into the perineural spaces of the fallopian canal and possibly into the nerve itself, presumably through dehiscences in the canal. Active therapy with appropriate antimicrobial drugs and myringotomy (when indicated) are usually adequate to control uncomplicated infections with a good prognosis for early recovery of facial function.

Chronic suppurative disease of the temporal bone when complicated by facial palsy is usually an indication for surgical intervention. In such cases the facial nerve trunk may be injured by compression by a keratoma (cholesteatoma) or by bacterial invasion from adjacent infected soft tissues or bone (Fig. 9.10).

D. MULTIPLE SCLEROSIS

Multiple sclerosis is a demyelinating disease process which involves primarily the white matter of the central nervous system with occasional encroachment upon the gray matter. Often the first symptoms consist of minor transient episodes of blurred vision, vertigo, cranial palsies, and awkwardness in the use of an extremity. Late in the course of the disease, when the classic Charcot's triad of nystagmus, scanning speech, and intention tremor are present, the diagnosis is more easily made. The irregular, widely distributed lesions create a diffuse set of neurological signs which include vertigo, nystagmus, hearing loss and tinnitus. The disease usually has its onset in the third and fourth decades of life, affects both sexes equally, and is a slowly disabling and fatal disorder with an average duration of 20 years.

Vertigo is present in about 30 percent (Bentzen et al., 1951) and nystagmus in 40 to 70 percent of the cases (National Multiple Sclerosis Society, 1947; Müller, 1949). The nystagmus may be horizontal, vertical, rotatory, or dissociated. Ataxic or dissociated nystagmus is manifested by a conjugate weakness with nystagmus of the out-turning eye (von Leden and Horton, 1948) and is considered to be pathognomonic for multiple sclerosis (Harris, 1944).

No consistent type of hearing loss has been described. Von Leden and Horton (1948) found progressive high-frequency hearing loss to be the most common finding. Frequently the hearing loss is of sudden onset. It is usually

Fig. 9.8: At the age of 32 this female patient complained of a mass in the left parotid gland. This was surgically excised, presumably incompletely, and diagnosed histologically as adenoid cystic carcinoma. She was asymptomatic until the age of 41 when she noted weakness and finally total paralysis of the left facial muscles. She received 5000r of irradiation therapy to the region of the left temporal bone. She was relatively well except for the facial palsy until the age of 45 when she complained of left ear pain and discharge. She received another 2200r of x-ray therapy to the left temporal bone. At no time did she show recurrence of neoplastic growth in the region of the parotid gland. She died at the age of 47 of direct extension of the malignant lesion into the posterior cranial fossa. Autopsy also revealed multiple distant metastases. Histological study shows extensive invasion and destruction of the left temporal bone by adenoid cystic carcinoma presumed to be of metastatic origin. The neoplastic tissue has destroyed the facial nerve by direct invasion throughout most of its course in the mastoid segment of the fallopian canal.

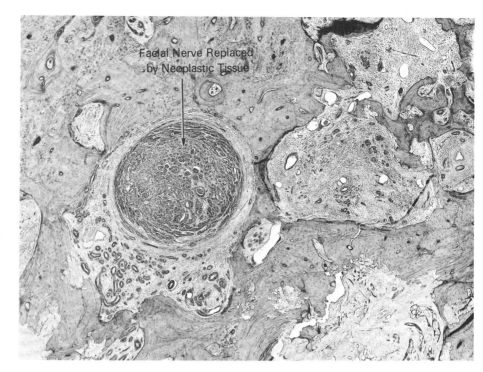

Fig. 9.9: Compression atrophy of the facial nerve from a metastatic growth of undifferentiated carcinoma in a 49-year-old female. The primary site of the malignancy was never determined, and the patient died of diffuse carcinomatosis five months after onset of facial paralysis.

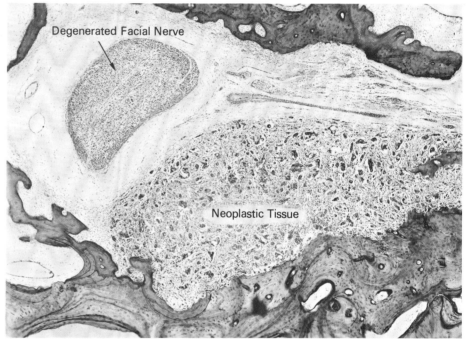

Fig. 9.10: Facial paralysis resulting from infection. This patient with severe uncontrollable diabetes mellitus developed osteitis of the temporal bone beginning at age 65 which progressed until the time of his death at age 69. He experienced total right facial paralysis at age 68. Histological study shows multiple inflammatory osteolytic lesions, one of which has invaded the descending part of the fallopian canal. The facial nerve is degenerated distal to this area.

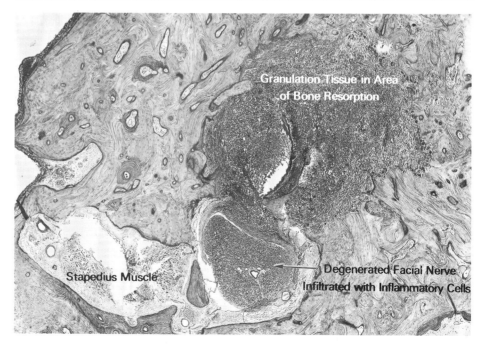

unilateral, most severe for the high frequencies, and followed by recovery after some days or weeks.

Citron et al. (1963) reported the auditory findings in a 16-year-old patient with multiple sclerosis who developed sudden profound hearing loss in the left ear. During a three-week period the hearing improved rapidly and returned to normal. They found that recovery of speech discrimination lagged behind the recovery of pure tone thresholds. Thus, at the time when pure tone thresholds first returned to normal, speech discrimination was still at the 40 percent level, following which it too reverted to normal within a few days. These findings are consistent with a neural (retrocochlear) lesion. It was the opinion of Citron et al. (1963) that the lesion was probably located in the cochlear nerve near the brain stem; however, Ward et al. (1965), commenting on this case, point out that the histological evidence currently available indicates that the lesions of multiple sclerosis commonly occur in the brain and spinal cord.

The pathological process appears to be a myelinoclasis resulting in isolated demyelinating areas mainly in the white matter. The destruction of myelin sheaths of the nerve fibers and interconnecting tracts is followed by glial replacement and eventual sclerotic plaque formation. The plaques are most numerous in the brain stem, pons, medulla, cerebral peduncles, and optic tracts. The spinal cord lesions are usually located in the lateral and posterior columns. Ward et al. (1965) studied the brains and temporal bones of a patient with multiple sclerosis who experienced a severe vertiginous attack 16 years prior to her death. The vestibular nerves and sense organs appeared normal. There were areas of focal demyelinization in the middle cerebellar peduncle and flocculo-nodular lobe which were interpreted to be responsible for the vertigo.

McMeekin et al. (1969) presented a clinicopathological study of a 34-year-old woman with multiple sclerosis which was activated following high-voltage X-radiation treatment of a glomus body tumor. The plaques, which were confined to the areas of radiation treatment, became symptomatic approximately six weeks following the completion of therapy and led to her early death.

E. ABERRANT INNERVATION SYNDROMES

The following two syndromes are presumed to occur because regenerating nerve fibers pursue aberrant courses and are of particular otological interest because of the surgical management which has been proposed.

1. FREY'S SYNDROME (GUSTATORY SWEATING)

Frey's syndrome is characterized by flushing and sweating in the area anterior to the auricle and on the cheek as a result of gustatory stimulation. The area corresponds to that region innervated by the auriculo-temporal branch of the trigeminal nerve. The syndrome usually develops some three to nine months following injury to the parotid gland. Spiro and Martin (1967) found the syndrome in 59 percent of 65 patients following superficial or total parotidectomy.

Although the condition has been recognized for more than a century (Baillarger, 1853), the first detailed description of the disorder and its relationship to the auriculo-temporal nerve was presented by Frey in 1923. List and Peet (1938) ascribed the condition to irritability of cholinergic fibers; however, Ford and Woodhall (1938) presented the "aberrant regeneration" theory which is generally accepted today (Laage-Hellman, 1958; Hemenway, 1960; Holloway and Singleton, 1967). Presumably both the secretory fibers to the parotid gland and the secreto-motor fibers to the sweat glands of the involved region of the face travel together for a short distance in the auriculo-temporal nerve. Injury to the nerve fibers in this region is followed by regeneration or sprouting of secretory nerve fibers into the empty axon sheaths of secreto-

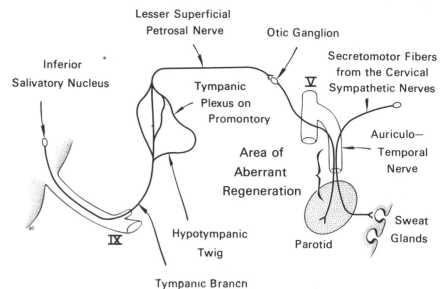

Fig. 9.11: Diagram showing probable neural pathways involved in Frey's syndrome (gustatory sweating).

motor nerve bundles which lead to the sweat glands (Fig. 9.11).

In an investigation of patients with Frey's syndrome, Ross (1970) has shown that electrical stimulation of the tympanic branch of the glossopharyngeal nerve results in gustatory sweating.

Surgical excision or cautery of the tympanic branch of the glossopharyngeal nerve is reported to be successful in relieving the condition (Golding-Wood, 1962). Ross (1970) has demonstrated that the hypotympanic twig of the tympanic nerve must be included in the resection to obtain a complete and permanent cure of gustatory sweating.

2. CROCODILE TEARING SYNDROME

Profuse tearing occurring with gustatory stimulation is known as the syndrome of crocodile tearing. The term derives from the popular legend that the crocodile sheds tears before devouring its prey.

This unusual condition has its onset several months following paralysis of the facial nerve due to Bell's palsy, herpes zoster, temporal bone fracture, or intracranial surgical trauma. Like Frey's syndrome, it is believed to be caused by misdirection of regenerating secretory nerve fibers. In this case the area of aberrant regeneration is probably located in the region where the lesser superficial petrosal and greater superficial petrosal nerves lie in close approximation. Regenerating or sprouting parotid secretory fibers in the lesser superficial petrosal nerve enter the greater superficial petrosal nerve and pass in empty axon sheaths of secreto-motor nerve bundles to reach the postsynaptic neurons in the sphenopalatine ganglion which supplies the lacrimal gland (Fig. 9.12). Successful treatment has been achieved by surgical resection of the tympanic branch of the glossopharyngeal nerve (Golding-Wood, 1962, 1963) and by section of the Vidian nerve (Chandra, 1967).

It is of interest that section of this nerve has also been used successfully in the treatment of chronic parotitis (Dishell, 1971).

Fig. 9.12: Diagram showing probable neural pathways involved in the syndrome of crocodile tearing.

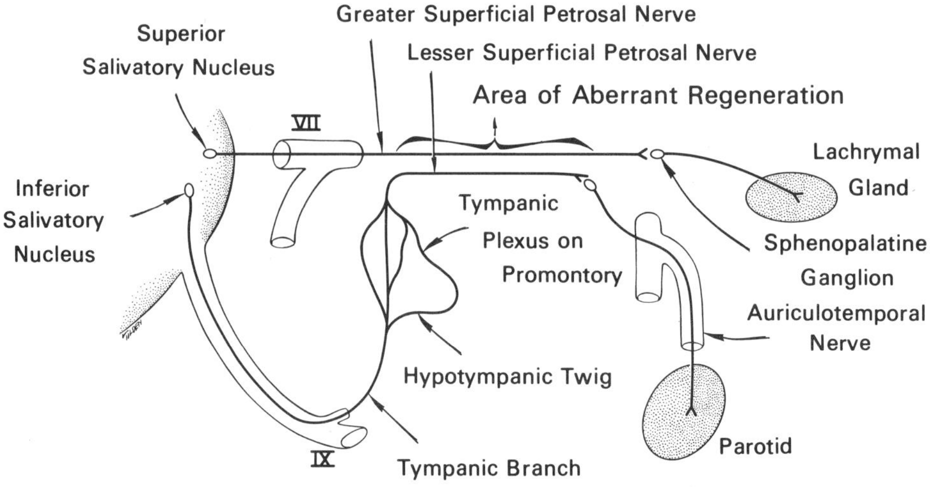

Fig. 9.13: At the age of 53 this patient experienced dysphagia followed by progressive paralysis of the muscles of the arms and neck. At 55 she had sudden profound left sensorineural hearing loss and vertigo. Examination revealed a total loss of hearing and absence of caloric responses in the left ear, as well as progressive weakness of the upper arms, hands, and neck. The clinical diagnosis was progressive cervical myelopathy of unknown cause. She experienced progressive weakness and deteriorated rapidly. She died at age 56 of terminal bronchopneumonia. Autopsy revealed destruction of neurons in the anterior horns and most of the posterior horns on both sides of the cervical spinal cord down to the VIIth and VIIIth cervical segments. The left cochlear nerve root showed marked fiber loss with phagocytosis of myelin breakdown products and nearly total disappearance of the nerve cells of the left ventral and dorsal cochlear nuclei. No definite changes were seen in the vestibular nuclei. An oat cell carcinoma was found in the right upper lobe bronchus with metastases to the hilar lymph nodes. Histological examination of the left temporal bone shows a total loss of cochlear neurons. Only scattered bundles of efferent fibers remain. The organ of Corti is atrophied in the basal 9 mm of the cochlea but appears normal elsewhere. The stria vascularis and limbus appear normal. The final diagnosis, carcinomatous encephalomyelitis, was made postmortem upon discovery of the oat cell carcinoma of the lung.

Fig. 9.14: Same case as Fig. 9.13. There is a total loss of neurons in both the superior and inferior divisions of the vestibular nerve of the left ear. The maculae and cristae appear normal except for complete loss of afferent nerve supply.

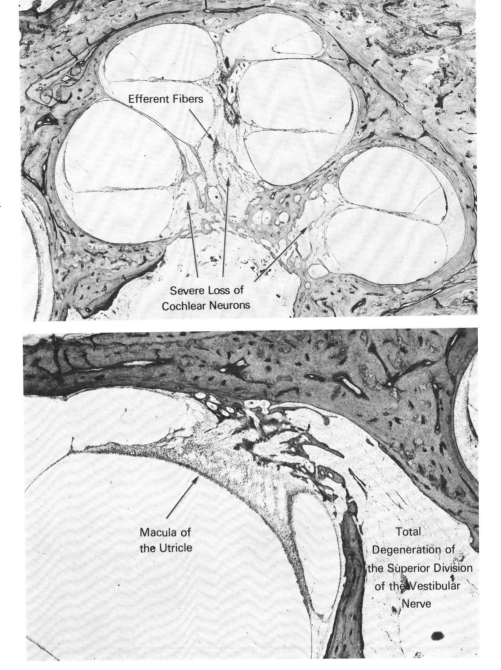

Efferent Fibers

Severe Loss of
Cochlear Neurons

Macula of
the Utricle

Total
Degeneration of
the Superior Division
of the Vestibular
Nerve

F. OTHER DISORDERS OF INNERVATION

1. CARCINOMATOUS ENCEPHALOMYELITIS

The association of carcinoma with a motor and sensory neuropathy of the lower brain stem and spinal cord is now well recognized (Henson et al., 1965). The most common neoplasm associated with this encephalomyelitis is bronchogenic oat cell carcinoma. The pathological changes are similar to those of anterior poliomyelitis; however, the clinical course is protracted. It is characterized usually by a slowly progressive involvement of neurons of the anterior and posterior horns of the cervical spinal cord and areas of the medulla oblongata (Castleman and McNeely, 1970). The facial, auditory, and vestibular nerves can be involved in this disease. The etiology has not been determined but is considered to be caused either by activation of latent viruses by the neoplastic disease or by an immune response mechanism (Figs. 9.13, 9.14).

2. GLIOMAS OF THE BRAIN STEM

Gliomas of the pons or cerebellar flocculus involve the facial and auditory pathways in their course in the brain stem. The vestibular pathways are less

Fig. 9.15: At the age of four this female patient first experienced pain in the left ear followed in two weeks by hearing loss and rapidly developing complete left facial paralysis. She next developed left VIth nerve palsy and ataxia. Audiometric studies showed a profound hearing loss in the left ear. Further investigation revealed a tumor in the left side of the pons and brain stem, and she received 4600r of x-ray therapy to the area. The cranial nerves, III to X inclusive, were progressively involved. Finally, she experienced involvement of the spinal, cerebellar, and pyramidal tracts and the medial lemniscus. Caloric tests were not performed. She died nine months after the onset of symptoms. Autopsy revealed diffuse cerebral edema, focal brain hemorrhages, cerebellar herniation, subarachnoid hemorrhage, and a neoplastic mass in the pons and brain stem region which was histologically compatible with astrocytoma. Histological study of the temporal bone reveals near total degeneration of the motor fibers of the facial nerve. The sensory component (nervus intermedius, geniculate ganglion, greater superficial petrosal nerve, chorda tympani nerve) appears normal. The hair cell populations of the organ of Corti and vestibular sense organs, as well as the cochlear and vestibular neurons, appear normal. The hearing loss and disequilibrium are presumably caused by involvement of the central auditory and vestibular neural pathways.

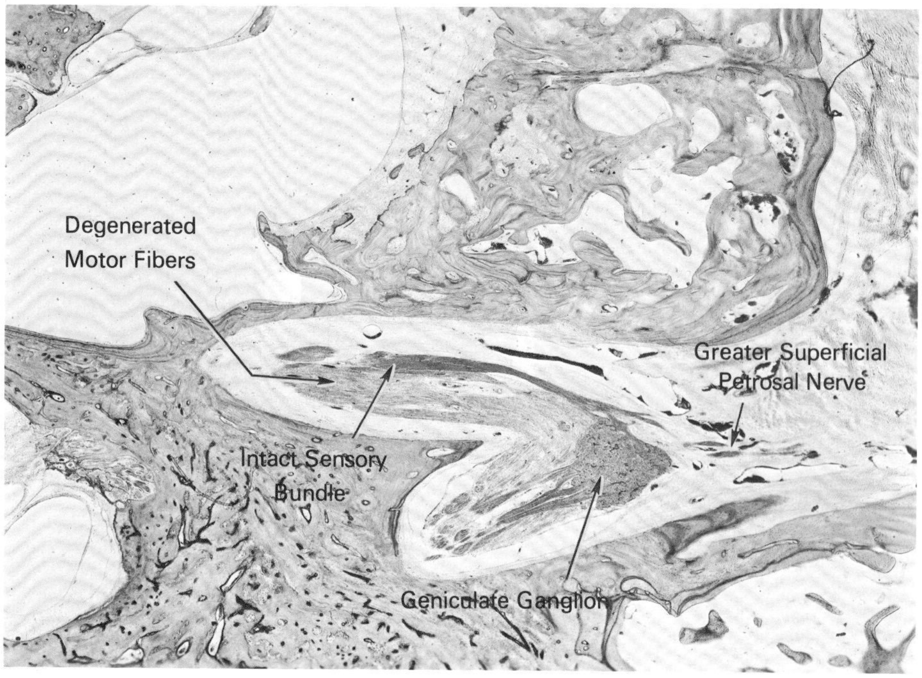

Fig. 9.16: Same case as Fig. 9.15. The facial nerve in its mastoid segment shows degeneration of the motor fibers and preservation of the sensory bundle.

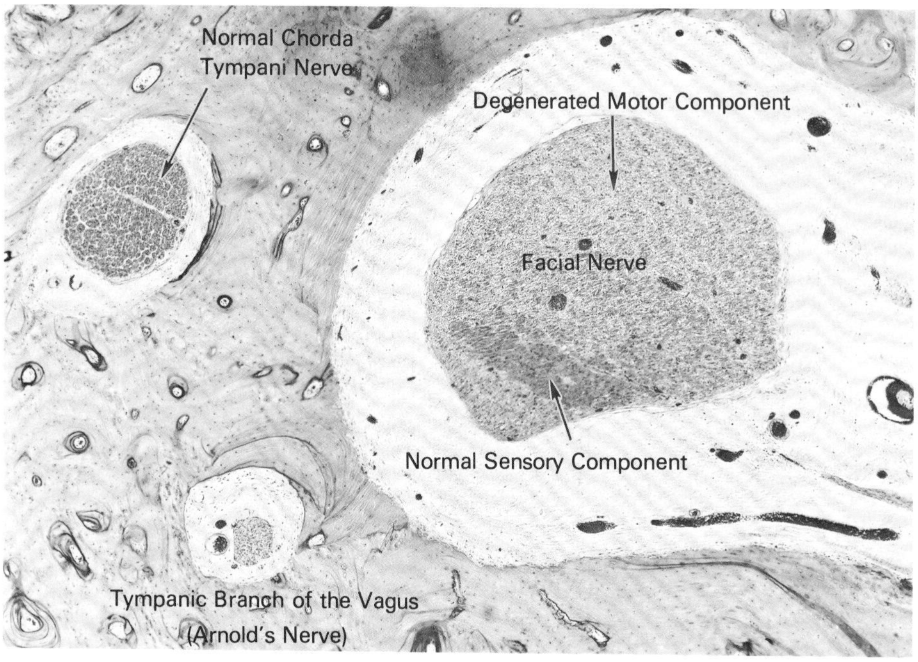

often involved. The types of gliomas in the order of frequency are astrocytomas, medulloblastomas, ependymomas, and glioblastomas. Early symptoms of the pontine gliomas are hearing loss and facial palsy. In these cases histological studies characteristically show a normal cochlear nerve, indicating that the hearing loss is caused by involvement of the second and third order neurons. The facial nerve shows loss of motor fibers with preservation of the sensory bundle (nervus intermedius and its branches) (Saito et al., 1970) (Figs. 9.15, 9.16).

3. TRAUMA TO THE CHORDA TYMPANI NERVE

Normally, after a nerve has been severed, the axons and myelin sheaths degenerate distal to the point of severance, following which Schwann cells proliferate and attempt to close the gap between the proximal and distal severed ends of the nerve. If the Schwann cells and regenerating axons are obstructed in their growth for any reason, such as connective tissue proliferation, they may proliferate locally into a snarled mass.

In transcanal and mastoid surgery the chorda tympani nerve is frequently injured or severed and may form small asymptomatic neuromas at the posterosuperior region of the tympanic annulus. In a study of the temporal bones of 14 ears in which the chorda tympani nerve had been surgically severed, Saito (1973) found four neuromas. In two the nerve was totally degenerated with no signs of regeneration, and in the remainder there were varying degrees of regeneration with nerve fibers extending into the tympanic membrane, subcutaneous layer of the external auditory canal, and into the severed distal stump of the nerve (Figs. 9.17, 9.18).

The ability of the regenerating chorda tympani nerve axons to find the distal segment of the nerve and re-innervate the submaxillary and sublingual glands seems confirmed by the clinical study of Wiberg (1971). He found that when the chorda tympani nerve was cut, the secretory response of the submaxillary gland was lost; but twelve months after injury it had recovered, on the average, to 25 percent of that of the opposite normal side.

Bull (1965) and Wiberg (1971), on the other hand, found little or no recovery of taste function in the involved area of the tongue following severance of the nerve. These authors also observed varying degrees of atrophy of the papillae of the anterior two-thirds of the tongue on the side of the lesion.

The incidence of impairment of subjective sense of taste following uni-

Fig. 9.17: Small amputation neuroma of the chorda tympani nerve in a 50-year-old man eight years following a surgical procedure (stapes mobilization) for otosclerosis. The nerve was totally transected at the time of surgery.

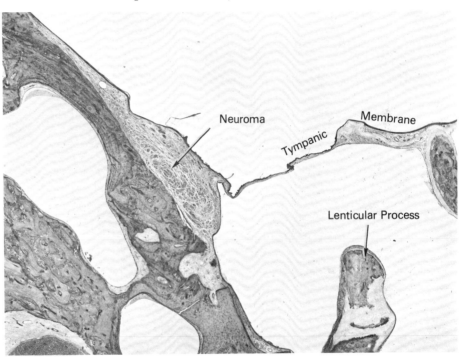

Fig. 9.18: Same case as Fig. 9.17. In a slightly more superior location there are numerous bundles of regenerating fibers of the chorda tympani nerve, some of which appear to have reinnervated the distal segment of the nerve.

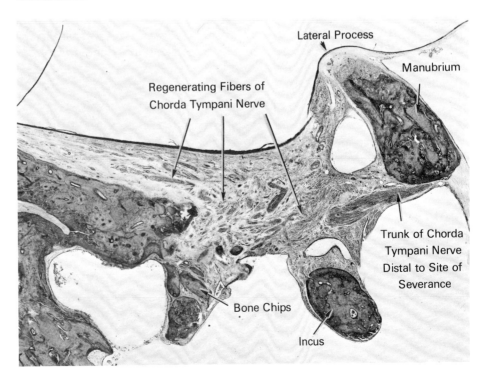

lateral division of the chorda tympani nerve varies considerably (Laumans and Jongkees, 1963; Moon and Pullen, 1963; Rice, 1963; Krarup, 1965; Roseburg, 1966; Jeppsson, 1969). Subjective recovery of taste sensation is accounted for by either adaptation (Diamant et al., 1959; Fortunato, 1959) or compensation from adjacent intact receptors (Gerhardt and Berndt, 1967).

Bull (1965) found that 78 percent of patients with bilateral injuries to the chorda tympani nerve complained of persisting diminution of taste. House (1963) and Moon and Pullen (1963) report bilateral section of the nerve may also result in complaints of dry mouth.

The evidence indicates, therefore, that regeneration of the chorda tympani nerve fibers can be expected even in the presence of total section but that the reinnervation is mainly to the submaxillary and sublingual salivary glands with very little, if any, reinnervation of the end-organs of taste.

References

Adour, K., and Bell, D., 1971: Incidence of diabetes mellitus in Bell's palsy. Lancet 2:168.

Adour, K., and Swanson, P., 1971: Facial paralysis in 403 consecutive patients, emphasis on treatment response in patients with Bell's palsy. Trans. Amer. Acad. Ophthal. Otolaryng. 75:1284.

Adour, K., Wingerd, J., Bell, D., Manning, J., and Hurley, J., 1972: Prednisone treatment for idiopathic facial paralysis (Bell's palsy). New Eng. J. Med. 287:1268.

Alexander, G., 1901–1902: Zur Klinik und pathologischen Anatomie der Sog, "rheumatischen" Facialislähmung. Arch. Psychiat. 35:778.

Alford, B., Jerger, J., Coats, A., Peterson, C., and Weber, S., 1973: Neurophysiology of facial nerve testing. Arch. Otolaryng. 97:214.

André-Thomas, 1907: Contribution à l'étude de l'anatomie pathologique de la paralysie faciale périphérique et de l'hemisphère faciale. (Trois cas suivis d'autopsie). Rev. neurol. 15:1273.

Baillarger, J., 1853: Mémoire sur l'oblitération du canal de sténon. Gaz. méd. Paris 23:194.

Ballance, C., and Duel, A., 1932: The operative treatment of facial palsy by the introduction of nerve grafts into the fallopian canal and by other intratemporal methods. Arch. Otolaryng. 15:1.

Barkas, W., 1895: Bilateral facial palsy as a sequence of influenza. Lancet 1:217.

Barré, J., and Reys, L., 1921: L'Encéphalite épidémique à Strasbourg; sa forme labyrinthique. Bull. méd. Paris 35:256.

Bell, C., 1833: The Nervous System of the Human Body. Duff Green, Washington, D.C.

Bentzen, O., Jelnes, K., and Thygesen, P., 1951: Acoustic and vestibular function in multiple sclerosis. Acta psychiat. scand. 26:265.

Blatt, I., and Freeman, J., 1966: Bell's palsy II: Pathogenetic mechanism of idiopathic peripheral facial paralysis. Trans. Amer. Acad. Ophthal. Otolaryng. 70:381.

Bull, T., 1965: Taste and the chorda tympani. J. Laryng. 79:479.

Burrowes, W., 1952a: Acute labyrinthitis. Brit. Med. J. 2:408.

Burrowes, W., 1952b: Acute labyrinthitis. Brit. Med. J. 2:1182.

Castleman, B., and McNeely, B., 1970: Case records of the Massachusetts General Hospital. New Eng. J. Med. 283:806.

Cawthorne, T., 1965: Idiopathic facial palsy: pathology and surgical treatment. Arch. Otolaryng. 81:494.

Chandra, R., 1967: Treatment of a case of crocodile-tears by Vidian neurectomy. J. Laryng. 81:669.

Charters, A., 1957: Epidemic vertigo in Kenya. E. African Med. J. 34:7.

Citron, L., Dix, M., Hallpike, C., and Hood, J., 1963: A recent clinico-pathological study of cochlear nerve degeneration resulting from tumor pressure and disseminated sclerosis, with particular reference to the finding of normal threshold sensitivity for pure tones. Acta oto-laryng. 56:330.

Coats, A., 1969: Vestibular neuronitis. Trans. Amer. Acad. Ophthal. Otolaryng. 73:395; Acta oto-laryng. Suppl. 251.

Collier, J., 1951: Discussion of paper presented by T. Cawthorne entitled: Pathology and surgical treatment of Bell's palsy. Proc. Roy. Soc. Med. 44:569.

Collier, J., 1954: Facial paralysis. In Modern Trends in Diseases of the Ear, Nose and Throat. Butterworth & Co., Ltd., London, p. 202.

Creaturo, N., 1950: Infectious mononucleosis and polyneuritis (Guillain-Barré syndrome). Report of a case of facial diplegia treated with 2,3 Dimercaptopropanol (BAL). J. Amer. Med. Assn. 143:234.

Dalsgaard-Nielsen, T., 1953: Further clinical studies on epidemic vertigo "Nevraxite Vertigineuse". Acta psychiat. scand. 28:263.

Dalton, G., 1960: Bell's palsy: Some problems of prognosis and treatment. Brit. Med. J. 1:1765.

Dejerine, J., and Theohari, A., 1897: Un Cas de paralysie faciale périphérique dite rhumatismale ou à frigore, suivi d'autopsie. C. R. Soc. Biol. 4:1033.

Diamant, H., Enfors, B., and Holmstedt, B., 1959: Salivary secretion in man elicited by means of stimulation of the chorda tympani. Acta physiol. scand. 45:293.

Dishell, W., 1971: Tympanic neurectomy in chronic parotitis. Arch. Otolaryng. 94:471.

Dix, M., and Hallpike, C., 1952: The pathology, symptomatology and diagnosis of certain common disorders of the vestibular system. Ann. Otol. Rhinol. Laryng. 61:987.

Djourno, A., Eyriès, C., and Vallancien, B., 1957: De l'excitation électrique du nerf cochléaire chez l'homme, par induction à distance, à l'aide d'un micro-bobinage inclus à demeure. C. R. Soc. Biol. 151:423.

Dott, N., 1963: Facial nerve reconstruction by graft bypassing the petrous bone. Arch. Otolaryng. 78:426.

Doyle, J., Doyle, J., Jr., and Trumbull, F., Jr., 1964: Electrical stimulation of eighth cranial nerve. Arch. Otolaryng. 80:388.

Drake, C., 1963: Intracranial facial nerve reconstruction. Arch. Otolaryng. 78:456.

Dreyfus, P., Hakim, S., and Adams, R., 1957: Diabetic ophthalmoplegia: Report of case with postmortem study and comments on vascular supply of human oculomotor nerve. Arch. Neurol. Psychiat. 77:337.

Fisch, U., and Esslen, E., 1972: Total intratemporal exposure of the facial nerve. Arch. Otolaryng. 95:335.

Ford, F., and Woodhall, B., 1938: Phenomena due to misdirection of regenerating fibers of cranial, spinal and automatic nerves. Arch. Surg. 36:480.

Fortunato, V., 1959: La Résection de la corde du tympan dans l'opération de Rosen. Acta oto-rhino-laryng. belg. 13:128.

Fowler, E., Jr., 1963: The pathologic findings in a case of facial paralysis. Trans. Amer. Acad. Ophthal. Otolaryng. 67:187.

Frey, L., 1923: Le Syndrome du nerf auriculo-temporal. Rev. neurol. 2:97.

Gerhardt, H., and Berndt, H., 1967: Zur Schädigung des Geschmackssines durch die Stapesoperation. Z. Laryng. Rhinol. Otol. 46:520.

Giancarlo, H., and Mattucci, K., 1970: Facial palsy, facial nerve decompression. Arch. Otolaryng. 91:30.

Golding-Wood, P., 1962: Tympanic neurectomy. J. Laryng. 76:683.

Golding-Wood, P., 1963: Crocodile tears. Brit. Med. J. 1:1518.

Gowers, W., 1893: A Manual of Diseases of the Nervous System, vol. I. P. Blakiston, Philadelphia, Pa., p. 229.

Greiner, G., Klotz, G., Gaillard, J., 1960: Le Traitement de la paralysie faciale après fracture du rocher. Librairie Arnette, Soc. Franc. Otolaryng., Paris.

Guilford, F., 1970: Surgical consideration in disorders of the horizontal and vertical portions of the facial nerve. Ann. Otol. Rhinol. Laryng. 79:241.

Hallpike, C., 1949: The pathology and differential diagnosis of aural vertigo. 4th International Congress on Otolaryngology, London, 2:514.

Hallpike, C., 1962: Vertigo of central origin. Proc. Roy. Soc. Med. 55:364.

Harris, W., 1944: Ataxic nystagmus: A pathognomonic sign in disseminated sclerosis. Brit. J. Ophthal. 28:40.

Harrison, M., 1962: Epidemic vertigo—vestibular neuronitis, a clinical study. Brain 85:613.

Hart, C., 1965: Vestibular paralysis of sudden onset and probably viral etiology. Ann. Otol. Rhinol. Laryng. 74:33.

Hemenway, W., 1960: Gustatory sweating and flushing: The auriculo-temporal syndrome—Frey's syndrome. Laryngoscope 70:84.

Henson, R., Hoffman, H., and Urich, H.,

1965: Encephalomyelitis with carcinoma. Brain 88:449.

Hilding, D., Kanda, T., and House, W., 1968: Vestibular neuronitis and small acoustic neuroma: Electron microscopic observations. Otolaryng. Clin. N. Amer., October, p. 305.

Hind, J., and Schuknecht, H., 1954: A cortical test of auditory function in experimentally deafened cats. J. Acoust. Soc. Amer. 26:89.

Holloway, R., and Singleton, G., 1967: Gustatory sweating. Eye, Ear, Nose, Throat Monthly 46:316.

House, H., 1963: Early and late complications of stapes surgery. Arch. Otolaryng. 78:606.

House, W., and Urban, J., 1973: Long term results of electrode implantation and electronic stimulation of the cochlea in man. Ann. Otol. Rhinol. Laryng. 82:504.

Jeppsson, P., 1969: Studies on the structure and innervation of taste buds. Acta oto-laryng. Suppl. 259.

Jongkees, L., 1961a: Über die intratemporalen Facialislähmungen und ihre chirurgische Behandlung (On intratemporal facial paralyses and their surgical treatment). Z. Laryng. Rhinol. Otol. 40:319.

Jongkees, L., 1961b: Quelques remarques sur les opérations de 26 malades avec paralysie faciale, causée par une fracture du rocher. Comptes rendus des Séances du 50e Congrès français d'Otorhinolaryngologie, Librairie Arnette, Paris, p. 62.

Joslin, E., Root, H., White, P., and Marble, J., 1959: The treatment of diabetes mellitus. 10th ed., Lea and Febiger, Philadelphia, Pa., p. 494.

Kattum, F., and Mündnich, K., 1957: Kritische Betrachtungen zur Neuronitis vestibularis (Hallpike). Z. Hals-Nas.-Ohrenheilk. 6:232.

Kerr, A., and Schuknecht, H., 1968: The spiral ganglion in profound deafness. Acta oto-laryng. 65:586.

Kettel, K., 1947: Bell's palsy: pathology and surgery. Arch. Otolaryng. 46:427.

Kettel, K., 1959: Bell's palsy. Chapter VI in Peripheral Facial Palsy: Pathology and Surgery. Charles C. Thomas, Springfield, Ill., p. 91.

Kettel, K., 1963: Surgery of the facial nerve. Arch. Otolaryng. 77:327.

Kley, W., 1961: Nervus facialis und Mittelohr. Z. Laryng. Rhinol. Otol. 40:409.

Korczyn, A., 1971: Bell's palsy and diabetes mellitus. Lancet 1:108.

Krarup, B., 1965: Kliniske Smagundersögelser. Med. Diss., Copenhagen.

Laage-Hellman, J., 1958: Gustatory sweating and flushing. Aetiological implications of latent period and mode of development after parotidectomy. Acta oto-laryng. 49:306.

Laumans, E., and Jongkees, L., 1963: On the prognosis of peripheral facial paralysis of endotemporal origin. Ann. Otol. Rhinol. Laryng. 72:307.

Leden, H. von, and Horton, B., 1948: Auditory nerve in multiple sclerosis. Arch. Otolaryng. 48:51.

Lindsay, J., and Hemenway, W., 1956: Postural vertigo due to unilateral sudden partial loss of vestibular function. Ann. Otol. Rhinol. Laryng. 65:692.

List, C., and Peet, M., 1938: Sweat secretion in man; sweat secretion of the face and its disturbances. Arch. Neurol. Psychiat. 40:443.

Mackiewicz, J., 1963: Vertigo epidemic. Pol Tyg. Lek 18:48.

Marshall, J., 1955: Epidemic vertigo (Letter to the Editor). Lancet 1:458.

McMeekin, R., Hardman, J., and Kempe, L., 1969: Multiple sclerosis after X-radiation: Activation by treatment of metastatic glomus tumor. Arch. Otolaryng. 90:617.

Mechelse, K., Goor, G., Huizing, E., Hammelburg, E., van Bolhuis, A., Staal, A., and Verjaal, A., 1971: Bell's palsy: Prognostic criteria and evaluation of surgical decompression. Lancet 2:57.

Melkersson, E., 1928: Et fall ay recidiverande facilspares i samband med angioneurotiskt öden. Hygiea 90:737.

Merifield, D., 1965: Self-limited idiopathic vertigo (epidemic vertigo). Arch. Otolaryng. 81:355.

Meulengracht, E., 1950: Correspondence. Brit. Med. J. 2:1493.

Michelson, R., 1971: The results of electrical stimulation of the cochlea in human sensory deafness. Trans. Amer. Otol. Soc. 59:152.

Miehlke, A., 1960: Die Chirurgie des Nervus Facialis. Urban and Schwarzenberg, Munich, Berlin.

Minkowski, 1891: Zur pathologischen Anatomie der rheumatischen Facialislähmung. Arch. Psychiat. 23:586.

Moon, C., Jr., and Pullen, E., 1963: Effects of chorda tympani section during middle ear surgery. Laryngoscope 73:392.

Morgenstein, K., and Seung, H., 1971: Vestibular neuronitis. Laryngoscope 81:131.

Müller, R., 1949: Studies in disseminated sclerosis. Acta med. scand. Suppl. 222.

National Multiple Sclerosis Society, 1947: Multiple sclerosis. Diagnosis and treatment. J. Amer. Med. Assn. 135:569.

Naufal, P., and Schuknecht, H., 1972: Vestibular, facial, and oculomotor neuropathy in diabetes mellitus. Arch. Otolaryng. 96:468.

Neff, W., 1947: The effects of partial section of the auditory nerve. J. Comp. Physiol. Psychol. 40:203.

Nylén, C., 1924: A case of affection of the otoliths. Acta oto-laryng. 6:113.

Otte, J., 1968: Estudio del ganglio espiral y su relacion con la discriminacion. Rev. Otorrinolaring. 28:89.

Patrick, H., 1916: Facial diplegia in multiple neuritis. J. Nerv. Ment. Dis. 44:323.

Pedersen, E., 1959: Epidemic vertigo. Clinical picture and relation to encephalitis. Brain 82:566.

Pedersen, E., 1961: Epidemic vertigo in Denmark. Wld. Neurology 2:212.

Pfaltz, C., 1955: Diagnose und Therapie der vestibulären Neuronitis. Pract. oto-rhino-laryng. 17:454.

Philipszoon, A., 1962: Nystagmus and Bell's palsy. Pract. oto-rhino-laryng. 24:233.

Pulec, J., 1969: Facial nerve grafting. Laryngoscope 79:1562.

Rice, J., 1963: The chorda tympani in stapedectomy. J. Laryng. 77:943.

Robert, F., and Pfaltz, C., 1970: Vestibuläre Funktionsstörungen bei idiopathischer Facialisparese (Lokalisations- und Kompensationsprobleme). Arch. Ohr. Nas.-Kehlk-Heilk. 197:183.

Root, H., 1933: Paralysis of external ocular muscles in diabetes. Med. Clin. N. Amer. 16:985.

Roseburg, B., 1966: Postoperative Befunde der Chorda tympani nach Otoskleroseoperationen. Hals-Nas.-Ohrenarzt 14:262.

Rosenthal, C., 1931: Klinisch-erbbiologischer Beitrag zur Konstitutionspathologie. Gemeinsames Auftreten von (rezidivierender familiärer) Facialislähmung, angioneurotischem Gesichtsödem und Lingua plicata in Arthritismus-Familien. Z. Neurol. Psychiat. 131:475.

Ross, J., 1970: The function of the tympanic plexus as related to Frey's syndrome. Laryngoscope 80:1816.

Saberman, M., and Tenta, L., 1966: The Melkersson-Rosenthal syndrome. Arch. Otolaryng. 84:292.

Sade, J., Levy, E., and Chaco, J., 1965: Surgery and pathology of Bell's palsy. Arch. Otolaryng. 82:594.

Saito, H., 1973: Regenerative types of the chorda tympani after severance. In press.

Saito, H., Ruby, R., and Schuknecht, H., 1970: Course of the sensory component of the nervus intermedius in the temporal bone. Ann. Otol. Rhinol. Laryng. 79:960.

Saunders, W., 1963: Viral infections and cranial nerve paralysis. Arch. Otolaryng. 78:85.

Saunders, W., and Lippy, W., 1959: Sudden deafness and Bell's palsy: A common cause. Ann. Otol. Rhinol. Laryng. 68:830.

Schuknecht, H.: Unpublished data.

Schuknecht, H., Neff, W., and Perlman, H., 1951: An experimental study of auditory damage following blows to the head. Ann. Otol. Rhinol. Laryng. 60:273.

Schuknecht, H., and Woellner, R., 1953: Hearing losses following partial section of the cochlear nerve. Laryngoscope 63:441.

Schulthess, G. von., 1961: Facialislähmungen nach Schädelbasisfrakturen. Z. Laryng. Rhinol. Otol. 40:404.

Schuring, A., and Saunders, W., 1964: Facial diplegia, a viral disease? Arch. Otolaryng. 80:103.

Sharp, C., Butterfield, W., and Keen, M., 1964: Diabetes survey in Bedford 1962. Proc. Roy. Soc. Med. 57:193.

Simmons, F., 1966: Electrical stimulation of the auditory nerve in man. Arch. Otolaryng. 84:2.

Spiro, R., and Martin, H., 1967: Gustatory sweating following parotid surgery and radical neck dissection. Ann. Surg. 165:118.

Spratt, I., and Hardin, R., 1957: The history of treated diabetes mellitus: A contrast of the young and the old. J. Iowa Med. Soc. 47:571.

Stahle, J., 1966: Vestibular neuritis. In The Vestibular System and Its Diseases. Edited by R. J. Wolfson, University of Pennsylvania Press, Philadelphia, Pa. p. 459.

Tomita, H., Hayakawa, W., and Hondo, R., 1972: Varicella-Zoster virus in idiopathic facial palsy. Arch. Otolaryng. 95:364.

Walford, P., 1952: An unusual epidemic (Letter to the Editor). Lancet 1:415.

Ward, P., Cannon, D., and Lindsay, J., 1965: The vestibular system in multiple sclerosis: A clinical-histopathological study. Laryngoscope 75:1031.

Wechsler, I., 1963: Clinical neurology with an introduction to the history of neurology. 9th ed., W. Saunders, Philadelphia, Pa.

Weiss, A., 1968: Neurological aspects of the differential diagnosis of vertigo. Ann. Otol. Rhinol. Laryng. 77:216.

Wever, E., and Neff, W., 1947: A further study of the effects of partial section of the auditory nerve. J. Comp. Physiol. Psychol. 40:217.

Wiberg, A., 1971: Function of the chorda tympani before and after operation for clinical otosclerosis. Med. Diss., Tryckeriaktiebolaget City, Umeå, Sweden.

Williams, S., 1963: Epidemic vertigo in children. Med. J. Austr. 2:660.

10 Disorders of Growth, Metabolism, and Aging

A. OTOSCLEROSIS

Otosclerosis is a disorder of the bony labyrinth and stapes known to affect only humans. The disorder causes hearing loss which usually has its onset in the second or third decade of life.

1. CLINICAL FEATURES

The foci of otosclerotic bone are symptomatically quiescent until the movement of the stapes is impaired by invasion of the stapediovestibular joint. Cawthorne (1955) reported that 70 percent of patients with clinical otosclerosis first noticed hearing losses between the ages of 11 and 30. Larsson (1960) found that only a small percentage of persons first noticed hearing loss before the age of 11 or after the age of 45.

Anamnestic data on the occurrence of hearing impairment in siblings, parents, or other near relatives of patients with otosclerosis are generally reported to be positive in about half the cases. Thus, Nager (1939) reported a positive family history in 58 percent of 1,146 cases, Cawthorne (1955) in 54 percent of 2,000 cases, Shambaugh (1949) in 54.5 percent of 2,000 cases, and Larsson (1960) in 49 percent of 262 cases.

In commenting on the incidence of otosclerosis, Guild (1944) emphasized the importance of distinguishing between clinical and nonclinical (histological) otosclerosis (Fig. 10.1). In temporal bone studies he found histological evidence of otosclerosis in 8.3 percent of 518 whites and 1 percent of 482 Negroes over the age of five years. The incidence of nonclinical otosclerosis in white populations was 11 percent of 200 temporal bone specimens studied by Weber (1935) and 12 percent of 100 cases studied by Engström (1940).

Otosclerosis usually involves both ears; however, in clinical studies, Nager (1939) found unilateral otosclerosis in 10.7 percent, Cawthorne (1955) in 13 percent, and Larsson (1960) in 15 percent.

Bauer and Stein (1924–1925) found the percentage of females affected to be 65 percent, Schmidt (1933), 72.5 percent, Nager (1939), 64 percent, Cawthorne (1955), 67 percent, and Shambaugh (1949), 68 percent. Studies on the sex incidence of histological (nonclinical) otosclerosis have failed to reveal any significant differences between males and females (Weber, 1935; Engström, 1940; Guild, 1944). It seems probable that the apparent sex difference in the incidence of clinical otosclerosis is due to the fact that women seek medical advice for otosclerosis about twice as frequently as men, and this may be related in some way to pregnancy. Schmidt (1933) reported that 19 of 25 females who were pregnant and had considerable hearing loss from otosclerosis, first noticed the loss during pregnancy. Nager (1939) stated that 30 percent of married women with otosclerosis showed an increased hearing loss as the result of pregnancy. Cawthorne (1955) found that 63 percent of his population of female patients with otosclerosis had the onset of deafness or the aggravation of their hearing loss during pregnancy. On the other hand, Walsh (1954) was unable to establish any relationship between pregnancy and increased hearing loss in women with otosclerosis.

Larsson (1960) states that the morbidity risk for siblings when one has otosclerosis is about 10 percent.

The primary symptom produced by the otosclerotic lesion is a conductive hearing loss, the magnitude of which is directly related to the degree of fixation of the stapes footplate. Typically the hearing loss reaches a maximum in the third decade of life after which there is little further change in the bone-air gap (Glorig and Gallo, 1962).

The early stages of otosclerosis may create mild degrees of fibrous fixation of the footplate and a bone-air gap of less than 30 db. Firm bony ankylosis of the anterior part of the footplate creates a conductive deficit of about 40 db and is the most common lesion encountered during surgery. When the entire circumference of the oval window is involved, the conductive deficit may be greater than 40 db (Figs. 10.2, 10.3).

It is very unusual to find bone-air gaps over 50 db, even with lesions that obliterate the oval window. Presumably, at these intensities sound is bone-conducted either through the ossicles or the skull. It is common for patients with otosclerosis to exhibit vestibular disturbances. Virolainen (1972) found the objective disturbances in order of frequency to be caloric hypoexcitability and elevated thresholds of angular acceleration and deceleration, directional preponderance, and positional nystagmus.

2. HISTOPATHOLOGY

Altmann (1962a), in a review of the histopathology of otosclerosis, has described the histogenesis and structure of the foci in the bony labyrinth.

Fig. 10.1: Nonclinical otosclerosis in a 39-year-old male. There is a small otosclerotic lesion at the anterior margin of the oval window which has not involved the annular ligament or footplate of the stapes.

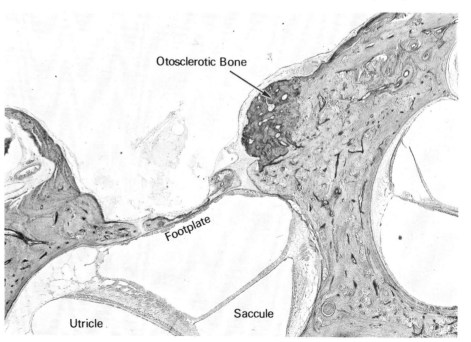

The studies of Politzer (1894), Siebenmann (1912), Manasse (1914), Wittmaack (1930), Mayer (1931), Greifenstein (1935), Weber (1935), Nager (1939), Guild (1944), and others have clarified the morphology and morphogenesis of otosclerosis to the extent that this is possible with light microscopy.

Four stages are generally recognized as occurring in the development and progression of the otosclerotic lesion:

(1) Destruction of enchondral bone with the formation of resorption spaces which contain a highly cellular fibrous tissue. On the basis of experimental evidence, Chevance et al. (1970) believe that the resorptive or lytic phase of the otosclerotic lesion is caused mainly by lysosomal hydrolases. With the aid of electron microscopy they have found cells containing numerous lysosomes in the areas of resorption. The lysosome is a single membrane-bound dense cytoplasmic particle containing numerous hydrolytic enzymes. These enzymes are capable of breaking down protein, DNA, RNA, and certain carbohydrates in an acid pH. It is possible that the cells containing these lysosomes are altered osteocytes or possibly histiocytes. Osteolysis (or osteolytic resorption) may also take place by osteoclastic activity (Fig. 10.4). In this case the osteoclasts act locally by absorbing calcium hydroxyapatite crystals by pinocytosis. It is also possible that osteoclasts exert activity through the use of hydrolytic enzymes such as acid phosphatase.

(2) Formation of mucopolysaccharide and osteoid deposits within the fibroblastic collagen of the resorption spaces leading to the production of immature basophilic bone.

(3) Repetition of the remodeling process of resorption and new bone formation through several generations with the development of a more mature acidophilic bone having a laminated matrix.

(4) Formation of a highly mineralized acidophilic bone having a mosaic-like appearance because of the irregular patterns of resorption and new bone formation associated with the deposition of fatty tissue in the marrow spaces.

The otosclerotic process may become quiescent at any time or may become reactivated. It is not unusual for an otosclerotic focus to contain both inactive and active regions (Fig. 10.5).

Growth may occur on a broad front or by finger-like projections. These finger-like resorption spaces become filled with bone which stains with hematoxylin and are termed "blue mantles" (Manasse, 1922; Weber, 1933) (Figs.

Fig. 10.2: Audiogram and cochlear chart showing a combined sensorineural and conductive hearing loss in a 74-year-old male with otosclerosis. Histological studies fail to show pathological changes adequate to explain the descending bone conduction threshold. See Fig. 10.3.

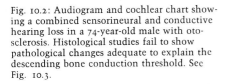
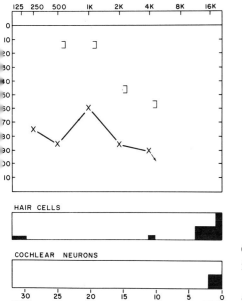

Fig. 10.3: Same case as Fig. 10.2. Histological study shows an otosclerotic lesion involving the bony labyrinth at the anterior margin of the oval window and the entire footplate of the stapes.

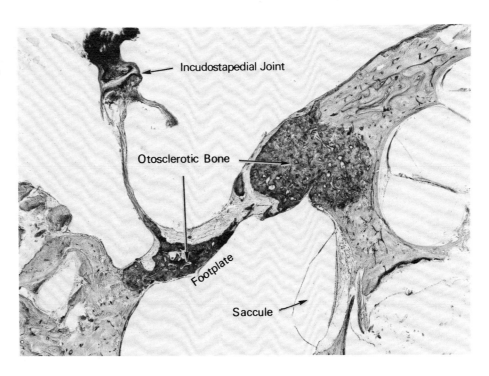

Fig. 10.4: Osteoclastic activity in an active otosclerotic lesion in the bony labyrinth at the anterior margin of the oval window in a 41-year-old male.

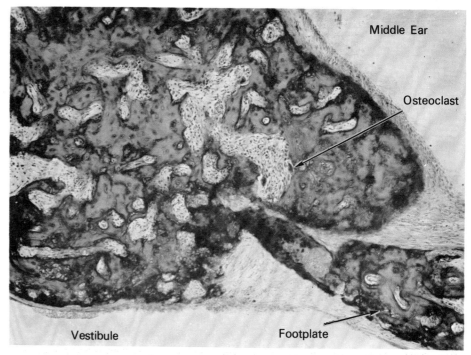

Fig. 10.5: There is a large otosclerotic lesion involving the lateral wall of the bony labyrinth and stapes footplate in a 75-year-old female. The otosclerotic bone shows a varied histological structure. Adjacent to the labyrinthine spaces the bone has a feathery appearance and stains deeply with hematoxylin. More peripherally there is a mosaic architecture with thick trabeculae staining with eosin.

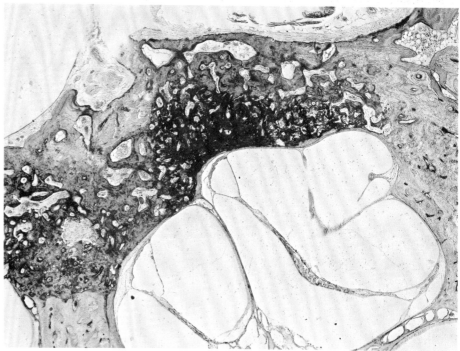

10.6, 10.7). Altmann (1962a) states that blue mantles may be found not only in direct continuity with otosclerotic foci but in other areas of the bony labyrinth of otosclerotic ears, particularly around the semicircular canals. Weber (1936) has pointed out that blue mantles should not be confused with "grenzscheiden," which are thin blue-staining membranes that normally cover the inner surfaces of the lacunae and canaliculae as well as the walls of vascular channels.

The formation of lamellar new bone in the inner ears of patients with otosclerosis has been described by Politzer (1894), Habermann (1904), Siebenmann (1912), Nager and Fraser (1938), and Rüedi (1963). Nager and Fraser (1938) showed that these deposits of new bone occur mainly in the scala tympani of the basal turn near large active foci of otosclerosis (Fig. 10.8). Rüedi (1963, 1969) has found shunts between the vascular system of the otosclerotic bone and the inner ear and suggested that venous stasis from these shunts might be responsible for sensorineural hearing loss.

Guild (1944) and Nylèn (1949) found that about 85 percent of otosclerotic foci are located in the oval window region. Other areas of predilection are

Fig. 10.6: Blue mantles in the enchondral bone surrounding the posterior semicircular canal in an 83-year-old woman with clinical otosclerosis. See Fig. 10.7.

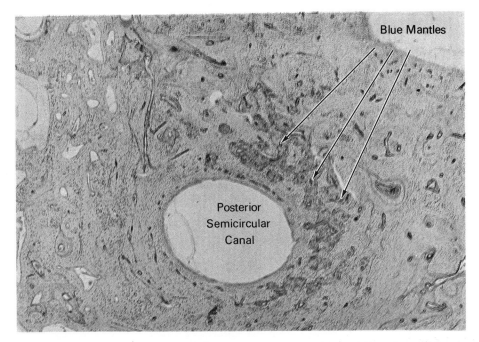

Fig. 10.7: High-power view of blue mantles shown in Fig. 10.6. Blue mantles consist of a uniform abnormal basophilic staining bone deposited primarily in the perivascular resorption spaces. Blue mantles should not be confused with the thin blue-staining membranes which normally cover the inner surfaces of the lacunae and canaliculae as well as the walls of the vascular channels and are termed *grenzscheiden*.

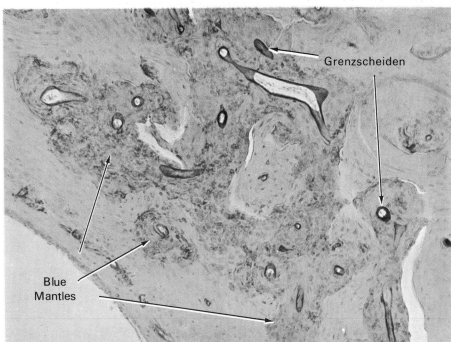

Fig. 10.8: In a 68-year-old female with clinical otosclerosis there is otosclerotic bone at the superior margin of the round window niche associated with lamellar new bone growth extending into the scala tympani. It is probable that some unexplained failures to improve hearing by the stapedectomy procedure are due to occlusion of the round window opening by extensive intrascalar growth of lamellar new bone.

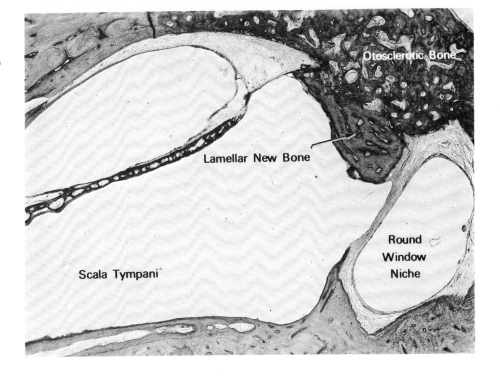

Fig. 10.9: The second most common site for otosclerosis is the bony margin of the round window as shown in this 53-year-old male. Experimental studies have shown that hearing is not affected unless the round window niche is completely obstructed. At the time of surgery it is sometimes impossible to determine with certainty whether the round window has an opening or is totally obstructed by otosclerotic bone.

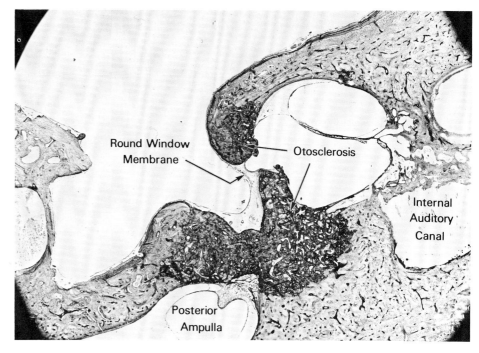

Fig. 10.10: Histological study of the temporal bone of a 69-year-old male with clinical otosclerosis demonstrates total obliteration of the round window opening. With massive lesions such as this, total occlusion of the round window can be readily determined at the time of surgery. Surgical removal of otosclerotic bone from this area is contra-indicated because of the high incidence of postoperative sensorineural hearing loss.

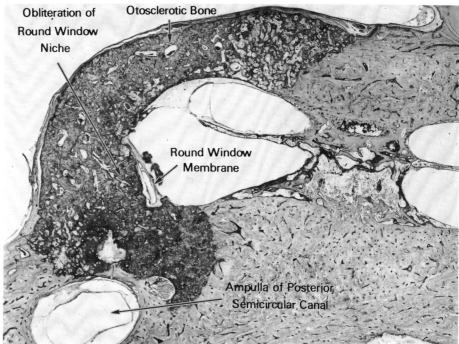

the round window niche (Figs. 10.9, 10.10), the anterior wall of the internal auditory canal (Fig. 10.11), and within the stapedial footplate. The otosclerotic growth may cause lateral displacement of the anterior margin of the stapes (Fig. 10.12). A large focus located primarily within the footplate may cause the stapes to be wedged into the oval window with very little or no involvement of the surrounding oval window margin (Fig. 10.13). Otosclerosis was restricted to the footplate in 12 percent of a series reported by Guild (1944) and 5 percent of those studied by Rüedi and Spoendlin (1957). The incus may be involved but it is extremely rare (Fig. 10.14).

As normal bone is replaced by otosclerotic bone the original anatomical configuration of the bony labyrinth is usually preserved. Actual invasion of the labyrinthine spaces is rare and occurs only in the most active lesions. Even the interscalar septa and part of the modiolus may be replaced by otosclerotic bone without invasion of the fluid spaces (Fig. 10.15). The ostia of the cribrose area which transmit the cochlear nerve fibers are rarely encroached upon, and the bony growth does not invade the internal auditory canal even in the most severe cases.

Young otosclerotic foci often contain fibrous areas with numerous small blood vessels. Mature lesions more often consist of dense bone with fewer

Fig. 10.11: The third most common site for the development of otosclerosis is in the anterior wall of the internal auditory canal as shown in the temporal bone of this 75-year-old female with clinical otosclerosis. Otosclerotic foci in this region appear to remain restricted to the bony wall and do not invade or narrow the internal auditory canal.

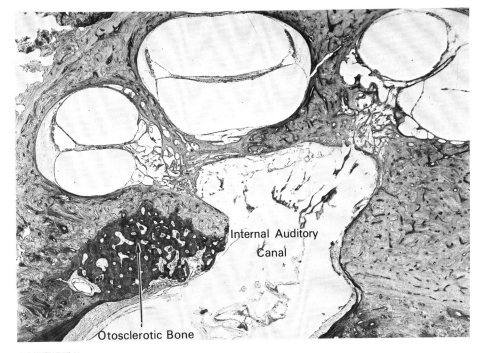

Fig. 10.12: In a 76-year-old female the footplate of the stapes is thickened by otosclerosis and its anterior margin is subluxated laterally. The small focus of otosclerosis at the anterior margin of the oval window does not appear to be in continuity with the footplate.

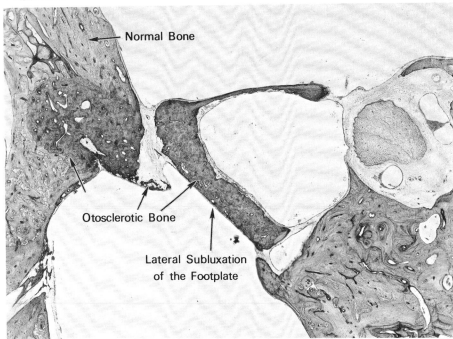

Fig. 10.13: The otosclerosis in this 84-year-old male is located primarily within the footplate of the stapes. There is involvement of only ½ mm to 1 mm of the margins of the oval window.

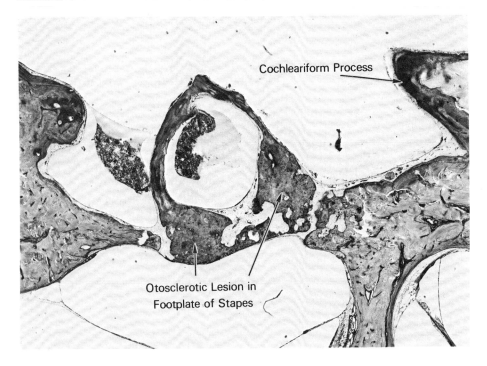

Fig. 10.14: Histological study of the right ear of a 72-year-old female shows an isolated otosclerotic lesion in the short process of the incus.

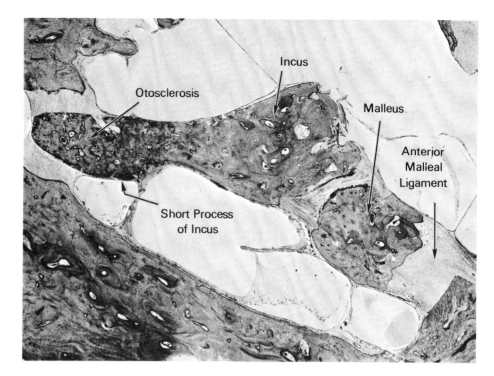

Fig. 10.15: This ear, from a 74-year-old patient, exhibits a large otosclerotic lesion involving the entire thickness of the bony labyrinth, extending into the interscalar septum between the first and second turn and into the modiolus. There are several large vascular channels within the otosclerotic lesion.

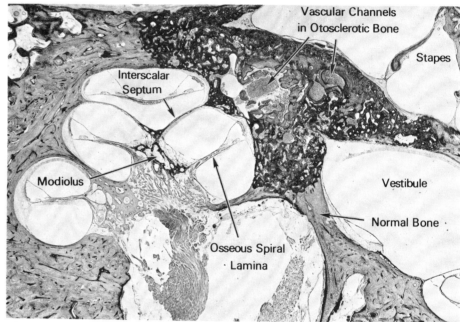

Fig. 10.16: A 75-year-old woman with clinical otosclerosis exhibits involvement of the full thickness of the bony labyrinth anterior to the oval window as well as obliteration of the oval window niche.

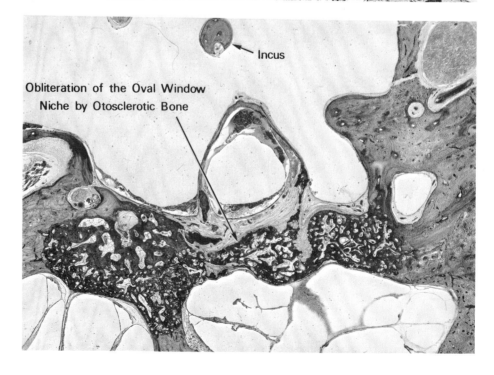

blood vessels, but in unusual cases, large vascular channels are present (Fig. 10.15). In some cases the oval window niche may become obliterated by otosclerotic bone (Fig. 10.16).

Many otologists are of the opinion that otosclerosis damages the inner ear to cause progressive sensorineural hearing loss (Altmann et al., 1966). In 1912 Siebenmann described the inner ear pathology in a 32-year-old woman with otosclerosis and suggested that these changes were due to an accumulation of the products of inflammation in the inner ear. Similarly in 1919, Wittmaack assumed that otosclerosis caused degeneration of the labyrinth by diffusion into the labyrinthine fluids of an acid liberated by the growth. Meurman and Wolff (1960) examined 163 patients under the age of 40 years who had clinical otosclerosis and found that 24.5 percent had an associated sensorineural hearing loss. Bosatra (1960) stated that 5 percent of temporal bones with otosclerotic foci showed involvement of the sensorineural structures. Wolff (1950) reported atrophy of the organs of Corti and cochlear neurons of the basal turns in temporal bones with otosclerosis.

Sataloff et al. (1964), in a study of patients with unilateral otosclerosis, compared the bone conduction levels in the involved ear with the air conduction levels in the normal ear and concluded that otosclerosis commonly causes a sensorineural impairment of more than 10 db for at least a three-octave range of higher frequencies. In a study of temporal bones of patients with otosclerosis, Keleman and Linthicum (1969) showed a positive correlation between the magnitude of sensorineural hearing loss and the severity of atrophic change in the spiral ligament. Sando et al. (1968), in a single temporal bone case report, showed focal loss of hair cells in the organ of Corti spatially related to areas of otosclerotic involvement of the bony labyrinth. Compere (1960) and Valvassori (1965) believe they can demonstrate radiologically the presence of otosclerosis of the bony labyrinth in some patients with pure sensorineural hearing loss.

Some investigations, on the other hand, have failed to establish a correlation between otosclerosis and sensorineural hearing loss. In a histological study Guild (1944) found that atrophy of cochlear neurons or organ of Corti occurred no more often in ears with otosclerotic foci than in ears free from otosclerosis. He found that when atrophy did occur in otosclerotic ears it was limited to the basal turn and differed in no way from the atrophy that is often seen in ears without otosclerosis. He concluded that the etiology of cochlear atrophy in ears without otosclerosis cannot, in most cases, be established and, therefore, it does not seem logical to attribute to otosclerosis the cochlear atrophy found in otosclerotic ears.

In 1962 Glorig and Gallo compared the audiometric data from patients with presbycusis, otosclerosis, noise-induced deafness and sensorineural hearing loss of unknown cause. Comparisons were made between bone conduction levels in patients with otosclerosis and air conduction levels in the general population. They assumed these comparisons to be valid because hearing losses found in the general population are overwhelmingly sensorineural. The number of flat audiometric patterns which they assumed to be due to conductive lesions was about 1 percent in a non-noise exposed population. The data indicated that otosclerosis does not increase sensorineural loss above that to be expected in the general population. Audiometric patterns for high frequencies in individuals with otosclerosis resembled closely those found in general and industrial populations. The only finding which might be in contradiction to these conclusions occurred in the group over 60 years of age where the sensorineural hearing loss for high frequencies was somewhat greater in patients with otosclerosis than in the general population.

A study of the temporal bones in the collection at the Massachusetts Eye and Ear Infirmary has shown that the inner ear structure most commonly affected by otosclerosis is the spiral ligament. This ligament forms the circumferential surface of the membranous labyrinth and lies in direct contact with the bony labyrinth. More than half of the patients with clinical otosclerosis had foci which were sufficiently large to involve the endosteal layer of the bony labyrinth, and in most of these there were atrophic changes in the spiral ligament more severe than normal for age. The earliest changes occurred in the areas adjacent to the otosclerotic bone and consisted of a loss of cellularity and deposition of a layer of collagen (Schuknecht and Gross, 1966) (Figs. 10.17, 10.18). Because the otosclerotic focus involved predominantly the lateral cochlear wall, the spiral ligament was involved most severely in the lateral arcs of each cochlear turn. Severe alterations in the bony labyrinth and spiral ligament may occur with no observable histological alterations in the structures of the cochlear duct (Fig. 10.19). It must be remembered that atrophy of the spiral ligament, most severe in the apical region, is a consistent finding in temporal bones without otosclerosis and constitutes one of the changes of aging. The evidence which indicates that otosclerosis aggravates this atrophy is that the changes are most severe in those regions where the spiral ligament is in contact with otosclerotic bone (Figs. 10.20, 10.21). There does not appear to be a consistent spatial relationship between areas of atrophy of the spiral ligament and atrophy of the organ of Corti; however, in exceptional cases the spiral ligament may become so greatly atrophied as to lead to rupture of the cochlear duct and profound deafness (Benitez and Schuknecht, 1962). The concept of "cochlear oto-

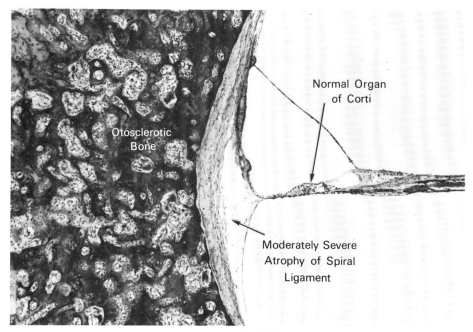

Fig. 10.17: This ear shows atrophy of the spiral ligament in the lateral part of the basal turn where the ligament is in contact with otosclerotic bone. See also Fig. 10.20.

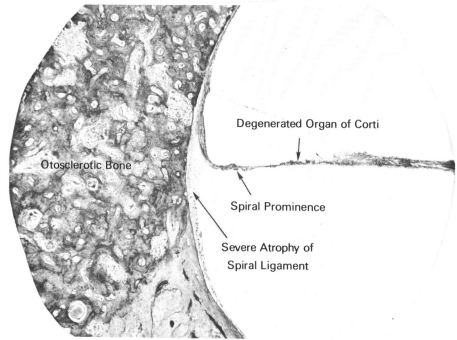

Fig. 10.18: This ear exhibited a profound sensorineural hearing loss. In the apical turn there is near total atrophy of the spiral ligament and degeneration of the organ of Corti. In other areas of the cochlea the basilar membrane is separated from the spiral ligament which may have been the basis for the profound hearing loss. See also Fig. 10.20.

Fig. 10.19: This patient had a long history of combined sensorineural and conductive hearing loss and died at the age of 74. Histological studies show a large otosclerotic lesion involving the lateral wall of the bony labyrinth and footplate of the stapes. This view from the middle turn of the cochlea shows irregular replacement of the endosteal layer of bone and atrophy of the spiral ligament. In spite of these changes the structures of the cochlear duct appear normal.

Fig. 10.20: This patient had a slowly progressive bilateral hearing loss beginning at the age of 23. At the age of 53 audiometric studies of the left ear (shown here) exhibited a combined sensorineural and conductive hearing loss. Histological studies show atrophy of the spiral ligament in the lateral parts of each cochlear turn where the ligament was in contact with the otosclerotic bone. See also Figs. 10.17 and 10.18.

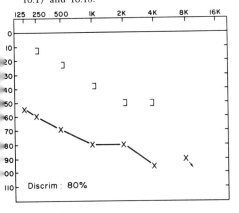

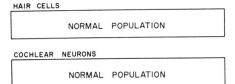

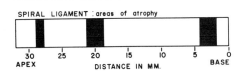

Fig. 10.21: View of entire cochlea of same patient as Fig. 10.20. The areas of most severe atrophy of the spiral ligament are located next to the otosclerotic bone.

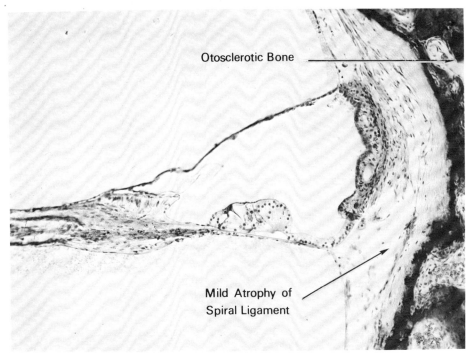

sclerosis," that is, pure sensorineural hearing loss caused by otosclerosis of the bony labyrinth *without stapes fixation*, has been the subject of much discussion (Shambaugh, 1965; Derlacki and Valvassori, 1965); however, this idea cannot be supported on the basis of histological studies. A study of the temporal bones of patients with pure sensorineural deafness of unknown cause has failed to show otosclerotic foci of significant incidence or size to explain the inner ear changes (Gross, 1969; Schuknecht and Kirchner, 1974).

3. SURGERY FOR OTOSCLEROSIS

a. Historical account

The first attempts to improve the hearing of patients with otosclerosis consisted of making fenestrae at various sites in the labyrinth. Holmgren's (1923, 1937) original attempts to maintain permanent fistulae were almost always unsuccessful; however, one patient apparently experienced improved hearing for more than nine months. Sourdille (1937) developed the first consistently successful operation for fenestration of the lateral semicircular canal;

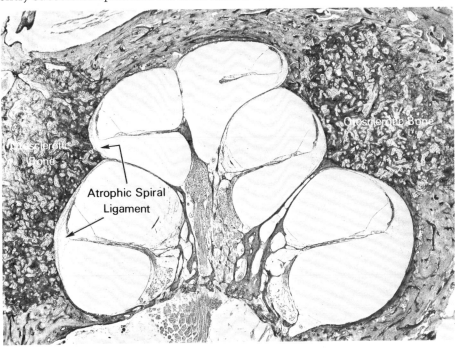

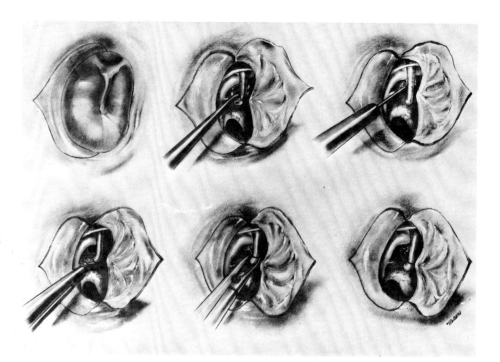

Fig. 10.22: Technique for stapedectomy as used by the author. After making incisions in the skin of the bony ear canal, a tympanomeatal flap is elevated to expose the posterior mesotympanum. The head and crural arch of the stapes is removed. The footplate is fractured and removed in pieces. A prosthetic replacement is constructed on a wire-bending die. This consists of a prosthesis made from 38 gauge (0.004 inch) stainless steel wire. It has a hook for attachment to the incus and a shaft measuring about 4.0 mm in length. It is tied to an autogenous graft of adipose tissue from the ear lobe measuring about 2 x 3 mm. This prosthesis is introduced with the adipose graft placed in the oval window and the hook on the incus where it is closed with a forceps. The tympanomeatal flap is then returned to its original position. When the footplate is greatly thickened by otosclerosis, a burr is used to saucerize the oval window area following which an opening measuring about 0.8 mm is made into the vestibule. A piston prosthesis made of a 38-gauge stainless steel wire shaft and hook and a teflon plunger of 0.6 mm diameter is then inserted.

however, it required a two-stage technique. Lempert (1941) later developed a successful one-stage operation.

Surgical approaches to the oval window area were attempted by Kessel (1876), Boucheron (1888), Miot (1890), Moure (1890), Jack (1892–1893), and Blake (1893); however, the results were inconsistent. Rosen (1953) revitalized interest in oval window surgery when he reported success with stapes mobilization. Hall and Rytzner (1957) had some success with stapedectomy; however, Shea (1958) developed the first consistently successful stapedectomy operation by substituting the stapes with a vein graft and polyethylene prosthesis.

b. Stapedectomy

There are two principal schools of thought regarding the best method of stapes surgery. One school prefers total or subtotal removal of the stapes bone followed by the introduction of a prosthesis of metal or plastic material (Shea, 1958, 1971; Kos, 1960; Schuknecht, 1960a, 1960b, 1962a, 1964a; House, 1962; McGee, 1962; Guilford, 1962) (Fig. 10.22). The other school prefers to avoid the introduction of artificial materials into the middle ear after total or partial dislocation or removal of the stapes. These surgeons utilize autogenous tissue grafts or reposition part of the stapes (capitulum and crus) to reconstitute the ossicular mechanism (Portmann, 1960; Hough, 1960; Zöllner, 1962; Antoli-Candela, 1962).

It appears that many different techniques can be used with success and that much depends upon the experience and technical skill of the surgeon (Schuknecht, 1971). By careful selection of candidates for surgery a high rate of success can be achieved (Fig. 10.23).

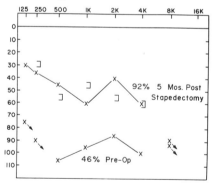

Fig. 10.23: Excellent improvement in pure tone thresholds and speech discrimination thresholds following stapedectomy in a patient with a severe combined sensorineural and conductive hearing loss.

Most studies which attempt to evaluate the long-term results of stapedectomy suffer from a lack of statistical validity. In a migrant population such as that found in the United States the number of patients available for follow-up study decreases rapidly as a function of time after surgery. Reports indicate that an initial bone-air gap of 10 db or better is achieved in about 80 to 90 percent of patients and that a sensorineural hearing loss associated with a loss of speech discrimination of 30 percent or more can be expected in 1 to 3 percent of the patients. Improvement is maintained at the 10 db bone-air gap level for five years in less than 70 percent of the patients (Bellucci, 1969; Antoli-Candela, 1969; House and Greenfield, 1969; McGee, 1969). A loss of speech discrimination of 10 to 30 percent can be expected in about 6 percent, simply as the result of improving sound transmission qualities of the middle ear (Feldman and Schuknecht, 1970). This is due to eliminating the

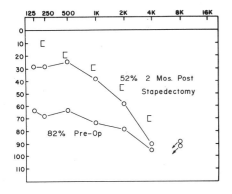

Fig. 10.24: Improvement in pure tone thresholds with loss of speech discrimination following stapedectomy. The loss in discrimination score is caused by converting a relatively flat preoperative threshold pattern to a descending postoperative pattern and is not the result of cochlear injury.

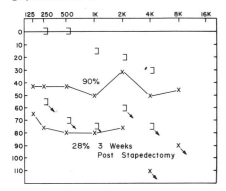

Fig. 10.25: Great decrease in pure tone threshold and speech discrimination following a stapedectomy procedure. Although the pathogenesis of this change is not known, it is presumed to be caused by either inflammation, biochemical changes, or toxic reaction to surgery rather than to bacterial invasion.

stiffness lesion in ears with descending bone conduction thresholds. Thus the audiometric pattern is altered so that a relatively flat preoperative air conduction threshold is converted to a descending postoperative air conduction threshold (Fig. 10.24). This occurs so consistently as to achieve a high level of predictability (Mock and Schuknecht, unpublished data). Losses of 30 percent or more in speech discrimination immediately following stapedectomy probably are caused by surgically induced degenerative changes in the sensory and neural structures (Fig. 10.25). Increased tinnitus is a consistent and annoying symptom for these patients and is a differentiating factor in determining whether the loss of speech discrimination is caused by an altered pattern of middle ear sound transmission or to a surgically induced cochlear lesion.

In a report of 154 revision operations for previously unsuccessful stapedectomies, Feldman and Schuknecht (1970) found the most common causes for failure to be host response to surgical trauma, 37 percent; prosthetic malfunctions, 32 percent; faulty ossicular management, 24 percent; and anatomical obstacles, 7 percent.

One of the most common early complications of stapedectomy is the reparative granuloma. It usually becomes manifest between the sixth to fifteenth day after surgery (Harris and Weiss, 1962; Lewis, 1962; Paparella et al., 1966; Kaufman and Schuknecht, 1967; Gacek, 1970). Kaufman and Schuknecht found ten granulomas in a total of 780 stapedectomies for an incidence of 1.3 percent. Three of these followed 170 fat-wire implants, and seven occurred after 610 Gelfoam-wire implants. The characteristic symptoms are a hearing loss (after an initial hearing gain) and/or dysequilibrium. Examination reveals an edematous, thickened, hyperemic skin flap and tympanic membrane. Prompt surgical removal of the granuloma and prosthesis and replacement with another graft and prosthesis are frequently successful in preventing a sensorineural hearing loss.

Stapedectomy frequently results in injury to the chorda tympani nerve at its exit at the iter chorda posterius and causes a loss or diminution of taste in the homolateral anterior two-thirds of the tongue and diminution of secretory function of the homolateral submaxillary and sublingual salivary glands. The symptoms usually are minimal and subside within a few weeks although permanent functional deficits can be expected. Saito (in press) has demonstrated that a small traumatic neuroma may form at the site of injury to this nerve (see Chapter 9F3, Trauma to the chorda tympani nerve).

A fistula of the oval window may be evident a few days or weeks following a stapedectomy or may be delayed for some weeks or months (Harrison et al., 1967; 1970; House, 1967; Hemenway et al., 1968; Arenberg and Shambaugh, 1969; Moon, 1970). The most characteristic symptoms are sensorineural hearing loss (often mild and sometimes fluctuating) and dysequilibrium of varying intensity occurring in the absence of any other findings. A review of the literature indicates that the incidence of perilymph fistula is related to the type of stapes replacement, the order of frequency being: (1) polyethylene tube and Gelfoam; (2) polyethylene tube and vein graft; (3) piston in a large opening; (4) piston in a small opening; (5) Gelfoam and wire prosthesis; and (6) tissue-wire prosthesis. The overall incidence of fistulae was reported to be 1.3 percent of 7,222 procedures by Harrison et al. (1970), and 2.5 percent of 1,784 procedures by Hemenway et al. (1968).

Sudden sensorineural hearing loss may occur some months or years following stapedectomy (Schuknecht, 1962b; Sale, 1969). This occurs more commonly following a traumatic stapedectomy or following a revision procedure. The pathogenesis and associated morphological changes resulting from this complication have not been fully elucidated. Other complications which have been described by Linthicum (1971) are regrowth of otosclerotic bone, resorption of the long process of the incus, ankylosis of the malleus, ankylosis of the incus, lateral location of the oval window membrane, foreign bodies in the vestibule, and adhesions in the vestibule.

Clinical studies suggest that stapedectomy does not render the ear more susceptible to injury from high-intensity noise (Ferris, 1965, 1967).

Suppurative labyrinthitis may occur as an early or late complication of stapedectomy (Lewis, 1961; Sheehy and House, 1962; Brown, 1967; Leonard, 1967; Matz et al., 1968) and death has been reported from this complication (Rutledge et al., 1963; Wolff, 1964; Palva et al., 1972) (Figs. 10.26, 10.27).

c. Histopathology of stapes surgery

Animal experiments. The success of surgery for otosclerosis depends in part on reparative reactions to surgical trauma, and these reactions can be studied in the normal animal ear. Experiments in which the stapedial footplate is fractured, displaced, or removed and replaced with various grafts and prostheses have provided useful information.

In the cat, fracture of a central portion of the footplate with only slight separation of the fragments usually results in fibrous union followed by bony healing (Singleton and Schuknecht, 1959). Bone chips introduced into the perilymphatic space of the vestibule become devitalized but create no osteogenic or fibrous tissue reaction and appear to behave as inert bodies (Schuknecht, 1962b).

Small fistulae of the oval windows heal with thin membranes (Fig. 10.28); however, large fistulae may remain open for long periods of time and provide a route for the development of meningitis (Schuknecht, 1962b, 1962c) (Fig. 10.29).

Surgical luxation and re-approximation of the articulating surfaces of the stapediovestibular joint are usually followed by healing with fibrous tissue without new bone formation. Direct trauma to the joint or to the periosteum adjacent to the joint frequently incites an osteogenic reaction followed by ankylosis of the footplate. Autogenous tissue grafts to the oval window (adipose tissue, mucous membrane, conjunctiva, connective tissue) consistently show tissue survival (Schuknecht et al., 1960) (Fig. 10.30), whereas homologous grafts tend to undergo progressive atrophy (Rutledge et al., 1965). Hayden and McGee (1965) demonstrated that traumatized autogenous adipose tissue, when transplanted, is transformed into fibrous tissue.

Gelfoam placed in the oval window following stapedectomy incites the following sequence of histological changes: (1) invasion with polymorphonuclear leucocytes and monocytes (24 hours); (2) fibroblastic proliferation within the Gelfoam (48 hours); (3) formation of an intact membrane on the vestibular surface of the Gelfoam (4 to 7 days); and (4) final resorption of the Gelfoam and replacement by a membrane of varying thickness (3 weeks) (Kylander, 1967) (Figs. 10.31, 10.32, 10.33).

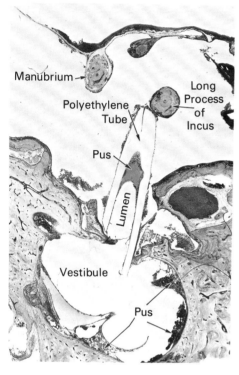

Fig. 10.26: A stapedectomy operation was performed on this patient with bilateral clinical otosclerosis at the age of 38. The operative procedure consisted of removing the capitulum and crura of the stapes and placing a polyethylene tube between the lenticular process and fragmented footplate. Two years later he developed an upper respiratory infection followed by ear pain, vertigo, and coma and died. Histological study shows the polyethylene tube extending from the lenticular process of the incus through the oval window into the vestibule. Collections of leucocytes are seen in the middle ear, within the lumen of the polyethylene tube, and throughout the perilymphatic spaces of the inner ear. Autopsy revealed purulent meningitis caused by Diplococcus pneumoniae. (Courtesy of Rutledge) See Fig. 10.27.

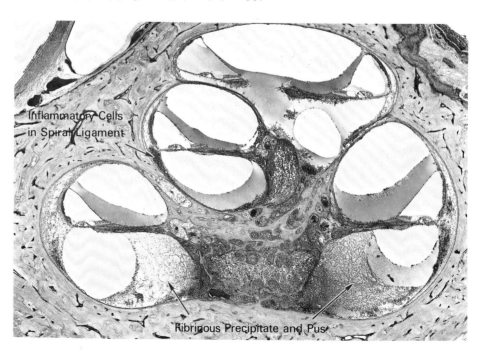

Fig. 10.27: Same ear as Fig. 10.26. This photomicrograph shows acute suppurative labyrinthitis as a delayed complication of stapes surgery for otosclerosis. Bacterial invasion of the inner ear occured through a fistula of the footplate. There is fibrinous precipitate and collections of leucocytes in the perilymphatic space. The patient died of pneumococcal meningitis four days after the onset of otitis media. (Courtesy of Rutledge)

Fig. 10.28: The footplate of the stapes of this cat was fractured by mechanical force with a small pick. The animal was killed four months later, and histological study shows that the fistula created by fracture dislocation has healed by the formation of a thin membrane consisting of a layer of regenerated epithelium on the middle ear surface and a layer of endosteum on the inner ear surface.

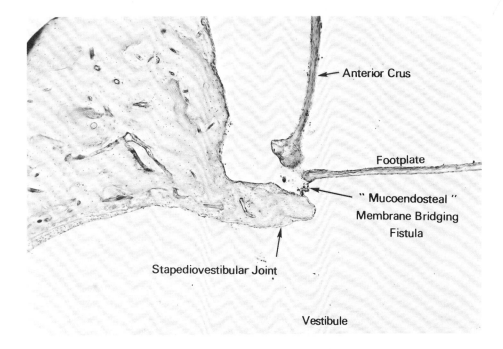

Fig. 10.29: Nine months after an experimental fracture of the footplate of the stapes this cat developed otitis media followed by meningitis. There is a purulent exudate extending from the middle ear through a perforation of the footplate into the perilymphatic space. The cochlear duct shows mild endolymphatic hydrops.

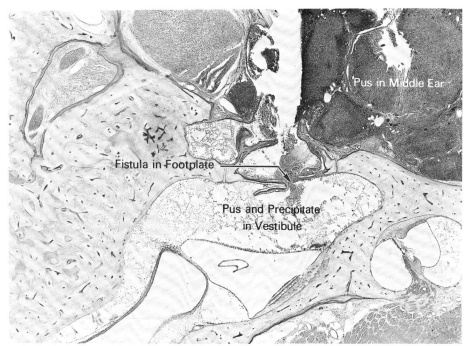

Fig. 10.30: In this cat a stapedectomy was performed, and an autogenous graft of subcutaneous adipose tissue was introduced into the oval window. After a survival time of three months the oval window is bridged by a viable fatty connective tissue graft covered on the middle ear surface by a layer of mucous membrane and on the vestibular surface by a layer of fibrous tissue.

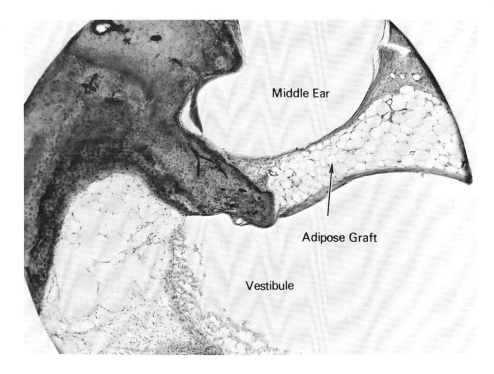

Fig. 10.31: In this squirrel monkey the stapes was removed and a pledget of Gelfoam placed in the oval window. After a survival period of 96 hours the Gelfoam is infiltrated with numerous polymorphonuclear leucocytes. No membrane has formed on the vestibular surface of the implant. There is a large amount of fibrinous precipitate in the perilymph of the vestibule.

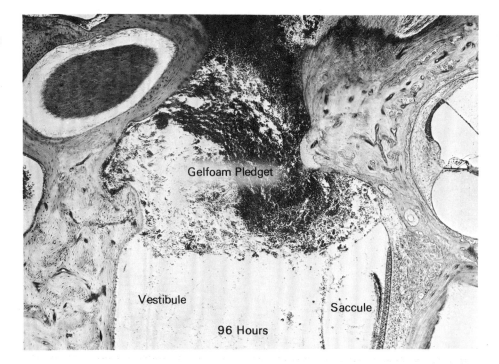

Fig. 10.32: The stapes was removed from this squirrel monkey and a pledget of Gelfoam placed in the oval window. After a survival time of one week there is partial resorption of the Gelfoam. Fibrous tissue has invaded the Gelfoam, and an intact membrane has formed on the vestibular surface. The perilymph contains a small amount of fibrinous precipitate.

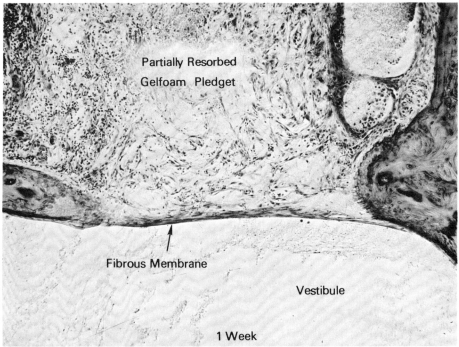

Fig. 10.33: Two weeks following stapedectomy and Gelfoam implant in this squirrel monkey, the Gelfoam has been completely resorbed and the oval window niche contains a mass of fibrous tissue. There is no fibrinous precipitate in the perilymph.

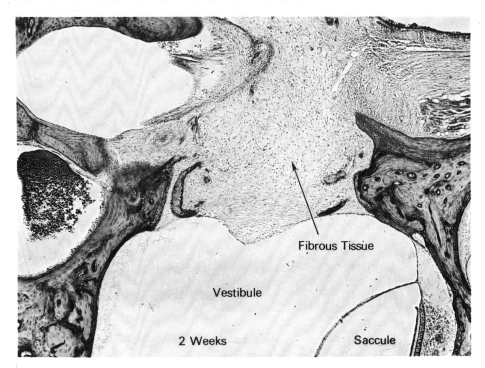

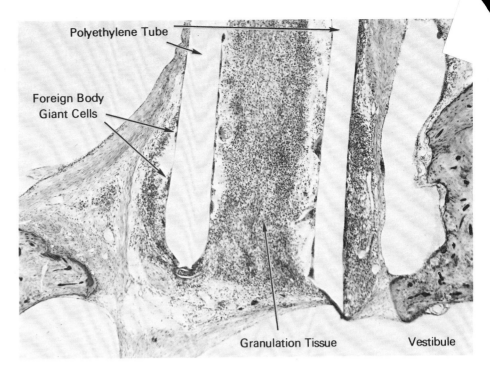

Fig. 10.34: In this cat the stapes was removed following which a graft of subcutaneous adipose tissue was placed in the oval window and a polyethylene tube was positioned between the incus and adipose graft. After a survival period of three months, histological studies show near total resorption of the adipose tissue. There is granulation tissue with foreign body giant cells surrounding the polyethylene tube.

Tantalum wire introduced into the middle ear and vestibule becomes ensheathed in thin membranes consisting of flat pavement-like epithelium without foreign body reaction (Schuknecht and Oleksiuk, 1960). Polyethylene prostheses on the other hand, incite foreign body reaction of varying intensities (Fig. 10.34).

Hohmann (1962) studied the inner ear reactions in a total of 64 animal ears in which Schuknecht and his colleagues had performed stapes surgery associated with the introduction of various types of grafts and implants. Many of these operations were designed purposely to provoke labyrinthine reactions; therefore, the incidence of complications would be greater than with uncomplicated stapes operations in human beings. Mild endolymphatic hydrops was the earliest and most common form of labyrinthine reaction to stapes surgery, occuring in 29 percent of the ears. Stimulation injury as evidenced by loss of hair cells of the organ of Corti in the upper basal turn occurred in 14 percent, serofibrinous labyrinthitis in 12 percent, and suppurative labyrinthitis in 3 percent.

Schuknecht and Tonndorf (1960) reported that inward displacement of part of the footplate can injure the organ of Corti. The location and morphological appearance of the lesion was identical to that which is known to occur as the result of high-intensity noise or blast-induced injury.

Human temporal bone studies. Since the advent of stapes mobilization (Rosen, 1953) and stapedectomy (Shea, 1958), numerous reports have appeared in the literature describing the findings in temporal bones of patients having had this type of surgery (Altmann and Basek, 1958; Lindsay et al., 1959; Altmann et al., 1960; Altmann, 1962b; Schuknecht et al., 1964; Baron and Lindsay, 1964; Reddy et al., 1966; Myers and Myers, 1968; Wolff et al., 1968; Igarashi et al., 1970; Subotić and Kaufman, 1971). These studies are providing useful information on the response of the human ear to surgical trauma and to its tolerance to prostheses.

Brief histories and histopathological findings in ears subjected to stapes surgery are seen in Figs. 10.35 to 10.55.

Stapedectomy is a technically difficult operative procedure, the success of which is directly related to the skills of the surgeon. The stapes must be removed without trauma to the middle and inner ear structures. The prosthesis must be of proper length, and the linkage to the incus must be stable. When properly executed, the stapedectomy procedure can be expected to provide long-term hearing gains (Shea, 1971).

Fig. 10.35: This patient first noted a hearing loss at the age of 35. The loss was progressive, and at the age of 41 a fenestration of the lateral semicircular canal was performed on the right ear. Auditory thresholds were improved but hearing was not restored to a practical hearing level. See also Figs. 10.36, 10.37, and 10.38.

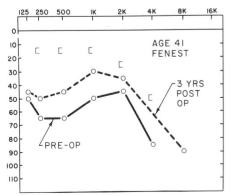

Fig. 10.36: Normal mastoid air cell system of patient's left ear for comparison with right ear shown in Fig. 10.37, which was subjected to the fenestration operation.

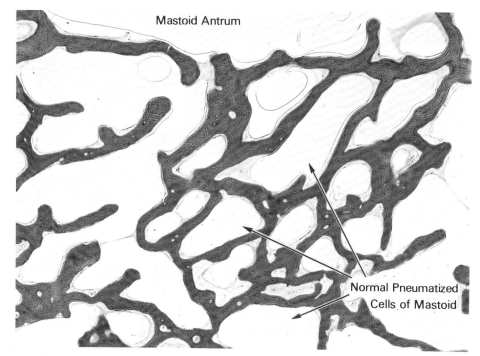

Mastoid Antrum

Normal Pneumatized Cells of Mastoid

Fig. 10.37: This photograph shows the periantral area of the right mastoid ten years following the fenestration operation (see Figs. 10.35, 10.36, and 10.38). In this procedure the mastoid air cell system is exenterated sufficiently to expose the superior part of the lateral semicircular canal. The posterior wall of the external auditory canal is removed, a tympanomeatal flap is laid into the epitympanum and over the lateral semicircular canal, and the remaining mastoid air cell system is left exposed to the external auditory canal. As shown in this view, the air cells normally become obliterated by proliferation of fibrous tissue and small central cystic spaces lined with epithelium. The surface of the mastoid bowl becomes lined with a more dense fibrous tissue covered with squamous epithelium derived as an ingrowth from the external auditory canal.

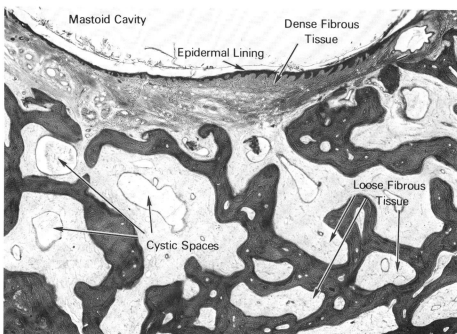

Mastoid Cavity

Dense Fibrous Tissue

Epidermal Lining

Loose Fibrous Tissue

Cystic Spaces

Fig. 10.38: Same case as Figs. 10.35, 10.36, and 10.37, fenestration of the lateral semicircular canal. Histological examination shows a wide bony opening which is bridged by a membrane consisting of a layer of connective tissue covered externally by a thin layer of squamous epithelium. This membrane represents part of the tympanomeatal flap which was transposed from the posterosuperior surface of the external auditory canal.

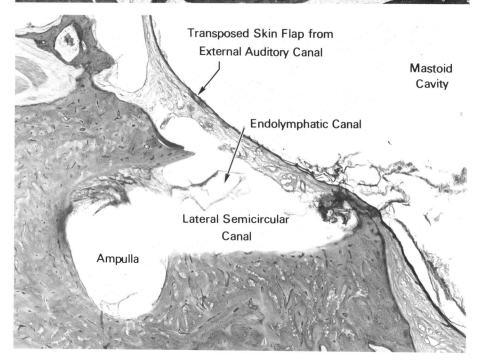

Transposed Skin Flap from External Auditory Canal

Mastoid Cavity

Endolymphatic Canal

Lateral Semicircular Canal

Ampulla

Fig. 10.39: At the age of 45 a partial stapedectomy operation was performed on this patient's left ear. The capitulum and crura were
removed; the posterior one-half of the footplate was mobilized and slightly depressed
into the vestibule. A 32-gauge stainless steel
wire prosthesis was introduced to bridge the
gap from the incus to the mobilized segment
of footplate. Auditory tests performed one
month later showed an improvement in auditory threshold. Although no further auditory
tests were performed it is known that the subjective improvement of hearing was maintained until the time of death six years later.
See Fig. 10.40.

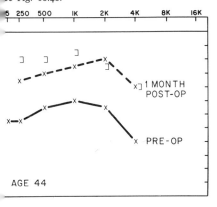

Fig. 10.40: See Fig. 10.39 for history. Histological study shows the anterior margin of the
footplate to be ankylosed by an otosclerotic
lesion. The posterior half of the footplate is
displaced slightly into the vestibule and the
surrounding gap bridged by a thin membrane.
The wire has been removed during preparation of the ear; however, the sheath of mucous membrane which enveloped the wire is
clearly visible.

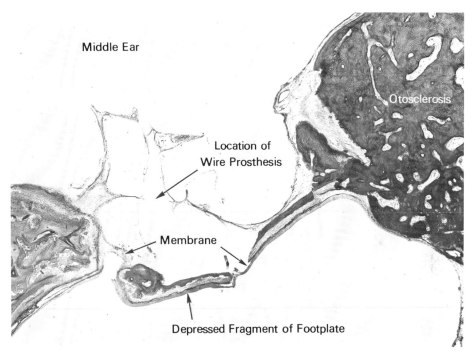

Middle Ear

Otosclerosis

Location of
Wire Prosthesis

Membrane

Depressed Fragment of Footplate

Fig. 10.41: This patient first experienced hearing loss at the age of 13. Examination at the
age of 54 revealed bilateral severe conductive
hearing loss with speech discrimination scores
of 98 percent on the right and 88 percent on
the left. A stapedectomy operation was performed on the right ear, and the stapes was
replaced with a prosthetic insert consisting of
adipose tissue and steel wire. Postoperative
audiometric tests revealed an excellent hearing gain which persisted until the time of her
death from myocardial infarction 21 months
after the operation. See Fig. 10.42.

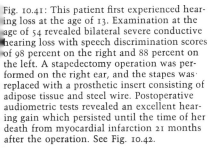
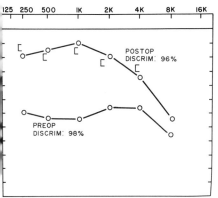

Fig. 10.42: See Fig. 10.41 for history. Histological study shows the stapes to be missing and the oval window niche to be filled with a soft tissue mass consisting principally of loose areolar connective tissue containing scattered fat cells. In the center of this tissue is a defect indicating the position of the stainless steel prosthesis which was removed prior to sectioning. There is an otosclerotic focus at the anterior margin of the oval window.

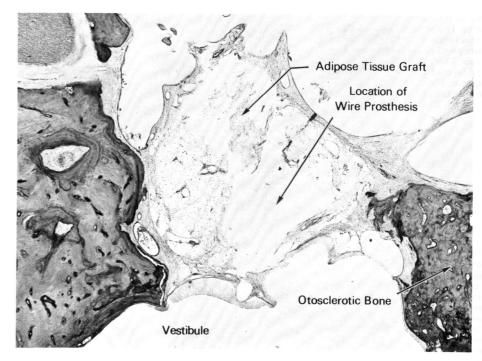

Fig. 10.43: This individual experienced a slowly progressive bilateral hearing loss beginning in adolescence and wore a hearing aid in the left ear. Examination at the age of 52 showed a bilateral combined sensorineural and conductive hearing loss and speech discrimination of 90 percent in both ears. A left stapedectomy operation was performed and the stapes replaced with a stainless steel prosthesis and adipose connective tissue graft from the ear lobe. Audiometric study six weeks later showed elimination of the conductive component of her hearing loss. No further hearing tests were performed, and she died nine years later at the age of 61. See Figs. 10.44 and 10.45.

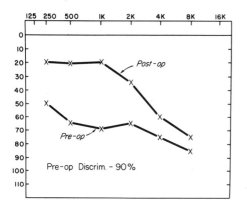

Fig. 10.44: See Fig. 10.43 for history. The graft consists of loose fibrous tissue with scattered islands of adipose tissue. Fragments of crura are seen on the anterior surface of the graft, and a focus of otosclerosis is seen at the anterior margin of the oval window. See Fig. 10.45.

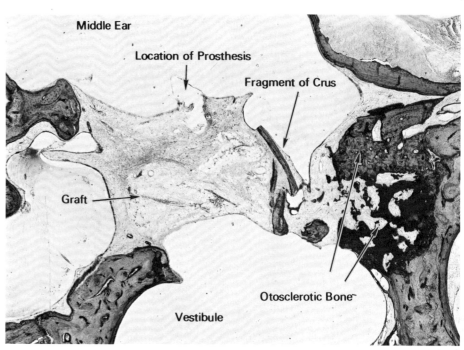

Fig. 10.45: Same case as in Figs. 10.43 and 10.44. This view shows the long process of the incus in the area where the loop of the steel wire prosthesis has been attached for nine years. There is resorption of some of the cortical layer of bone on the medial surface and some new bone formation on the lateral surface of the process.

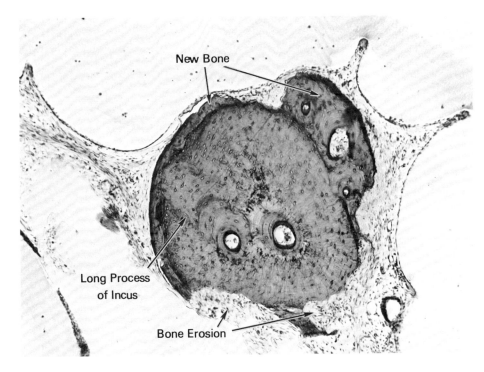

Fig. 10.46: This patient had a slowly progressive bilateral hearing loss first noticed at the age of 20. Audiometric studies at the age of 75 revealed a bilateral combined sensorineural and conductive hearing loss. At that age a left stapedectomy was performed and the stapes was replaced with a Gelfoam-steel wire prosthesis. She experienced a good gain in pure tone thresholds, however, the speech discrimination score, which was 64 percent prior to surgery, diminished to 32 percent. She died of myocardial infarction four months after surgery. Although histological study showed patchy atrophy of the stria vascularis and partial loss of sensory cells and cochlear neurons in the basal turn, there was no clear pathological explanation for the discrimination loss which followed surgery. See Fig. 10.47.

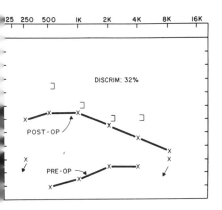

Fig. 10.47: For history see Fig. 10.46. Histological study shows a small otosclerotic focus at the anterior margin of the oval window. The stapes is missing, and the oval window is bridged by a membrane of fibrous tissue averaging about 1 mm in thickness. The position occupied by the steel prosthesis is marked by channels lined with a thin membrane extending toward the incus.

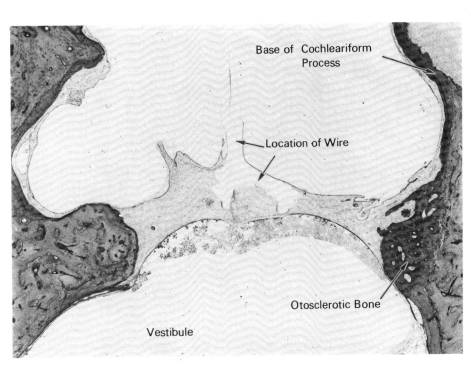

Fig. 10.48: This patient with a severe combined sensorineural and conductive hearing loss of long duration was subjected to a left stapedectomy at the age of 80. The stapes was removed and replaced by a Gelfoam-steel wire prosthesis. He experienced an excellent hearing gain which was particularly useful with a hearing aid. He died of intestinal infarction nine months later. Histological study shows a moderate diffuse loss of hair cells, a slight loss of cochlear neurons in the basal turn, and areas of strial atrophy in the 20 and 30 mm regions. See Fig. 10.49.

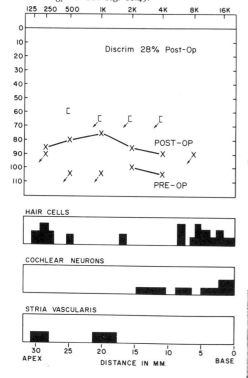

Fig. 10.49: See Fig. 10.48 for history. The tympanic membrane is thickened, and the posterosuperior part of the bony tympanic annulus has been surgically removed. The stapes has been surgically removed except for a small fragment of the anterior crus. The oval window is bridged by a membrane which varies from 1/2 mm to 1 mm in thickness.

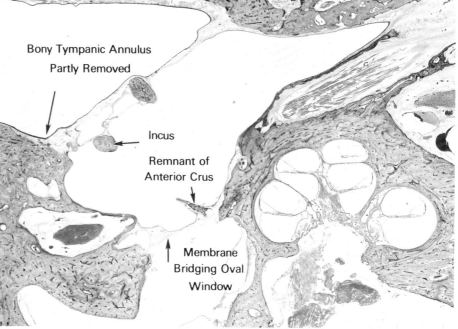

Bony Tympanic Annulus
Partly Removed

Incus

Remnant of
Anterior Crus

Membrane
Bridging Oval
Window

Fig. 10.50: At about the age of 20 the patient first noted hearing loss. The deafness was slowly progressive and at the age of 66 a right stapedectomy was performed. The stapes was replaced with a Gelfoam-wire prosthesis. He experienced a good gain in hearing which persisted until the time of his death four years later. See Fig. 10.51.

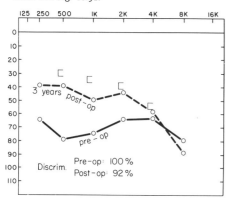

Fig. 10.51: Photograph showing the prosthesis in place. See Fig. 10.50 for history. Photomicrograph is shown in Fig. 10.52.

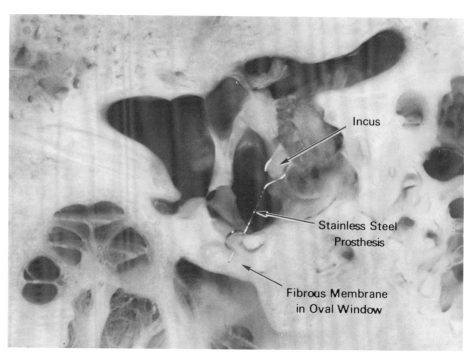

Incus

Stainless Steel
Prosthesis

Fibrous Membrane
in Oval Window

Fig. 10.52: Same case as Figs. 10.50 and 10.51. Histological study shows the oval window bridged by a fibrous membrane varying from 0.2 mm to 0.4 mm in thickness. There is an otosclerotic focus at the anterior margin of the oval window.

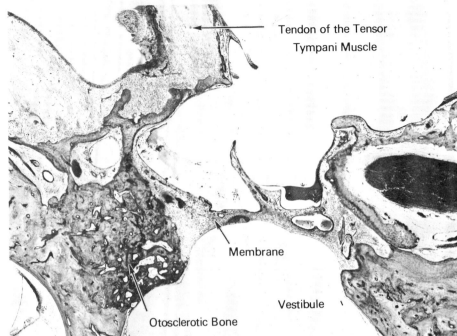

Fig. 10.53: This patient first noted bilateral hearing loss at the age of 25 and at the age of 41 began using a hearing aid in his right ear. At the age of 60 a stapedectomy procedure was performed in his right ear. The stapes was replaced with a Gelfoam-wire prosthesis. He experienced a good hearing gain and died two years later of myocardial infarction. See Figs. 10.54 and 10.55.

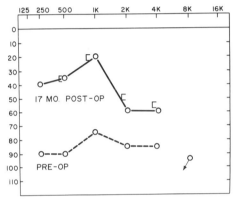

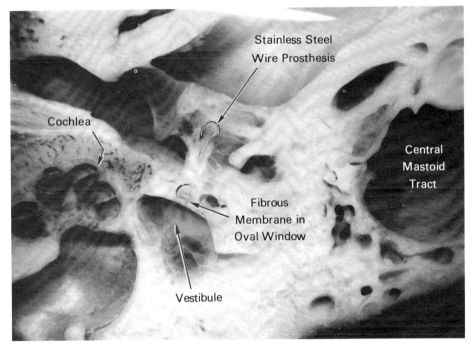

Fig. 10.54: Photograph showing the prosthesis in place. See Fig. 10.53 for history and Fig. 10.55 for photomicrograph.

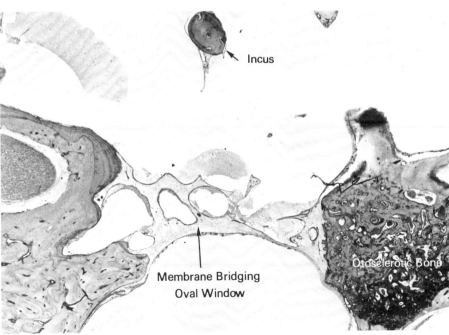

Fig. 10.55: Same case as Figs. 10.53 and 10.54. Histological study of the right ear shows the oval window bridged by a fibrous membrane. In its thinnest areas the membrane is 6 to 10 cell layers in thickness. The incus appears normal. There is an otosclerotic focus at the anterior margin of the oval window.

B. PAGET'S DISEASE

Although it was Czerny (1873) who named this disorder osteitis deformans, it was Sir James Paget (1877, 1882) who correlated and described in detail the clinical and pathological features of this disease. Since his description, no one has suggested a better name for the disorder than "Paget's disease." There is no evidence that the basic pathology is inflammatory, nor is the disease deforming in the majority of cases. The disorder seems to be restricted to humans, and males are affected more frequently than females in a ratio of 4:1.

Plausible and bizarre theories of etiology have been advanced although most now have only an historical interest. Among the etiologies proposed by different authors are syphilis, neurotrophic conditions, endocrine dysfunction, auto-immune phenomena, vascular lesions, and inflammatory disorders. Although it is difficult to study the hereditary aspects of Paget's disease because of its occurance so late in life, there is evidence that it is inherited as a sex-linked recessive gene (Ashley Montagu, 1949), or more probably as a simple autosomal mendelian dominant gene (McKusick, 1966). The full clinical picture of the patient with an enlarged skull and progressive kyphosis with shortening of stature is rarely seen. A subclinical form of the disease is more common, and the areas most frequently involved are the skull, spine, pelvis, femur, and tibia.

Hearing loss was described in Paget's early papers and discussed subsequently in more detail by Mayer (1917), Nager (1919), Wyllie (1923), Weber (1930), Brunner (1931), and Tamari (1942). Since that time there have been many reports on the nature of deafness occurring in Paget's disease. Many patients with Paget's disease demonstrate a skull prominence and tortuosity of the terminal branches of the superficial temporal artery. Although hypertrophy of the anterior branch of the superficial temporal artery is not pathognomonic of Paget's disease, its occurrence associated with deafness should make the clinician aware of the possibility of Paget's disease. Original investigators suggested that narrowing of the internal auditory canal and the nerve channels in the bony modiolus with pinching of the nerve fibers might account for the sensorineural hearing loss; however, histological studies do not support this hypothesis.

In a study of 236 cases of Paget's disease, Davies (1968) described the high incidence of a progressive combined sensorineural and conductive hearing loss. His findings were consistent with the reports of others showing a slowly progressive sensorineural hearing loss worse for the high frequencies. The bone-air gap averaged about 30 db for females and 20 db for males and was consistently greater at 500 Hz. Studies by Davies (1968) and Clemis et al. (1967) have shown relatively good speech discrimination scores and positive SISI scores, indicating a disorder of the sense organ rather than of the cochlear neurons. Roentgenologic studies by tomograms have shown the initial osteolytic and resorptive phase of Paget's disease to be most pronounced in the petrous apex so that the semicircular canals and cochlea become unusually well visualized. Periosteal bone is first attacked and later the denser enchondral bone is involved. As the disease progresses, the cochlea and lateral and superior semicircular canals are less well visualized on tomograms although the ossicles appear normal. In more advanced stages the bony labyrinth and internal auditory canal cannot be identified, and in this stage the hearing loss is usually moderately severe, although still serviceable. Invagination of the occipital condyle (basilar impression) is frequent. Due to excessive softening and twisting of the base of the skull, there is sometimes an upward tilting of the petrous apices and internal auditory canals. Because 30 to 50 percent of the bone calcium in a local area must be altered before radiological changes are evident, a patient may have Paget's disease without evidence of x-ray involvement.

Paget's disease may exhibit a variable histological picture because of differences in the ratio of osteoclastic and osteoblastic activity, the speed of the regenerative and destructive processes, and the frequency of local remissions.

Local differences in the rates of osteoblastic and osteoclastic activity are responsible for the development of porotic and sclerotic areas, frequently observed in adjacent areas (Fig. 10.56). The mosaic pattern of Paget's disease is due to irregular and curved cement lines within the bony tissues and the irregular notches and depressions on the surface of the bone trabeculae. The peculiar bony architecture is caused by pronounced osteoclastic absorption of old and fully calcified bone with the deposition of new osteoid layers calcifying in the normal fashion (Fig. 10.57). If the resorptive process is halted at a certain stage and then followed by new bone formation, a cement line develops to mark the point of application of new bone upon the old. Subsequently, further resorptive changes may occur so that the architecture of a given area is further disturbed. Increased vascularity and fibrosis of the intertrabecular spaces may also occur.

The pagetic changes are most marked in areas best supplied with marrow tissue, these being the petrous apex area, the peritubal area, and the peripheral areas of the mastoid. The bony labyrinths, due to their almost marrowless structure, are the last to be involved and then only in the most severe cases (Figs. 10.58, 10.59).

The conductive-type deafness which is present in many patients with ad-

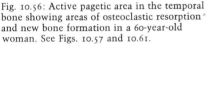

Fig. 10.56: Active pagetic area in the temporal bone showing areas of osteoclastic resorption and new bone formation in a 60-year-old woman. See Figs. 10.57 and 10.61.

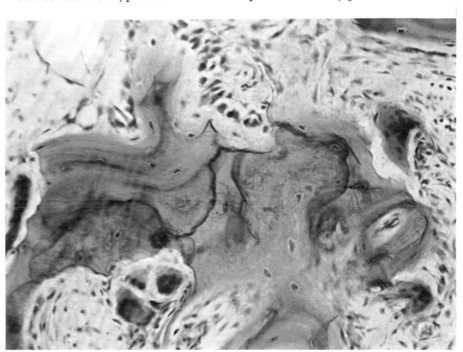

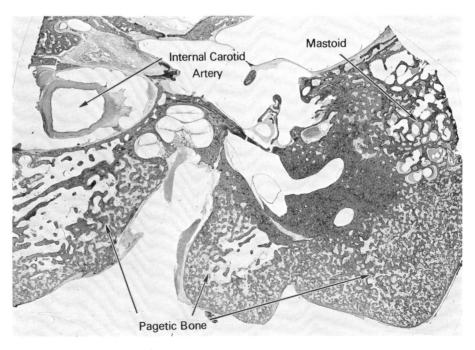

Fig. 10.57: Same case as Fig. 10.56. In spite of involvement of the walls of the internal auditory canal, there is no narrowing of its lumen. See also Fig. 10.61.

Internal Carotid Artery

Mastoid

Pagetic Bone

Fig. 10.58: Active Paget's disease with extensive involvement of the bony labyrinth in an elderly male (age unknown). The homogeneous network of fine bony spicules is separated by loose cellular fibrous tissue containing numerous osteoblasts and multinucleated osteoclasts. The auditory and vestibular sense organs and nerves appear normal.

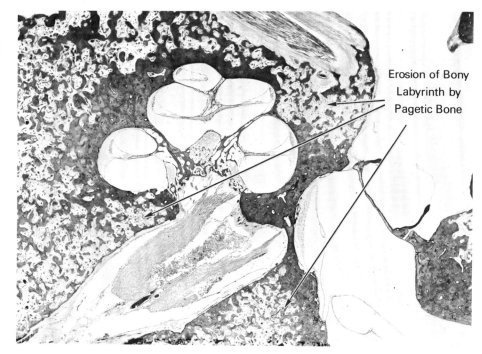

Erosion of Bony Labyrinth by Pagetic Bone

Fig. 10.59: Asymptomatic Paget's disease in a 70-year-old male. There is a protuberance of pagetic bone at the posterior margin of the internal auditory canal. The mastoid is enlarged by pagetic bony growth. See Fig. 10.60.

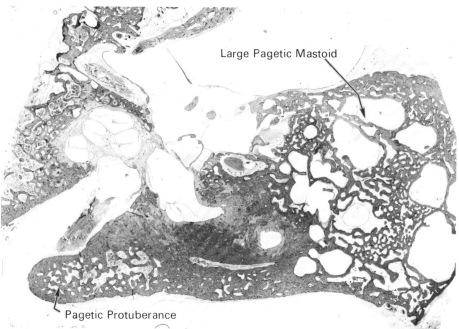

Large Pagetic Mastoid

Pagetic Protuberance

vanced Paget's disease of the skull is presumed to be caused by encroachment of pagetic bone on the ossicles, in either the epitympanum or oval window area. A review of the literature reveals reports of histological studies of 28 temporal bones showing Paget's disease. Only two revealed pagetic changes in the stapes footplate and only one in the annular ligament (Jenkins, 1923; Nager and Meyer, 1932; Anson and Wilson, 1937; Waltner, 1965; Davies, 1968). In histological studies from eight patients, Davies found pagetic changes in some of the ossicles and in some cases bone spurs in the attic region which were in proximity to the ossicles. Although firm histological documentation is still lacking, it seems probable that the conductive hearing loss is due to a combination of pagetic changes in the ossicles, pagetic spurs in the epitympanum interfering with ossicular motion, and fibrotic or bony change in the annular ligament.

Kornfeld (1967) studied seven temporal bones of patients affected with Paget's disease and found histopathologic changes which he interpreted as atrophy of the stria vascularis as well as thrombosis, micro-aneurysms, and inorganic deposits in the strial vessels in areas adjacent to pagetic bone. Rüedi (1968) also described these changes and found, in addition, the presence of shunts connecting the blood vessels of the diseased pagetic bone with those

Fig. 10.60: Same case as Fig. 10.59. The dense trabeculae are composed of both old and new bone and separated by spaces containing active hemopoietic bone marrow. There is severe loss of cochlear neurons throughout the basal turn of the cochlea and degeneration of the organ of Corti in the basal 7 mm of the cochlea. The organ of Corti and cochlear neurons appear normal in the remainder of the cochlea. It cannot be determined whether these inner ear changes are related to the Paget's disease.

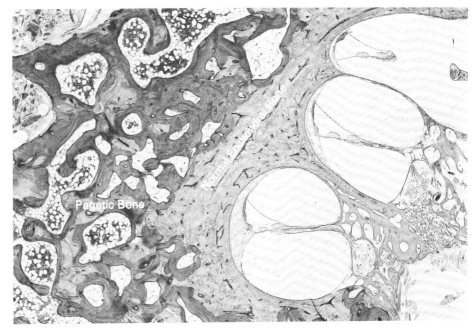

Fig. 10.61: Same case as Figs. 10.56 and 10.57. Extensive pagetic involvement of the bony labyrinth has caused atrophy of the membranous lateral and posterior semicircular canals. The canals are shrunken, exhibit basophilic staining, and in some areas are surrounded by fibrous tissue. Shrinking has resulted in displacement of the membranous canals to the internal surfaces of the bony canals. The ampullae and cristae appear normal.

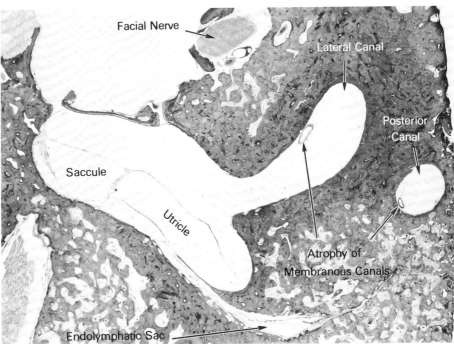

of the spiral ligament. Specimens studied by Schuknecht (unpublished data) do not show these changes in the vascular system.

The specimens in the collection at the Massachusetts Eye and Ear Infirmary show varying degrees of atrophy of the structures of the cochlear duct and nerve, most severe in the basal turns of the cochleae (Fig. 10.60). The sensorineural hearing loss is characterized by a descending audiometric pattern and is presumed to be caused by some form of toxic effect by the pagetic disease of the bony labyrinth, similar to that observed in otosclerosis.

Degenerative changes in the membranous labyrinth may occur in ears exhibiting severe destructive lesions of the bony labyrinth. Atrophy of the membranous lateral and posterior semicircular canals was observed in one specimen (Fig. 10.61). In a 79-year-old patient with profound hearing loss, Lindsay and Lehman (1969) found pagetic destruction of the bony labyrinth with invasion of the inner ears, fractures, and degeneration of the membranous labyrinths.

The medical treatment of Paget's disease with cortisone and fluorides has not been impressive and probably is of little value. The success of reconstructive middle ear surgery for correction of the conductive deafness would seem to be compromised by the lack of a consistent predictable bony involvement of the sound transmitting structures (Davies, 1970).

C. OSTEOGENESIS IMPERFECTA (VAN DER HOEVE'S SYNDROME—BLUE SCLERAE, FRAGILE BONES AND DEAFNESS)

Adair-Dighton (1912) first described deafness with blue sclerae and multiple fractures in 14 persons from four generations; however, van der Hoeve and de Kleyn (1918) are credited with the most detailed early description of this syndrome. It has been described as occurring in congenital and retarded forms. In the congenital form, there may be multiple fractures in utero, in which case the infant is usually born dead. In the retarded form, the disorder manifests itself at a later age and is featured by the occurrence of relatively painless fractures following minor trauma. The long bones usually have slender shafts and often show abrupt widening near the epiphyses. The bones of the lower limbs often show an anterior bowing resulting in adults with short legs as compared to the length of the upper limbs. Kyphoscoliosis and pectus excavatum are common. The teeth may be fragile, and caries and discoloration are common. The joint capsules are weak.

The basic pathology seems to be a disorganization of the collagen structure of bone (Engfeldt et al., 1954). It appears that collagen does not mature beyond the reticulin stage. Mineral studies of the bone have shown calcium and phosphorus to be normal (Albright and Reifenstein, 1948). The laying down of inorganic salts in a faulty framework results in weak, soft bones.

Osteogenesis imperfecta appears to be transmitted as an autosomal dominant character. Approximately one-half of all the offspring of an affected parent will inherit the disease, although the severity of the signs and symptoms varies widely with each case. It is known that the disease can "skip" a generation, indicating the extreme variation in genetic expressivity.

Stoller (1962) made a genetic study covering five generations and including a total of 58 individuals. Of this group 26 (68.4 percent) had blue sclerae; 18 (47.3 percent) had fractures; and 11 (28.9 percent) had hearing losses.

The theory has been advanced that osteogenesis imperfecta and otosclerosis are based upon a common genetic abnormality and that otosclerosis occurring alone is a local manifestation of osteogenesis imperfecta (Wullstein et al., 1960; Oglivie and Hall, 1962). This idea finds support in the fact that many patients with otosclerosis exhibit blue sclerae without evidence of fragile bones.

The hearing loss found in osteogenesis imperfecta is clinically indistinguishable from otosclerosis. Characteristically a conductive hearing loss begins shortly after puberty when fractures become less frequent. The incidence of sensorineural hearing loss associated with conductive loss appears to be more common than when otosclerosis occurs alone.

Temporal bone studies from patients with osteogenesis imperfecta and deafness are currently lacking, and information on the nature of the pathology of the bony labyrinth is based mainly on observations made at the time of surgery and small fragments removed from the oval window area during the course of stapedectomy. Many surgeons (Clerc and Deumier, 1958; Wullstein et al., 1960; Shea et al., 1963; Patterson and Stone, 1970; Schuknecht, unpublished data) have reported that the bone found in the oval window resembles otosclerotic bone. A frequent finding is soft vascular bone, often filling the oval window niche and often covered by a thickened, highly vascular layer of mucoperiosteum. Other surgeons (Sooy, 1960; Opheim, 1968) failed to find gross otosclerosis in the stapes or bony labyrinth of patients with hearing loss associated with osteogenesis imperfecta. Opheim (1968) was the first to emphasize that the conductive hearing loss in patients with osteogenesis imperfecta may sometimes be caused by fibrous degeneration of the crura of the stapes as the result of generalized skeletal disease. Atrophy of the crura occurring either alone or in association with a bony growth in the oval window has been reported by Hall and Røhrt (1968), Bretlau et al. (1970), and Patterson and Stone (1970).

Altmann (1962a) and Altmann and Kornfeld (1967) were unable to find histological evidence of otosclerosis in the temporal bones of five patients with congenital osteogenesis imperfecta.

It appears at this time, therefore, that these patients frequently have a bony lesion of the oval window and footplate which is similar or identical to otosclerosis; however, many have an associated atrophy of the crural arch. In unusual cases crural atrophy is the only pathological change to account for the conductive hearing loss.

D. FIBROUS DYSPLASIA OF THE TEMPORAL BONE

Fibrous dysplasia of the temporal bone was reported by Weil in 1922 and later was described in detail by Lichtenstein and Jaffe in 1942 when they coined the term "fibrous dysplasia."

For many years fibrous dysplasia was not distinguished from hyperparathyroidism. The lesions of these two disorders are pathologically and radiologically similar and were formerly known as "osteitis fibrosa cystica." In the past, many patients with fibrous dysplasia were subjected to fruitless surgical explorations for parathyroid tumors (Pritchard, 1951); however, the differentiation of isolated fibrous dysplasia from that associated with parathyroidism can usually be made by blood chemistry studies, for in simple fibrous dysplasia the serum calcium, serum phosphorus, and alkaline phosphatase are within normal limits. Occasionally the polyostotic type of fibrous dysplasia occurs in a form known as Albright's syndrome (Albright et al., 1937), which is characterized by multiple involvement of the long bones, pigmentation of the skin, and precocious puberty in females.

Fibrous dysplasia of bone usually first becomes manifest during childhood or early adult life and the lesions grow slowly. The polyostotic type characteristically involves the long bones and rarely the skull. The monostotic type may occur in the long bones, facial bones, or membranous bones. Involvement of the temporal bone manifests itself as a swelling in the region of the mastoid and external auditory canal (Schlumberger, 1946; Towson, 1950; Brunner, 1952; Kearney, 1959; Sussman, 1961; Basek, 1967; Shiffman and Aengst, 1967; Cohen and Rosenwasser, 1969; Tembe, 1970; Sharp, 1970). The history of a painless swelling associated with the characteristic radiographic appearance and biopsy are adequate to differentiate the condition from Ollier's (1899, 1900) enchondromatosis, von Recklinghausen's disease, Paget's disease, Hand-Schüller-Christian disease, and other bone tumors.

The histological appearance is quite characteristic, consisting of replacement of marrow with fibrous tissue containing spicules of bone undergoing resorption and formation (Fig. 10.62). Active osteoblastic and osteoclastic

Fig. 10.62: Fibrous dysplasia of bone. There are spicules of bone undergoing resorption and formation in a cellular fibrous stroma.

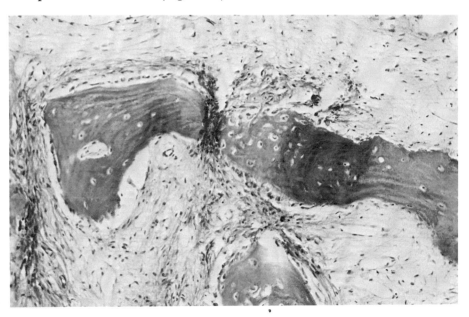

activity is usually present, and islands of cartilage may be observed. The connective tissue component may become extremely cellular and at times have a whorled arrangement and be confused with sarcoma. As the lesions enlarge, the bony cortex becomes thinner; however, the histological structure of the cortex usually remains normal.

Lichtenstein and Jaffe (1942) suggest that the disease is a congenital anomaly manifested by perverted activity of specific bone-forming mesenchyme. Murray et al. (1946) believe that the lesions are due to an extraskeletal congenital disorder of calcium and phosphorus metabolism. Schlumberger (1946) concludes that monostotic fibrous dysplasia is unrelated to Albright's syndrome and probably represents a disturbance of the normal reparative processes following bone injury.

Fibrous dysplasia is a chronic, slowly progressive growth, and although it is not self-limiting, it tends to show less activity in older patients. Because these lesions may become cosmetically deforming, most authorities believe that they should be surgically removed as thoroughly as possible.

Fibrous dysplasia has a female sex preponderance in a ratio of three to one. The onset is usually in childhood, and the lesions, when multiple, are often unilateral.

Schwartz and Alpert (1964) reviewed the literature and found reports of 28 cases of malignant transformation of fibrous dysplasia and concluded that the rate of malignant change is 0.4 percent or about 400 times the spontaneous rate for *de nova* bone sarcoma. Radiotherapy appears to have a predisposing propensity to malignant degeneration as 12 of the 29 cases studied by Schwartz and Alpert (1964) had received irradiation an average of 14 years before the malignant change. Gross and Montgomery (1967) reported an additional case of malignant degeneration of fibrous dysplasia of the maxilla 19 years after treatment with 2,400 rads of low voltage x-ray therapy. It would appear prudent at the present time to consider radiation therapy as contraindicated for the treatment of fibrous dysplasia.

E. OSTEOPETROSIS (ALBERS-SCHØNBERG DISEASE (1904, 1907); MARBLE BONE DISEASE)

Osteopetrosis is a rare bone disorder which occurs both as a clinically benign, dominantly-inherited form and a malignant recessively-inherited form (Johnson et al., 1968). The abnormal bone growth is characterized by a failure of resorption of calcified cartilage and primitive bone. A persistence of mineralized cartilage and osteoid tissue interferes with the formation of adult bone and crowds the area where resorption should produce a medullary cavity (Fig. 10.63).

Among the most common symptoms of the malignant recessive form are optic atrophy, splenomegaly, hepatomegaly, poor growth, frontal bossing, fractures, loss of hearing, mental retardation, and facial palsy. Children with this disorder usually die at an early age from anemia or secondary infection. There is no known recessive case that has survived past the age of twenty.

Histological studies of temporal bones of infants with this disease show the bony labyrinths and ossicles to consist principally of dense calcified cartilage (Myers and Stool, 1969). The mastoids are nonpneumatized, and the stapes persist in fetal form (Figs. 10.64, 10.65).

Many patients with the benign dominantly-inherited form of the disease are asymptomatic, and diagnosis is made by radiologic study alone. Most of these patients can be expected to survive to old age (Ellis and Jackson, 1962; Higinbotham and Alexander, 1941). The most frequent complaints are easy fracturing of bone and bone pain. Some develop osteomyelitis of the mandible as the result of tooth infections. In unusual cases the skull lesion interferes with the mechanisms of cerebrospinal fluid resorption and venous drainage, causing progressive increase in intracranial pressure, headaches,

Fig. 10.63: Osteopetrosis. The enchondral bone consists predominantly of calcified cartilage which appears as irregular round and ovoid forms staining various shades of blue with hematoxylin and having sharp outlines. They contain one or more ill-defined inclusion bodies presumed to be nuclei. These forms are located in a pale blue matrix containing very few blood vessels. There are scattered spicules of lamellar bone particularly around the vascular channels. See Figs. 10.64 and 10.65.

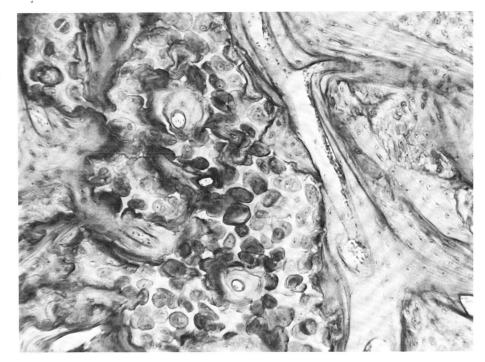

Fig. 10.64: The diagnosis of osteopetrosis was made on this white male infant at the time of birth. Soon after birth he experienced repeated grand mal seizures and exhibited poor feeding and growth. Mental retardation, deafness, and blindness were apparent at the age of one. He suffered from persistent anemia, fractured left femur, and recurrent episodes of aspiration pneumonia, the last of which terminated in death at the age of 15 months. The stapes has a fetal form and is made up of calcified cartilage. The enchondral layer of the bony labyrinth exhibits a sharp staining differentiation from the surrounding bone. The enchondral layer is composed of interconnected strands and islands of irregularly shaped basophilic forms which are the size of cartilage cells, some of which contain round structures presumed to be nuclei. This abnormal bone is separated by small islands of fibrous stroma containing blood vessels and an irregular interconnected lacework of lamellar bone. The organ of Corti is atrophied throughout; however, the population of cochlear neurons appears to be normal. The cristae, maculae, and vestibular nerves appear normal. See Figs. 10.63 and 10.65.

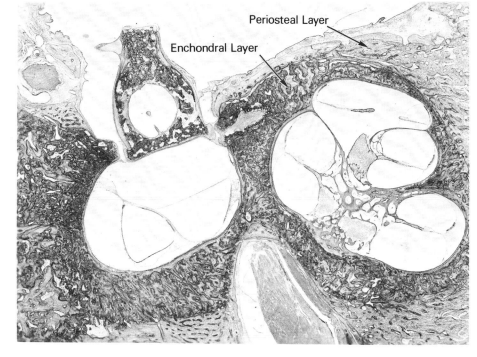

Periosteal Layer

Enchondral Layer

Fig. 10.65: Osteopetrosis. Same specimen as Figs. 10.63 and 10.64 showing a higher-power view of the stapes. It has retained its fetal form and consists predominantly of calcified cartilage.

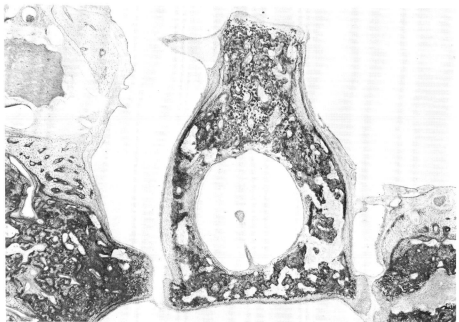

Fig. 10.66: Osteopetrosis. Thickening of the base of the skull in a 21-year-old male who died suddenly from increased intracranial pressure. Two other siblings of four also had the disease and died in a similar manner at ages 26 and 30. (Courtesy of Hammersma)

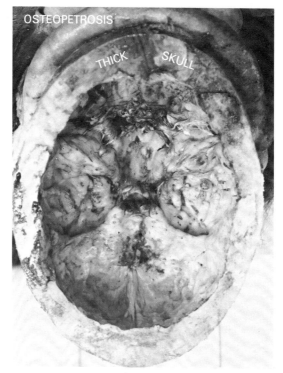

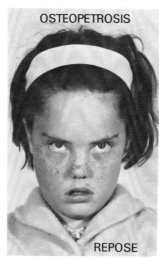 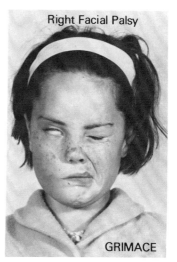

Fig. 10.67: Osteopetrosis. At birth this patient had unilateral facial nerve paralysis from which she recovered within four months. She subsequently had numerous attacks of facial palsy involving both sides independently. Radiologic studies at the age of nine revealed osteopetrosis. The photograph taken at age 11 of her face at repose (left) and a grimace (right) shows a right facial palsy. A decompression of the mastoid segment of the right facial nerve was performed; however, another attack of right facial paralysis occurred at the age of 14. She also exhibited a 40 db conductive hearing loss in both ears and narrowed external auditory canals. (Courtesy of Hammersma)

and sudden death. As the skull thickens there is narrowing of the foramina for the cranial nerves. The nerves most frequently affected are the optic, trigeminal, facial, and auditory. The overall dimensions of the skull are often increased, and in adults the calvarium can be 3 cm in thickness (Fig. 10.66). Macrocephaly and enlargement of the mandible becomes evident in the teenager. The patient usually grows very tall and exhibits clubbing of the long bones and proptosis due to thickening of the orbital bones. Most of the patients exhibit normal intelligence.

Recurring facial palsies involving one or both sides is a frequent manifestation of this disease (Fig. 10.67). Any child or young adult with recurring facial palsies should have radiologic studies as a routine diagnostic evaluation to determine the possible existence of osteopetrosis. The facial palsies behave identically to Bell's palsy, having an acute onset with varying degrees of recovery but with a tendency toward progressive residual weakness following each episode. Decompression of the mastoid segment of the facial nerve (Yarington and Sprinkle, 1967; Hamersma, 1970) have not arrested the attacks of facial palsy; however, total intratemporal decompression of the nerve as performed by House and Fisch (quoted by Hamersma, 1970) may meet with more success.

Deafness is of the combined sensorineural and conductive type and is caused by interference with ossicular movement by osteopetrotic bone (Jones and Mulcahy, 1968; Hamersma, 1970). Although Haynes (quoted by Hamersma, 1970) found conductive deafness in an 11-year-old patient to be due to a fixed stapes in a narrow oval window niche, it has not been established that this is the usual lesion. The cause for the sensorineural hearing loss is not clear. Jones and Mulcahy (1968) explored one ear of a patient with osteopetrosis and bilateral conductive hearing loss and found the oval window niche to be filled with ivory-like bone.

F. EXOSTOSES OF THE EXTERNAL AUDITORY CANAL

Exostoses arise as new growths of bone from the osseous portion of the external auditory canal. The bone is of periosteal origin and is formed in layers suggesting a periodic growth pattern (Figs. 10.68, 10.69, 10.70). In affected individuals the exostoses usually are multiple and bilateral. They may arise from any portion of the external auditory canal with no apparent site of predilection. They may appear as discrete, round, ovoid, or elongated excrescences with small, almost pedunculated bases, or as diffuse bulges of ivory-like bone. They are limited to the external auditory canal. Any bony growths which extend beyond this region, for example, into the mastoid, must be considered to be osteomas of neoplastic origin.

Exostoses have been reported to be more common in males (Hrdlicka, 1935; Fenner, 1939) and apparently demonstrate racial differences in incidence (Roche, 1964). It is now generally accepted that the most common cause is swimming in cold water (Field, 1893; van Gilse, 1938; Adams, 1951a, 1951b). Gregg and Bass (1970) found exostoses in 5.4 percent of 483 adult Indian skulls removed from burial sites in South Dakota. Harrison (1951) found the incidence of exostoses in a male population in England to be 0.7 percent and noted that all cases occurred in individuals giving a history of regular swimming. In an experiment on human volunteers he studied the comparative duration of erythema of the skin of the external auditory canal following irrigation with water of different temperatures. Utilizing irrigation times of 15 seconds, the average duration of erythema with water at 40°C was one minute, and with water at 15°C was 45 minutes. He also demonstrated that individuals with already existing small exostoses had longer periods of post-irrigation erythema than individuals with normal canals. Fowler and Osmun (1942) irrigated the external canals of a guinea pig for a total of 1,172 hours with water at 19°C and produced fibrous proliferation in the subcutaneous tissues with scattered islands of osteoid tissue.

Exostoses remain asymptomatic unless they cause retention of water or epithelial debris in the depths of the canal, in which case they may cause hearing loss. At first the hearing loss is fluctuating in behavior and may be associated with external otitis. Fluctuating hearing loss may also be caused by contact of the growth with the tympanic membrane or manubrium. Total occlusion of the external auditory canal is rare.

If the growths produce symptoms, they may be removed surgically. Skin grafting may be required to prevent postoperative stenosis of the external auditory canal.

G. HISTIOCYTOSIS

Letterer-Siwe disease, Hand-Schüller-Christian disease, and eosinophilic granuloma are believed to be clinical gradations of expression of the same basic disorder, that being an inflammatory reticuloendotheliosis (Jaffe and Lichtenstein, 1944, 1947; Lichtenstein, 1953).

Letterer-Siwe's disease (Letterer, 1924; Siwe, 1933) is a rapidly fatal condition usually occurring before the age of two. The principal clinical manifestations are enlargement of the liver, spleen, lymph nodes, secondary anemia, cutaneous eruption, destructive skeletal lesions, especially in the skull, and a rapidly downhill, acute febrile course. The temporal bone pathology of an infant with this rapidly fatal disease was reported by Lopez-Rios et al. (1968) (Fig. 10.71).

The term "Hand-Schüller-Christian disease" (Hand, 1893; Schüller, 1915; Christian, 1920) originally was applied to those cases in which the triad of diabetes insipidus, exophthalmos, and calvarial defects were present. Diabetes insipidus and exophthalmos are due to involvement of the sphenoid bone and the bones of the orbit and represent only a small part of the usual involvement. The skull lesions may involve the temporal bone, resulting in disturbances in and around the ear before other symptoms occur (Tos, 1966, 1969). Otorrhea and roentgen findings of a destructive lesion of the temporal bone may be the only early symptoms (Fig. 10.72). Mastoidectomy is frequently performed in these cases before the nature of the lesion is suspected. Because irradiation therapy is the treatment of choice for uncomplicated lesions, the importance of making an early diagnosis is obvious. Hand-Schüller-Christian disease usually appears in childhood but may occur in the second or third decade of life or even later. About 15 to 30 percent terminate fatally. In addition to the skull lesions there may be osteolytic lesions in the long bones, scapula, and ribs, and diffuse infiltrative lesions of the liver and spleen, resulting in enlargement of those organs. The heart, lungs, meninges, brain, and spinal cord may also be sites of infiltrations. The principal feature of the lesions is the presence in them of sheets of histiocytes, many of which contain lipid (cholesterol and cholesterol esters) and some of which unite to form multinucleated cells. Commonly there are areas containing numerous polymorphonuclear leucocytes, predominantly eosinophiles, and areas of necrosis and hemorrhage (Fig. 10.73).

Schuknecht and Perlman (1948) reported two cases of Hand-Schüller-Christian disease involving the temporal bone. One case was a 30-year-old male with otorrhea, vertigo, tinnitus, and loss of hearing with a positive fistula test. The other was a 22-year-old male with ottorrhea, severe vertigo with sudden onset, and eventual total loss of cochlear and vestibular function. Mastoid surgery was performed on both patients before the diagnosis was made. Similar cases have been reported by Greifenstein (1932), Rosenwasser (1940), Chisolm (1954), Shea (1938), and Osborne et al. (1944). Tos (1966) reviewed five hundred cases of Hand-Schüller-Christian disease reported in the literature and found 60 cases with auditory and vestibular symptoms probably due to involvement of the inner ear. Hudson and Kenan (1969) found temporal bone destruction and aural discharge in 6 of 16 patients with Hand-Schüller-Christian disease.

Eosinophilic granuloma is the mildest form of the disorder and usually appears as one or more benign lesions of the skeleton without visceral, neural, or cutaneous involvement (Johnson and Zonderman, 1946). It usually occurs in children or young adults, with onset before the age of 30 in 80 percent of the cases. The most commonly affected areas are the long bones, skull, ribs, and vertebrae. The usual presenting symptoms are pain and tenderness. Radiologically, the lesions appear as sharply delineated radiolucent zones in the bone (Lichtenstein and Jaffe, 1940). The microscopic picture is that of sheets of histiocytes with one or two nuclei, and scattered collections of small eosinophiles with lobulated, indented, or round nuclei. Areas of necrosis and hemorrhage are found, and giant cells may be present.

The small temporal bone lesions of Hand-Schüller-Christian disease and eosinophilic granuloma may produce no symptoms; however, as the lesion grows in size there may be pain, swelling, hearing loss, vertigo, facial palsy, involvement of cranial nerves in the jugular foramen, and secondary infection with otorrhea. It is common for granulations to appear in a fistula in the posterior wall of the external auditory canal. When this condition is found in the presence of an intact tympanic membrane, it is strongly suggestive of eosinophilic granuloma or Hand-Schüller-Christian disease. The diagnosis can usually be made by microscopic examination of a biopsy specimen. Another

Fig. 10.68: Asymptomatic exostoses of the anterior and posterior walls of the external auditory canal of a 75-year-old male.

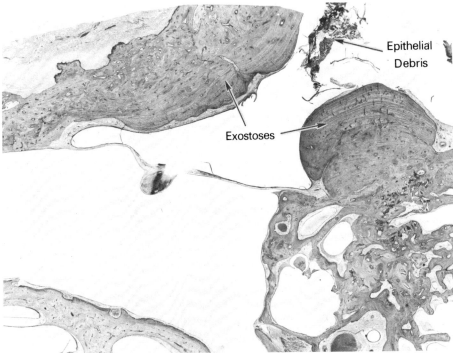

Exostoses

Epithelial Debris

Fig. 10.69: Asymptomatic exostoses of the anterior wall of the external auditory canal of a 61-year-old male. See Fig. 10.70.

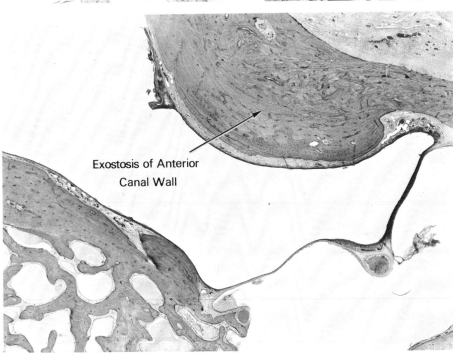

Exostosis of Anterior Canal Wall

Fig. 10.70: High-power view of exostoses shown in Fig. 10.69. Exostoses appear to form by the periodic laying down of strata of bone as the result of recurring irritation of the periosteum, the most common cause being cold water swimming. This laminated bone may subsequently undergo partial remodeling with the development of a mosaic pattern of lamellar bone.

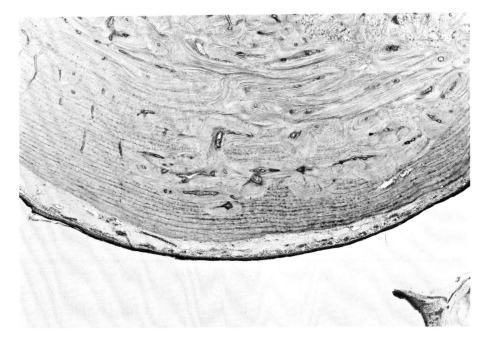

clue to diagnosis is radiological evidence of bone destruction greater than that which is consistent with suppurative disease. When the nature of the lesion is suspected, a search should be made for other skeletal or visceral lesions. Surgery is indicated for biopsy diagnosis and for drainage of infected areas, but the therapy of choice is irradiation.

H. HYPOTHYROIDISM

It is the general impression of clinicians that the hypothyroid state is associated with hearing loss. Batsakis and Nishiyama (1962) report that about half of patients with hypothyroidism experience hearing improvement upon treatment with thyroid extract. Apparently the hearing losses may be conductive, sensorineural, or a combination of both. Cody (1971) reported the findings in a 78-year-old woman with hypothyroidism and sensorineural hearing loss who experienced improvement in pure tone threshold and speech discrimination scores when treated with desiccated thyroid.

Although it is the general impression of clinicians that the hypothyroid state is associated with hearing loss, a review of the literature fails to provide convincing documentation of a causal relationship. Well-controlled studies are needed to answer this question.

I. DIABETES MELLITUS

The most specific major vascular alteration occurring in association with diabetes mellitus is narrowing of the lumens of the arterioles, capillaries, and venules by hypertrophy and proliferation of the intimal endothelium and by deposition of lipids. These disseminated vascular changes have a devastating effect on the retina and renal glomerulus, as well as many other tissues, and may precede the appearance of a clinically recognizable metabolic derangement. Arteriolosclerosis is a second common vascular alteration in diabetes. It is presumed to be the result of hypertension, which is commonly associated with diabetes and thus is not a direct consequence of the metabolic disorder. Arteriolosclerosis involves the small arteries and arterioles throughout the body and is characterized by intimal fibrosis without endothelial proliferation. A third vascular change in diabetes is atherosclerosis. It affects the larger blood vessels and is associated with an increased incidence of cerebral, coronary, and peripheral vascular disease. It is characterized by thickening, hyalinization, and calcification of the intima and atrophy of the arterial wall without endothelial proliferation.

It is reasonable to expect that diffuse vascular pathology, such as that occurring in diabetes mellitus, will involve the inner ear. Several recent reports suggest that this is true. Jorgensen (1961) studied the temporal bones of 32 diabetics and found a high incidence of PAS-positive thickening of the capillary walls, particularly in the stria vascularis. These changes were most severe in patients who also exhibited diabetic retinopathy and nephropathy. Jorgensen and Buch (1961) examined 60 diabetic patients and found that 28 had hearing losses. There was no distinct correlation between the duration of the diabetes and the degree of hearing loss; however, the loss was more severe in the older patients and in patients exhibiting diabetic retinopathy. In patients under 40 there was a positive correlation between hearing loss and nephropathy. No correlation was found between the degree of hearing impairment and diabetic neuropathy or blood pressure. In most of the patients hearing loss was bilateral and progressive. Three patients had sudden hearing losses and nine experienced vertigo. Gladney and Shepherd (1970), have implicated subclinical diabetes as a cause for auditory and vestibular dysfunction.

Costa (1967), working with Alloxan-induced diabetic albino rats, found

Fig. 10.71: Letterer-Siwe disease. This 23-month-old infant developed bilateral otorrhea and profound hearing loss, and the diagnosis was made by a biopsy of tissue from the ear canal. The child died, in spite of radiotherapy. Histological study shows an extensive destructive lesion involving the posterior part of the right temporal bone. The mastoid bone and the bony labyrinth surrounding the canals are destroyed and replaced by friable vascular granulation tissue consisting of histiocytes, eosinophils, monocytes, polymorphonuclear leukocytes, and foam cells with areas of necrosis and hemorrhage. The perilymphatic and endolymphatic spaces contain fibrinous precipitate with large numbers of monocytes and polymorphonuclear leukocytes. The organ of Corti and vestibular sense organs appear normal. (Courtesy of Lopez-Rios, Benitez, and Vivar)

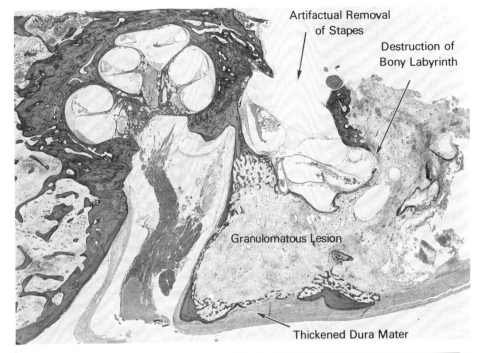

Fig. 10.72: Bilateral involvement of the mastoids with Hand-Schüller-Christian lesions in a two-year-old infant. The diagnosis was made by histological study of granulation tissue removed from the right external auditory canal. These lesions healed after radiation therapy. See Fig. 10.73.

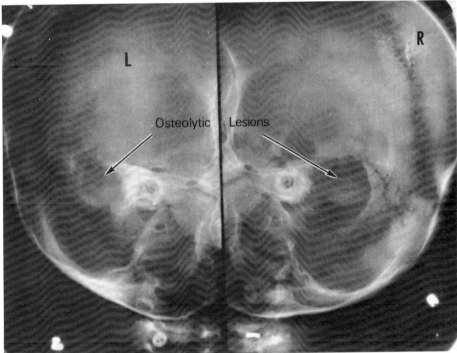

Fig. 10.73: Same case as Fig. 10.72. Granulation tissue removed from the external auditory canal shows a dense sheet of histiocytes with a few foam cells and numerous eosinophils consistent with Hand-Schüller-Christian disease.

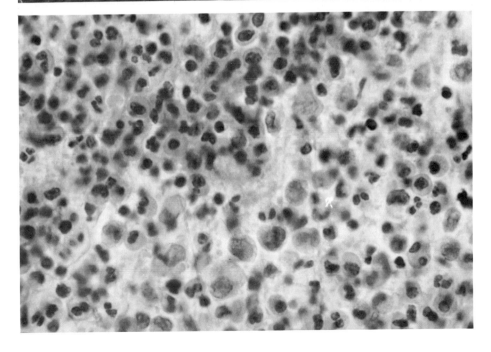

PAS-positive deposits in the vascular walls of the small vessels of the inner ears. Cojazzi and Bötner (1950), working with Alloxan-induced diabetes in rabbits, found similar changes in the stria vascularis and degenerative changes in Scarpa's ganglia and vestibular nerve fibers. Makishima and Tanaka (1971) found a severe loss of cochlear neurons, most severe in the basal turn, in the temporal bones of four diabetic individuals. The blood vessels in the internal auditory canals, modioli, and striae vasculares showed hyalinization and narrowing.

The collection of temporal bones at the Massachusetts Eye and Ear Infirmary reveals 11 sets of specimens from individuals ranging in age from 49 to 87 with diabetes mellitus and a clinical history of hearing loss. Temporal bones were taken only from individuals with hearing losses; therefore, these data have no significance regarding the incidence of deafness in diabetes. The five who were tested exhibited bilateral losses of varying magnitude, worse for the high frequencies. Histological studies show all 11 to have neuronal degeneration of varying degrees, most severe in the basal turns. Six showed moderate to severe strial atrophy and four showed atrophy of the spiral ligaments. The temporal bones of all 11 individuals also showed atrophy of the spiral ligament. The temporal bones of all 11 individuals showed greater intimal thickening and PAS deposits in the capillaries and arterioles than that found in nondiabetics with hearing losses of similar magnitude. From these studies it seems that there are no pathological changes except those occurring in the small vessels which are specific for diabetes mellitus. Although clinical impressions support this contention, there are, in fact, no really convincing statistical data to show an increase in hearing loss.

Hypoglycemia has also been correlated with hearing loss. Weille (1968) pointed out that 42 percent of patients with Ménière's disease who were evaluated with glucose tolerance tests showed hypoglycemia at some point in the test. This was compared to a 15 percent incidence of hypoglycemia in glucose tolerance tests in patients with other diagnoses. Parkin and Tice (1970) performed a careful study of the relationship of hypoglycemia to hearing in a patient who complained of fluctuation in his hearing before meals. The studies demonstrated a hearing loss during the hypoglycemic state which was reversed when normal glucose levels were attained. It could not be established, of course, that the hypoglycemic state was of etiologic significance to the inner ear disorder, which was presumed to be Ménière's disease.

J. PRESBYCUSIS

Biologic aging appears to be a physiologic process engendered by the genotype and the adaptive norm of the species. Superimposed on the inherited processes seems to be the gradual accumulation of errors in DNA, which is probably related to a decline in normal mechanisms of repair. Each member of a species appears to be a distinct chemical entity, owing in part to subtle variants in many genes. Several genes may work in concert to determine the rate of aging. Aging of the whole body, and of specific organs as well, proceeds along an uneven front, occurring sooner in some cells and later in others (Goldstein, 1971).

The auditory system, like all systems of the body, exhibits senescent changes with the passage of time. By the fourth decade of life there already is decreased efficiency of some organs and of the individual as a whole. In the fifth decade the reduction in efficiency becomes apparent, and the further passage of time brings a cascade of senile changes which usually terminate in death during the seventh and eighth decades of life. It is known that with increasing age there is decreased ability of certain cell systems to undergo mitosis (Needham, 1950; Bullough, 1949). There are decreases in nuclear proteins in certain systems (Andreasen, 1943), accumulations of pigment and other insoluble compounds in the cytoplasm (Simms and Stolman, 1937; Ishii et al., 1967), and chemical changes in the intercellular fluid (Lansing, 1952). The structural aspects of aging for many organ systems appears in a book edited by Bourne (1961).

It is now quite clear that aging cannot be accounted for on the basis of changes in one system—for example, the cardiovascular system. Although there is a popular cliché that man is as old as his arteries, there is not a satisfactory parallelism between vascular age and senility. The study of aging changes in individual cells is complicated by the fact that the cellular populations of many organs are replaced during the life of the individual; furthermore, there is difficulty in distinguishing the normal changes of aging from alterations caused by injury or disease.

The term "presbycusis" implies a hearing loss caused by the degenerative changes of aging. The time of onset and rate of progression vary widely. The durability of the auditory mechanism like other body systems is determined in great part by genetic factors and by the physical stress it is subjected to during a lifetime. Environmental factors such as climate and diet (Rosen and Olin, 1965; Rosen, 1966) may be of some importance. It is frequently impossible to make a clear distinction between hereditary deafness and presbycusis.

Studies by Nixon et al. (1962) indicate that aging causes a slight impairment in the transmission of high frequencies through the middle ear. The loss involves principally the frequencies above 2,000 Hz and reaches a magnitude of about 12 db for 4,000 Hz at age 55. They stated that the tympanic membrane thickens and looses its elasticity with aging and that the ossicular system, along with its ligaments and muscles, undergoes degenerative changes with aging. They reasoned that these changes contributed to a gradual diminishing of the mechanical integrity of the ossicular articulations with dissipation of vibratory energy at these junctures. It should be pointed out, however, that this hypothesis of laxity or decreased stiffness is not consistent with the histological changes observed in the joints of the aging ear. Belal and Stewart (1974) have shown that the arthritic changes occurring in the ossicular articulations progress toward fibrous and calcific fixation and, in the most severe cases, to eventual ankylosis. Furthermore, these changes appeared to have no significant effect on hearing. At this time, therefore, it appears that aging has only a minimal effect on middle ear function and that presbycusis is predominantly a phenomenon of the sensory and neural structures.

The cells of the auditory sense organ and neural pathways belong to the group of body cells which have been termed "fixed postmitotics." Other cells in this group are cardiac and skeletal muscle cells, odontoblasts, bone cells, and rod and cone cells. They are the most highly differentiated cells in the body. After specialized function has been established for them, they cannot reproduce and therefore can pursue only the course of aging and dying. For them the length of individual cell life is not determined by stimulation or inhibition of mitotic activity but by ability to maintain their characteristic structural organization in the continual adaptation they must make to changes in the tissue fluid environment.

Since Zwaardemaker (1899) first described the clinical manifestations of high-tone deafness from aging, there have been many reports on this condition. Crowe et al. (1934) and Saxén (1937, 1952) recognized two types of presbycusis, the pathology in one involving mainly the organ of Corti and in the other the cochlear neurons. In a study of animal and human ears, Schuknecht, in 1955, confirmed and further elucidated these changes in the sensory and neural structures.

A third type of inner ear conductive deafness was first proposed by Mayer (1919-20) and subsequently alluded to by Crowe et al. (1934), Glorig and Davis 1961), and Nixon et al. (1962). Subsequently, Schuknecht and Igarashi (1964) and Schuknecht (1964b) provided further indirect evidence in support of an inner ear conductive deafness. They also described a fourth type of presbycusis due to atrophy of the stria vascularis which they then termed "meta-

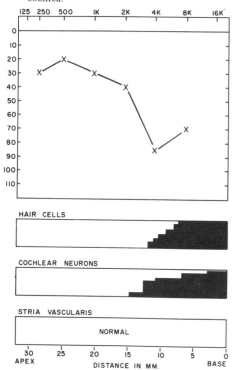

Fig. 10.74: Sensory presbycusis. Abrupt high-tone hearing loss (bilateral, symmetrical) in a 79-year-old man. There is severe atrophy of the organ of Corti with loss of hair cells and cochlear neurons at the basal end of the cochlea.

Fig. 10.75: Audiogram and cochlear reconstruction showing hair cells population of the right ear of a 70-year-old man who had a bilateral symmetrical high-frequency hearing loss. The loss of hair cells is most severe at the basal end of the cochlea. The loss of cochlear neurons is interpreted to represent secondary neural degeneration—that is, secondary to atrophy of supporting cells of the organ of Corti.

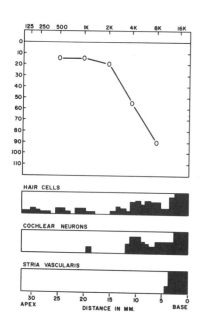

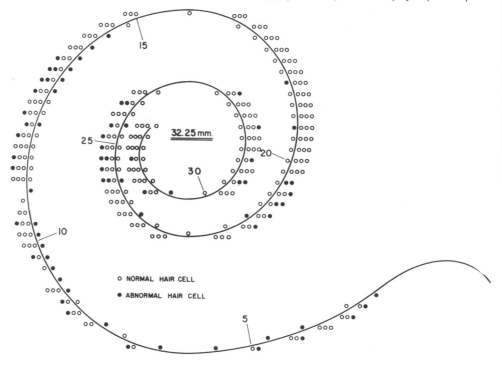

bolic" presbycusis. In 1967, Schuknecht also described a type of presbycusis which is characterized by atrophy of the spiral ligament and rupture of the cochlear duct; however, it now seems more logical to consider this pathological change as an unusual catastrophic end result in inner ear conductive deafness.

Thus, we can currently identify four types of presbycusis based on the selective atrophy of different morphological structures in the cochlea. These structures may be involved individually or in combination. When occurring in pure form, each is manifested by a characteristic pattern of functional disturbance which can be identified by medical history, otologic examination, and auditory testing. The audiometric pattern once established is commonly retained throughout life (Dayal and Nussbaum, 1971). The hearing losses are usually symmetrical in the two ears and slowly progressive. There appear to be no therapeutic measures which alter the course of presbycusis.

1. SENSORY PRESBYCUSIS

This well-documented disorder is characterized by atrophy of the organ of Corti in the basal end of the cochlea and is manifested by abrupt high-tone hearing loss (Fig. 10.74). The degenerative change usually begins in middle age but may already be evident in childhood (Guild, 1950). The condition progresses very slowly, and even in advanced age (Johnsson and Hawkins, 1972a) the lesion frequently is limited to a few millimeters of the basal end of the cochlea and therefore may not affect hearing for the speech frequencies (Figs. 10.75, 10.76). Light microscopic studies show atrophy of both supporting cells (pillars, Deiters', Hensen's) and hair cells. The earliest change is slight distortion and flattening of the organ of Corti. This is followed by loss of supporting and sensory cells (Figs. 10.77,10.78). Eventually the organ of Corti appears as an undifferentiated epithelial mound on the basilar membrane and may eventually disappear completely from the basal end of the cochlea. There is a concomitant loss of cochlear neurons which parallels closely the spatial distribution and magnitude of atrophy of the supporting cells of the organ of Corti. This loss of neurons is presumed to be a consequence of injury to the afferent nerve endings and is termed secondary neural degeneration (see Chapter 9A2, Secondary neural degeneration).

The cause for the degeneration of the sensory cells is not clearly known; however, microscopists observed long ago that lipofuscin accumulates in the tissues of aged individuals; hence its popular synonym "wear and tear" pigment and its German name "abnutzungspigment" (Lubarsch, 1902; Sehrt,

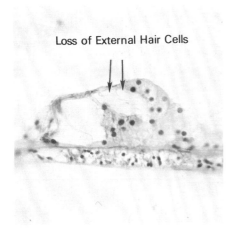

Fig. 10.76: Same case as shown in Fig. 10.75. This view shows the loss of external hair cells in the 8 mm region of the cochlea.

Loss of External Hair Cells

Fig. 10.77: Behavioral audiogram and charts of cochlear pathology on an aged cat with an abrupt high-frequency hearing loss. There is severe degeneration of both the sensory and supporting cells of the organ of Corti as well as cochlear neurons in the basal 14 mm of the cochlea. The findings are characteristic of the sensory type of presbycusis. See Fig. 10.78.

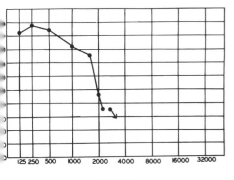

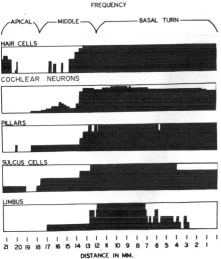

Fig. 10.78: Photomicrographs showing atrophy of the sensory cells and supporting cells of the organ of Corti in the basal turn of the cochlea of an aged cat. The findings are characteristic of sensory presbycusis. Same ear as Fig. 10.77.

1904; Hueck, 1912). Ishii et al. (1967) have shown that lipofuscin granules accumulate in the apical cytoplasm of all epithelial cells within the cochlear duct and vestibular sense organs of the aging ear (Fig. 10.79). It was not demonstrable in individuals under the age of six years, but increased in quantity as a function of age. The location of the lipofuscin granules correlated with the location of lysosomes and was therefore assumed to be a waste product of lysosomal activity (Fig. 10.80). Lysosomes are rich in acid hydrolases, at least sixteen different enzymes having been identified in them (DeDuve, 1963). Bennett (1956) was the first to suggest that insoluable end products of metabolism accumulate in lysosomes. It would seem reasonable that these changes are a reflection of exhaustion of enzymatic activity leading to decreased cell function and eventually to death of the cell.

2. NEURAL PRESBYCUSIS

It is now well established that a loss of neuronal population in the central nervous system begins early in life and continues until the death of the individual (Brody, 1955). These degenerative changes vary in time of onset and are controlled principally by genetic factors. Neural presbycusis may begin at any age, but it seems that there is little or no affect on hearing until late in life when the population of neural units falls below that required for effective transmission, integration, and decoding of the patterns of neural flow. Pestalozza and Shore (1955), Goetzinger et al. (1961), Hinchcliffe (1962), Jerger (1968), and others have described the psychoacoustic features of this type of presbycusis. A loss in population of cochlear neurons in the presence of a functional endorgan creates a distinctive pattern of auditory dysfunction characterized by a loss of speech discrimination which is relatively more severe than the hearing loss for pure tones. The progressive loss of speech discrimination in the presence of stable pure tone thresholds has been termed phonemic regression (Gaeth, 1948). Palva and Jokinen (1970) found the speech discrimination scores of patients over 60 years of age to be better in the left ear and attributed this to cerebral dominance becoming manifest as the result of degenerative change in the auditory pathways. Elderly patients with rapidly progressive neural presbycusis often demonstrate associated diffuse degenerative changes of the central nervous system exhibited by motor weakness and lack of coordination, tremors, irritability, loss of memory, and intellectual deterioration. Because of poor speech discrimination, patients with neural presbycusis find amplification to be of limited value.

The temporal bones of these individuals reveal a loss in population of cochlear neurons often involving the entire cochlea but consistently more

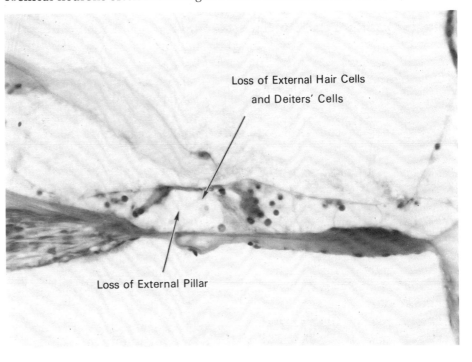

Loss of External Hair Cells and Deiters' Cells

Loss of External Pillar

Fig. 10.79: Electron micrograph of the external hair cells from the cochlea of a 63-year-old man. Lipofuscin granules are concentrated in the cytoplasm of the apical region of the cells. These lipofuscin granules contain large homogeneous oval masses, banded structures and numerous small dense granules. (Courtesy of Ishii)

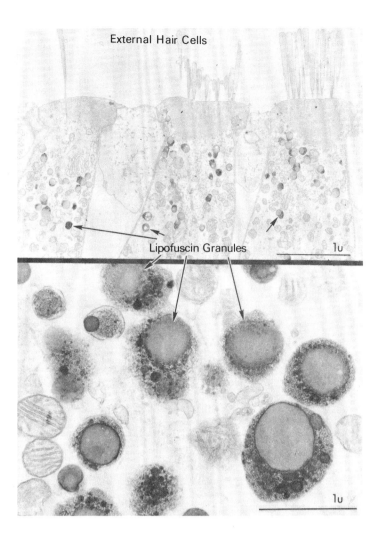

External Hair Cells

Lipofuscin Granules

1u

1u

Fig. 10.80: This view shows the organ of Corti of a 91-year-old man as viewed under the ultraviolet microscope. Lipofuscin granules with strong yellow autofluorescence are located in the apical zones of the hair cells, pillar cells, Hensen's cells, Deiters' cells, and Claudius cells, the normal location for lysosomes. The granules are assumed to be a waste product of lysosomal activity. (Courtesy of Ishii)

Fig. 10.81: Neural presbycusis. This patient experienced bilateral progressive hearing loss, worse in the left ear, during the later years of life and died at the age of 75. Histological study of the left ear shows a severe loss of cochlear neurons in the basal 15 mm of the cochlea. See Fig. 10.82.

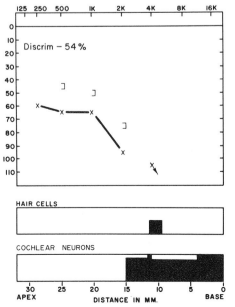

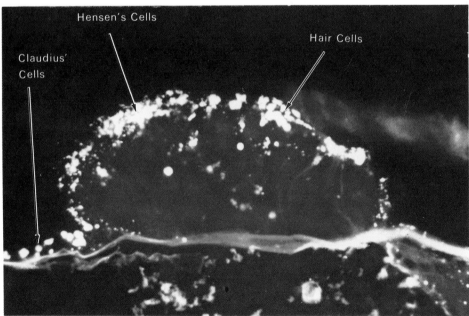

Hensen's Cells

Claudius' Cells

Hair Cells

severe in the basal turn (Guild et al., 1931). Probably there is also a loss of neurons in the higher auditory pathways. Histological studies are needed to verify this possibility. The loss of nerve fibers in the basal turn of the aging ear is particularly well demonstrated in surface preparations (Bredberg, 1968).

Otte (1968) correlated cochlear neuronal populations with speech discrimination scores and found that losses of neurons restricted to the basal turns, even when severe, had little if any detrimental effect on speech discrimination. Losses in the apical region, on the other hand, were closely correlated with poor speech discrimination. This observation reflects the fact that the apical region of the cochlea is important for the analysis of frequencies in the speech range of 500 to 2,000 Hz (Figs. 10.81 to 10.88).

Fig. 10.82: For history see legend, Fig. 10.81. This photomicrograph from the 12 mm region shows a near total loss of cochlear neurons. The organ of Corti and other structures of the cochlear duct appear normal.

Fig. 10.83: Neural presbycusis (in association with sensory and possible cochlear conductive deafness). At the age of 70 this patient complained of bilateral hearing loss. Audiometric tests at the age of 80 revealed bilateral symmetrical hearing loss characterized by modestly descending audiometric patterns. He died at the age of 81. Histological studies show small areas of hair cell loss in the basal ends of the cochleae and in the 10 to 15 mm regions; however, the most striking change is a diffuse loss of cochlear neurons, most severe in the basal ends. See Fig. 10.84.

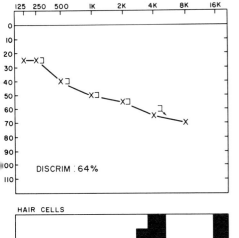

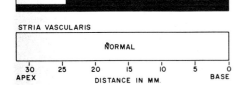

Fig. 10.84: For history see legend, Fig. 10.83. The midmodiolar section of the left ear shows a severe loss of cochlear neurons in the basal end of the cochlea. Atrophy of the organ of Corti in the middle part of the basal turn is consistent with stimulation injury (acoustic trauma). The occupation of this individual is not known.

Fig. 10.85: Neural presbycusis. Midmodiolar section of the cochlea of a 90-year-old woman who experienced a slowly progressive hearing loss for many years. Audiometric studies showed a bilateral symmetrical pure tone threshold loss of 50 to 70 db. There is a diffuse loss of over 75 percent of the cochlear neurons throughout the cochlea. There is atrophy of the organ of Corti only in the extreme basal end of the cochlea. Elsewhere the organ of Corti and other structures of the cochlear duct appear normal.

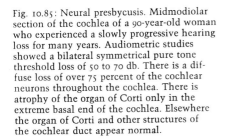

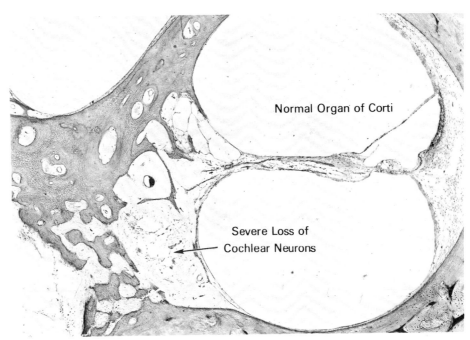

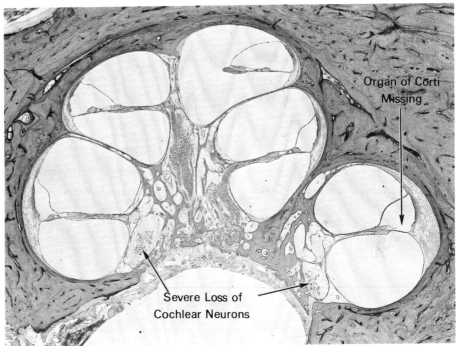

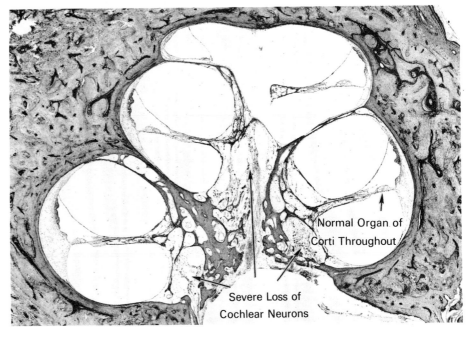

Atrophy of the stria vascularis is a common pathological entity often affecting several members of a family (Fig. 10.89). Typically the hearing loss has an insidious onset in the third to sixth decades of life and progresses slowly. The clinical feature which distinguishes it from other types of presbycusis is the flat audiometric pattern usually associated with an excellent speech discrimination score. Speech discrimination scores are usually normal until the threshold elevation exceeds 50 db. The findings indicate that ears with pure strial atrophy, when stimulated within their sensitivity ranges, are capable of accurate stimulus coding. Although the SISI test commonly is positive, these patients do not complain of discomfort for loud sounds or of distortion. They respond well to the use of amplification and may be given a good prognosis for continued useful hearing (Schuknecht, 1964a; Schuknecht and Ishii, 1966).

Typically, there is patchy atrophy of the stria vascularis in the middle and apical turns of the cochlea (Johnsson and Hawkins, 1972b). There may be partial or complete loss of strial cells, sometimes with cystic structures and occasionally with basophilic deposits (Figs. 10.90 to 10.98).

Takahashi (1971) studied, by electron microscopy, the stria vascularis

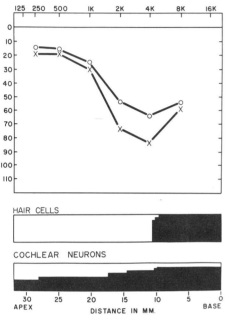

Fig. 10.86: Neural presbycusis (in association with sensory presbycusis and possibly with cochlear conductive presbycusis). At the age of 71 this man complained of having had a hearing loss for many years. Audiometric tests showed a bilateral hearing loss worse for the high frequencies. He died at the age of 80. The cochlear chart below is for the left ear and shows a loss of 90 percent of the neurons in the basal turn, 60 percent in the middle turn, and 40 percent in the apical turn. There is a total loss of hair cells in the basal 11 mm of the cochlea.

Fig. 10.87: See audiogram and cochlear chart of the left ear in Fig. 10.86. There is a severe loss of neurons throughout the cochlea. Except for loss of hair cells in the basal 11 mm of the cochlea, all structures of the cochlear duct appear normal.

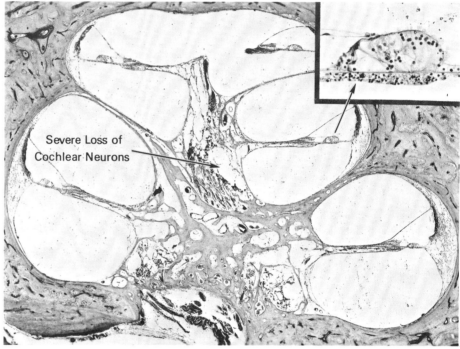

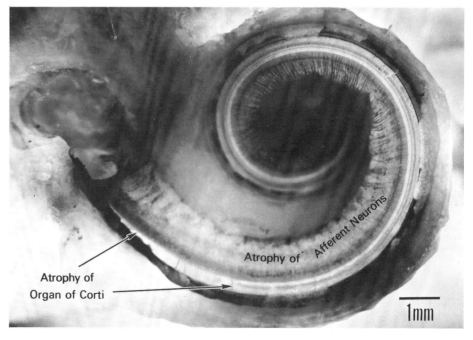

Fig. 10.88: Surface preparation of the cochlea of a 72-year-old male. The apical turn and part of the middle turn have been removed. There is a severe loss of afferent nerve fibers in the basal turn. The organ of Corti is severely degenerated at the basal end. (Courtesy of Johnsson)

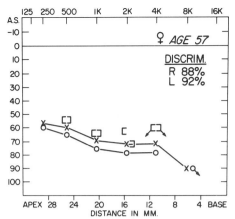

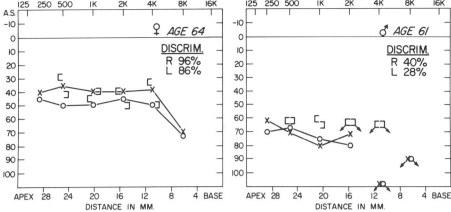

Fig. 10.89: Strial presbycusis (clinical impression). Audiograms of three siblings showing bilateral sensorineural hearing losses characterized by flat audiometric patterns. Speech discrimination scores are excellent in two and diminished in one. The findings are consistent with presbycusis due to atrophy of the stria vascularis.

Fig. 10.90: Strial presbycusis. This patient first noted hearing loss at the age of 49. At the age of 62 audiometric studies showed a bilateral hearing loss. The pure tone thresholds exhibited flat audiometric patterns. Speech discrimination was excellent. There is a slight loss of cochlear neurons throughout the basal 20 mm of the cochlea; however, the most striking change is patchy atrophy of the stria vascularis, most severe in the apical half of the cochlea.

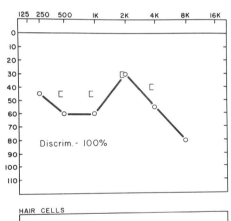

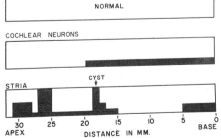

Fig. 10.91: For history see legend, Fig. 10.90. This photomicrograph from the 18 mm region shows a cystic structure replacing the atrophied stria vascularis. There is normal population of hair cells in the organ of Corti.

in individuals over the age of 60. He demonstrated two types of atrophy: (1) a patchy type most severe in the apical and extreme basal regions and (2) a diffuse type often showing normal strial thickness with large intercellular spaces which might not be visible by light microscopy. Kimura and Schuknecht (1970) found similar atrophic changes in the ears of patients with Ménière's disease and assumed they represented alterations of aging rather than Ménière's disease (Fig. 10.99). The three cell layers of the stria are involved in varying degrees and combinations; however, the marginal cells appear to be most severely affected. In some regions of atrophy the stria consists of only a layer of basal cells aligning the endolymphatic space. The guinea pig is the only animal other than the human being which has been found to show strial atrophy (Fig. 10.100).

Possibly the loss of strial tissue affects some quality of endolymph which results in a detrimental influence on the physical and chemical processes by which energy is made available to the sense organ. Experimental observations permit several interesting speculations on the functional significance of the stria vascularis.

First, the stria vascularis appears to be the source of the positive 80 mv DC potential of the scala media. Davis et al. (1958) observed in guinea pigs that degeneration of the stria vascularis following cochlear venous obstruction caused marked lowering or absence of the DC endolymphatic potential. In subsequent experiments Tasaki and Spyropoulos (1959) and Misrahy et al. (1958) have used electrodes to explore the walls of the scala media and determined that the stria vascularis is the only area from which a positive DC potential can be recorded.

Second, the stria vascularis has long been thought to be the site of endolymph formation (Nachlas and Lurie, 1951). Von Fieandt and Saxén (1936),

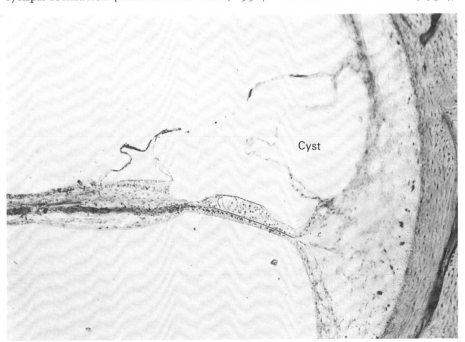

Fig. 10.92: Strial presbycusis. At the age of 76 this patient complained of slowly progressive hearing loss of more than 10 years' duration. Audiometric tests revealed a bilateral symmetrical hearing loss exhibiting flat threshold patterns. He died at the age of 89. Histological studies show patchy atrophy of the stria vascularis in the apical halves of the cochleae.

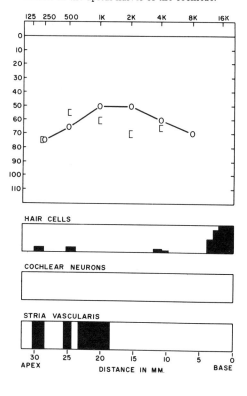

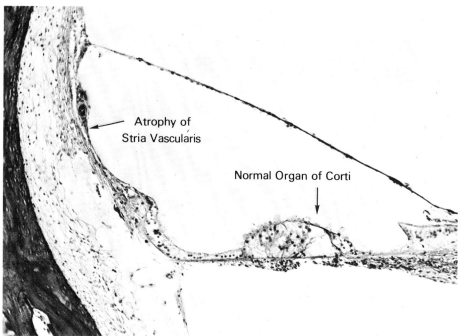

Fig. 10.93: For history see legend, Fig. 10.92. Photomicrograph from the 25 mm region shows severe atrophy of the stria vascularis. The population of hair cells is normal. The alteration in the tectorial membrane is probably an artifact of preparation.

Fig. 10.94: Strial presbycusis. At the age of 68 this woman had bilateral symmetrical hearing losses exhibiting flat threshold patterns with relatively good speech discrimination scores. She died at the age of 72. Histological studies show severe patchy atrophy of the stria vascularis throughout the cochleae, most severe in the apical regions. See Figs. 10.95 and 10.96.

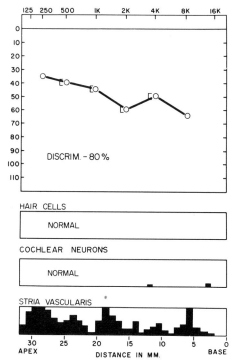

Fig. 10.95: For history see legend, Fig. 10.94. This photomicrograph from the basal turn shows the atrophied stria vascularis to be replaced by a faintly basophilic homogeneous deposit, encapsulated by a single layer of cells. The other structures of the cochlear duct are normal.

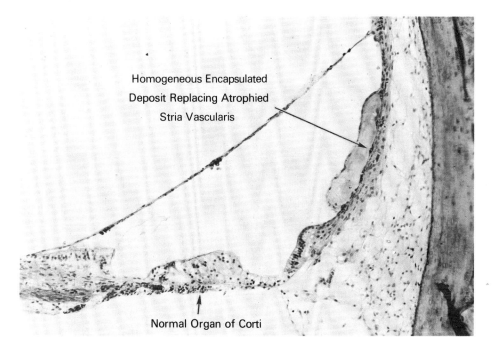

Homogeneous Encapsulated

Deposit Replacing Atrophied

Stria Vascularis

Normal Organ of Corti

Fig. 10.96: Same case as Figs. 10.94 and 10.95. In this view from the middle turn, about 50 percent of the stria vascularis is atrophied and replaced by an encapsulated cystic structure containing a homogeneous basophilic substance.

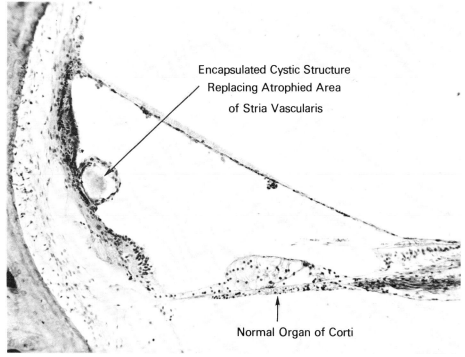

Encapsulated Cystic Structure

Replacing Atrophied Area

of Stria Vascularis

Normal Organ of Corti

Fig. 10.97: Strial presbycusis. Audiometric tests at the age of 64 showed this woman to have a bilateral symmetrical sensorineural hearing loss. At the age of 68 the hearing loss had progressed and was now worse in the left ear. She died three months after the last test. Histological study of the left ear (shown here) shows patchy areas of atrophy of the stria vascularis in the apical half of the cochlea. There is a small region of atrophy of the hair cells and cochlear neurons at the extreme basal end of the cochlea and slight loss of external hair cells in the 7–14 mm region and at the extreme apex. See Fig. 10.98.

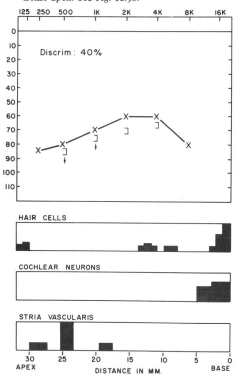

Fig. 10.98: For history see legend, Fig. 10.97. Photomicrograph showing the stria vascularis to be normal in the 12 mm region and totally atrophied in the 23 mm region. The organ of Corti and other structures of the cochlear duct appear normal.

using the light microscope, and more recently Engström et al. (1955) and Smith (1957), using the electron microscope, have shown that the stria vascularis has morphological features consistent with secreting organs in other parts of the body. Smith has shown that the marginal cells which face the endolymph surround the capillary networks with their basal surfaces exhibiting numerous extensions and infoldings of the basal plasma membrane which interdigitate with other cells, including the capillary endothelial cells. The implication of a secreting function is found in the fact that this type of structure is present in kidney tubules, serous alveoli, choroid plexus, ciliary bodies, and secretory ducts of the submaxillary gland (Pease, 1955).

Third, the tissues of the stria vascularis contain large amounts of oxidative enzymes which are required for glucose metabolism and which may be essential for the production of energy to support cochlear function (Vosteen, 1961).

These observations assign an important functional role to the stria vascularis. It seems reasonable that atrophy of this important structure should lead to hearing loss.

4. COCHLEAR CONDUCTIVE PRESBYCUSIS

Although cochlear conductive presbycusis is not yet a proven pathological entity, it seems an appropriate explanation for that type of hearing loss which is characterized by the descending audiometric pattern for bone conduction. Cochlear conductive deafness usually first becomes evident in middle age and exhibits bilateral symmetrical threshold losses showing straight-line descending audiometric patterns. The speech discrimination scores are inversely related to the steepness of the threshold gradient, and this determines, in great part, the effectiveness of amplification. Microscopic studies of cochleae exhibiting descending threshold patterns usually fail to reveal morphological changes in the sensory or neural structures adequate to explain the hearing losses (Figs. 10.101, 10.102). It is proposed, therefore, that the hearing loss is due to a disorder in motion mechanics of the cochlear duct.

It is tempting to try to relate such linear decrements of function to the physical-anatomical gradients which determine the resonance characteristics of the cochlear duct, e.g., the width and thickness of the basilar membrane. The greatest threshold loss is for high frequencies which have their locus of action in the basal end of the cochlea where the basilar membrane

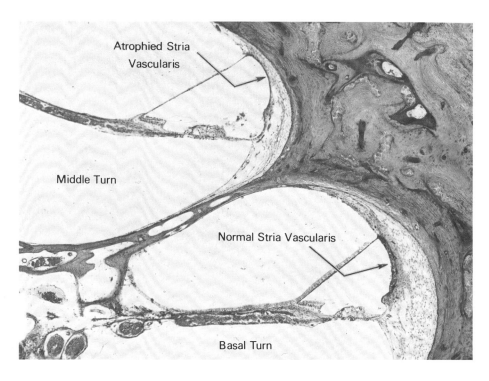

Fig. 10.99: These transmission electron micrographs show the stria vascularis in surgical specimens removed during labyrinthectomy for Ménière's disease. It is assumed, but not certain, that these changes represent atrophy of aging rather than alterations associated with Ménière's disease.

Age 61. The basal cell extends to the luminal surface in an area where the marginal and intermediate cells are atrophied. Lipofuscin granules have accumulated in some of the strial cells.

Age 80. The marginal cells are flattened and in some areas abut directly onto the basal cells.

Age 39. The intermediate and marginal cells have degenerated, and the basal cells line the endolymphatic space.

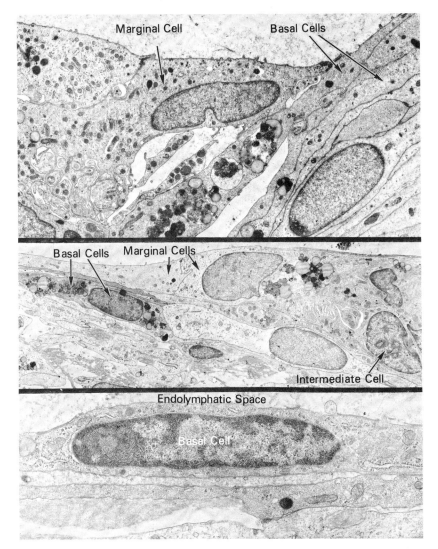

Fig. 10.100: Guinea pig. There is atrophy of the stria vascularis in the fourth turn of the cochlea.

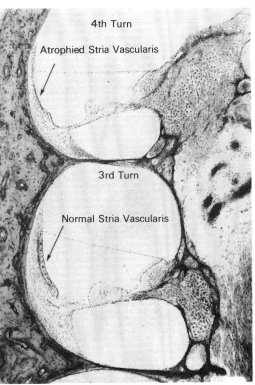

is thicker and narrower, whereas the least loss is for low frequencies which act mainly upon the apical region of the cochlea where this membrane is thinner and wider.

The notion that the deafness in these patients might be due to a disorder of the brain or auditory nerve is untenable. Two bodies of evidence are pertinent:

(a) Patients with bilateral slowly progressive deafness with descending audiometric patterns for bone conduction characteristically manifest serviceable speech discrimination which is indicative of a cochlear rather than a neural lesion.

(b) It has been demonstrated that lesions of the auditory neural pathways have a greater effect on speech discrimination than on pure tone thresholds (Walsh and Goodman, 1955). Lesions which involve the cochlear nerve, such as vestibular schwannoma and multiple sclerosis, characteristically create loss of speech discrimination with relatively less loss for pure tone thresholds (Citron et al., 1963). Animal experiments have shown that bilateral ablation of the auditory cortices does not alter pure tone thresholds (Neff, 1967); and as much as 75 percent of cochlear neurons can degenerate in an area of the cochlea without affecting the pure tone thresholds for frequencies located in those areas (Schuknecht and Woellner, 1955).

In 1919–1920 Mayer suggested that impaired hearing of old age might be due to stiffening of the basilar membrane and supported his thesis with histological sections which he interpreted as showing calcification of the basilar membrane. Crowe et al. (1934) found partial atrophy of the cochlear nerve to the basal turn to be a prominent lesion in the majority of ears with descending audiometric thresholds but noted that "some ears with the gradual type of loss do not have sufficient degree of nerve atrophy to explain the impairment of hearing." They also reported finding hyalinization and deposition of calcium salts in the basilar membrane at the basal end of the cochlea to be more common in patients with descending audiometric patterns than in normal ears or ears with abrupt high-tone hearing losses. Covell and Rogers (1957) and Pestalozza et al. (1957), in studies on senile guinea pigs, found that the losses in cochlear microphonic response were greater than could be attributed to hair cell changes and suggested that conductive lesions might be present.

Glorig and Davis (1961) accept the idea of an inner ear conductive impairment as being perfectly logical. In support of this concept they observed that loudness recruitment is absent in many cases of presbycusis.

Nomura (1970) found neutral fat and cholesterol in the filamentous structure of the pars pectinata of the basilar membrane in 9 of 20 aged patients. He considered this lipidosis of the basilar membrane to represent an alteration of aging which might cause presbycusis. Kraus (1970) has recently shown that the basilar membrane of guinea pigs exhibits a decrease in density as a

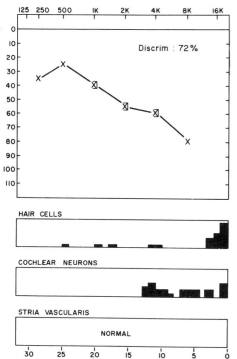

Fig. 10.101: Cochlear conductive presbycusis. Audiometric studies at the age of 66 show this man to have bilateral sensorineural hearing terns. He died at the age of 68. Both ears show slight loss of hair cells and cochlear neurons in the basal ends of the cochleae, but these changes are inadequate to explain the hearing loss. Left ear shown. See Fig. 10.102.

Fig. 10.102: For history see legend, Fig. 10.101. Left ear. All structures of the cochlear duct (as well as cochlear neurons) were normal in the 15 mm region of the cochlea, which serves the 2,000 Hz frequency for which the patient exhibited a 50 db hearing loss.

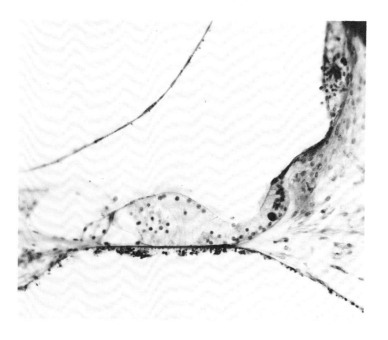

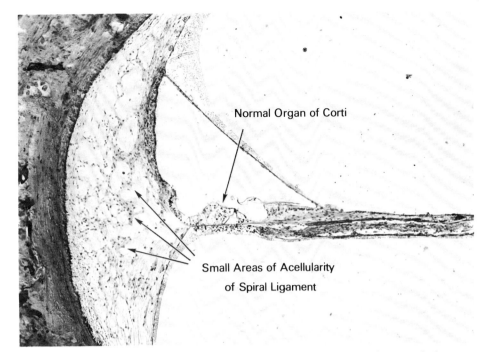

Normal Organ of Corti

Small Areas of Acellularity
of Spiral Ligament

Fig. 10.103: The cochleae of this 77-year-old woman who had no history of hearing loss show small areas of acellularity in the spiral ligament in the basal turns considered to be normal for age. The organ of Corti and other structures of the cochlear duct appear normal. See Fig. 10.106.

Fig. 10.104: At the age of 49 this man had a bilateral high-frequency hearing loss exhibiting descending threshold patterns, slightly worse on the right side. He died four years later. See Fig. 10.105.

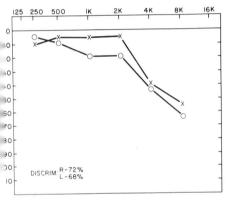

DISCRIM: R - 72%
         L - 68%

function of aging, which supports the concept of a physico-chemical alteration in its structural characteristics.

The only pathological change which is found consistently in ears exhibiting descending threshold patterns is atrophy of the spiral ligament greater than that found in normal ears of the same age (Wright and Schuknecht, 1972).

Atrophic changes in the spiral ligament begin in childhood and progress throughout the life of the individual. When these changes occur in moderate degree they are compatible with normal hearing. The changes appear to be as consistent a function of aging as those which occur, for example, in the skin. The atrophy is most severe in the apical region of the cochlea and is progressively less severe toward the basal end (Schuknecht, 1967). The earliest alteration is a loss of fibrocytes in the region adjacent to the attachment of the basilar membrane (Fig. 10.103). As the atrophy progresses, a zone of acellularity develops in the midportion of the spiral ligament (Figs. 10.104, 10.105). There appears to be a loss of fibrocytes as well as a migration of fibrocytes toward the margins of the ligament. With further change two distinct zones are seen, a larger internal zone, remarkable for its acellularity and cystic spaces, and an external smaller zone containing scattered fibrocytes in a fibrillar stroma (Fig. 10.106). Commonly there is a dense layer of closely packed fibrocytes at the interface between these zones. All of these changes can be found in normal-hearing ears but are more frequent in ears exhibiting descending audiometric patterns (Wright and Schuknecht, 1972).

As the spiral ligament shrinks, the configuration of the cochlear duct is altered. Commonly the basilar membrane retains its continuity with the structures of the lateral wall by a thin layer of ligamentous tissue which converts the cochlear duct from a triangular to a flattened shape (Fig. 10.107). Sometimes the basilar membrane separates from the lateral wall by a break in the area between the basilar crest and the spiral prominence. This brings the endolymphatic space into continuity with cystic spaces in the spiral ligament. When this happens the only remaining connection of the basilar membrane with the bony cochlear wall is a thin layer of spiral ligament tissue bordering the scala tympani (Fig. 10.108).

The functional effects of lesions of this type are not currently known. Specimens from patients with accurate auditory tests are needed to answer this question.

Clinical observations have shown that ears with chronic suppurative disease exhibit an increased incidence of sensorineural hearing loss characterized by a descending audiometric pattern for bone conduction (Paparella et al., 1970) (Fig. 10.109). Paget's disease is another disorder which is frequently associated with this type of hearing loss (see Paget's Disease, this chapter).

Fig. 10.105: For history see legend, Fig. 10.104. The spiral ligament in the 18 mm area of the right ear shows large areas of acellularity. All structures of the cochlear duct and the cochlear neuronal population appear normal.

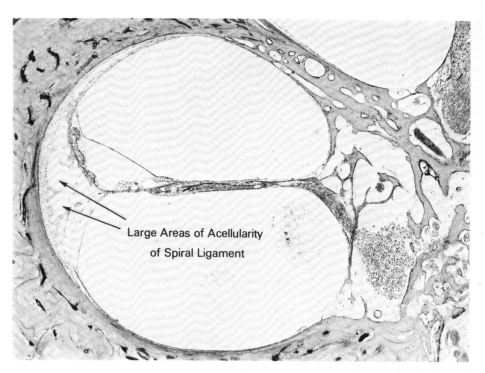

Large Areas of Acellularity
of Spiral Ligament

Fig. 10.106: The spiral ligaments in the middle turns of the cochleae of this 77-year-old woman whose hearing status is unknown show external zones with normal cellularity and larger internal zones which are nearly devoid of cells. There is a dense layer of cells in the interface between these two zones. These changes are normal for age. See Fig. 10.103.

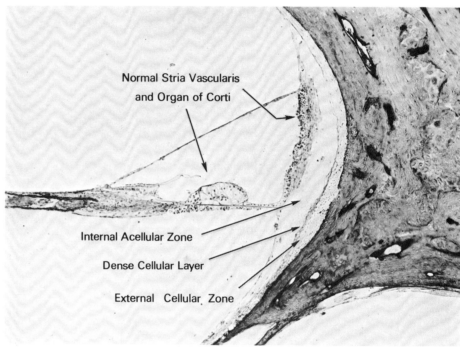

Normal Stria Vascularis
and Organ of Corti

Internal Acellular Zone

Dense Cellular Layer

External Cellular Zone

Fig. 10.107: The auditory function of this 36-year-old male is not known. Both ears of this individual show severe atrophy of the spiral ligaments in the 20 to 32 mm regions. The basilar membrane has retained its connection to the spiral prominence by a thin layer of ligamentous tissue.

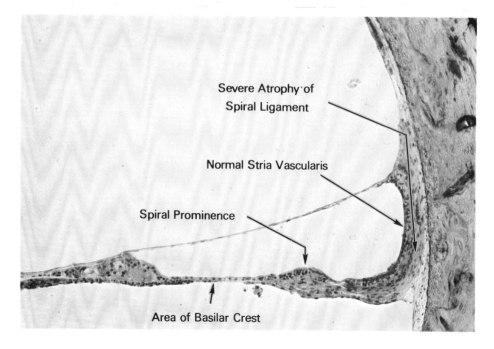

Severe Atrophy of
Spiral Ligament

Normal Stria Vascularis

Spiral Prominence

Area of Basilar Crest

Fig. 10.108: This view shows the cochlear duct of a 63-year-old woman whose hearing status is unknown. Histological study of both ears shows severe atrophy of the spiral ligaments, most severe in the middle and apical turns. In the apical turn of the ear shown there is an area of discontinuity of the lateral wall of the cochlear duct between the basilar crest and spiral prominence. Except for moderate compression artifact, the organ of Corti and stria vascularis appear normal. The histological appearance suggests that this discontinuity occurred before death; however, the possibility of an artifactual rupture of an atrophied spiral ligament caused by the shrinking effect of fixative solutions cannot be ruled out.

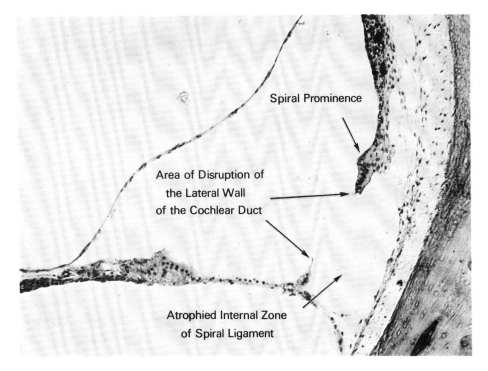

Spiral Prominence

Area of Disruption of
the Lateral Wall
of the Cochlear Duct

Atrophied Internal Zone
of Spiral Ligament

Fig. 10.109: Descending bone conduction thresholds in an ear with chronic otitis media. This female experienced bilateral recurring acute otitis media in childhood and chronic suppurative otitis media throughout adult life. A left radical mastoidectomy was performed at the age of 58. Audiometric studies showed progressive bilateral sensorineural and conductive hearing loss. She died at the age of 67. Histological studies show perforations of the tympanic membranes and advanced fibrocystic sclerosis of the middle ears. Both cochleae show a loss of hair cells and cochlear neurons at the basal ends and moderate atrophy of the spiral ligaments.

Otosclerosis is considered by many clinicians to cause sensorineural hearing loss (Fig. 10.110). Certainly the spiral ligament undergoes atrophic changes in areas where it abuts otosclerotic bone, and severe atrophy may lead to rupture of the cochlear duct. In this chapter, see Otosclerosis.

It seems plausible that these diseases cause an acceleration of those atrophic changes normally occurring in the supportive tissue which determine, in part at least, the motion mechanics of the cochlear duct.

Rupture of the cochlear duct and profound hearing loss appear to be the ultimate, but rare, end result of advanced atrophy of the spiral ligament. Although more documentation is needed, several specimens in the collection at the Massachusetts Eye and Ear Infirmary support this contention (Figs. 10.111 to 10.114). In assessing morphological changes of this magnitude it is important to consider the possible role of postmortem autolysis and preparation artifact as causes for the changes. Controlled studies on postmortem autolysis have failed to show changes of the type shown in these ears. The spiral ligament and basilar membrane are much less affected by postmortem changes than the other structures of the cochlea (see Chapter 1D, Postmortem Autolysis). Furthermore, changes of this type have not been seen as a preparation artifact in other ears prepared by the same method.

Although cochlear conductive presbycusis and spiral ligament presbycusis were designated previously as separate entities it now seems more likely that atrophy of the spiral ligament is but one of the pathological changes that lead to cochlear conductive deafness. The concept that atrophic changes can cause alterations in the physical properties of the cochlear duct must remain hypothetical, until it is demonstrated that there are alterations in mass, stiffness, or friction of this structure.

Finally, it seems clear that whereas the cochleae of many individuals exhibit a rather pure atrophy of one of the four types described here, there are some which show a combination of these types. In the latter instance, the functional deficits from each appear to be additive (Figs. 10.115, 10.116).

K. THE DYSEQUILIBRIUM OF AGING

Clinical experience has shown that many aging individuals experience a loss of equilibratory function. The condition may be viewed as the vestibular counterpart of the deafness of aging (presbycusis). The clinical manifestations suggest that there are four types of dysequilibrium of aging, that

125 250 500   1K   2K   4K   8K   16K

4 YEARS
POST-OP
RADICAL MAST.

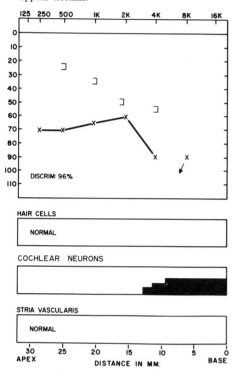

Fig. 10.110: Cochlear conductive presbycusis and neural presbycusis in association with otosclerosis. This female first complained of hearing loss at the age of 15. Audiometric tests at the ages of 49, 67, and 75 revealed bilateral progressive sensorineural and conductive hearing loss (left ear shown here). She died two weeks after the final test. Histological studies show bilateral otosclerosis with stapes fixation without involvement of the endosteal layers of the cochlear walls. Both ears show a partial loss of cochlear neurons in the basal 14 mm of the cochleae and moderate atrophy of the spiral ligaments; however, the structures of the cochlear ducts appear normal.

Fig. 10.111: Cochlear conductive presbycusis in association with sensory and strial presbycusis. This man experienced a progressive hearing loss from the age of 70 until the time of his death at the age of 78. No audiometric studies were performed. Histological examination reveals severe atrophy of the spiral ligaments and striae vasculares through the apical halves of the cochleae. The left ear is shown here. Both ears exhibit rupture of the cochlear ducts in the middle turns where the spiral ligaments are totally missing. The apical displacement of the osseous spiral lamina of the middle turn is an artifact following decalcification. There is a loss of 25 to 40 percent of the cochlear neurons throughout the basal turns but the populations in the middle and apical turns are normal. There is severe atrophy of the organs of Corti in the basal ends and scattered loss of hair cells throughout the remainder of the cochleae. The severe atrophy of the spiral ligaments and rupture of the cochlear ducts are presumed to be an antemortem pathological change rather than preparation artifact.

the pathological change is located in the vestibular sense organs in three and in the vestibular neural pathways in one, and that they may occur individually or in combination. One of these, cupulolithiasis of aging, is supported by pathological documentation; however, the others evolve purely from clinical observations.

(1) Cupololithiasis of aging is manifested by severe vertiginous episodes of short duration, precipitated by certain head positions. Aging is but one of several etiologies for the cupololithiasis syndrome. Usually the syndrome is self-limiting. When it develops insidiously in an aged individual with no obvious inciting factor such as head injury, it tends to be persistent and may exist throughout the remainder of life. Because the attacks may be of sudden onset and cause falling, it is a particularly serious malady for aged individuals. Pathological studies have shown that the disorder is caused by deposits on the cupula of the posterior semicircular canal. It is presumed that the deposits consist of insoluble products generated by atrophic changes in the pars superior (utricle and semicircular canals). These products settle into the most dependent part of the pars superior, the ampulla of the posterior semicircular canal, and become fixed to the cupula. The deposits are presumed to have a specific gravity greater than endolymph and therefore are capable of producing cupular deflections when head position is changed relative to the direction of gravitational force. For a detailed description see Chapter 12B, Cupulolithiasis.

(2) Ampullary dysequilibrium of aging is characterized by vertigo associated with angular head movements. These individuals experience a sensation of rotatory movement of the field of vision with certain head movements which excite the cristae. For example, when turning quickly to the right or left, or on extension or flexion of the head, a sense of rotation may persist for one or more seconds after the movement has been completed. Some individuals complain that a sensation of downward movement continues for several seconds after a stooping movement has been completed. Associated eye movements are fleeting and difficult to observe. Although the sensation of dysequilibrium is usually momentary, a severe angular stimulus can be followed by a sensation of unsteadiness for several hours. Although pathological documentation is lacking, it seems possible that the disorder is caused by degenerative changes in the ampullary mechanism of the semicircular canals. This theoretical explanation derives some support from the observation that there is a decreased vestibular re-

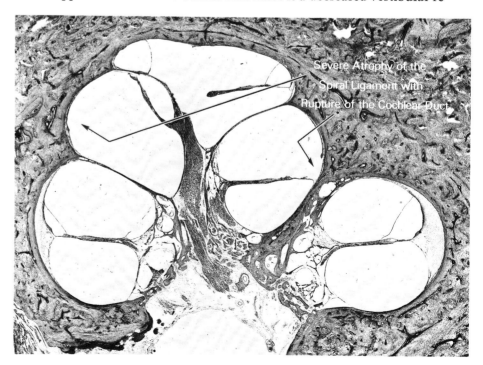

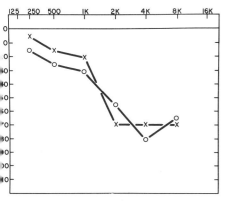

Fig. 10.112: Cochlear conductive presbycusis. At the age of 78 this man exhibited a bilateral hearing loss characterized by descending threshold patterns. See Fig. 10.113.

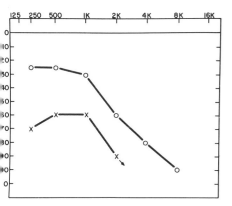

Fig. 10.113: Same case as Fig. 10.112. One year later the loss was much worse, particularly on the left. He died at the age of 80. His relatives reported that during the last six weeks of life he was "stone deaf." See Fig. 10.114.

Fig. 10.114: Same case as Figs. 10.112 and 10.113. Left ear shown. There is severe atrophy of the spiral ligament throughout the apical half of the cochlea. The cochlear duct is ruptured in the middle turn. In the region of the rupture the osseous spiral lamina is displaced toward Reissner's membrane, and it presumably is an artifact caused by the pull of Reissner's membrane following decalcification. The organ of Corti shows moderately severe autolysis. It is severely atrophied in the basal turn with scattered hair cell loss in the middle and apical turns. There is a severe loss of cochlear neurons in the basal 15 mm of the cochlea.

sponse to rotation and caloric stimulation as a function of aging in healthy individuals (Allard, 1938; Okano, 1938; Arslan, 1957; Bruner and Norris, 1971). Furthermore, the so-called pigment of aging, lipofuscin granules, have been demonstrated in the hair cells and supporting cells of the cristae of aged individuals (Ishii et al., 1967) (Figs. 10.117, 10.118, 10.119). Thus, degenerative changes in the sensory epithelium, possibly associated with alterations in the cupular mechanism, are a possible cause for the ampullary dysequilibrium of aging.

(3) Macular dysequilibrium of aging is characterized by vertigo precipitated by changing head position relative to the direction of gravitational force, after the head has been maintained in a position for some time. For example, upon attempting to arise from bed, the sensation of dysequilibrium may be so pronounced that sitting up may have to be accomplished in stages. Some individuals with this disorder must sit on the edge of the bed for some minutes before attempting to walk. Orthostatic hypotension may cause a similar type of sensation but is usually accompanied by other signs of intracranial ischemia and visual blackout. The caloric responses of individuals exhibiting macular dysequilibrium of aging are usually normal for age. It would seem reasonable to assume that these symptoms may be caused by degenerative changes in the otolithic membranes or sensory epithelia of the utricle and saccule.

In support of this contention is the observation that both animals and human subjects with the sensory type of presbycusis frequently exhibit atrophy of the saccule (Schuknecht et al., 1965; Johnsson and Hawkins, 1969). The alterations consist of loss of hair cells and supporting cells, atrophy of the otolithic membrane, and collapse of the saccular wall (Figs. 10.120, 10.121). In a more recent study Johnsson (1971) observed the vestibular system by the technique of *in situ* microdissection in the temporal bones of 24 individuals with presbycusis. He found varying degrees of degeneration of the saccular nerve network and its neuroepithelium and severe to total loss of otoconia in individuals over the age of 60 years. There was comparable but less severe loss of utricular otoconia. Specimens from individuals under the age of 30 years, with few exceptions, displayed a continuous layer of otoconia in the otolithic membrane (Fig. 10.122).

(4) Vestibular ataxia of aging is manifested by a constant sensation of

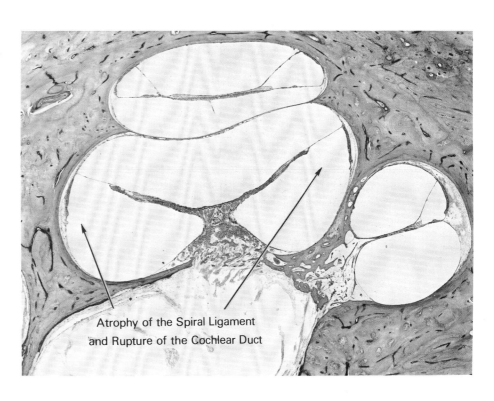

Atrophy of the Spiral Ligament and Rupture of the Cochlear Duct

Fig. 10.115: Presbycusis of multiple pathological types. This man experienced bilateral progressive sensorineural hearing loss throughout his adult life. When he died at the age of 88, he was severely deaf. Final audiometric tests (right ear shown here) revealed bone conduction thresholds at 55 to 70 db and air conduction thresholds at 75 to 80 db. The speech discrimination score (PB max) was zero. Incidentaly, the long process of the incus was resorbed, and the tympanic membrane was in contact with the stapes. See Fig. 10.116.

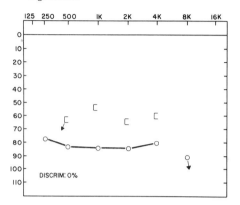

Fig. 10.116: For history see legend, Fig. 10.115. Both cochleae (right ear shown here) show severe atrophy of the spiral ligaments throughout the apical halves of the cochleae and atrophy of the organs of Corti and cochlear neurons throughout the basal halves of the cochleae. Throughout the apical halves there is also extensive atrophy of the striae vasculares and tectorial membranes. In some areas in the right ear the tectorial membrane is displaced into the angle between the limbus and Reissner's membrane.

dysequilibrium on ambulation. There is no unsteadiness when sitting or standing but when walking there is inability to control the center of gravity. Walking is accomplished with a hesitancy, with frequent side steps, and with a fixed head position to gain optimum advantage of visual points of reference. It occurs predominantly in the seventh and eighth decades of life. The caloric responses of these patients are usually normal for age. Although there is no pathological documentation for vestibular ataxia, the symptoms suggest a loss of vestibular control over the lower limbs. Possible sites for the lesion are the vestibular nerves, the medial, lateral, or descending vestibular nuclei, the

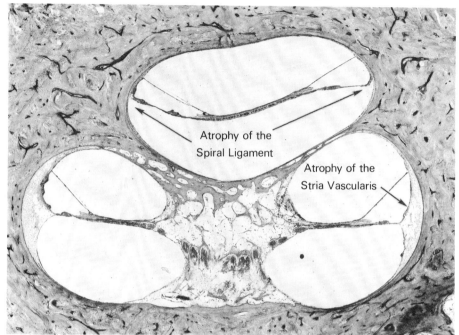

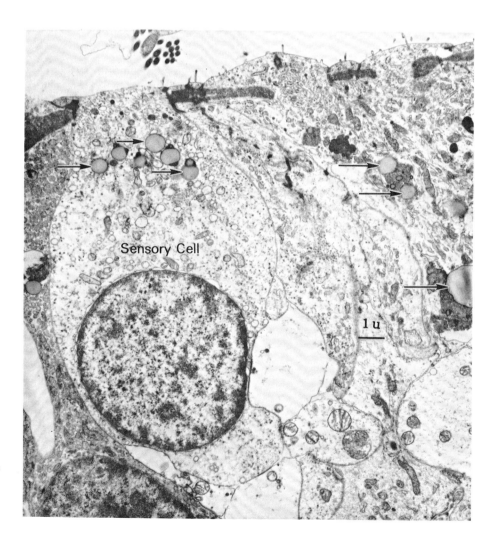

Fig. 10.117: Transmission electron micrograph showing lipofuscin granules (arrows) in the apical zones of the hair cells and supporting cells of the crista ampullaris of an aged individual. (Courtesy of Ishii)

descending medial longitudinal fasciculi, and the vestibulospinal tracts (see Chapter 2E2, Vestibular pathways). Vestibular tests, as currently used, do not provide distinct differentiation of sensory from neural lesions or of the level of lesions in the vestibular neural pathways. Vestibular ataxia may be considered to be the vestibular counterpart of neural presbycusis. The disorder frequently persists for the remainder of the life of the individual.

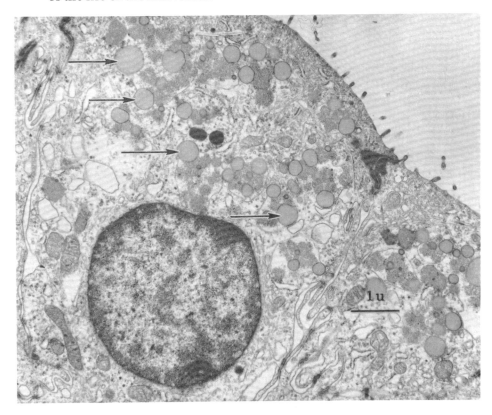

Fig. 10.118: Transmission electron micrograph showing numerous lipofuscin granules (arrows) in the apical area of an epithelial cell in the transitional zone of the crista of an aged individual. (Courtesy of Ishii)

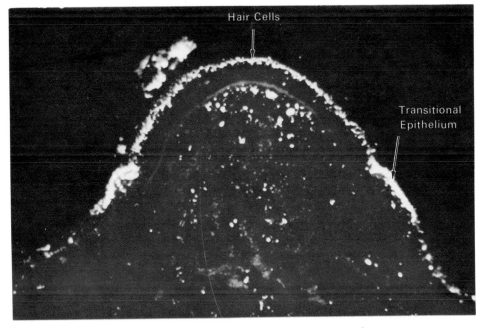

Fig. 10.119: Fluorescent granules in the crista ampullaris of an 80-year-old man. These granules become more numerous and larger with aging. They are assumed to be composed of lipofuscin and are the end product of deterioration of lysosomal activity. (Courtesy of Ishii)

Fig. 10.120: This individual had a moderate bilateral subjective loss of hearing in old age and died at the age of 85. Right ear shown here. In addition to degenerative changes in the cochlea there is severe atrophy of the saccule. The wall of the saccule has collapsed and is adherent to a degenerated otolithic membrane. There is disruption of the sensory epithelium in one area and a loss of about 50 percent of the hair cells throughout the saccule.

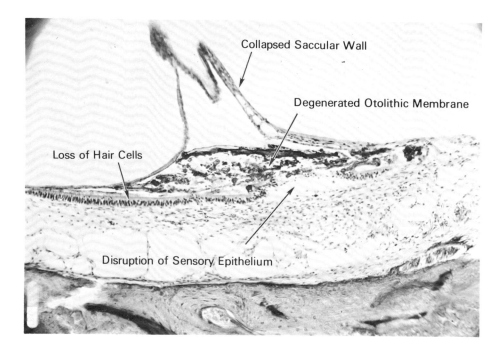

Fig. 10.121: These views show the saccules of a 20-year-old dog and a 19-year-old cat, both of which suffered progressive bilateral hearing loss during the later years of life and were severely deaf at the time of death. Both show bilateral severe atrophy of the organ of Corti and cochlear neurons as well as atrophy of the saccules. In the dog the sensory epithelium of the saccule is flattened. The supporting cells are shrunken, and there is loss of about half of the hair cells. The otolithic membrane is atrophied and displaced toward the posterior margin of the macula. The saccular nerve appears normal. In the cat there is a loss of about half of the hair cells and supporting cells of the saccular macula. The otolithic membrane, saccular wall, and saccular nerve appear normal. In both animals the utricular maculae and the cristae are normal.

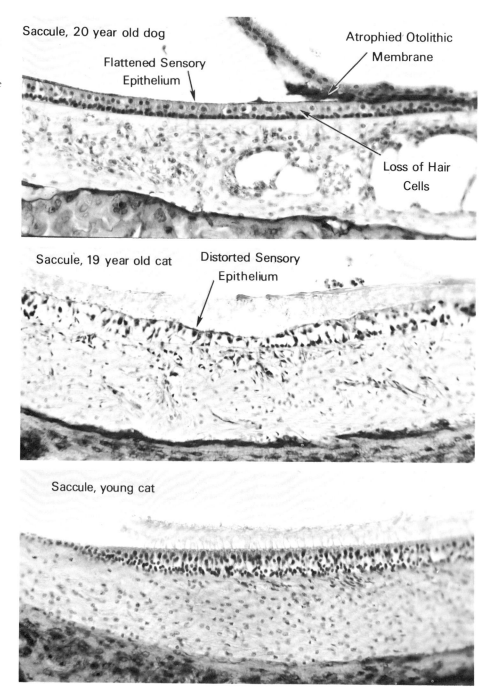

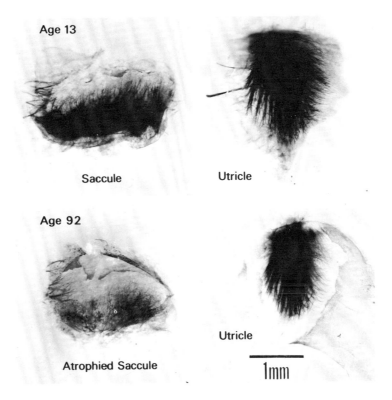

Fig. 10.122: Surface preparations of the saccules and utricles from individuals aged 13 and 92. The sensory epithelium and otolithic membranes have been removed and osmic tetroxide used to stain the nerve fibers. There is severe loss of nerve fiber population in the saccule of the 92-year-old individual. (Courtesy of Johnsson)

Age 13

Saccule   Utricle

Age 92

Atrophied Saccule   Utricle

1mm

References

Adair-Dighton, C., 1912: Four generations of blue sclerotics. Ophthalmoscope 10:188.

Adams, W., 1951a: The aetiology of swimmer's exostoses of the external auditory canals and of associated changes in hearing. Part I. J. Laryng. 65:133.

Adams, W., 1951b: The aetiology of swimmer's exostoses of the external auditory canals and of associated changes in hearing. Part II. J. Laryng. 65:232.

Albers-Schönberg, H., 1904: Röntgenbilder einer seltenen Knochenerkrankung. Münch. med. Wschr. 51:365.

Albers-Schönberg, H., 1907: Eine bisher nicht beschriebene Allgemeinerkrankung des Skelettes im röntgenbild. Fortschr. Röntgenstr. 11:261.

Albright, F., Butler, A., Hampton, A., and Smith, P., 1937: Syndrome characterized by osteitis fibrosa disseminata, areas of pigmentation and endocrine dysfunction, with precocious puberty in females. New Eng. J. Med. 216:727.

Albright, F., and Reifenstein, E., 1948: The parathyroid glands and metabolic bone disease. Bailière, Tindall & Cox, London.

Allard, A., 1938: Contribution à l'étude de la sensibilité de l'appareil semi-circulaire, par la méthode des petites stimulations post-rotatoires primaires, réalisées au moyen du fauteuil Buys-Ryliint. Ann. Otol. Rhinol. Laryng. (Paris) 1:417.

Altmann, F., 1962a: Histopathology and etiology of otosclerosis: A critical review. Chap. 2 in Otosclerosis: Henry Ford Hospital International Symposium. Edited by H. F. Schuknecht. Little, Brown, Boston, Mass., pp. 15–42.

Altmann, F., 1962b: Histopathology of stapes surgery. Chap. 29 in Otosclerosis: Henry Ford Hospital International Symposium. Edited by H. F. Schuknecht. Little, Brown, Boston, Mass., pp. 351–357.

Altmann, F., and Basek, M., 1958: Histological examination of a case of otosclerosis fifteen months after stapesmobilization operation. Arch. Otolaryng. 68:314.

Altmann, F., Basek, M., and Hough, J., 1960: Otosclerosis with bilateral stapes mobilization: Histological and clinical considerations. Arch. Otolaryng. 72:147.

Altmann, F., and Kornfeld, M., 1967: Osteogenesis imperfecta and otosclerosis: New investigations. Ann. Otol. Rhinol. Laryng. 76:89.

Altmann, F., Kornfeld, M., and Shea, J., 1966: Inner ear changes in otosclerosis: Histopathological studies. Ann. Otol. Rhinol. Laryng. 75:5.

Andreasen, E., 1943: Studies on thymolymphatic system: quantitative investigations on thymolymphatic system in normal rats at different ages, under normal conditions and during inanition and restitution after starvation. Acta path. microbiol. scand. Suppl. 49:1.

Anson, B., and Wilson, J., 1937: Structural alterations in the petrous portion of the temporal bone in osteitis deformans. Arch. Otolaryng. 25:560.

Antoli-Candela, F., 1962: Audiosurgery of the stapes and oval window in clinical otosclerosis. Chap. 37 in Otosclerosis. Edited by H. F. Schuknecht. Little, Brown, Boston, Mass., pp. 457–473.

Antoli-Candela, F., 1969: Long-term results in stapedectomy. Arch. Otolaryng. 89:412.

Arenberg, I., and Shambaugh, G., Jr., 1969: Fistulae with off-center prosthesis. Arch. Otolaryng. 90:275.

Arslan, M., 1957: The senescence of the vestibular apparatus. Pract. oto-rhino-laryng. 19:475.

Ashley Montagu, M., 1949: Paget's disease (osteitis deformans) and heredity. Amer. J. Hum. Genet. 1:94.

Baron, S., and Lindsay, J., 1964: Stapedectomy with fat graft and polyethylene strut: A case report. Arch. Otolaryng. 80:128.

Basek, M., 1967: Fibrous dysplasia of the middle ear. Arch. Otolaryng. 85:4.

Batsakis, J., and Nishiyama, R., 1962: Deafness with sporadic goiter. Arch. Otolaryng. 76:401.

Bauer, J., and Stein, C., 1924–1925: Vererbung und Konstitution bei Ohrenkrankheiten. Beiträge zur klinischen Konstitutionspathologie. Ztschr. f.d. ges. Anat. 2 Abt. 10:483.

Belal, A., and Stewart, T., 1974: Pathological changes in the middle ear joints. Ann. Otol. Rhinol. Laryng. 83:159.

Bellucci, R., 1969: Survey of stapes surgery: Five-year study. Arch. Otolaryng. 89:408.

Benitez, J., and Schuknecht, H., 1962: Otosclerosis: A human temporal bone report. Laryngoscope 72:1.

Bennett, H., 1956: A suggestion as to the nature of the lysosome. J. Biophys. Biochem. Cytol. 2, Suppl. 185.

Blake, C., 1893: Stapedectomy and other middle ear operations. Trans. Amer. Otol. Soc. 5:464.

Bosatra, A., 1960: Otosclerosis of the inner ear: A clinical study. J. Laryng. 74:209.

Boucheron, E., 1888: La Mobilisation de l'étrier et son procédé opératoire. Un. Med., Paris, 46:412.

Bourne, G., 1961: Structural Aspects of Aging. Hafner Publishing Co., New York.

Bredberg, G., 1968: Cellular pattern and nerve supply of the human organ of Corti. Acta oto-laryng. Suppl. 236.

Bretlau, P., Jørgensen, M., and Johansen, H., 1970: Osteogenesis imperfecta: Light and electron microscopic studies of the stapes. Acta oto-laryng. 69:172.

Brody, H., 1955: Organization of the cerebral cortex: III. Study of aging in human cerebral cortex. J. Comp. Neurol. 102:511.

Brown, J., 1967: Meningitis following stapes surgery: The pathway of spread to the intracranial cavity. Laryngoscope 77:1295.

Bruner, A., and Norris, T., 1971: Age-related changes in caloric nystagmus. Acta oto-laryng. Suppl. 282.

Brunner, H., 1931: Die Beteiligung der Innenohrkapsel . . . Z. Hals-Nas.-Ohrenheilk. 30:128.

Brunner, H., 1952: Fibrous dysplasia of facial bones and paranasal sinuses. Arch. Otolaryng. 55:43.

Bullough, W., 1949: Age and mitotic activity in the male mouse, Mus musculus L. J. Exp. Biol. 26:261.

Cawthorne, T., 1955: Otosclerosis. J. Laryng. 69:437.

Chevance, L., Bretlau, P., Jørgensen, M., and Causse, J., 1970: Otosclerosis: An electron microscopic and cytochemical study. Acta oto-laryng. Suppl. 272.

Chisolm, J., 1954: Otorhinologic aspects of Hand-Schuller-Christian's disease. Laryngoscope 64:486.

Christian, H., 1920: Defects in membranous bones, exophthalmos and diabetes insipidus: An unusual syndrome of dyspituitarism. Med. Clin. N. Amer. 3:849.

Citron, L., Dix, M., Hallpike, C., and Hood, J., 1963: A recent clinico-pathological study of cochlear nerve degeneration resulting from tumor pressure and disseminated sclerosis, with particular reference to the finding of normal threshold sensitivity for pure tones. Acta oto-laryng. 56:330.

Clemis, J., Boyles, J., Harford, E., and Petasnick, J., 1967: The clinical diagnosis of Paget's disease of the temporal bone. Ann. Otol. Rhinol. Laryng. 76:611.

Clerc, P., and Deumier, R., 1958: La Surdité dans les dysplasies osseuses et les dysmorphies crânio-faciales. Ann. Otol. Rhinol. Laryng. (Paris) 75:852.

Cody, D., 1971: Rehabilitation for sensorineural hearing loss, I., Chap. 23 in Clinical Otology, An International Symposium. Edited by M. Paparella, A. Hohmann, and J. Huff, C. V. Mosby Co., St. Louis, Mo., pp. 211-223.

Cohen, A., and Rosenwasser, H., 1969: Fibrous dysplasia of the temporal bone. Arch. Otolaryng. 89:447.

Cojazzi, L., and Bötner, V., 1950: Le alterazioni istologiche dell'orecchio interno nel diabete sperimentale da allossana. Riv. Crit. Clin. Med. 50, Suppl. 2:266.

Compere, W., 1960: Radiologic findings in otosclerosis. Arch. Otolaryng. 71:150.

Costa, O., 1967: Inner ear pathology in experimental diabetes. Laryngoscope 77:68.

Covell, W., and Rogers, J., 1957: Pathologic changes in the inner ears of senile guinea pigs. Laryngoscope 67:118.

Crowe, S., Guild, S., and Polvogt, L., 1934: Observations on pathology of high-tone deafness. Bull. Johns Hopkins Hosp. 54:315.

Czerny, V., 1873: Eine lokale Malacie des Unterschenkels. Wien. med. Wschr. 23:895.

Davies, D., 1968: Paget's disease of the temporal bone: A clinical and histopathological survey. Acta oto-laryng. Suppl. 242.

Davies, D., 1970: The temporal bone in Paget's disease. J. Laryng. 84:553.

Davis, H., Deatherage, B., Rosenblut, B., Fernandez, C., Kimura, R., and Smith, C., 1958: Modification of cochlear potentials produced by streptomycin poisoning and by extensive venous obstruction. Laryngoscope 68:596.

Dayal, V., and Nussbaum, M., 1971: Patterns of puretone loss in presbycusis: A sequential study. Acta oto-laryng. 71:382.

DeDuve, C., 1963: The lysosome concept. In Lysosomes. Ciba Foundation Symposium. Edited by A. V. S. de Reuk and M. P. Cameron, Little, Brown, Boston, Mass., pp. 1–31.

Derlacki, E., and Valvassori, G., 1965: Clinical and radiological diagnosis of labyrinthine otosclerosis. Laryngoscope 75:1293.

Ellis, P., and Jackson, W., 1962: Osteopetrosis. Amer. J. Ophthal. 53:943.

Engfeldt, B., Engström, A., and Zetterström, R., 1954: Biophysical studies of the bone tissue in osteogenesis imperfecta. J. Bone Jt. Surg. 36B:654.

Engström, H., 1940: Über das Vorkommen der Otosklerose nebst experimentellen Studien über chirurgische Behandlung der Krankheit. Acta oto-laryng. Suppl. 43.

Engström, H., Sjöstrand, F., and Spoendlin, H., 1955: Feinstruktur der Stria vascularis beim Meerschweinchen. Pract. oto-rhinolaryng. 17:69.

Feldman, B., and Schuknecht, H., 1970: Experiences with revision stapedectomy procedures. Laryngoscope 80:1281.

Fenner, F., 1939: The Australian aboriginal skull: Its nonmetrical morphological characters. Roy. Soc. South Austr. Trans. 63:248.

Ferris, K., 1965: On the temporary effect of industrial noise on the hearing at 4000 c/s of stapedectomized ears. J. Laryng. 79:881.

Ferris, K., 1967: A further study on the temporary effect of industrial noise on the hearing of stapedectomized ears at 4000 cps. J. Laryng. 81:613.

Fieandt, H. von, and Saxén, A., 1936: Beiträge zur Histologie der Stria vascularis und der Prominentia spiralis bei Säugern (Hund und Mensch). Z. Anat. EntwGesch. 106:424.

Field, G., 1893: A Manual of Diseases of the Ear, 4th ed. Baillière, Tindall and Cox, London, p. 83.

Fowler, E., Jr., and Osmun, P., 1942: New bone growth due to cold water in the ears. Arch. Otolaryng. 36:455.

Gacek, R., 1970: The diagnosis and treatment of poststapedectomy granuloma. Ann. Otol. Rhinol. Laryng. 79:970.

Gaeth, J., 1948: Study of phonemic regression in relation to hearing loss. Thesis, Northwestern University, Chicago, Ill.

Gilse, P. van, 1938: Des observations ultérieures sur la genèse des exostoses du conduit externe par l'irritation d'eau froide. Acta oto-laryng. 26:343.

Gladney, J., and Shepherd, D., 1970: Labyrinthine dysfunction in latent and early manifest diabetes: A preliminary report. Ann. Otol. Rhinol. Laryng. 79:984.

Glorig, A., and Davis, H., 1961: Age, noise and hearing loss. Ann. Otol. Rhinol. Laryng. 70:556.

Glorig, A., and Gallo, R., 1962: Comments on sensorineural hearing loss in otosclerosis. Chap. 4 in Otosclerosis. Edited by H. F. Schuknecht. Little, Brown, Boston, Mass., p. 63–78.

Goetzinger, C., Proud, G., Dirks, D., and Embrey, J., 1961: Study of hearing in advanced age. Arch Otolaryng. 73:662.

Goldstein, S., 1971: The biology of aging. New Eng. J. Med. 285:1120.

Gregg, J., and Bass, W., 1970: Exostoses in the external auditory canals. Ann. Otol. Rhinol. Laryng. 79:834.

Greifenstein, A., 1932: Die Mitbeteiligung des Gehörorgans, der Nebenhöhlen und der Kiefer bei der Schüller-Christianschen Krankheit, nebst einer neuen eigenen Beobachtung. Arch. Ohr. Nas.-KehlkHeilk. 132:337.

Greifenstein, A., 1935: Vergleichende Untersuchungen zur Histologie der Otosklerose. Arch. Ohr. Nas.-KehlkHeilk. 139:14.

Gross, C., 1969: Sensori-neural hearing loss in clinical and histologic otosclerosis. Laryngoscope 79:104.

Gross, C., and Montgomery, W., 1967: Fibrous dysplasia and malignant degeneration. Arch. Otolaryng. 85:653.

Guild, S., 1944: Histologic otosclerosis. Ann. Otol. Rhinol. Laryng. 53:246.

Guild, S., 1950: The progression of impaired hearing for high tones during childhood. Laryngoscope 60:885.

Guild, S., Crowe, S., Bunch, C., and Polvogt, L., 1931: Correlations of differences in density of innervation of the organ of Corti with differences in the acuity of hearing, including evidence as to the location in the human cochlea of the receptors for certain tones. Acta oto-laryng. 15:269.

Guilford, F., 1962: Experiences in the surgery of otosclerosis. Chap. 42 in Otosclerosis. Edited by H. F. Schuknecht. Little, Brown, Boston, Mass. pp. 523–541.

Habermann, J., 1904: Zur Pathologie der sogenannten Otosklerose. Arch. Ohr. Nas.-KehlkHeilk. 60:37.

Hall, A., and Rytzner, C., 1957: Stapedectomy and autotransplantation of ossicles. Acta oto-laryng. 47:319-324.

Hall, J., and Røhrt, T., 1968: The stapes in osteogenesis imperfecta. Acta oto-laryng. 65:345.

Hamersma, H., 1970: Osteopetrosis (marble bone disease) of the temporal bone. Laryngoscope 80:1518.

Hand, A., 1893: Polyuria and tuberculosis. Arch. Pediat. 10:673.

Harris, I., and Weiss, L., 1962: Granulomatous complications of oval window fat grafts. Laryngoscope 72:870.

Harrison, D., 1951: Exostosis of the external auditory meatus. J. Laryng. 65:704.

Harrison, W., Shambaugh, G., Jr., Derlacki, E., and Clemis, J., 1967: Perilymph fistula in stapes surgery. Laryngoscope 77:836.

Harrison, W., Shambaugh, G., Jr., Derlacki, E., and Clemis, J., 1970: The perilymph fistula problem. Laryngoscope 80:1000.

Hayden, R., and McGee, T., 1965: Traumatized oval window fat grafts. Arch. Otolaryng. 81:243.

Hemenway, W., Hildyard, V., and Black, F., 1968: Post stapedectomy perilymph fistulas in the Rocky Mountain area: The importance of nystagmography and audiometry in diagnosis and early tympanotomy in prognosis. Laryngoscope 78:1687.

Higinbotham, N., and Alexander, S., 1941: Osteopetrosis: Four cases in one family. Amer. J. Surg. 53:444.

Hinchcliffe, R., 1962: Anatomical locus of presbycusis. J. Speech Hearing Dis. 27:301.

Hoeve, J. van der, and de Kleyn, A., 1918: Blaue Sclera, Knochenbrüchigkeit und Schwerhörigkeit. Arch. Ophtal. (Berlin) 95:81.

Hohmann, A., 1962: Inner ear reactions to stapes surgery (animal experiments). Chap. 25 in Otosclerosis: Henry Ford Hospital International Symposium. Edited by H. F. Schuknecht. Little, Brown, Boston, Mass., pp. 305–317.

Holmgren, G., 1923: Some experiences in the surgery of otosclerosis. Acta oto-laryng. 5:460.

Holmgren, G., 1937: The surgery of otosclerosis. Ann. Otol. Rhinol. Laryng. 46:3.

Hough, J., 1960: Partial stapedectomy. Trans. Amer. Otol. Soc. 48:170.

House, H., 1962: Experiences with stapes surgery. Chap. 36 in Otosclerosis: Henry Ford Hospital Symposium. Edited by H. F. Schuknecht. Little, Brown, Boston, Mass., pp. 447–456.

House, H., 1967: The fistula problem in otosclerosis surgery. Laryngoscope 77:1410.

House, H., and Greenfield, E., 1969: Five-year study of wire loop-absorbable gelatin sponge technique. Arch. Otolaryng. 89:420.

Hrdlička, A., 1935: Ear exostoses. Smithsonian Misc. Collection 93:1.

Hudson, W., and Kenan, P., 1969: Otologic manifestations of histiocytosis X. Laryngoscope 79:678.

Hueck, W., 1912: Pigmentstudien. Beitr. path. Anat. 54:68.

Igarashi, M., Guilford, F., and Alford, B., 1970: Bilateral vein graft stapedectomy. Acta oto-laryng. 69:94.

Ishii, T., Murakami, Y., Kimura, R., and Balogh, K., Jr., 1967: Electron microscopic and histochemical identification of lipofuscin in the human inner ear. Acta oto-laryng. 64:17.

Jack, F., 1892–1893: Remarkable improvement in hearing by removal of the stapes. Trans. Amer. Otol. Soc. 5:284, 5:474.

Jaffe, H., and Lichtenstein, L., 1944: Eosinophilic granuloma of bone. Arch. Path. 37:99.

Jaffe, H., and Lichtenstein, L., 1947: Eosinophilic granuloma of bone. J. Amer. Med. Assn. 135:935.

Jenkins, G., 1923: Otosclerosis and osteitis deformans. J. Laryng. 38:344.

Jerger, J., 1968: Review of diagnostic audiometry. Ann. Otol. Rhinol. Laryng. 77:1042.

Johnson, C., Lavy, D., Lord, T., Vellias, F., Merritt, A., and Deiss, W., 1968: Osteopetrosis. Medicine 47:149.

Johnson, C., and Zonderman, B., 1946: Eosinophilic granuloma. Ann. Otol. Rhinol. Laryng. 55:938.

Johnsson, L., 1971: Degenerative changes and anomalies of the vestibular system in man. Laryngoscope 81:1682.

Johnsson, L., and Hawkins, J., Jr., 1969: Nerve degeneration and vascular changes in Corti's organ based on surface preparations of the human cochlea. Excerpta med. Internat. Congr. Series 206, Proc. 9th Internat. Congr. Oto-rhino-laryng.

Johnsson, L., and Hawkins, J., Jr., 1972a: Sensory and neural degeneration with aging, as seen in microdissections of the human inner ear. Ann. Otol. Rhinol. Laryng. 81:179.

Johnsson, L., and Hawkins, J., Jr., 1972b: Symposium on basic ear research. II. Strial atrophy in clinical and experimental deafness. Laryngoscope 82:1105.

Jones, M., and Mulcahy, N., 1968: Osteopathia striata, osteopetrosis, and impaired hearing. Arch. Otolaryng. 87:116.

Jorgensen, M., 1961: The inner ear in diabetes mellitus. Arch. Otolaryng. 74:373.

Jorgensen, M., and Buch, N., 1961: Studies on inner-ear function and cranial nerves in diabetics. Acta oto-laryng. 53:350.

Kaufman, R., and Schuknecht, H., 1967: Reparative granuloma following stapedectomy: A clinical entity. Ann. Otol. Rhinol. Laryng. 76:1008.

Kearney, H., 1959: Fibrous dysplasia of the temporal bone. Laryngoscope 69:571.

Kelemen, G., and Linthicum, F., Jr., 1969: Labyrinthine otosclerosis. Acta oto-laryng. Suppl. 253.

Kessel, J., 1876: Über das Ausschneiden des Trommelfelles und Mobilisieren des Steibügels. Arch. Ohr. Nas.-Kehlk Heilk. 11:199.

Kimura, R., and Schuknecht, H., 1970: The ultrastructure of the human stria vascularis. Part II. Acta oto-laryng. 70:301.

Kornfeld, M., 1967: Pathological changes in the stria vascularis in Paget's disease. Pract. oto-rhino-laryng. 29:406.

Kos, C., 1960: Results of stapes mobilization and vein plug stapedioplasty. J. Amer. Med. Assn. 174:2187.

Kraus, H., 1970: Quantitativ-cytochemische Untersuchungen am Innenohr junger und seniler Meerschweinchen. Acta oto-laryng. Suppl. 278.

Kylander, C., 1967: Reparative processes following stapedectomy and gelfoam implant. Ann. Otol. Rhinol. Laryng. 76:346.

Lansing, A., 1952: Cowdrey's Problems of Aging. 3rd ed. Williams & Wilkins, Baltimore, Md.

Larsson, A., 1960: Otosclerosis: A genetic and clinical study. Acta oto-laryng. Suppl. 154.

Lempert, J., 1941: Fenestra nov-ovalis: A new oval window for the improvement of hearing in cases of otosclerosis. Arch. Otolaryng. 34:880.

Leonard, J., 1967: Prophylactic antibiotics in human stapedectomy. Laryngoscope 77:663.

Letterer, E., 1924: Aleukämische Reticulose. Ztschr. f. Path. 30:377.

Lewis, M., Jr., 1961: Inner ear complications of stapes surgery. Laryngoscope 71:377.

Lewis, M., Jr., 1962: Sudden inner ear deafness after stapedectomy. A surgical emergency. Southern Med. J. 55:744.

Lichtenstein, L., 1953: Histiocytosis X—integration of eosinophilic granuloma of bone, "Letterer-Siwe disease", and "Schüller-Christian disease", as related manifestations of single nosologic entity. Arch. Path. 56:84.

Lichtenstein, L., and Jaffe, H., 1940: Eosinophilic granuloma of bone, with report of a case. Amer. J. Path. 16:595.

Lichtenstein, L., and Jaffe, H., 1942: Fibrous dysplasia of bone. Arch. Path. 33:777.

Lindsay, J., Hilding, A., McLaurin, J., Keeler, N., and House, H., 1959: Histopathologic changes following fenestration and stapes mobilization. Trans. Amer. Acad. Ophthal. Otolaryng. 63:187.

Lindsay, J., and Lehman, R., 1969: Histopathology of the temporal bone in advanced Paget's disease. Laryngoscope 79:213.

Linthicum, F., Jr., 1971: Histological evidence of the causes of failure in stapes surgery. Ann. Otol. Rhinol. Laryng. 80:67.

Lopez-Rios, G., Benitez, J., and Vivar, G., 1968: Histiocytosis: Histopathological study of the temporal bone. Ann. Otol. Rhinol. Laryng. 77:1171.

Lubarsch, O., 1902: Ueber fetthaltige Pigmente. Zbl. allg. Path. path. Anat. 13:881.

Makishima, K., and Tanaka, K., 1971: Pathological changes of the inner ear and central auditory pathways in diabetics. Ann. Otol. Rhinol. Laryng. 80:218.

Manasse, P., 1914: Über Ossifikationsanomalien im menschlichen Felsenbein und ihre Beziehungen zur sogenannten Osteosklerose. Arch. Ohr. Nas.-KehlkHeilk. 95:145.

Manasse, P., 1922: Neue Untersuchungen zur Otosklerosenfrage. Z. Ohrenheilk. 82:76.

Matz, G., Lockhart, H., and Lindsay, J., 1968: Meningitis following stapedectomy. Laryngoscope 78:56.

Mayer, O., 1917: Untersuchungen über die Otosklerose. Alfred Hölder, Vienna, Leipzig, 80 pp.

Mayer, O., 1919–1920: Das anatomische Substrat der Alterschwerhörigkeit. Arch. Ohr. Nas.-KehlkHeilk. 105:1.

Mayer, O., 1931: Die Ursache der Knochenneubildung bei der Otosklerose. Acta oto-laryng. 15:35.

McGee, T., 1962: Techniques and experiences with stapedectomy and metal implant. Chap. 39, in Otosclerosis. Edited by H. F. Schuknecht. Little, Brown, Boston, Mass., pp. 489–496.

McGee, T., 1969: Fat-and-wire stapedectomy surgery: Long-term follow-up study. Arch. Otolaryng. 89:423.

McKusick, V., 1966: Hereditable Disorders of Connective Tissue, 3rd ed. C.V. Mosby Co., St. Louis, Mo.

Meurman, O., and Wolff, H., 1960: High-tone loss in otosclerosis. Acta oto-laryng. 51:229.

Miot, C., 1890: De la mobilisation de l'étrier. Rev. Laryng. 10:113, 145, 200.

Misrahy, G., De Jonge, B., Shinabarger, E., and Arnold, J., 1958: Effects of localized hypoxia on electrophysiological activity of cochlea of the guinea pig. J. Acoust. Soc. Amer. 30:705.

Mock, M., and Schuknecht, H. (unpublished data).

Moon, C., 1970: Perilymph fistulas complicating the stapedectomy operation: A review of forty-nine cases. Laryngoscope 80:515.

Moure, E., 1890: De la mobilisation de l'étrier. Rev. Laryng. 10:225.

Murray, R., Kirkpatrick, H., and Forrai, E., 1946: Case of Albright's syndrome (osteitis fibrosa disseminata). Brit. J. Surg. 34:48.

Myers, E., and Myers, D., 1968: Stapedectomy in advanced otosclerosis: A temporal bone report. J. Laryng. 82:557.

Myers, E., and Stool, S., 1969: The temporal bone in osteopetrosis. Arch. Otolaryng. 89:460.

Nachlas, N., and Lurie, M., 1951: The stria vascularis: Review and observations. Laryngoscope 61:989.

Nager, F., 1919: Ueber die Mitbeteiligung des Felsenbeines bei Osteitis deformans (Paget). Zeitschr. f. Ohrenh. 78:195.

Nager, F., 1939: Zur klinik und pathologischen Anatomie der Otosklerose. Acta oto-laryng. 27:542.

Nager, F., and Fraser, J., 1938: On bone formation in the scala tympani of otosclerotics. J. Laryng. 53:173.

Nager, F., and Meyer, M., 1932: Die Erkrankungen des Knochensystems und ihre Erscheinungen an der Innenohrkapsel des Menschen. S. Karger, Berlin, pp. 124.

Needham, A., 1950: Growth and regeneration rates in relation to age in the crustacea. J. Geront. 5:5.

Neff, W., 1967: Auditory discriminations affected by cortical ablations. In Chapter 16, Sensorineural Hearing Processes and Disorders. Edited by A. B. Graham. Little, Brown, Boston, Mass., pp. 201.

Nixon, J., Glorig, A., and High, W., 1962: Changes in air and bone conduction thresholds as a function of age. J. Laryng. 76:288.

Nomura, Y., 1970: Lipidosis of the basilar membrane. Acta oto-laryng. 69:352.

Nylén, B., 1949: Histopathological investigations on the localization, number, activity and extent of otosclerotic foci. J. Laryng. 63:321.

Ogilvie, R., and Hall, I., 1962: On the aetiology of otosclerosis. J. Laryng. 76:841.

Okano, H., 1938: Klinisch-statistische Untersuchungen der japanischen Greise in dem oto-rhino-laryngologischen Gebiete. J. Otorhinolaryng. Soc. Jap. 44:1.

Ollier, L., 1899: Dela dyschondroplasie. Bull. Soc. Chir. Lyon 3:22.

Ollier, L., 1900: Dyschondroplasie. Lyon Med. 93:23.

Opheim, O., 1968: Loss of hearing following the syndrome of Van der Hoeve-de Kleyn. Acta oto-laryng. 65:337.

Osborne, R., Freis, E., and Levin, A., 1944: Eosinophilic granuloma of bone presenting neurologic signs and symptoms. Arch. Neurol. Psychol. 51:452.

Otte, J., 1968: Estudio del ganglio espiral y su relacion con la discriminacion. Rev. Otorinolaring. 28:89.

Paget, J., 1877: On a form of chronic inflammation of bones (osteitis deformans). Medico-Chirurgical Trans. 60:37.

Paget, J., 1882: Additional cases of osteitis deformans. Medico-Chirurgical Trans. 65:225.

Palva, A., and Jokinen, K., 1970: Presbyacusis. V. Filtered speech test. Acta oto-laryng. 70:232.

Palva, T., Palva, A., and Kärjä, J., 1972: Fatal meningitis in a case of otosclerosis operated upon bilaterally. Arch. Otolaryng. 96:129.

Paparella, M., Brady, D., and Hoel, R., 1970: Sensori-neural hearing loss in chronic otitis media and mastoiditis. Trans. Amer. Acad. Ophthal. Otolaryng. 74:108.

Paparella, M., Lim, D., Sugiura, S., and Bolz, A., 1966: Inner ear pathology after experimental stapedectomy. Arch. Otolaryng. 84:154.

Parkin, J., and Tice, R., 1970: Hypoglycemia and fluctuating hearing loss. Ann. Otol. Rhinol. Laryng. 79:992.

Patterson, C., and Stone, H., 3rd, 1970: Stapedectomy in Van der Hoeve's syndrome. Laryngoscope 80:544.

Pease, D., 1955: Electronmicroscopy of vascular bed of kidney cortex. Anat. Rec. 121:701.

Pestalozza, G., Davis, H., Eldredge, D., Covell, W., and Rogers, J., 1957: Decreased bio-electric potentials in the ears of senile guinea pigs. Laryngoscope 67:1113.

Pestalozza, G., and Shore, I., 1955: Clinical evaluation of presbycusis on the basis of different tests of auditory function. Laryngoscope 65:1136.

Politzer, A., 1894: Über primäre Erkrankung der knöchernen Labyrinthkapsel. Z. Ohrenheilk. 25:309.

Portmann, M., 1960: Procedure of "interposition" for otosclerotic deafness. Laryngoscope 70:166.

Pritchard, J., 1951: Fibrous dysplasia of bones. Amer. J. Med. Sci. 222:313.

Reddy, J., Sataloff, J., and Liu, J., 1966: Histopathological changes following bilateral stapedectomy. Arch. Otolaryng. 84:165.

Roche, A., 1964: Aural exostoses in Australian aboriginal skulls. Ann. Otol. Rhinol. Laryng. 73:82.

Rosen, S., 1953: Mobilization of the stapes to restore hearing in otosclerosis. N.Y. J. Med. 53:2650.

Rosen, S., 1966: Hearing studies in selected urban and rural populations. Trans. N.Y. Acad. Sci. 29:9.

Rosen, S., and Olin, P., 1965: Hearing loss and coronary heart disease. Bull. N.Y. Acad. Med. 41:1052; also in Arch. Otolaryng. 82:236.

Rosenwasser, H., 1940: Lipoid granulomatosis (Hand-Schüller-Christian disease) involving the middle ear and temporal bone. Arch. Otolaryng. 32:1045.

Rüedi, L., 1963: Pathogenesis of otosclerosis. Arch. Otolaryng. 78:469.

Rüedi, L., 1968: Are there cochlear shunts in Paget's and Recklinghausen's disease? Acta oto-laryng. 65:13.

Rüedi, L., 1969: Otosclerotic lesion and cochlear degeneration. Arch. Otolaryng. 89:364.

Rüedi, L., and Spoendlin, H., 1957: Die Histologie der otosklerotischen Stapesankylose im Hinblick auf die chirurgische Mobilisation des Steigbügels. Bibl. oto-rhino-laryng. Fasc. 4:1.

Rutledge, L., Lewis, M., and Sanabria, F., 1963: Fatal meningitis related to stapes operation: Report of a case with temporal bone study. Arch. Otolaryng. 78:637.

Rutledge, L., Sanabria, F., Tabb, H., and Igarashi, M., 1965: Experimental fat grafts and teflon pistons in cats. Arch. Otolaryng. 81:570.

Saito, H. (in press): Post-traumatic regeneration of the chorda tympani nerve.

Sale, C., 1969: Bilateral deafness due to stapes surgery. Arch. Otolaryng. 90:467.

Sando, I., Hemenway, W., Hildyard, V., and English, G., 1968: Cochlear otosclerosis: A human temporal bone report. Ann. Otol. Rhinol. Laryng. 77:23.

Sataloff, J., Farb, S., Menduke, H., and Vassallo, L., 1964: Sensori-neural hearing loss in otosclerosis. Trans. Amer. Acad. Ophthal. Otolaryng. 68:243.

Saxén, A., 1937: Pathologie und Klinik der Altersschwerhörigkeit nach Untersuchungen von H. von Fieandt und Arno Saxen. Acta oto-laryng. Suppl. 23.

Saxén, A., 1952: Inner ear in presbyacusis. Acta oto-laryng. 41:213.

Schlumberger, H., 1946: Fibrous dysplasia of single bones (monostotic fibrous dysplasia). Milit. Surg. 99:504.

Schmidt, E., 1933: Erblichkeit und Gravidatät bei der Otosklerose. Arch. Ohr. Nas.-KehlkHeilk. 136:188.

Schuknecht, H., 1955: Presbycusis. Laryngoscope 65:402.

Schuknecht, H., 1960a: Substituting steel wire in surgery for otosclerosis. Michigan Hearing, Autumn, p. 10.

Schuknecht, H., 1960b: Film: Stapedectomy and graft-prosthesis operation. Acta otolaryng. 51:241.

Schuknecht, H., 1962a: Stapedectomy operation for hearing loss from otosclerosis. Sound 1:16.

Schuknecht, H., 1962b: Sensorineural hearing loss following stapedectomy. Acta oto-laryng. 54:336.

Schuknecht, H., 1962c: Bone and soft tissue repair following stapes surgery (animal experiments). Chap. 28 in Otosclerosis. Edited by H. F. Schuknecht. Little, Brown, Boston, Mass., p. 337.

Schuknecht, H., 1964a: A new stapedectomy prosthesis. Arch. Otolaryng. 80:474.

Schuknecht, H., 1964b: Further observations on the pathology of presbycusis. Arch. Otolaryng. 80:369.

Schuknecht, H., 1967: The effect of aging on the cochlea. Chap. 29 in Sensorineural Hearing Processes and Disorders. Edited by A. B. Graham. Little, Brown, Boston, Mass., p. 393.

Schuknecht, H., 1971: Stapedectomy. Little, Brown, Boston, Mass., 119 pp.

Schuknecht, H.: Unpublished data.

Schuknecht, H., and Gross, C., 1966: Otosclerosis and the inner ear. Ann. Otol. Rhinol. Laryng. 75:423.

Schuknecht, H., and Igarashi, M., 1964: Pathology of slowly progressive sensorineural deafness. Trans. Amer. Acad. Ophthal. Otolaryng. 68:222.

Schuknecht, H., Igarashi, M., and Gacek, R., 1965: The pathological types of cochleo-saccular degeneration. Acta oto-laryng. 59:154.

Schuknecht, H., and Ishii, T., 1966: Hearing loss caused by atrophy of the stria vascularis. Jap. J. Otol. Tokyo 69:1825.

Schuknecht, H., and Kirchner, J., 1974: Cochlear otosclerosis: fact or fantasy. Laryngoscope. In press.

Schuknecht, H., McGee, T., and Colman, B., 1960: Stapedectomy. Ann. Otol. Rhinol. Laryng. 69:597.

Schuknecht, H., McGee, T., Igarashi, M., Fujita, S., and Davison, R., 1964: Stapedectomy: Postmortem studies. Arch. Otolaryng. 79:437.

Schuknecht, H., and Oleksiuk, S., 1960: The metal prosthesis for stapes ankylosis. Arch. Otolaryng. 71:287.

Schuknecht, H., and Perlman, H., 1948: Hand-Schüller-Christian disease and eosinophilic granuloma of the skull. Ann. Otol. Rhinol. Laryng. 57:643.

Schuknecht, H., and Tonndorf, J., 1960: Acoustic trauma of the cochlea from ear surgery. Laryngoscope 70:479.

Schuknecht, H., and Woellner, R., 1955: An experimental and clinical study of deafness from lesions of the cochlear nerve. J. Laryng. 69:75.

Schüller, A., 1915: Über eigenartige Röntgenstr. 23:12.

Schwartz, D., and Alpert, M., 1964: The malignant transformation of fibrous dysplasia. Amer. J. Med. Sci. 247:1.

Sehrt, E., 1904: Zur Kenntnis der fetthaltigen Pigmente. Virchow Arch. path. Anat. 17:248.

Shambaugh, G., Jr., 1949: Fenestration operation for otosclerosis: Experimental investigations and clinical observations in 2,100 operations over a period of ten years. Acta oto-laryng. Suppl. 79.

Shambaugh, G., Jr., 1965: Clinical diagnosis of cochlear (labyrinthine) otosclerosis. Laryngoscope 75:1558.

Sharp, M., 1970: Monostotic fibrous dysplasia of the temporal bone. J. Laryng. 84:697.

Shea, J., 1938: Xanthomatosis (Schüller-Christian's disease): A report of a case with radiosensitive pathology in the mastoid. Laryngoscope 48:589.

Shea, J., Jr., 1958: Fenestration of the oval window. Ann. Otol. Rhinol. Laryng. 67:932.

Shea, J., 1971: A 15-year report on fenestration of the oval window. Trans. Amer. Acad. Ophthal. Otolaryng. 75:31.

Shea, J., Smyth, G., and Altmann, F., 1963: Surgical treatment of the hearing loss associated with osteogenesis imperfecta tarda. J. Laryng. 77:679.

Sheehy, J., and House, H., 1962: Causes of failure in stapes surgery. Laryngoscope 72:10.

Shiffman, F., and Aengst, F., 1967: Fibrous dysplasia of temporal bone. Arch. Otolaryng. 86:528.

Siebenmann, F., 1912: Totaler knöcherner Verschlus bei der Labyrinthfenster und Labyrinthitis serosa infolge progressiver Spongiosierung. Verh. dtsch. Ges. Otol. 20:267.

Simms, H., and Stolman, A., 1937: Changes in human tissue electrolytes in senescence. Science 86:269.

Singleton, G., and Schuknecht, H., 1959: Experimental fracture of the stapes in cats. Ann. Otol. Rhinol. Laryng. 68:1069.

Siwe, S., 1933: Die Reticuloendotheliose—ein neues Krankheitsbild unter den Hepatosplenomegalien. Z. Kinderheilk. 55:212.

Smith, C., 1957: Structure of the stria vascularis and the spiral prominence. Ann. Otol. Rhinol. Laryng. 66:521.

Sooy, F., 1960: The management of middle ear lesions simulating otosclerosis. Ann. Otol. Rhinol. Laryng. 69:540.

Sourdille, M., 1937: New technique in the surgical treatment of severe and progressive deafness from otosclerosis. Bull. N. Y. Acad. Med. 13:673.

Stoller, F., 1962: The ear in osteogenesis imperfecta. Laryngoscope 72:855.

Subotić, R., and Kaufman, R., 1971: Human temporal bone findings post stapedectomy: A review of ten cases. Acta otolaryng. 71:385.

Sussman, H., 1961: Monostotic fibrous dysplasia of the temporal bone: Report of a case. Laryngoscope 71:68.

Takahashi, T., 1971: The ultrastructure of the pathologic stria vascularis and spiral prominence in man. Ann. Otol. Rhinol. Laryng. 80:721.

Tamari, M., 1942: Histopathologic changes of the temporal bone in Paget's disease. Ann. Otol. Rhinol. Laryng. 51:170.

Tasaki, I., and Spyropoulos, C., 1959: Stria vascularis as source of endocochlear potential. J. Neurophysiol. 22:149.

Tembe, D., 1970: Fibro-osseous dysplasia of temporal bone. J. Laryng. 84:107.

Tos, M., 1966: A survey of Hand-Schüller-Christian's disease in otolaryngology. Acta oto-laryng. 62:217.

Tos, M., 1969: Facial palsy in Hand-Schüller-Christian's disease. Arch. Otolaryng. 90:563.

Towson, C., 1950: Monostotic fibrous dysplasia of the mastoid and the temporal bone. Arch. Otolaryng. 52:709.

Valvassori, G., 1965: Radiologic diagnosis of cochlear otosclerosis. Laryngoscope 75:1563.

Virolainen, E., 1972: Vestibular disturbances in clinical otosclerosis. Acta otolaryng. Suppl. 306.

Vosteen, K., 1961: Neue Aspekte zur Biologie und Pathologie des Innenohres. Arch. Ohr. Nas.-KehlkHeilk. 178:1.

Walsh, T., 1954: The effect of pregnancy on the deafness of otosclerosis. Trans. Amer. Acad. Ophthal. Otolaryng. 58:420.

Walsh, T., and Goodman, A., 1955: Speech discrimination in central auditory lesions. Laryngoscope 65:1.

Waltner, J., 1965: Stapedectomy in Paget's disease. Arch. Otolaryng. 82:355.

Weber, M., 1930: Otosclerosis in its histogenic relations to osteodystrophia fibrosa (ostitis fibrosa). Arch. Otolaryng. 11:1.

Weber, M., 1933: The blue mantles in otosclerosis: A contribution to the pathology of the labyrinthine capsule. Ann. Otol. Rhinol. Laryng. 42:438.

Weber, M., 1935: Otosklerose und Umbau der Labyrinthkapsel. Offizin Poeschel und Trepte, Leipzig, 52 pp.

Weber, M., 1936: Zur Frage des Erbganges des Otosklerose. Erbbl. Hals Nas. Ohrenarzt Hft. 1:3, 3:42.

Weil, A., 1922: Pubertas praecox und Knochenbrühigkeit. Klin. Wschr. 1:2114.

Weille, F., 1968: Hypoglycemia in Ménière's disease. Arch. Otolaryng. 87:555.

Wittmaack, K., 1919: Die Otosklerose auf Grund eigener Forschungen. G. Fischer, Jena, 188 pp.

Wittmaack, K., 1930: Über die sogenannte experimentelle Hühnerotosklerose. Acta oto-laryng. 14:228.

Wolff, D., 1950: Otosclerosis: Hypothesis of its origin and progress. Arch. Otolaryng. 52:853.

Wolff, D., 1964: Untoward sequelae eleven months following stapedectomy. Ann. Otol. Rhinol. Laryng. 73:297.

Wolff, D., Schuknecht, H., and Bellucci, R., 1968: Otosclerosis and multiple surgery in the temporal bone. Ann. Otol. Rhinol. Laryng. 77:37.

Wright, J., and Schuknecht, H., 1972: Atrophy of the spiral ligament. Arch. Otolaryng. 96:16.

Wullstein, H., Ogilvie, R., and Hall, I., 1960: Van der Hoeve's syndrome in mother and daughters. J. Laryng. 74:67.

Wyllie, W., 1923: The occurrence in osteitis deformans of lesions of the central nervous system with a report of four cases. Brain 46:336.

Yarington, C., and Sprinkle, P., 1967: Facial palsy in osteopetrosis. Relief by endo-temporal decompression. J. Amer. Med. Assn. 202:549.

Zöllner, F., 1962: Stapedectomy: Reconstruction with vein graft and bone strut. Chap. 46 in Otosclerosis. Edited by H. F. Schuknecht. Little, Brown, Boston, Mass., p. 603.

Zwaardemaker, H., 1891: Der Verlust an höhen Tönen mit zunehmendem Alter: Ein neues Gesetz. Arch. Ohr. Nas.-Kehlk-Heilk. 32:53.

11 Neoplastic Growth

A. PRIMARY NEOPLASMS

1. EPIDERMOID CARCINOMA

The clinical and pathological features of epidermoid carcinoma of the ear have been known for many years (Politzer, 1883; Kretschmann, 1886). There have been numerous reports since that time (Broders, 1921; Yates, 1936; Figi and Hempstead, 1943; Lewis, 1960) indicating the relatively good prognosis for carcinomas of the auricle and external auditory canal and poor prognosis for carcinoma of the middle ear and mastoid. Lewis (1960), in assaying a group of 150 cases, found the origin of the lesion to be the auricle in 60 percent, the external auditory canal is 28 percent, and the middle ear and mastoid in 12 percent. Among 212,000 cases of otologic disease seen between 1905 and 1924 at the Manhattan Eye, Ear and Throat Hospital, Robinson (1931) found neoplasms in only 48 cases for a ratio of 1:4000. Schall (1935) examined the diagnoses of 90,040 patients with ear disorders in a twelve-year period at the Massachusetts Eye and Ear Infirmary and found only 15 with neoplasms for an incidence of 1:6000. Towson and Shofstall (1950) determined the incidence of carcinoma of the middle ear and mastoid in all ear conditions to be 1:5000 to 1:20,000.

Lewis (1960) reported that two-thirds of the epidermoid carcinomas of the auricle were the basal cell type and one-third of the squamous cell type, which is consistent with the incidence of these lesions elsewhere on exposed skin surfaces of the body. In contrast, three-fourths of the widely invasive lesions of the auditory canal and middle ear were of the squamous cell type with 11 percent having already metastasized to neck nodes by the time of the patient's hospital admission (Figs. 11.1, 11.2).

The most common symptoms of epidermoid carcinoma of the middle ear and mastoid are otorrhea (often hemorrhagic), hearing loss, pain, facial paralysis, mastoid swelling, and vertigo. Lewis (1960) found that 40 percent of cases gave a history of otorrhea from one to fifty years' duration with the onset in some cases dating back to early childhood.

Fig. 11.1: This patient first experienced pain and bloody discharge from the left ear at the age of 55. Biopsy revealed a well differentiated squamous cell carcinoma. In spite of x-ray therapy, partial surgical excision, cryosurgical treatment, and methatrexate therapy, she died of the disease one year later. Histological study shows an invasive squamous cell carcinoma of the temporal bone. The bony labyrinth is surrounded by neoplastic tissue. The membranous labyrinth shows severe endolymphatic hydrops and severe degeneration of the organ of Corti and vestibular sense organs. The histological picture is that of strands and islands of epithelial cells with numerous scattered keratin masses and pearls. See also Fig. 11.2.

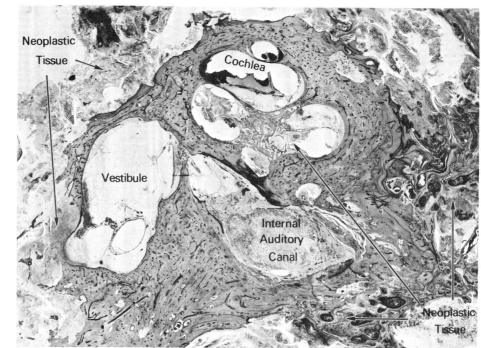

Fig. 11.2: Same case as Fig. 11.1. This view shows squamous cell carcinoma invading Rosenthal's canal, the modiolus, the scala tympani, and the scala vestibuli. There is endolymphatic hydrops and severe degeneration of all structures of the cochlear duct.

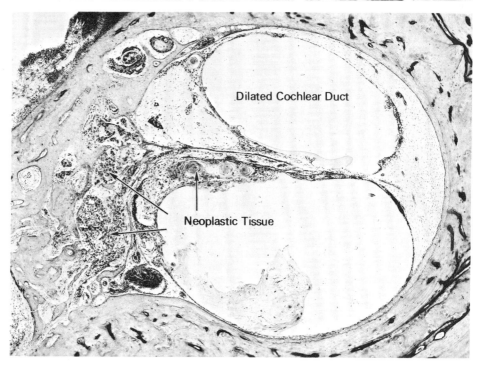

Fig. 11.3: Surgical specimen showing squamous cell carcinoma in the external auditory canal invading the mandibular fossa and parotid gland. The patient died of the disease at the age of 47, eleven months after surgery. The most medial part of the mandibular fossa contains an abscess. The lateral part of the external auditory canal contains viable neoplastic tissue, the central part contains a plug of degenerating keratinizing neoplastic tissue, and the medial part contains a keratin mass.

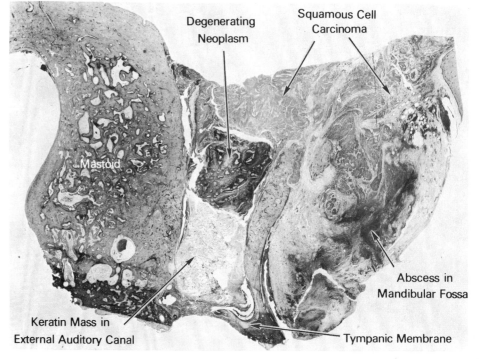

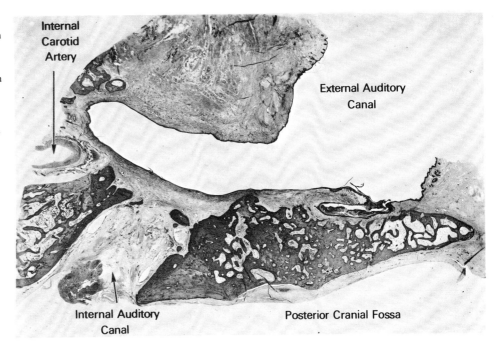

Internal
Carotid
Artery

External Auditory
Canal

Internal Auditory
Canal

Posterior Cranial Fossa

Fig. 11.4: At the age of 72 this patient noted bleeding from the right ear. Biopsy of tissue in the ear canal revealed squamous cell carcinoma. She was given x-ray therapy; however, viable tumor tissue remained and she developed right facial paresis. A radical resection of the temporal bone was performed, following which she experienced vertigo and total facial paralysis but made an uneventful and rapid recovery. She died of myocardial infarction five years later at the age of 78. Histological study of the autopsy specimen reveals most of the temporal bone to have been surgically removed. The external auditory canal, middle ear, mastoid, and bony labyrinth are missing. The posteromedial wall of the petrous bone is about 1 cm in thickness and is intact except for a small area at the sigmoid sulcus. The area of the sigmoid sinus is occupied by dense fibrous tissue and presumably is obliterated. The internal auditory canal contains fibrous tissue and several large vessels. Bundles of nerve fibers in the internal auditory canal probably derive from the facial nerve. The petrous apex is normal and contains bone marrow. The carotid artery is normal. The area previously occupied by the middle ear and bony labyrinth consists of a cavity lined with squamous epithelium. The cartilaginous external auditory canal is displaced medially into the surgical defect. Nowhere is there evidence of squamous cell carcinoma.

In advanced cases the facial nerve and inner ear are destroyed by tumor invasion (Scott and Colledge, 1939; Bradley and Maxwell, 1954; Sorensen, 1960). Diagnosis can usually be made by biopsy through the external auditory canal.

Treatment consists of surgery alone or in combination with preoperative or postoperative irradiation. Early lesions of the pinna may be excised by means of a wedge or V-shaped incision. Larger lesions may necessitate removal of the auricle and adjacent regions. Early lesions of the external auditory canal may be treated by sleeve resection and split thickness skin grafting. Subtotal resection of the temporal bone may be indicated in more advanced cases. Involvement of the middle ear and mastoid, when amenable to surgery, requires temporal bone resection. This is a formidable procedure requiring a combination of intracranial and extracranial en bloc resection. Cryosurgery has been used successfully for palliation of recurrent lesions (Miller et al., 1972). In analyses of the results of temporal bone resection, Lewis (1960) reports a 31 percent three-year cure rate for 13 cases, and Conley (1965) a 25 percent five-year cure rate for 35 cases (Figs. 11.3 and 11.4).

2. ADENOID CYSTIC CARCINOMA

Adenoid cystic carcinoma of the external auditory canal and middle ear is a rare malignant growth arising from apocrine, seromucinous or salivary gland tissue. The principal clinical features are pain, slow relentless growth, recurrence following surgical removal, and eventual distant metastases. Histologically, the tumor commonly presents a "Swiss cheese" pattern, with the cells forming cylinders, many of which have hollow centers. Some of the cystic spaces contain acidophilic mucoid material. The tumor cells are small, uniform in size, and have large nuclei. Occasionally, the histological pattern is that of anastomosing cords or sheets of cells or solid nests of cells with little tendency to form patterns. The intervening stroma is frequently dense and fibrous and may show hyaline changes. The microscopic differential diagnosis includes basal cell carcinoma, ceruminoma, mucoepidermoid tumor, and the usual adenocarcinomas. (Furstenberg, 1924; Lukens, 1936; Warren and Gates, 1941).

Pulec et al. (1963) reported on their experiences with 21 cases of adenoid cystic carcinoma of the external auditory canal which were treated at the Mayo Clinic. They found that radiotherapy provided short-term palliation only and that wide excision of the tumor area was the therapy of choice. One of their patients developed a local recurrence and pulmonary metastases 15 years after apparently adequate treatment. Their patients lived an average of 16.5 years (range 6 to 29 years) from the onset of symptoms to death.

417   Neoplastic Growth

Fig. 11.5: This photomicrograph shows an invasive embryonal rhabdomyosarcoma in a surgical specimen of the temporal bone. Symptoms were first noted at the age of 4, and in spite of 6,000 rads of high-voltage radiation therapy and administration of Actinomycin D and vincristine, recurrence of the tumor was noted two years later. Temporal bone resection was performed but the patient died of diffuse metastases two months following surgery. The specimen includes the mastoid, tympanic, and petrous bones, and part of the mandibular fossa. Neoplastic tissue is seen in the middle ear and external auditory canal, as well as in the anterior part of the mastoid. The facial nerve is partly degenerated, and the chorda tympani nerve is destroyed. (Courtesy of Jaffe) See Fig. 11.6.

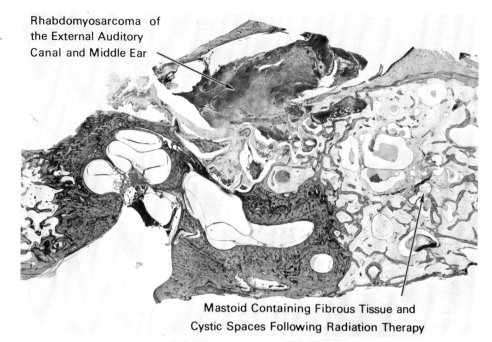

Rhabdomyosarcoma of the External Auditory Canal and Middle Ear

Mastoid Containing Fibrous Tissue and Cystic Spaces Following Radiation Therapy

Fig. 11.6: Same case as Fig. 11.5. This embryonal rhabdomyosarcoma is characterized histologically by scattered small round cells with pyknotic nuclei in scanty cytoplasm in a loose, myxomatous matrix. There are a few scattered large round cells with granular acidophilic cytoplasm. (Courtesy of Jaffe)

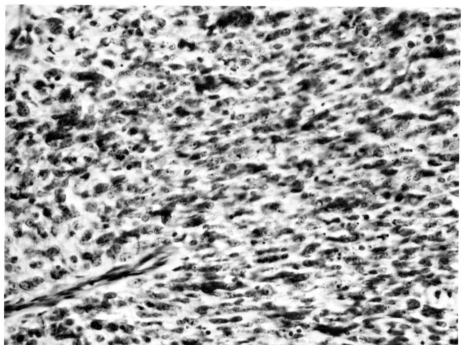

3. SARCOMA

a) *Embryonal rhabdomyosarcoma*

Rhabdomyosarcoma of the head and neck region is almost exclusively a disease of children with the common sites of origin being orbit, oral cavity, nose, pharynx, and middle ear (Friedmann et al., 1965).

Embryonal rhabdomyosarcoma of the middle ear is nearly always fatal (Alexy, 1968; Jaffe et al., 1971). Only recently has long-term survival been reported following radiation therapy (Conte and Sagerman, 1971). Although the histogenesis of these tumors is uncertain, they appear to recapitulate in an abortive form the embryonic development of skeletal muscle from primitive myotonal segments or, less often, from mesenchymal derivatives (Schuman, 1966).

The tumor usually occurs in the first decade of life, with the highest incidence in children under the age of 5. The initial symptoms frequently consist of bleeding from the ear or otorrhea, often associated with facial paralysis. In most instances, the first mode of therapy has been mastoidectomy. The neoplastic growth often is found to extend beyond the confines of the middle ear to involve the petrous apex and often the posterior or middle cranial fossae. Karatay (1949) and Myers et al. (1968) observed that the neoplasm grows along the fallopian canal and internal auditory canal to reach the posterior cranial fossa.

In the final stage of the disease there is extensive regional spread as well as distant metastases. (Figs. 11.5 and 11.6)

Schuman (1966) described two types of embryonal rhabdomyosarcoma. The *botryoid type* is characterized histologically by scattered small round cells or stellate cells with pyknotic nuclei and scanty cytoplasm in a loose myxomatous matrix. The stellate cells are connected by long fibrillary processes in a fine reticular syncytium sometimes resembling myxoid liposarcoma without a definite vascular pattern. In addition to indifferent mesenchymal cells, rhabdomyoblastic elements are usually recognizable. These consist of large round cells with granular or homogeneous acidophilic cytoplasm, halo cells, and elongated spindle forms in which longitudinal and cross striations are sometimes discernable. *Embryonal alveolar rhabdomyosarcoma* presents a variety of histological patterns merging imperceptibly with each other. The prevailing pattern is alveolar, but pseudorosettes may form about the blood vessels or may be aligned in papillary formation. Characteristic cells are likely to be large, oval, or rounded in uninuclear forms with scanty cytoplasm resembling reticulin cells; however, among them are many cells with marginal chromatic nuclei and strongly acidophilic cytoplasm in which myofibrils are discernible. There may also be isolated polyhedral and giant cells sometimes with dense nuclear chromatin and a vacuolated granular or homogeneous cytoplasm in which transverse striations can often be demonstrated.

Friedmann and Bird (1969) have presented an elaborate classification of histological types of rhabdomyosarcomas based on the electron microscopic observations of experimentally produced tumors.

b) Chondrosarcoma

Neoplasms of cartilaginous origin make up about 33 percent of primary tumors of bone. The differentiation of chondroma from chondrosarcoma can be very difficult (Dahlin, 1957). The differential criteria are based on subtle changes in cell nuclei and chondrocytes. Despite the benign microscopic appearance, the clinical course may be characterized by early pulmonary metastases (Lindbom et al., 1961). Rapid growth and the radiologic appearance of an osteolytic lesion with irregular borders indicate malignant behavior (O'Neal and Ackerman, 1952; Wronski et al., 1964). Chondrosarcoma is predominantly a disease of adults in the age range of 25 to 50 years. The histological picture is that of clusters and strands of rounded stellate cells with single and double nuclei having the usual characteristics of chondroblasts distributed in a mucoid and myxomatous matrix (Anderson, 1966). The tumor is often composed of small lobules separated by loose fibrous stroma. Frequently there is cyst formation, hemorrhage, necrosis, and focal calcification. Chondrosarcoma occurring in the region of the apex of the petrous bone is shown in Figs. 11.7 and 11.8.

c) Osteogenic sarcoma

Osteogenic sarcoma is the most common primary malignant neoplasm of bone, with about 75 percent of the tumors occurring in patients between the ages of 10 and 25 years. This neoplasm arises most commonly in the metaphyseal ends of the shafts of long bones, particularly the lower ends of the femur, upper end of the tibia, and upper end of the humerus. There are two main histological types: (1) *sclerosing osteogenic sarcoma*, which produces a calcifying osteoid matrix; and (2) *osteolytic osteogenic sarcoma*, which produces little or no recognizable bone. Osteogenic sarcoma occurring as a primary tumor of the temporal bone is rare. In a review of 430 cases treated at the Mayo Clinic, Coventry and Dahlin (1957) found only three involving the skull. Osteosarcoma of the temporal bone in a patient with multiple hereditary osteochondromatosis is shown in Figures 11.9 and 11.10.

4. GLOMUS BODY TUMOR

Glomus bodies in the region of the middle ear were first described by Guild (1941) as small masses of epithelioid-like cells with a rich vascular supply located near or within the adventitia of the jugular bulb. Later he also reported finding these bodies of tissue along the course of the tympanic branches of the IXth and Xth cranial nerves (Guild, 1953) (Fig. 11.11). Rosenwasser (1945) first identified these glomus bodies as the site of origin for neoplastic disease. Since that time numerous reports of glomus body tumors of this region have appeared in the literature (Lattes and Waltner, 1949; Simpson and Dallachy, 1958; Ash et al., 1964).

Glomus bodies of the jugular and tympanic regions, as well as those in association with the carotid bifurcation and vagus nerve (Burman, 1955; Trail and Chambers, 1970) are classified as paraganglionic tissue which is derived from the ganglionic neural crest. Watzka (1943) divided paraganglionic tissue into two groups: (1) chromaffin epinephrine-producing paraganglionic tissue, and (2) nonchromaffin non-epinephrine-producing paraganglionic tissue. Watzka (1943) and LeCompte (1951) place the jugular and tympanic

Fig. 11.7: Chondromyxosarcoma of the temporal bone. At the age of 24 this woman first noted hearing loss in the right ear. Examination revealed a fluid-filled middle ear which was treated by the introduction of a ventilating tube through the tympanic membrane. Two years later (age 26) she had evidence of a destructive lesion of the right temporal bone associated with multiple right cranial nerve palsies and left hemiparesis. At this time there was a tumor in the inferior part of the right middle ear which on biopsy showed chondromyxosarcoma. At the age of 27, a craniotomy was performed and part of the tumor was removed; however, she died twelve days later of aspiration pneumonia. Histological study of the right temporal bone shows a large neoplasm which has destroyed the petrous apex and invaded the infralabyrinthine area as well as the inferior part of the middle ear. Occlusive compression of the internal carotid artery is presumed to have caused the left hemiparesis. There is also occlusive compression of the eustachian tube accounting for the fluid in the middle ear. The bony labyrinth shows areas of erosion; however, the endosteal layer is intact and the sensory and neural structures appear normal. The facial nerve is degenerated beyond the level of the second genu. See also Fig. 11.8.

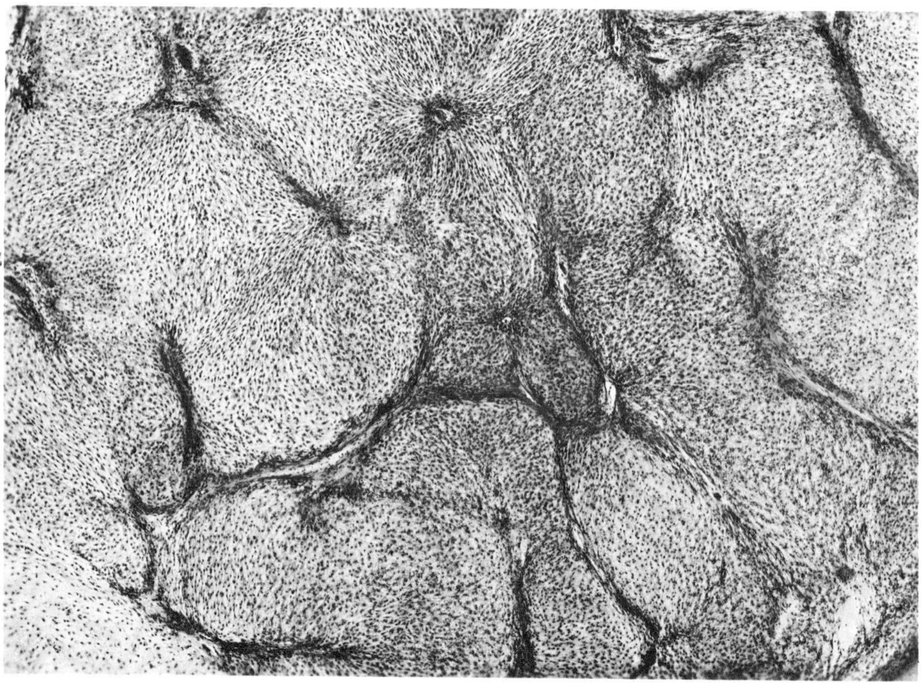

Fig. 11.8: Chondromyxosarcoma. Same case as Fig. 11.7. There are lobules of tumor separated by a loose fibrous stroma. The tumor is composed of rounded stellate cells having single or double nuclei lying in a myxomatous matrix.

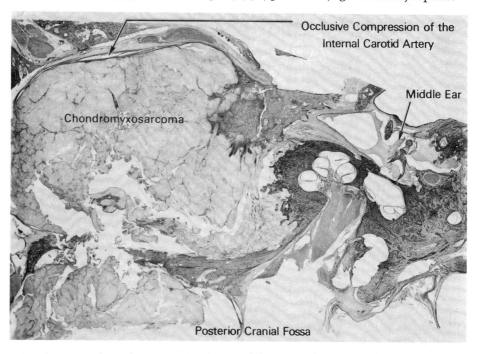

glomus bodies as well as the carotid and vagal glomus bodies in group 2. Carotid and vagal bodies are known to have a chemoreceptor function sensitive to changes in oxygen tension; however, there is no evidence that the glomus bodies of the jugular and tympanic region have such a function.

Rauch (1969) suggests that the term "nonchromaffin" be dispensed with since the chromaffin tumor of the suprarenal gland is termed pheochromocytoma rather than paraganglioma. Furthermore, the term "chemodectoma" is not appropriate (Mulligan, 1950), as very few paraganglioma, particularly those located in the jugular or tympanic areas, deliver significant quantities of humorally active substances.

Tumors of these paraganglionic bodies, which arise in the region of the middle ear cleft, are generally referred to as glomus jugulari tumors. Symptoms most frequently begin in middle age with a high proportion of reported cases occurring in caucasian females. Hearing loss was present as an initial symptom in 91 percent of the cases reported by Alford and Guilford (1962) and in 100 percent of the cases reported by McCabe and Fletcher (1969). The hearing loss may be conductive, sensorineural, or combined. Pulsating tinnitus occurs in over half of the cases, and pain in about 25 percent of cases. Vertigo occurs in about 25 percent because of invasion of the inner ear. With increasing growth the tumor may extend into the infralabyrinthine region, the petrous apex region, the mastoid, the external auditory canal, and jugular

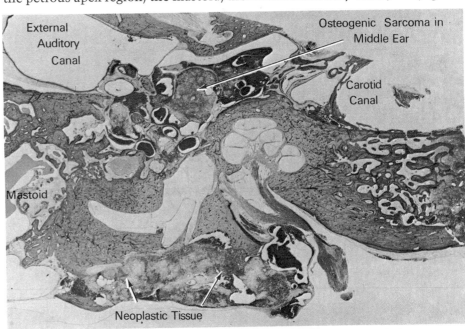

Fig. 11.9: Osteogenic sarcoma of the temporal bone. This patient was born of a family which for four generations had numerous members with deforming osteochondromatoses. From the age of 3 he exhibited multiple exostoses of the extremities and at the age of 21 developed a mass of rapidly increasing size in the left mastoid and suboccipital region. Biopsy showed the tumor to be an osteoblastic osteogenic sarcoma. In spite of 8,000r of x-ray therapy the tumor continued its rapidly invasive behavior and the patient died three months after treatment. Histological studies show extensive invasion of the mastoid, middle ear, and inferior part of the bony labyrinth. The tumor bulges into the postero-inferior part of the internal auditory canal and into the posterior cranial fossa. It is lobulated, containing solidly cellular areas alternating with cystic regions and large vascular spaces. There is severe endolymphatic hydrops, and a fine fibrillar precipitate is seen throughout the endolymphatic system. There is near total loss of hair cells of the organ of Corti; however, the cochlear neurons appear normal. The vestibular sensory and neural structures appear normal. (Courtesy of Dahlin) See also Fig. 11.10.

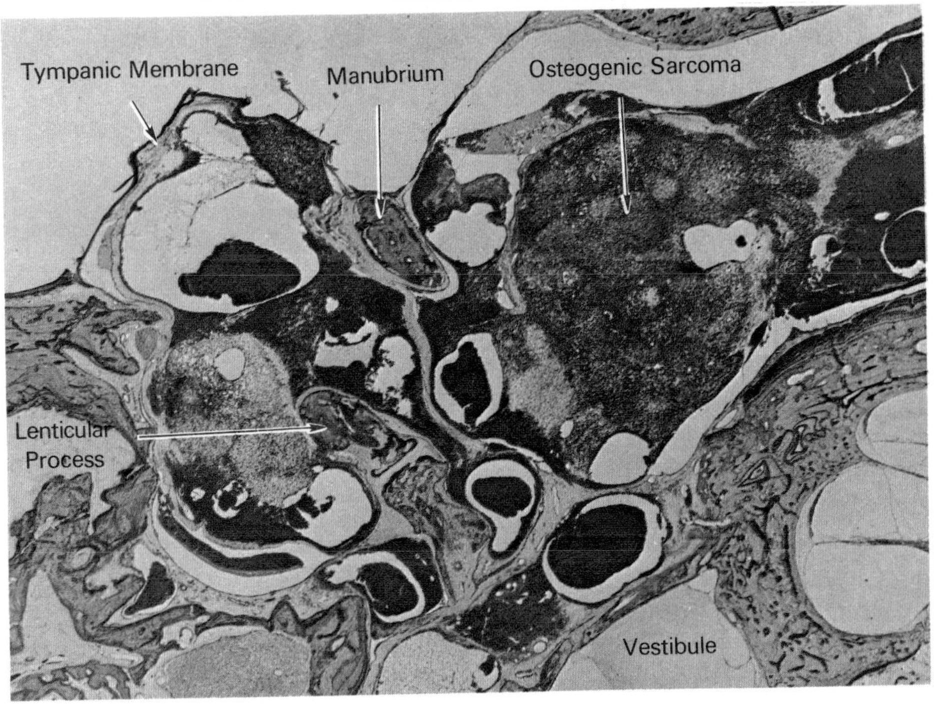

Fig. 11.10: Osteogenic sarcoma. Same case as Fig. 11.9. Neoplastic tissue fills the middle ear and is causing lateral displacement of the posterior part of the tympanic membrane. (Courtesy of Dahlin)

Fig. 11.11: Glomus body located on the promontory of the cochlea in close association with the tympanic branch of the glossopharyngeal nerve.

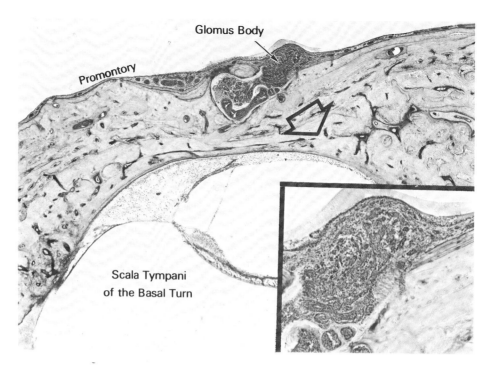

Fig. 11.12: Retrograde jugulography demonstrates a filling defect of the jugular bulb indicating that the glomus body tumor has extended into the vein. See Fig. 11.13.

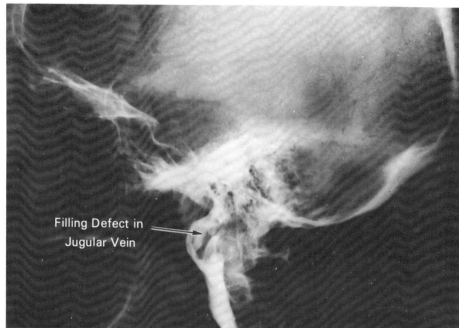

Fig. 11.13: Same case as Fig. 11.12. Carotid angiography shows a vascular flush characteristic of a glomus body tumor. This tumor was partly removed surgically, following which it was treated with 4,500 rads of cobalt therapy.

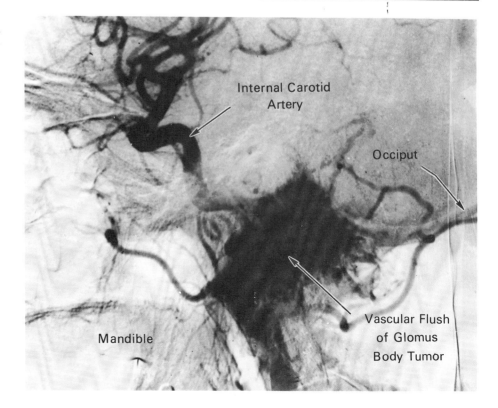

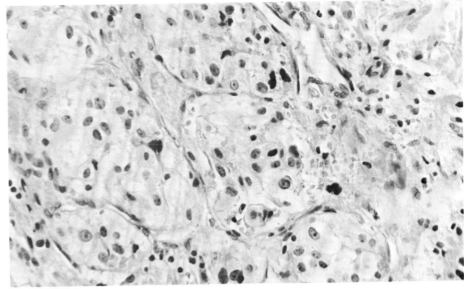

Fig. 11.14: Glomus body tumor (jugular bulb area). Nests of epithelioid cells are surrounded by reticulin fibers of the subendothelial layers of the vascular spaces to form alveolar-like patterns.

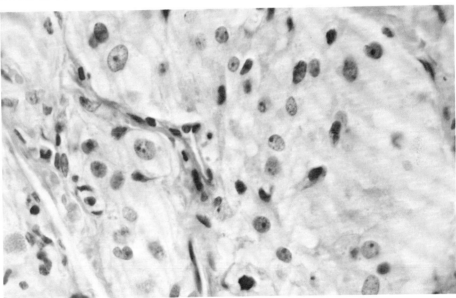

Fig. 11.15: Glomus body tumor from the region of the jugular bulb. The epithelioid cells are of varying size, round or polyhedral in shape, with abundant clear or granular acidophilic cytoplasm which is sometimes vacuolated.

foramen involving the IXth, Xth, XIth, and XIIth cranial nerves (Myers et al., 1971). McCabe and Fletcher (1969) found that at least one cranial nerve palsy existed in 44 percent of their patients. Distant metastases may occur but are uncommon (Taylor et al., 1965).

Otological examination typically reveals a reddish-blue pulsating mass behind the inferior portion of the tympanic membrane. With more extensive growths, tumor tissue may be visualized in the floor of the external auditory canal. The tumor is extremely vascular and biopsy frequently results in profuse hemorrhage. Retrograde venography frequently reveals tumor extending into the lumen of the jugular bulb (Gejrot and Laurén, 1964a, 1964b; Gejrot, 1964a, 1964b) (Fig. 11.12). Carotid arteriography characteristically shows a vascular flush at the tumor site (Fig. 11.13).

Marshall and Horn (1961) divided the tumor into three histological types: (1) a predominantly cellular tumor, (2) a mixed cellular and vascular type, and (3) a predominantly vascular type. Although mitotic figures are rare, cells containing two or more nuclei are occasionally encountered.

Histologically there are nests of epithelioid cells of varying size, round or polyhedral in shape with abundant clear or granular acidophilic cytoplasm which is sometimes vacuolated. These cells are in close contact with the endothelium of the thin-walled blood vessels or sinusoids. There is much variability in the proportion and size of the blood vessels within the same tumor and between different tumors. Reticulin fibers from the subendothelial layers of vascular spaces spread out to surround groups of epithelioid cells, thus forming an alveolar-like pattern (Figs. 11.14 and 11.15).

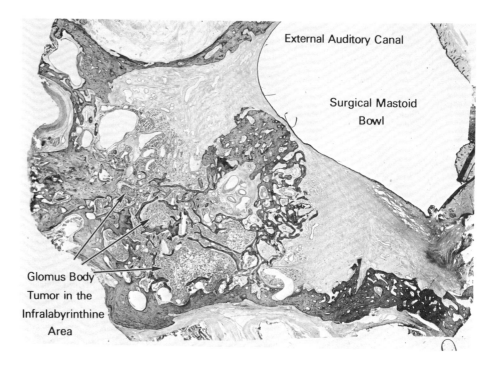

External Auditory Canal

Surgical Mastoid Bowl

Glomus Body Tumor in the Infralabyrinthine Area

Fig. 11.16: Glomus body tumor of the hypotympanic region. This patient, who survived 19 years with the tumor, typifies the chronicity with which glomus body tumor may manifest itself. At the age of 54 she first complained of pulsating tinnitus and hearing loss in the right ear. Examination revealed a reddish mass behind the right tympanic membrane. An attempted middle ear biopsy was unsuccessful because of profuse bleeding. A radical mastoidectomy revealed a vascular tumor in the middle ear and mastoid antrum which was partially removed. Histological studies confirmed the diagnosis of glomus body tumor. The patient was quite well until age 63, when she noted the insidious onset of right facial weakness and pain in the area of the right ear. Biopsy of tissue in the hypotympanum demonstrated recurring glomus body tumor, and roentgen studies showed a destructive lesion of the base of the skull. Radiation therapy was given in a dosage of 4,000r (200 kv) and she had no further special complaints referable to her ear and no clinical evidence of recurring glomus body tumor until she died at the age of 73 of bronchopneumonia complicating cerebral hemorrhage. Histological studies of the right temporal bone reveal extensive neoplastic tissue in the inferior part of the petrous bone with finger-like projections extending into the petrous apex, infralabyrinthine area, anterior part of the mastoid, hypotympanum, and posterior mesotympanum. The histological pattern is typical of glomus body tumor.

Kawabata et al. (1969), in a study of the ultrastructural appearance of the tumor, found the neoplastic cells to contain a large number of membrane-bounded electron-dense granules and a well-developed Golgi apparatus.

McCabe and Fletcher (1969) recommended that the form of treatment be determined by the size and location of the tumor; thus, purely tympanic tumors should be removed via the transcanal approach. Tympano-mastoid tumors should be treated by radical mastoidectomy and followed by radiation therapy if excision is incomplete, and petrosal and extrapetrosal tumors should be treated by radiation therapy after biopsy. Using the treatment as outlined, they reported the results of 32 cases with follow-up periods varying from five to nineteen years. They found 7 patients without tumor and 22 with tumor but without evidence of growth. Three died of rapid extratemporal spread or metastases to brain, bone or viscera. Two-thirds of the group living with tumor had multiple cranial nerve palsies.

There seems to be general agreement that surgery alone is often inadequate to control the tumor and that radiation in combination with surgery is required to effect long-term survival (Dill, 1959; Grubb and Lampe 1965; Rosenwasser, 1968) (Fig. 11.16).

Gejrot (1965) performed retrograde jugulography on 12 cases and found intravascular growth in six. He advised that such cases be treated by excision of the jugular bulb along with radical mastoidectomy and described the technique for this surgical procedure.

5. CERUMINOMA

The dermal layer of the cartilaginous part of the external auditory canal contains hair follicles, sebaceous glands, and ceruminous glands (modified sweat glands). The ceruminous glands are histologically similar to the apocrine sweat glands of the axilla and genital region. These glands, like sweat glands elsewhere in the body, have a two-layered epithelial structure consisting of an inner oxyphilic columnar layer and an outer myoepithelial layer. Johnstone et al. (1957) pointed out that neoplasms of these glands (ceruminomas) cannot be differentiated histologically from sweat gland tumors occurring elsewhere in the body and suggested they be termed hidradenomas. O'Neill and Parker (1957) shared this viewpoint and termed them sweat gland tumors of the external auditory canal. Because of the specific location of these tumors in the external auditory canal and their origin from these modified sweat glands, otologists will probably continue to identify them as ceruminomas.

The characteristic clinical feature is a mass in the external auditory canal.

It is covered with a layer of squamous epithelium and is usually asymptomatic until it causes obstruction of the external auditory canal. Growth is extremely variable but usually is slow and progressive until a visible swelling is produced in the region of the ear.

Histologically the tumor consists of acidophilic cells which either surround lumens or are arranged in solid cords and bordered by a few inconspicuous myoepithelial cells (Figs. 11.17, 11.18, 11.19). There is a variable amount of interglandular stroma. Occasionally the tumors exhibit histologic similarities to adenoma, mixed tumors, and adenoid cystic carcinoma.

Incomplete removal leads to recurrence (Johnstone et al., 1957). Successful treatment consists of wide excision of the tumor (Naessen, 1965; Juby, 1957). Although there have been no recorded cases of metastases from ceruminomas, local aggressiveness or invasion must be equated with malignancy (Batsakis et al., 1967).

6. VESTIBULAR SCHWANNOMA

Schwannomas are neoplasms which arise from the Schwann sheath cells of the cranial and spinal nerve roots as well as peripheral nerves. They occur mainly on sensory nerves of which the vestibular is the most frequently involved. The vagus and glossopharyngeal nerves and the roots of motor nerves are more apt to be involved in the multiple manifestations of von Recklinghausen's disease.

These tumors have variously been termed neuromas, neurilemmomas, neurofibromas, and perineural fibroblastomas. This confusion regarding terminology has evolved because one group of investigators believes the tumors arise from Schwann cells and another believes they are of fibroblastic origin. Penfield (1927) attributed these encapsulated growths on the nerves to fibroblastic proliferation and named them perineural fibroblastomas. The term "neurinoma" as proposed by Verocay (1910) signifies a proliferation of nerve fibers which is clearly incorrect. Stout (1935) suggested the term "neurilemmoma," thereby indicating that these tumors arise from the sheath of Schwann; however, Young (1942) believes that the term "neurilemma" should be applied only to the inner endoneurium or sheath of Plenk-Laidlaw which forms a basement membrane to the Schwann cells. Since we are concerned with multiplication of cells rather than membranes, the term "neurilemmoma" is inappropriate.

Electron microscopic studies of these tumors have demonstrated morphological characteristics which are typical for Schwann cells. The cells are surrounded by a basement membrane and in the spaces between cells there is a moderate amount of collagen and numerous cross-striated (Luse) bodies (Luse, 1960; Raimondi et al., 1962; Hilding and House, 1965).

For most cranial nerves the Schwann cells ensheath the axons from the point at which the latter penetrate the pia mater to their terminations. The supporting elements in the proximal part of the nerve root are neuroglial and the zone at which neuroglial tissue ends and Schwann sheath cells begin is termed the glial-Schwann sheath junction.

The Schwann cells are regarded by many as homologous with the oligodendroglia of the central nervous system as both are concerned with the maintenance of the myelin sheath. It is generally assumed that the Schwann cells are derived from the neural crest and thus are of neuroectodermal origin.

It is abundantly clear that nearly all of the schwannomas arising in the internal auditory canal take origin from the vestibular nerves. The tumor occasionally takes origin from the facial nerve and in rare instances from the cochlear nerve (Nager, 1964a).

In a histological study of 250 temporal bones removed at autopsy, Hardy and Crowe (1936) found six minute vestibular schwannomas which apparently had not caused clinical symptoms and had not been observed at autopsy because of their small size. Subsequently, Leonard and Talbot (1970) described four asymptomatic schwannomas in 883 temporal bones in the Johns Hopkins collection. These small tumors have also been described by Henschen (1915),

Fig. 11.17: Ceruminoma of the external auditory canal. The tumor cells have an irregular adenoid arrangement with luminal and cystic spaces of varying size. There is a surface layer of squamous epithelium. (Courtesy of Friedmann)

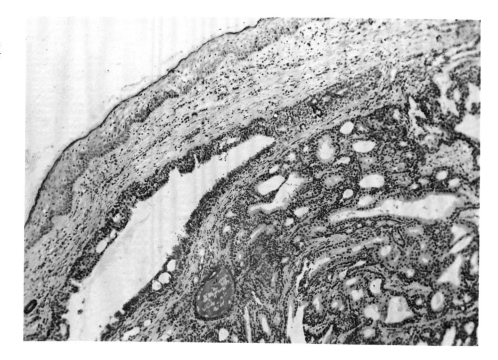

Fig. 11.18: Ceruminoma of the external auditory canal. The densely acidophilic cells are arranged in cords, or in tubular formations of varying size, and are separated by a dense fibrous stroma. (Courtesy of Friedmann)

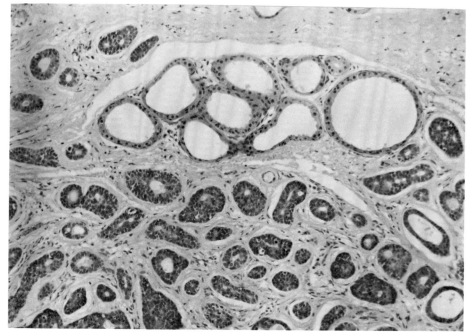

Fig. 11.19: Ceruminoma of the external auditory canal. The cellular pattern consists of lumens and clefts lined by inner oxyphilic columnar cells and outer myoepithelial cells. The intervening stroma of this particular tumor is sparse. (Courtesy of Friedmann)

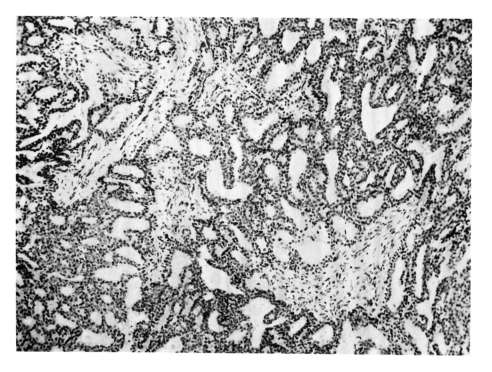

Fig. 11.20: Vestibular schwannoma. An incidental finding in the right temporal bone of this 84-year-old man is a small schwannoma arising in the superior division of the vestibular nerve. The patient had no symptoms referable to this tumor. The vestibular nerve fibers cross over the surface of the tumor and appear to be intact.

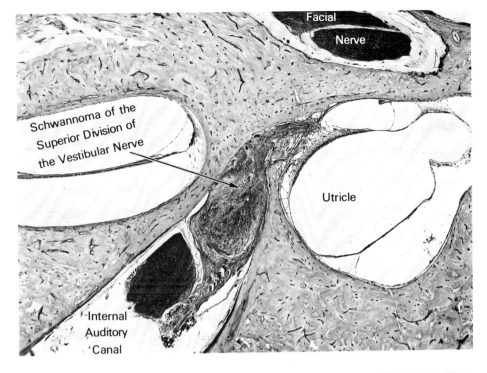

Fig. 11.21: Vestibular schwannoma. This 49-year-old man had a small asymptomatic schwannoma arising from the inferior division of the vestibular nerve. There is no degeneration of nerve fibers.

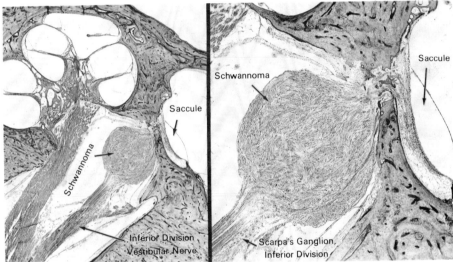

Fig. 11.22: Vestibular schwannoma. A small asymptomatic schwannoma located on the superior division of the vestibular nerve occured as an incidental finding in the temporal bone of this 57-year-old man. There is partial degeneration of the vestibular nerve fibers. (Courtesy of Rüedi)

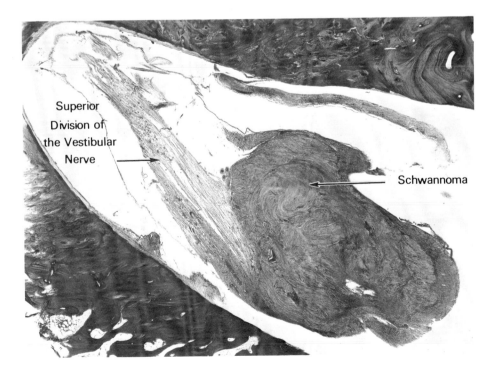

Marx (1926), and Lange (1929). In the collection of 900 temporal bones at the Massachusetts Eye and Ear Infirmary, three small asymptomatic vestibular schwannomas were found on the superior division of the nerve (Figs. 11.20, 11.21, 11.22).

Schwannomas may arise anywhere between the glial-Schwann sheath junction and the cribrose areas. There is no evidence to support the idea that schwannomas arise predominantly at the glial-Schwann sheath junction.

Henschen (1915) and Skinner (1929) have an embryologic explanation for the common locus of occurrence in the internal auditory canal. During embryonic growth the acoustical-facial ganglion arises medial and ventral to the auditory vesicle, with the facial portion differentiating early and the remaining cell mass eventually dividing into the vestibular and cochlear ganglia. These cells give rise to the bipolar ganglia of the vestibular and cochlear nerves and to their Schwann sheath cells. The bipolar ganglion cells send fibers to the auditory vesicle peripherally and to the brain stem centrally. The growing fibers are accompanied by neurilemmal cells but outgrow them. When the nerve fibers reach the brain stem, glial fibers grow out peripherally to meet the Schwann sheath cells. Inasmuch as the vestibular fibers reach the brain stem at an earlier age than the cochlear fibers, the glial cells migrate out further along the vestibular division than along the cochlear division. This is thought to result in a disordered arrangement and apparent excess of sheath cells in the vestibular nerve as compared to the cochlear nerve, and predisposes the vestibular nerve to develop schwannomas.

The distance from the brain stem to the glial-Schwann sheath junction in the VIIIth nerve complex is about 10 to 13 mm in the male and about 7 to 10 mm in the female, being somewhat more distal in the vestibular than the cochlear nerve.

Vestibular schwannomas account for about 8 to 10 percent of all intracranial tumors (Walshe, 1931; Cushing, 1935; Olivecrona, 1940; Zülch, 1957) and about 78 percent of all tumors in the cerebellopontine angle (Gonzalez-Revilla, 1948).

Erickson et al. (1965), in a study of 129 subjects with vestibular schwannomas, found the mean age at hospital admission to be 45.1 years and the mean duration of symptoms to be 4.6 years. Olsen and Horrax (1944) found the average duration of symptoms prior to correct diagnosis in 54 cases to be about two years.

These tumors are generally slow-growing, although hemorrhage, cyst formation, and edema may provide clinical evidence of increased rate of growth. Olivecrona (1950) concluded that growth may be self-limiting. He observed that 50 percent of 83 patients remained symptom-free in spite of only partial removal of the tumor.

Pathological characteristics. Vestibular schwannomas are usually firm, circumscribed, and encapsulated and when small, they are round or ovoid in shape. Larger tumors tend to become lobulated, then protrude from the internal auditory meatus into the cerebellopontine angle, and when fully developed produce deformation of the brain stem and adjacent cerebellum. As the tumor enlarges, adjacent nerve roots are stretched over the surface of the mass or are incorporated into it and the internal auditory canal becomes enlarged and funnel-shaped as the result of pressure erosion of bone (Figs. 11.23, 11.24).

Edematous portions of the tumor may be watery, cystic, and soft, whereas cellular areas may appear rubbery. The cut surfaces often show a variegated color pattern. Recent hemorrhage is dark red; old hemorrhage is brown; xanthomatous foci are dull yellow and calcified areas appear whitish. Degenerative changes within the tumor probably explain some of the fluctuations in clinical symptomatology. Edema and hemorrhage tend to produce sudden enlargement, whereas degeneration and fibrosis results in shrinkage of the mass.

Microscopic sections of vestibular schwannomas frequently show vascular changes such as acute necrosis of the endothelium and perivascular tissue, organized and recanalized thrombi, aneurysmal dilatations simulating hemangioma, acute hemorrhage, and aggregates of homosiderin granules indicative of old hemorrhage (Dykstra, 1964).

Antoni, in a 500-page monograph published in 1920, divided these tumors into two types: *Type A* is composed of compact tissue of merging and diverging streams of elongated spindle cells, usually with fairly large nuclei, with the tendency for the nuclei to be aligned in straight or curved rows with the long axes parallel to one another, thus resulting in a palisading pattern. At times the arrangement of nuclei and fibers creates formations simulating tactile corpuscles known as Verocay bodies (Figs. 11.25, 11.26). *Type B* is a degenerate form which often is intermingled with Type A but may be well demarcated. It is characterized by loose texture and polymorphism of tumor cells. There are two subgroups of Type B (Nager, 1969). One shows fatty degeneration leading to a characteristic honeycombed appearance of large pale tumor cells with small pyknotic nuclei (Fig. 11.27). The other form shows transformation of tumor tissue into hyaline masses in which case the cell content is often reduced to such an extent that only a few stellate tumor cells remain embedded in the amorphous hyaline substance (Fig. 11.28). Murray (1942) and Stout (1949) demonstrated that distinctive forms of Schwann cells

Fig. 11.23: Vestibular schwannoma. At the age of 63 the patient reported having a severe hearing loss in the left ear. He had no other symptoms, and no otologic examinations were performed. He died of cardiac failure 18 years later at the age of 81. Histological studies show a schwannoma occupying a large part of the internal auditory canal. The vestibular nerves are displaced inferiorly and are incorporated into the tumor mass with about 25 percent of the neurons remaining. The cochlear nerve is also displaced inferiorly with about 50 percent of the neurons remaining. There is a near total loss of external hair cells of the organ of Corti although some internal hair cells remain. The maculae of the utricle and saccule appear normal, but about 25 percent of the hair cells appear to be missing in the cristae. There is a granular and fibrinous acidophilic precipitate in both the perilymphatic and endolymphatic spaces. The facial nerve is displaced anteriorly and stretches over the surface of the tumor in the shape of a thin ribbon. See also Fig. 11.24.

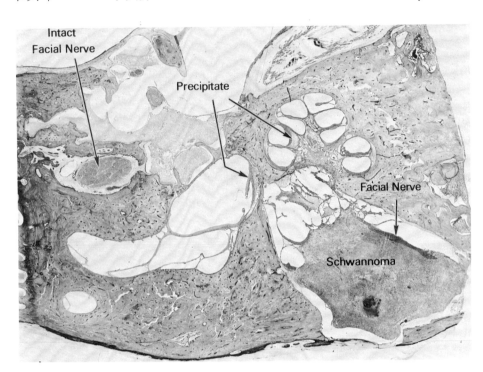

Fig. 11.24: Same case as Fig. 11.23. The vestibular schwannoma has compressed the facial nerve into the shape of a thin ribbon. Facial motor function was normal.

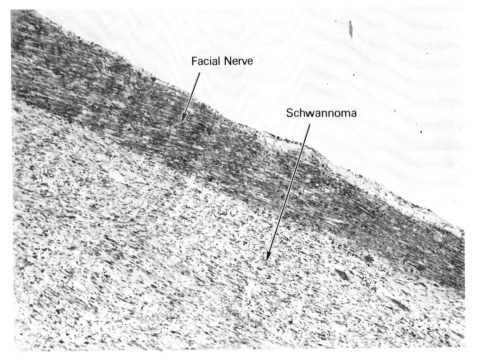

Fig. 11.25: Vestibular schwannoma, Antoni type A. The tumor is composed of compact and interwoven bundles of long or oval cells. In some areas the cells are arranged in whorls and in other areas there is a parallel alignment of the nuclei (palisading). (Courtesy of Nager)

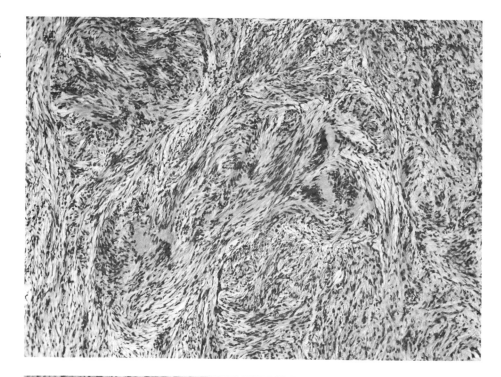

Fig. 11.26: High-power view of vestibular schwannoma, Antoni type A, showing whorled arrangement and palisading of nuclei.

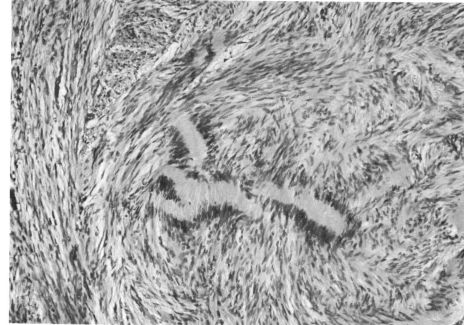

Fig. 11.27: Vestibular schwannoma, Antoni type B, subgroup 1. The tissue shows a loose texture and polymorphic appearance and is characterized by fatty degeneration. The accumulation of lipids within the cell causes it to swell and leads to the characteristic honeycombed appearance of the tumor cells. There are small pyknotic nuclei, either centrally or eccentrically located. (Courtesy of Nager)

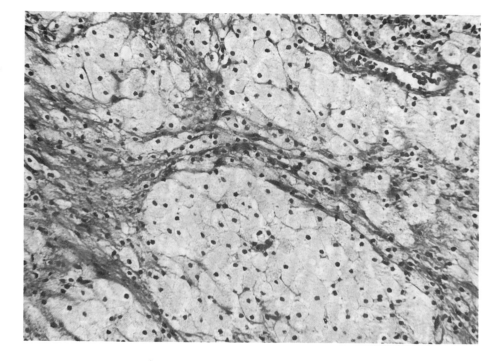

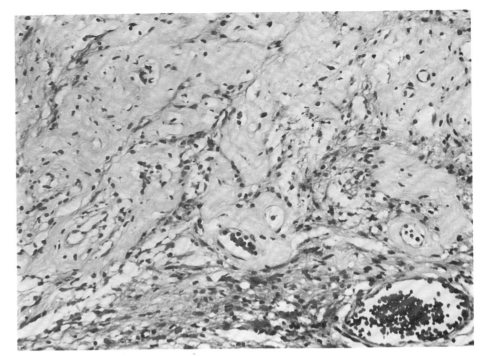

Fig. 11.28: Vestibular schwannoma, Antoni type B, subgroup 2. The tumor is transformed into hyaline masses with the cell content greatly reduced. Subgroups 1 and 2 of the Antoni B type may occur side by side in the same tumor. (Courtesy of Nager)

Fig. 11.29: Malignant transformation of vestibular schwannoma. At the age of 9 this patient developed symptoms of an expanding lesion of the posterior cranial fossa. In spite of partial removal through a posterior craniotomy approach and radiotherapy, the tumor continued to grow and she died eight months later. Histological examination of the right temporal bone reveals a schwannoma which appears to arise from the inferior division of the vestibular nerve, causing displacement of the superior division and the cochlear nerve. The tumor is encapsulated, and the cellular structures are arranged in whorls, strands, and sheaths with palisading of nuclei characteristic of Antoni type A. There is an estimated 50 percent loss of vestibular neurons and 90 percent loss of cochlear neurons. The hair cell populations of the organ of Corti and vestibular sense organs appear normal. The inferior part of the schwannoma is in continuity with a growth which has invaded the medial, apical, and inferior parts of the petrous bone. It has destroyed the anterior and inferior walls of the internal auditory canal and extends laterally into the protympanum and hypotympanum. This mass is highly cellular but shows a slight tendency toward palisading and formation of whorls. The nuclei are less elongated and more hyperchromatic than the adjacent Antoni type A tumor. There are numerous mytotic figures. See also Figs. 11.30, 11.31, and 11.32.

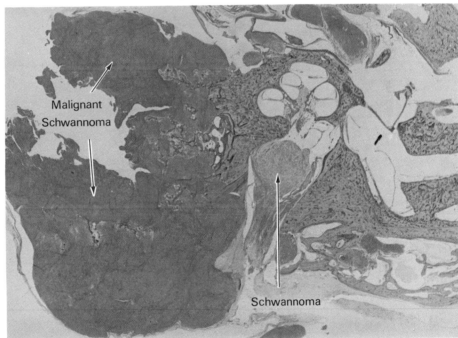

Fig. 11.30: Same case as Figs. 11.29, 11.31, and 11.32. This view shows the schwannoma, Antoni type A, in the internal auditory canal and the malignant schwannoma in the region of the petrous apex.

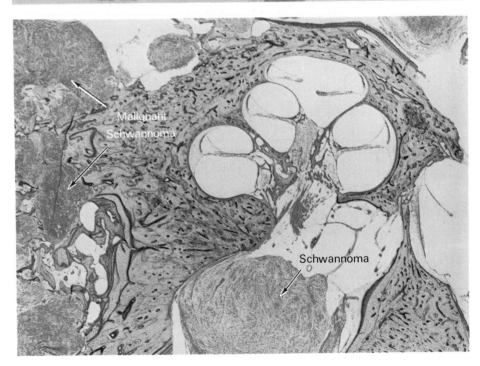

Fig. 11.31: Same case as Figs. 11.29, 11.30, and 11.32. The schwannoma in the internal auditory canal has the cytological characteristics of Antoni type A.

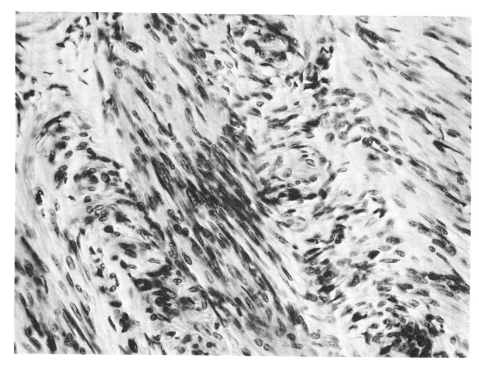

Fig. 11.32: Same case as Figs. 11.29, 11.30, and 11.31. The tumor of the petrous apex region is composed of densely packed pleomorphic cells with small irregularly shaped hyperchromatic nuclei and numerous mitotic figures.

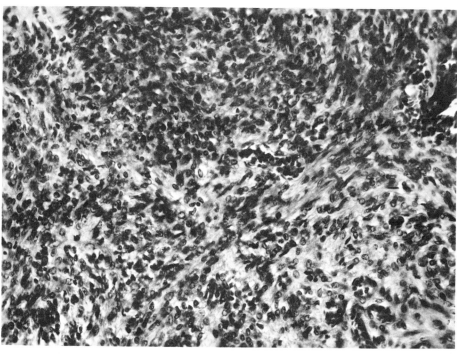

Fig. 11.33: The audiograms of these three individuals with surgically and histologically proven vestibular schwannomas demonstrate the characteristic elevation of air and bone conduction thresholds, absence of loudness recruitment, and severe loss of speech discrimination.

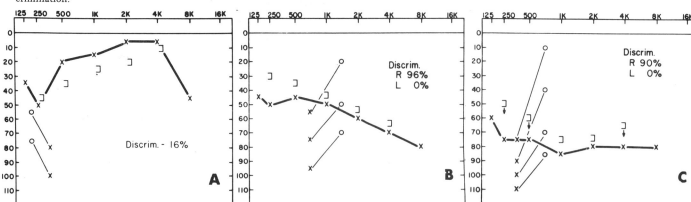

can be cultured from both the Antoni A and Antoni B tumor tissue.

Although it is extremely rare, it is possible for the tumor to transform from the typical slow-growing schwannoma into a rapidly invasive malignant growth (Figs. 11.29 to 11.32).

Pathophysiology. Clinical and histological studies indicate that there are at least three mechanisms responsible for auditory and vestibular dysfunction: (1) *Destruction of cochlear and vestibular nerve fibers.* A common auditory manifestation is a loss of speech discrimination out of proportion to the pure tone threshold loss (Fig. 11.33). This finding correlates with animal experiments (Schuknecht and Woellner, 1955) which have shown that up to 75 percent of the nerve fibers can be lost without creating pure tone threshold losses, providing the organ of Corti is intact. The functional implication is that only a few nerve fibers are needed to transmit pure tone stimuli of threshold magnitude whereas many fibers are necessary to carry the complex neural patterns of speech. The auditory symptoms usually are slowly progressive until there is a total loss of hearing for pure tones as well as for speech. The vestibular manifestations of a loss of nerve fibers are decreased threshold sensitivity and diminished amplitude of response on vestibular stimulation (caloric tests). The relationship of nerve fiber population to test response characteristics has not been clearly determined for the vestibular system (Litton and McCabe, 1966). (2) *Destruction of the sense organs.* In addition to destroying nerves in the internal auditory canal, the tumor may cause degenerative changes in the membranous labyrinth (De Moura, 1967; De Moura et al., 1969). There may be atrophy or complete loss of the organ of Corti. Usually the change is most severe in the basal turn. The maculae and cristae are less often involved. In exceptional cases the initial auditory manifestations indicate sensory rather than neural involvement (Figs. 11.34, 11.35). It is probable that structural changes such as shrinking of the sense organs or loss of sensory or supporting cells are secondary to impairment of blood supply as the result of compression or invasion of arteries in the internal auditory canal. (3) *Biochemical disturbances in the fluids of the inner ear.* Changes in the staining characteristics of the perilymph are a well-known phenomenon with vestibular schwannomas (Dix and Hallpike, 1950; Schuknecht, 1966). The high protein content of the perilymph has subsequently been confirmed by Silverstein and Schuknecht (1966). It is probable that biochemical alterations in the inner ear fluids are responsible, in part at least, for the hearing losses showing flat audiometric patterns and loudness recruitment.

Symptoms. The progressive growth of a schwannoma of the internal auditory canal and cerebellopontine angle produces a sequence of symptoms

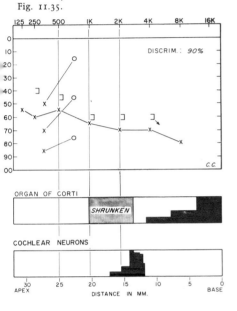

Fig. 11.34: Vestibular schwannoma in a 57-year-old female. The audiometric tests show a sensorineural hearing loss characterized by a flat threshold pattern, loudness recruitment, and relatively good speech discrimination. The patient died three days following partial intracapsular removal through a suboccipital craniotomy approach. Autopsy revealed severe edema of the brain, left temporal pressure cone, and infarction of the left cerebellar hemisphere. Histological studies of the temporal bone show a partial loss of hair cells in the basal 12 mm region of the cochlea and a shrunken organ of Corti in the 13 to 20 mm region. A loss of cochlear neurons was found only in the 12 to 17 mm region. There were no morphological alterations to explain the hearing loss for frequencies below 1,000 Hz. The clinical manifestations and histological findings in this case demonstrate a sensory disorder of the cochlea, probably caused by circulatory and biochemical alterations. See Fig. 11.35.

Fig. 11.35: Same case as Fig. 11.34. The tumor fills the internal auditory canal and shows areas of hemorrhage, edema, and necrosis. There is a partial loss of cochlear neurons in the 12 to 17 mm region and atrophy of the organ of Corti in the 13 to 20 mm region.

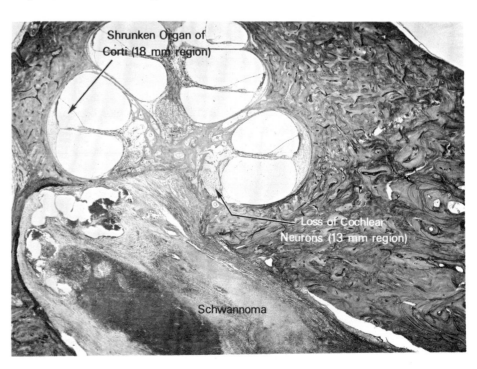

which tend to occur in the following order: (1) *Loss of hearing and disequilibrium* (Table 11.1). Either the auditory or the vestibular symptoms may be the first to appear. Auditory symptoms consist of tinnitus and hearing loss, which the patient may not notice for some months or years after onset. The main vestibular symptoms are unsteadiness, but occasionally frank vertigo, associated with nausea, may occur. Ordinarily the disequilibrium is more constant and prolonged and not as abrupt and episodic as in Meniere's disease. When destruction of the vestibular nerve has occurred very slowly, it is possible for vestibular function to be completely destroyed with little or no symptoms, which attests to the great adaptability of the vestibular system. In rare cases

Table 11.1 Vestibular Schwannoma
Frequency of Auditory and Vestibular Symptoms

	Number	Tinnitus and deafness %	Disequilibrium %	Nystagmus and impaired caloric responses %
Edwards and Paterson (1951)	157	99	42	98
Olsen and Horrax (1944)	54	93	31	97
Gonzalez-Revilla (1947)	145	99	41	87
Cushing (1917)	30	100	—	63
Pool and Pava (1957)	122	92	58	99
Erickson et al. (1965)	129	98.6	6.45	99

the first symptom may be a rather sudden and severe attack of vertigo with complete compensation taking place over a period of weeks (Hallberg et al., 1959). (2) *Headaches*. Headaches are a common symptom of large vestibular schwannomas and are usually either occipital or frontal in location and aggravated by stooping, straining, or sneezing. (3) *Cerebellar symptoms*. A growing tumor in the cerebellopontine angle will, in time, exert pressure on the adjacent cerebellar hemisphere, resulting in incoordination of movement and nystagmus. Incoordination affects the lower limbs more than the upper limbs and tends to become more severe as the tumor enlarges. When walking the patient tends to fall to the side on which the tumor is located. Nystagmus is commonly in the horizontal plane with the slow component to the side of the lesion. Rarely the nystagmus may be vertical in direction. Nystagmus is believed to be caused by involvement of the corticocerebellar fibers which pass in the middle of the cerebellar peduncle, or to involvement of the vestibular nerves. (4) *Involvement of adjacent cranial nerves*. Apart from the cochlear and vestibular nerves, the two cranial nerves most commonly involved are the Vth and VIIth. The VIth, IXth, and Xth nerves may become involved in terminal stages. The Vth nerve is compressed against the pons and midbrain by the enlarging tumor, which may result in stabbing paroxysmal pain followed by numbness and paresthesias of the face. Cushing (1935) found corneal insensitivity on the ipsilateral side in 76 percent of cases. Corneal insensitivity in association with ipsilateral deafness suggests the presence of a cerebellopontine angle tumor. In addition, impairment of pressure, touch sensation, and pain are often found over all three divisions of the Vth nerve. Involvement of the VIIth nerve is less common than the Vth and occurs later in the course of the disease. The symptoms consist of partial or complete paralysis and occasionally spasms of the facial muscles. The IXth and Xth nerves may be involved late in the disease and give rise to loss of pharyngeal reflexes and laryngeal paralysis, resulting in dysphagia and dysphonia. Sometimes there is impaired sensation of the tragus and the postauricular region on the affected side. Paralysis of the IVth nerve causes diplopia due to paralysis

Fig. 11.36: This case is presented in detail as it demonstrates the difficulty which may be encountered in the clinical differentiation of vestibular schwannoma and Ménière's disease. At age 53 the patient first noted hearing loss in his right ear. An audiogram six months later showed a severe hearing loss in the right ear for frequencies above 2,000 Hz. During this period he had occasional fleeting sensations of unsteadiness, particularly on arising in the morning. Ice water caloric test revealed severe decreased vestibular response on the right. Radiological studies, including laminograms of the temporal bone, appeared normal. Six months later, audiometric studies of the right ear showed a pure tone loss of about 60 db for all frequencies and a speech discrimination score of 44 percent. After another six months there was profound hearing loss in the right ear with no speech reception and no caloric response to ice water. Neurological examination was negative, except for the VIIIth nerve findings. Pantopaque studies showed less filling and irregularity of contour of the cerebellopontine cistern and internal auditory canal on the right side in comparison to the left. Analysis of fluid removed from the vestibule of the labyrinth showed sodium at 60 mEq., potassium at 100 mEq., and protein at 1,630 mg %. The high potassium level was consistent with Ménière's disease, and the elevated protein was suggestive of vestibular schwannoma; therefore, the findings were considered to be inconclusive.

At age 55, 2½ years after the hearing loss was first noticed, a translabyrinthine exploratory operative procedure was performed to determine the possible existence of a vestibular schwannoma. A tumor was not found; however, postoperative hemorrhage occurred and the patient died three days later.

Autopsy revealed partial surgical ablation of the right cerebellar hemisphere with postoperative bleeding, bilateral uncal and cerebellar grooving, bilateral bronchopneumonia, and terminal esophageal perforation and mediastinitis. The right temporal bone was removed for histological study. See Figs. 11.37 and 11.38.

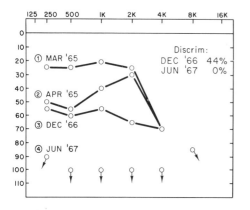

of the lateral rectus muscle. (5) *Elevated intracranial pressure.* With continued growth of the tumor there may be obstruction to the outflow of cerebrospinal fluid resulting in internal hydrocephalus causing headache, diplopia, papilledema and vomiting, and eventually cerebellar and respiratory crises and death.

Diagnosis and treatment. The diagnosis of vestibular schwannoma can be made with a high degree of certainty by history, otological and neurological examinations, and a battery of tests (Pulec and House 1964; Hambley et al, 1964; Crabbe, 1966). The examination should include auditory and vestibular testing and an evaluation of cranial nerve function. Radiologic studies should include views of the petrous pyramids with particular reference to the internal auditory canals, laminography or polytomography, and contrast dye studies of the internal auditory canals and cerebellopontine angles. Cerebrospinal fluid should be studied with special reference to its protein content. In the presence of small tumors the cerebrospinal fluid may be normal. When the diagnosis is in doubt an evaluation of the protein and electrolyte concentrations of inner ear fluid can be helpful (Silverstein and Schuknecht, 1966).

Ménière's disease presenting atypical symptoms may be difficult to differentiate from vestibular schwannoma. A mistaken diagnosis can lead to inappropriate surgical management. For a case in point see Figs. 11.36, 11.37, and 11.38.

Based on the incidence of the two disorders it seems obvious that Ménière's disease and vestibular schwannoma will, in rare cases, occur coincidentally in

Fig. 11.37: Same case as Figs. 11.36 and 11.38. Serial sections of the right temporal bone show a large surgical defect due to the translabyrinthine surgical procedure performed three days before death. The entire mastoid and approximately the posterior half of the petrous portion of the temporal bone are missing. The mastoid air cell system, the semicircular canals, and most of the vestibule of the inner ear have been removed. The posterior wall of the internal auditory canal has been removed except for the bony margin of the internal auditory meatus. The nerves of the internal auditory canal (including the facial) are missing, presumably due to avulsion at the time of autopsy. The facial nerve is intact throughout the remainder of its course.

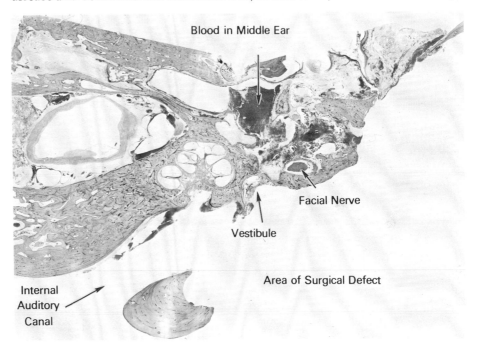

Fig. 11.38: Same case as Figs. 11.36 and 11.37. The morphological changes in the cochlea are typical of Ménière's disease. In all turns of the cochlea there is severe endolymphatic hydrops. Reissner's membrane has herniated through the helicotrema into the scala tympani of the apical and middle turns of the cochlea. The supporting cells of the organ of Corti are intact throughout; however, only 10 percent of the normal population of hair cells can be identified throughout the cochlea. There appears to be a slight loss of cochlear neurons in the basal turn but the population in the remainder of the cochlea appears to be normal. The nuclei are pale and swollen and presumably are in an early stage of degeneration. The tectorial membrane is missing in the basal turn and is displaced onto the limbus in the middle turn and part of the apical turn. There is a small amount of fresh blood in the cochlear duct of the basal and apical turns, and there is precipitate in the perilymphatic space of the middle and apical turns.

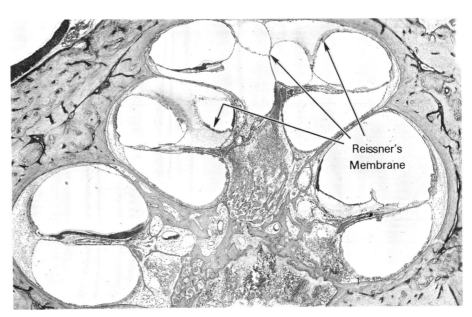

the same ear. De Moura (1968) presented such a case (Fig. 11.39). In the early part of this century the surgical removal of acoustic tumors was associated with a high rate of morbidity and mortality (Cushing, 1917). To reduce the mortality most surgeons resorted to the technique of intracapsular removal. Dandy (1934) reported, however, that the recurrence rate was high and that a second operation was a formidable procedure. He stressed total removal at the first operation and introduced the concept of unilateral suboccipital craniectomy with total tumor removal. Possibly at that time he was dealing with smaller, more favorably located lesions than earlier pioneers in the field. In 1950, Pennybacker and Cairns reported that even though it was then possible to make earlier diagnoses of these tumors, they were difficult to reach at the time of surgery and the postoperative neurological deficits were often so great that the advantages of early surgical removal were compromised.

Although approaches to the cerebellopontine angle through the temporal bone had been advocated long ago (Panse, 1904; Quix, 1911; Schmiegelow, 1915), the procedure failed to gain popularity because of technical difficulties (House and House, 1964). This situation was improved with the development of modern otologic surgery. The dilemma created by the mortality of untreated tumors and the morbidity of surgical removal has been rather effectively resolved by the surgical innovations of House and associates (House, 1961, 1964a, 1964b; Hitselberger and House, 1966).

A system of operations has been developed to cope with these tumors at each stage of their development. The middle fossa approach is designed for tumors confined to the internal auditory canal (Glasscock, 1969), the translabyrinthine approach for tumors which have extended outside the canal but are not associated with elevated intracranial pressure, and the combined suboccipital-petrosal approach for large tumors which have extended below the jugular bulb and are associated with elevated intracranial pressure.

For removal of large tumors, a two-stage approach may be used (Montgomery et al., 1966; Ojemann et al., 1972). The first procedure is performed by the translabyrinthine route at which time much of the tumor is removed and the facial nerve is identified and tagged. The second stage is an approach through the posterior cranial fossa in which an attempt is made to remove the remainder of the tumor while dissecting it away from the previously tagged facial nerve.

These procedures have resulted in greatly decreased morbidity and mortality and take advantage of the capability for early diagnosis.

7. VON RECKLINGHAUSEN'S DISEASE

Von Recklinghausen's disease is of interest to the otologist because of the high incidence in this disease of bilateral vestibular schwannomas (Figs. 11.40, 11.41, 11.42). It is a widely spread hamartoblastomatosis of connective and

Fig. 11.39: Vestibular schwannoma associated with Ménière's disease. At the age of 38 this male experienced severe vertiginous episodes with nausea, vomiting, and right hearing loss. He died at the age of 84 (46 years later) of adenocarcinoma of the colon. Histological studies of the right temporal bone reveal a tumor in the scala tympani of the basal turn having the typical histological characteristics of schwannoma, Antoni type A. The contents of the internal auditory canal were avulsed at the time of autopsy and are not available for study. There is a severe loss of cochlear neurons, suggesting that there may have been a tumor within the internal auditory canal. There is severe endolymphatic hydrops involving the entire membranous labyrinth. (Courtesy of DeMoura, 1968)

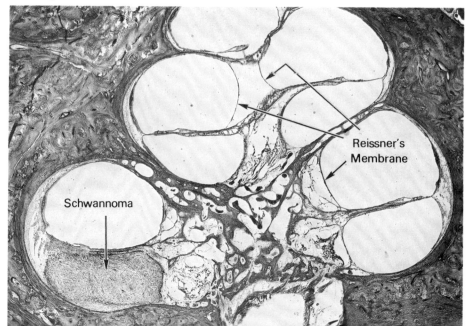

Reissner's Membrane

Schwannoma

Fig. 11.40: Von Recklinghausen's disease in a 31-year-old female. This patient had bilateral vestibular schwannomas causing profound loss of auditory and vestibular function in both ears. She died seven days following suboccipital craniotomy for removal of the tumor on the left side. The photomicrograph of the right temporal bone shows the neoplasm partially filling the internal auditory canal and extending through the cribrose areas into the basal turn of the cochlea and into the vestibule. There is atrophy of the organ of Corti in the 10 to 16 mm region with preservation of the sensory and neural elements elsewhere. The neurons of the superior division of the vestibular nerve are destroyed; however, the population of hair cells in the maculae and cristae appear normal. The perilymph stains with eosin, suggesting an elevation of protein concentration. (Courtesy of Benitez et al., 1967)

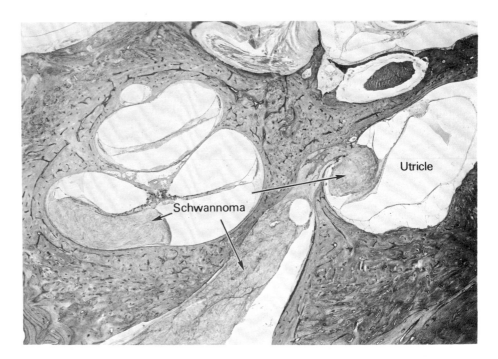

Fig. 11.41: Von Recklinghausen's disease. This patient, whose father and sister died of von Recklinghausen's disease, first noted hearing loss at the age of 44. Audiometric studies at yearly intervals showed a progressive loss of pure tone thresholds, speech discrimination scores, and caloric responses in both ears. He died at the age of 48, and autopsy revealed bilateral vestibular schwannomas and multiple schwannomas involving the nerves of the cauda equina. This view of the left temporal bone shows a large schwannoma occupying the internal auditory canal. The inner ear shows severe degeneration of sensory and neural structures and an acidophilic precipitate throughout the perilymphatic spaces. See also Fig. 11.42. (Courtesy of DeMoura et al.,

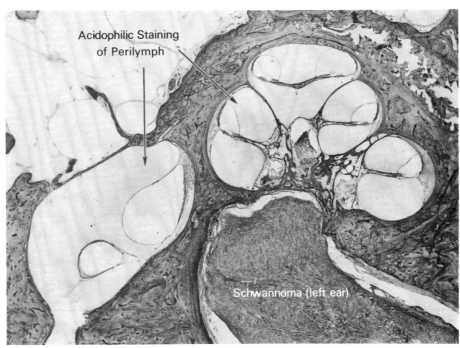

Fig. 11.42: Same case as Figure 11.41. The schwannoma on the right ear is nearly identical to that of the left.

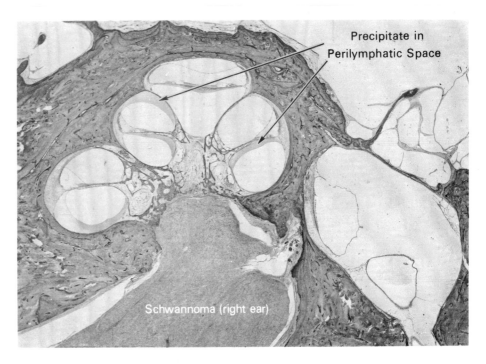

neural tissues showing a female preponderance. In its full-blown manifestation the disorder exhibits schwannomas of myelinated and nonmyelinated nerves, racemose angiomas, pigmented nevi, and a variety of intracranial tumors including meningiomas, spongioblastomas, and ependymomas. Less frequently there are vascular tumors of the nervous system, glial tumors of the retina, ganglioneuromas, and pheochromocytomas (Nager, 1964a).

In a significant number of patients, bilateral vestibular schwannomas are the principal manifestations of von Recklinghausen's disease (Gardner and Frazier, 1930; Gardner and Turner, 1940). Vestibular schwannomas occur in about 5 percent of reported cases of the disease and when present are nearly always bilateral. A young person who develops a unilateral vestibular schwannoma and who has a family history of von Recklinghausen's disease has a great possibility of eventually acquiring bilateral schwannomas. Young et al. (1970) studied a kindred including 97 individuals with definite or possible bilateral vestibular schwannomas and found the trait to be an autosomal dominant inheritance with high penetrance. The onset of symptoms in their cases was at about age 20, and survival without surgery varied from 2 to 42 years. Severe accidents, including drowning, were a common occurrence and may have been caused by the neurological deficits experienced by these patients. On the basis of natural history and genetic etiology, bilateral vestibular schwannoma must be considered as an entity distinct from unilateral vestibular schwannoma.

8. FACIAL NERVE NEOPLASMS

In an extensive review of facial nerve tumors, Pulec (1969) found reports of 74 intratemporal facial nerve schwannomas, 6 neurofibrosarcomas, 2 meningiomas, and 1 angiofibroma. He reported the findings in 11 additional cases, 10 of which were facial nerve schwannomas and 1 a cavernous hemangioma.

Small unsuspected facial nerve schwannomas have been found during surgical procedures (Plester, 1959) and at autopsy (Greifenstein, 1936; Kos, 1940). Saito and Baxter (1972) found five of these tumors in 600 temporal bones in the collection at the Massachusetts Eye and Ear Infirmary. The clinical records revealed that one of these five patients had slight facial weakness on the involved side. Their histological studies confirmed the generally held belief that these tumors arise from the sensory component of the facial nerve, for in two of their cases the tumor had a close anatomical relationship with the sensory bundle (Fig. 11.43). Two of these tumors occurred in the internal auditory canal and contained geniculate ganglion neurons intermingled with the tumor tissue (Fig. 11.44).

The most common symptom of facial nerve schwannoma is facial palsy, and although the history of slow progression of the palsy should be adequate to differentiate the disorder from Bell's palsy (Smith et al., 1971), the latter diagnosis is frequently made. Shambaugh et al. (1969) found that radiologic examination is of great assistance in making the diagnosis of schwannoma of the facial nerve.

Pulec (1972) reported on the surgical removal of 8 facial nerve schwannomas. He explored the nerve via the mastoid approach for neoplasms in the middle ear and mastoid segments, via the middle fossa approach for neoplasms involving the nerve in the internal auditory canal, and via the translabyrinthine approach when cochlear and vestibular function were useless. Resection of the involved segment of nerve followed by nerve graft or anastomosis resulted in good recovery of facial function.

9. OTHER TUMORS OF THE CEREBELLOPONTINE ANGLE

In addition to vestibular schwannoma there is a large variety of neoplasms, cysts, aneurysms, and granulomas which may be found in the cerebellopon-

Fig. 11.43: Schwannoma of the facial nerve. This small schwannoma is located in the vertical portion of the facial nerve of a 70-year-old woman. The sensory bundle is degenerated distal to the tumor, suggesting that the tumor originated from the sensory bundle.

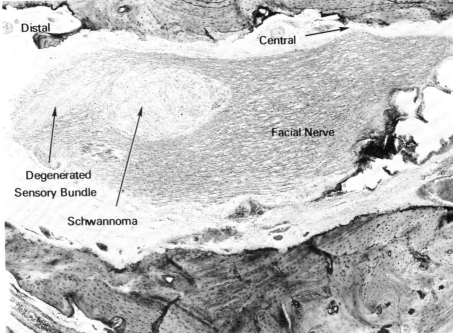

Fig. 11.44: Schwannoma of the facial nerve. This small asymptomatic tumor lies within the facial nerve trunk in the internal auditory canal and measures 3.5 mm in its greatest diameter. Aberrant neurons of the geniculate ganglion are intermingled with the tumor cells. Female, age 74.

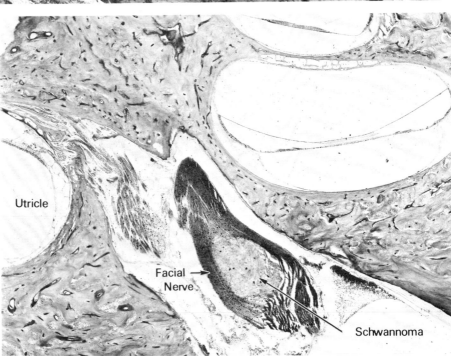

tine angle. The pathological identity of these lesions should be determined, if possible, before surgical removal is attempted. This can usually be done by history, examination, and a variety of tests including radiological studies.

Gonzalez-Revilla (1948) reviewed the pathological characteristics of 205 tumors occurring in the cerebellopontine angles of patients admitted to the Johns Hopkins Hospital between 1926 and 1945. He found that 78 percent were vestibular schwannomas, 6.3 percent were meningiomas, 6.3 percent were primary cholesteatomas, 5.9 percent were glomus body tumors, and the remaining 3.5 percent were abscesses and miscellaneous tumors.

Tumors which are less commonly encountered in the cerebellopontine angle include teratomas, schwannomas of cranial nerves other than the vestibular, osteomas, lipomas, sarcomas, and metastatic tumors. Other space-occupying lesions which must be considered are abscesses, tuberculomas, gummas, fungus lesions, aneurysms, and arachnoid cysts.

Epidermoid and dermoid cysts (primary keratomas) arise from congenital epithelial inclusion rests in the region of the petrous apex and frequently encroach upon the cerebellopontine angle. They are slowly growing tumor masses which commonly become symptomatic before the age of 20 and

Fig. 11.45: Meningioma. This woman died at the age of 75 of myocardial infarction. Post-mortem studies revealed an asymptomatic psammomatous meningioma of the petrous ridge. See Fig. 7.46.

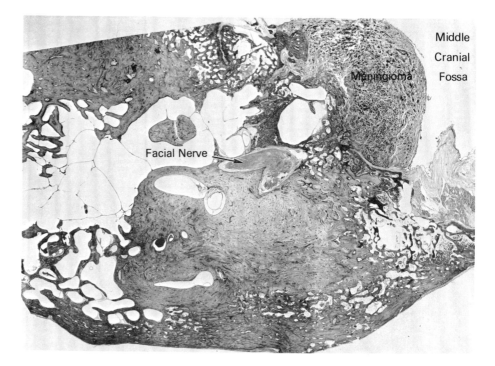

Fig. 11.46: Same case as Fig. 11.45, showing cytological detail of psammomatous meningioma. There are clusters of cells separated by varying amounts of stroma. The cells are similar to those of the outer layer of arachnoid, having moderately chromatic oval and round nuclei and finely granular cytoplasm. They are arranged in whorls in the center of which are irregularly round structures of varying size having a central hyaline mass and surrounding concentric lamellar calcifications typical of psammoma bodies.

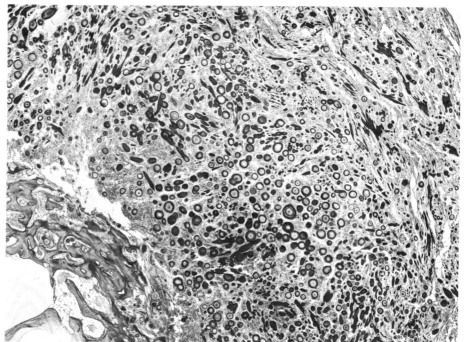

require surgical intervention before the age of 40. Epidermoid cysts have a delicate, whitish shiny capsule of epidermis resembling mother of pearl, a smooth or lobulated surface, and contain glistening, friable, whitish material. Dermoid cysts, on the other hand, have a firm capsule with hair follicles, sebaceous and sweat glands (Nager, 1969), and contain a greasy mass which may include hair. The radiologic appearance is that of a destructive lesion of the petrous apex. An interesting clinical feature of these lesions is that they tend to produce spasms of the facial muscles (facial tic) as an early sign. Radiologic studies of the posterior cranial fossa with contrast dyes often reveal a distinctive scalloped surface contour (Hitselberger and Gardner, 1968).

Gliomas which arise in the pons or cerebellar flocculus may extend into the cerebellopontine angle. The types in the order of occurrence are astrocytomas, medulloblastomas, ependymomas, and glioblastomas (Gonzalez-Revilla, 1947).

Meningiomas are believed to arise from the arachnoid villi, the cell of origin being the arachnoidal fibroblast. The arachnoid villi are bulbous extensions of the arachnoid into the venous sinuses and are concerned with the transfer of cerebrospinal fluid into the venous system. Meningiomas frequently arise on the posterior aspect of the petrous pyramid in relation to the sigmoid and petrosal sinuses and may encroach on the cerebellopontine angle (Nager, 1964b; Igarashi et al., 1971). The ratio of meningioma to vestibular schwannoma has been reported to be 1:12 (House, 1964b). Meningiomas are usually grayish-white and nodular and are firmly attached to the dura. They displace but do not invade brain tissue. In the posterior fossa, the lobulated (en-globe) type is more common than the flat (en-plaque) type. Calcification within the tumor is common and, when dense enough to be visualized by roentgen films, constitutes an important diagnostic feature. They frequently excite osteoblastic reaction in adjacent bone. Most meningiomas of the petrous pyramid contain a rich blood supply and may surround vessels that are vital to the brain stem (Costellano and Ruggiero, 1953) and may make surgical removal very hazardous.

Meningiomas may be classified into meningotheliomatous, psammomatous, and fibroblastic types (Robbins, 1962). The meningotheliomatous type consists of clusters of cells, appearing almost identical with the outer layer of arachnoid, and contains varying amounts of stroma. In the psammomatous type the cells are arranged in whorls in the centers of which are small deposits of hyalin which are formed in concentric lamellar fashion. These structures may become calcified and are known as psammoma bodies. They are thought to take their origin in degenerating cells in the centers of the whorls (Figs. 11.45, 11.46). The fibroblastic meningoma has the appearance of fibroblastic tumors elsewhere in the body.

B. METASTATIC NEOPLASMS

Metastatic involvement of the temporal bone by malignant tumors usually occurs in association with a more diffuse hematogenous dissemination. Schuknecht et al. (1968) reviewed the previously published reports of metastatic malignant tumors to the temporal bone and found the most common sites of origin in order of frequency to be breast, kidney, lung, stomach, larynx, prostate, and thyroid gland. It is probable that metastatic involvement of the temporal bone is much more common than is suggested by reports in the literature. Metastatic involvement of the temporal bone may occur as the first evidence of malignant disease (Figs. 11.47, 11.48). More often, temporal bone involvement occurs late in the course of the disease and the symptoms are overshadowed by the primary growth or by other metastatic lesions (Figs. 11.49, 11.50, 11.51). Proctor and Lindsay (1947) hypothesize that sluggish blood flow in the sinusoidal capillaries of bone marrow favors deposition of tumor cells in these areas.

Tumor cells deposited in the temporal bone behave no differently from tumor cells deposited elsewhere. They may proliferate rapidly or remain dormant for many years only to grow later, possibly after the primary tumor has been cured and thus present as an isolated metastatic growth (Fig. 11.52). Although metastatic lesions usually resemble the primary tumor in histologic appearance they are often less well differentiated. Only in a few histologic types, such as renal cell carcinoma, are they sufficiently differentiated to permit a determination of the probable site of origin (Figs. 11.53, 11.54).

Metastatic tumors of the temporal bone, like tumors elsewhere in the skeleton, may be predominantly osteolytic or may invoke new bone formation. In the beginning all metastatic lesions are destructive, but some are followed by bone repair. Metastases from carcinoma of the prostate often are characterized by osteoblastic activity, possibly because these tumor cells are rich in phosphatase. Mammary carcinoma often incites new bone formation. Metastatic lesions which have existed for a long period of time are more often associated with osteoblastic activity.

The enchondral layer of the bony labyrinth appears to resist neoplastic invasion (Nager, 1938); therefore, involvement of the inner ear is uncommon.

Fig. 11.47: At the age of 69 the patient noted sudden hearing loss in the right ear which progressed to profound deafness over a period of three days. Five days later she developed a loss of hearing in the left ear which progressed to profound deafness in two days. Roentgenograms revealed a mass in the right lung, and biopsy of a right axillary lymph node showed squamous cell carcinoma. Two weeks later she experienced right facial weakness which progressed to total paralysis over a period of five days. Her condition deteriorated rapidly, and she died of complications of bronchogenic carcinoma one month following the onset of sudden deafness. The left internal auditory canal is filled with a combination of viable and necrotic tumor tissue and remnants of nerve trunks. There is partial degeneration of the sense organs and precipitate in the perilymphatic spaces. See Fig. 11.48.

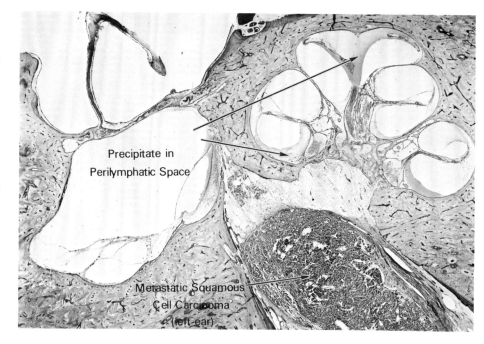

Fig. 11.48: Same case as Fig. 11.47. In the right ear there is neoplastic tissue filling the internal auditory canal. The motor division of the facial nerve is severely degenerated; however, the sensory bundle is intact. There is a severe loss of hair cells in all sense organs and a moderate loss of cochlear and vestibular neurons.

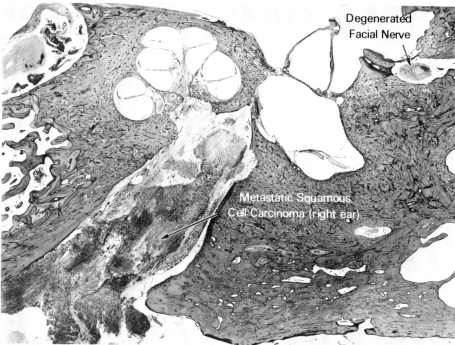

Fig. 11.49: Metastatic carcinoma of the temporal bone from a primary lesion in the esophagus. At the age of 65 this patient noted dysphasia and four months later developed a progressive right facial palsy. Biopsy of an esophageal lesion revealed undifferentiated carcinoma. He then experienced disequilibrium and right hearing loss and died six months later of diffuse carcinomatosis. Histological studies of the temporal bone show multiple osteolytic metastatic lesions involving the posterior wall of the petrous bone and internal auditory canal. The tumor invades the cochlear, vestibular, and facial nerves. There is severe degeneration of the sensory and neural elements of the membranous labyrinth associated with scattered hemorrhages in the endolymphatic and perilymphatic spaces. See Figs. 11.50 and 11.51.

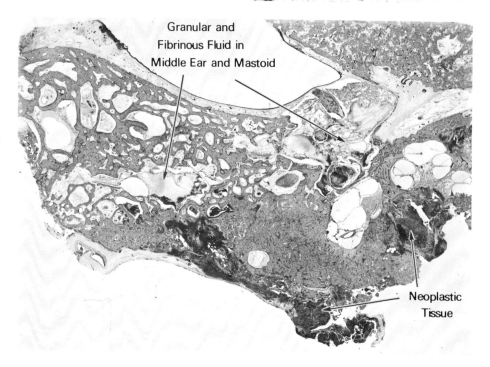

Fig. 11.50: Same case as Figs. 11.49 and 11.51. Neoplastic cells are seen in the internal auditory canal, marrow spaces of the bony labyrinth, and in the scala tympani of the basal turn.

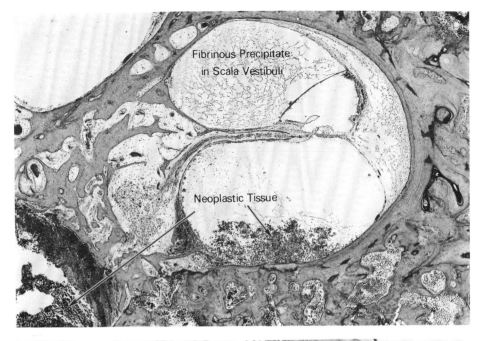

Fig. 11.51: Same case as Figs. 11.49 and 11.50. The neoplastic growth has partly destroyed the bony labyrinth and invaded the facial nerve. The inner ear shows scattered hemorrhages and precipitate.

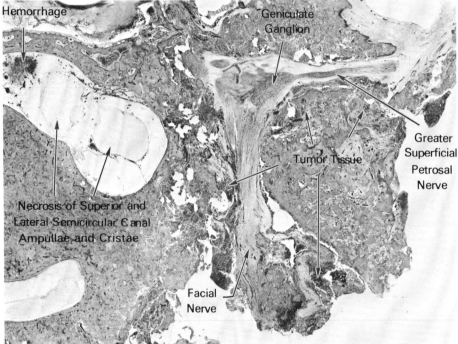

Fig. 11.52: Metastatic adenocarcinoma. At the age of 60 this patient had bilateral mastectomies for adenocarcinoma. Fifteen years later, at the age of 75, she suddenly developed right facial weakness, hearing loss, and vertigo. She had spontaneous nystagmus to the left, no caloric response to ice water stimulation on the right, and profound right hearing loss. Radiologic studies revealed a destructive lesion of the right petrous bone. She died of diffuse carcinomatosis nine months after the onset of otologic symptoms. Histological studies show neoplastic tissue characteristic of adenocarcinoma in the marrow spaces of the petrous apex, as well as the mastoid, tensor tympani muscle, and submucosa of the middle ear. Neoplastic tissue fills the internal auditory canal and has partially destroyed the cochlear, vestibular, and facial nerves. There is a severe loss of hair cells and cochlear neurons throughout the basal turn. The vestibular sense organs appear normal.

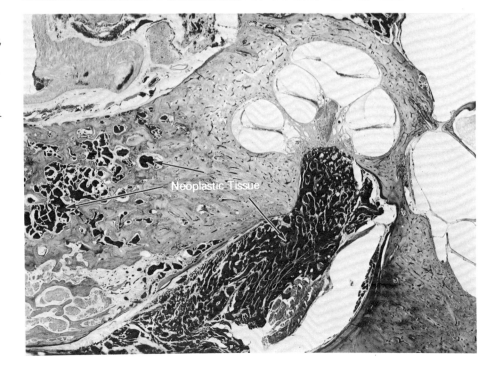

Fig. 11.53: Metastatic renal cell carcinoma of the temporal bone in association with Lindau-von Hippel disease (von Hippel, 1904; Melmon and Rosen, 1964). (This case was reported in the New England Journal of Medicine, Weekly Clinicopathological Exercises, 275: 950–959, Oct. 27, 1969). At the age of 17 this patient first noticed progressive loss of vision in the left eye, and a diagnosis of Lindau-von Hippel disease was made. The disorder was progressive, and at the age of 21 he became totally blind. At the age of 38 he developed left facial weakness and noted decreased hearing in the left ear. At the age of 40 he complained of pain in the region of his neck, and angiograms showed a right cerebellar lesion which by craniotomy was determined to be a cerebellar hemangioblastoma. At the age of 48 there was a polypoid mass in the left external auditory canal which biopsy showed to be metastatic renal cell carcinoma. Audiometric studies showed a total hearing loss in the left ear and normal hearing in the right. Roentgenograms revealed a destructive lesion of the left temporal bone. He died of hemorrhage from esophageal varices at the age of 48, thirty-one years after the first symptoms of Lindau-von Hippel disease. Histological studies of the left temporal bone reveal extensive destruction of the bony labyrinth, external auditory canal, and petrous apex by neoplastic growth. The cochlea, vestibule, and canals are extensively destroyed with only remnants of the bony and membranous labyrinths remaining. See also Fig. 11.54.

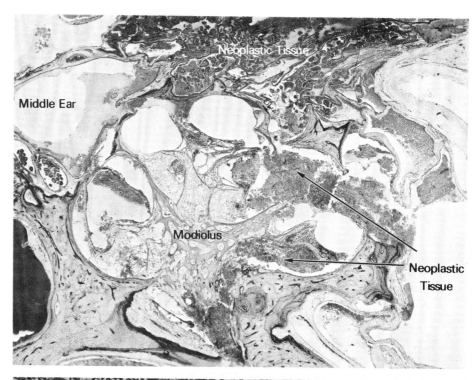

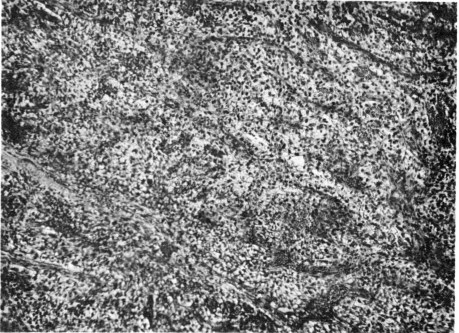

Fig. 11.54: Same case as Fig. 11.53. The tumor cells resemble cuboidal tubular epithelium, having round, small, regular nuclei and granular pink cytoplasm with great regularity and constancy of cytological detail. Some areas have predominantly clear cells with complete vacuolization of the cytoplasm.

The symptoms depend, of course, upon the location and size of the metastases. If they involve the external auditory canal, middle ear, mastoid, or eustachian tube, the patient experiences conductive deafness and pain. Lesions which involve the petrous bone and internal auditory canal may produce sensorineural hearing loss, vertigo, and facial paralysis.

The internal auditory canal appears to be a common site for metastatic growth. In this site the tumor cells frequently invade and destroy the cochlear, vestibular, and facial nerve trunks and often extend along the nerve bundles as far as the cribrose areas. The inner ear may be invaded by this route (Harbert et al., 1969) (Figs. 11.55, 11.56).

C. OTHER NEOPLASTIC DISEASES

1. LEUKEMIA

Leukemia is a disease characterized by greatly increased production of white blood cells, the failure of many of the cells to reach maturity, and the

Fig. 11.55: At the age of 59, the patient had a radical mastectomy for a small adenocarcinoma. One month later she experienced nausea, dizziness, headache, ataxia and deafness. Pneumoencephalogram revealed a left cerebellar space-occupying lesion which was treated by irradiation. She died one year later of generalized carcinomatosis. Histological study of the left ear reveals nests and columns of tumor cells within the vestibular and cochlear nerve trunks. See Fig. 11.56.

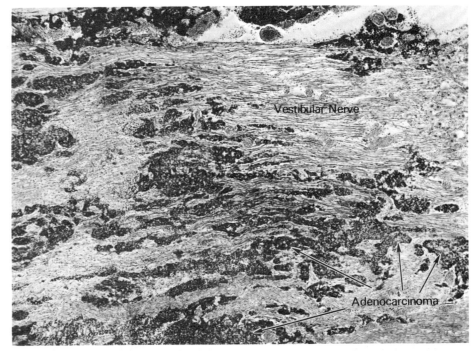

Fig. 11.56: Same case as Fig. 11.55. Metastatic adenocarcinoma is found throughout the cochlear and vestibular nerve trunks extending into the cribrose areas but not into the inner ear.

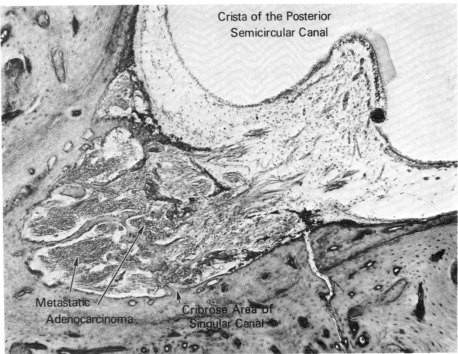

deposition of such cells not only at the normal sites of their formation but also in the interstices of organs where they are not ordinarily found. Abnormal leukemic cells usually appear in large numbers in the circulating blood. The types commonly recognized are (1) myeloid leukemia, (2) lymphatic leukemia, and (3) monocytic leukemia (Anderson, 1966).

All varieties may occur in acute, subacute, or chronic forms and all are characterized by hemorrhagic tendency and severe anemia. The disorder is slightly more common in males.

Deafness in leukemia was first described by Donné (1844) and then by Vidal (1856). The first histological account of leukemia of the inner ear was presented by Politzer (1884). His patient experienced bilateral severe deafness one year prior to death, and histological examination revealed degeneration of the membranous labyrinths and new bone growth in the cochleas.

Schwabach (1897) and Alexander (1906) performed histological studies on temporal bones of leukemic patients and stressed the high incidence of involvement of the middle and inner ears. Numerous studies since that time (Fraser, 1928; Druss, 1945; Hallpike and Harrison, 1950; Schuknecht et al., 1965; Zechner and Altmann, 1969) have shown that leukemic involvement

445   Neoplastic Growth

of the temporal bone takes two main forms: (1) leukemic infiltration and (2) hemorrhage.

A uniform finding in the temporal bones of patients dying of leukemia is intense infiltration and replacement of the bone marrow by leukemic cells (Fig. 11.57). The tympanic membrane and the mucous membrane of the pneumatized spaces of the temporal bone may be thickened by leukemic infiltrates (Fig. 11.58). The remaining spaces often contain an inflammatory exudate with free-floating leukemic cells. Infiltrates are also frequently found in the perilymphatic spaces of the inner ear. Lowered resistance of the individual frequently leads to secondary bacterial infection of the middle ear and mastoid.

Hemorrhages are commonly found in association with leukemic infiltrates (Fig. 11.59). In the middle ear and mastoid these may consist of isolated small hemorrhages or massive hemorrhage. Hemorrhage into the inner ear may result in sudden hearing loss and/or disequilibrium. Hallpike and Harrison (1950) found extensive leukemic infiltrates and hemorrhage in the vestibular labyrinth of a 43-year-old leukemic patient who had experienced a sudden vertiginous episode ten days prior to death. Schuknecht et al. (1965) found a massive hemorrhage in the cochlea and vestibular labyrinth of an 11-year-old patient with acute leukemia who experienced sudden profound hearing loss and vertigo six days prior to death (see Chapter 8A2, Hemorrhage into the inner ear).

In a study of 148 cases of leukemia, Druss (1945) found hearing loss in 25 cases (16.8 percent) of which 9 (6 percent) were of the sensorineural type.

2. MULTIPLE MYELOMA

Multiple myeloma is a distinctive malignant disease of the skeleton having pathological and clinical features which differentiate it from other disorders of myeloid formative tissue. This disease is characterized by decline of hemoglobin and erythrocyte values, depletion of leukopoietic marrow, myeloma cells in blood smears and biopsy tissue, hypercalcemia, and Bence-Jones proteinuria. Marrow obtained by sternal puncture is often of great value in establishing the diagnosis. The majority of patients are in the age range between 40 and 60 years with a slightly higher incidence in males. The progress of the disease is variable, with the average patient surviving about two years. Eventually almost every bone in the body, including the calvarium, may become involved; however, sites of predilection are the vertebral column and long bones. The presence of numerous rounded, punched-out rarifications of the calvarium is strong presumptive evidence for multiple myeloma.

The characteristic histological picture is that of large aggregates or sheets of compact cells without any discernible intercellular material and without conspicuous supporting stroma. The tumors can be fitted into two general cytologic types, one having uniform small cells representing plasma cells, and the other dominated by larger cells which generally exceed the myoblast in size and show abundant cytoplasm and large, round, pale, stippled nuclei. In any particular tumor site one may find both histologic types.

The temporal bone is frequently involved in the terminal stages of the disease and shows replacement of bone marrow with myeloma cells, infiltrates in the mucous membrane, and discrete punched-out lesions of the bony structures (Fig. 11.60).

Any symptoms referable to temporal bone involvement are overshadowed by the manifestations of diffuse skeletal disease (Lichtenstein and Jaffe, 1947).

3. TERATOMA

Teratomas are true tumors composed of various tissues of ectodermal, mesodermal, and entodermal origin showing a haphazard organization, having no useful function, and occurring in an area foreign to the one in which

Fig. 11.57: Acute myelogenous leukemia in a 38-year-old male. There are extensive leukemic infiltrates into the tympanic membrane and mucous membrane of the middle ear. The middle ear space contains exudate with numerous free-floating leukemic cells. The bone marrow is replaced by leukemic cells, and there is hemorrhage into the central mastoid tract. The inner ear appears normal.

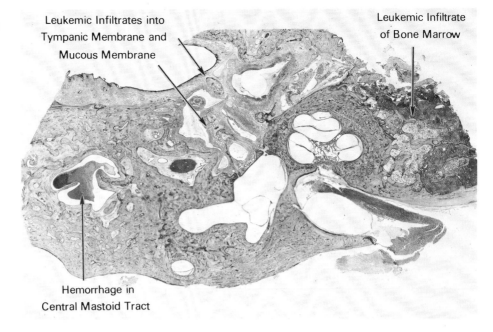

Leukemic Infiltrates into
Tympanic Membrane and
Mucous Membrane

Leukemic Infiltrate
of Bone Marrow

Hemorrhage in
Central Mastoid Tract

Fig. 11.58: Acute lymphatic leukemia in a 9-year-old male. This patient complained of ear pain, was found to have a hyperemic tympanic membrane and tender mastoid and was given antibiotic therapy. He died ten days later. Histological study shows the tympanic membrane and the mucous membrane of the middle ear to be thickened by infiltration with lymphocytes, edema, and hypervascularity. There is exudate in the middle ear containing numerous small round cells and a few polymorphonuclear leucocytes. There are hemorrhages in the inner ear. See also Fig. 11.59.

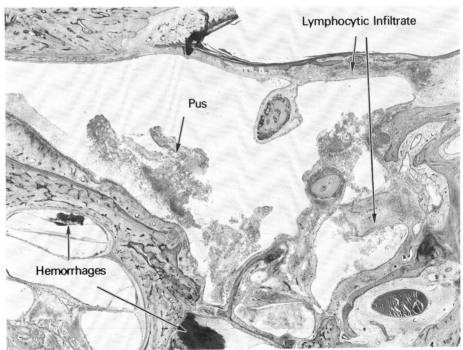

Lymphocytic Infiltrate

Pus

Hemorrhages

Fig. 11.59: Same case as Fig. 11.58. There are hemorrhages in the scala vestibuli of the apical turn, the perilymphatic space of the vestibule, and in the macula sacculi. The sensory and neural structures appear normal. This individual did not complain of hearing loss or vertigo; however, these symptoms, if present, could have been masked by the more severe systemic manifestations of the disease.

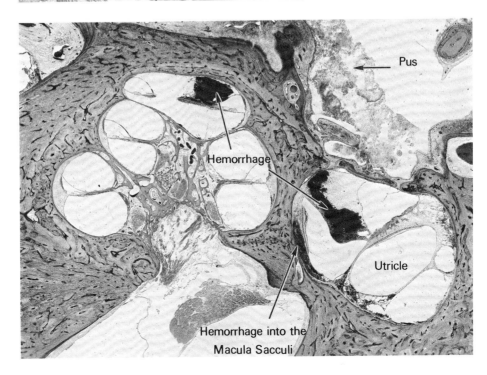

Pus

Hemorrhage

Utricle

Hemorrhage into the
Macula Sacculi

447   Neoplastic Growth

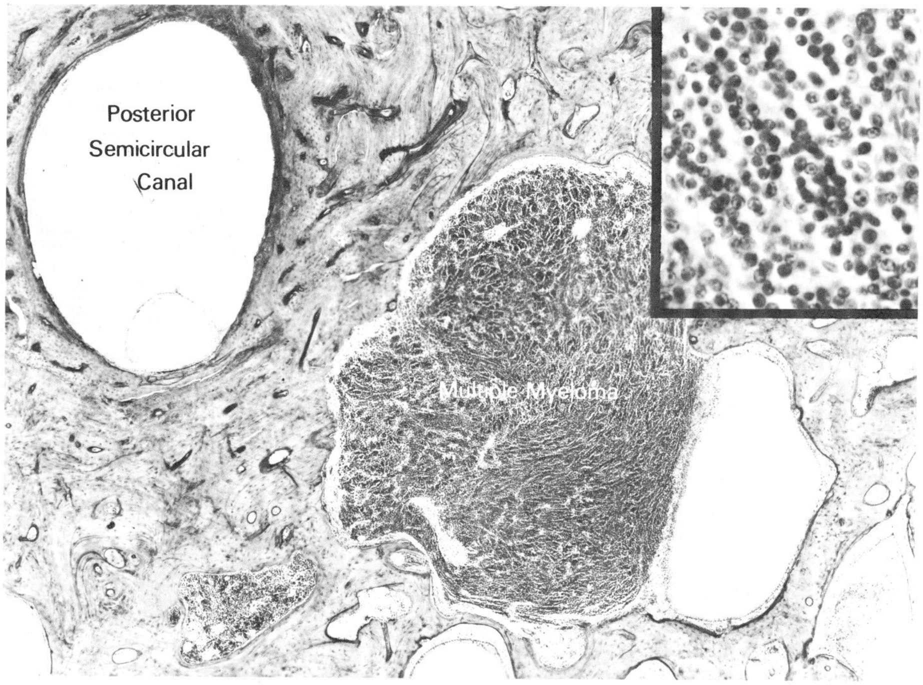

Fig. 11.60: Multiple myeloma involving the temporal bone. At the age of 66 this woman first complained of back pain and was found to have myeloma involving the sacrum. The disease subsequently became disseminated, and she received chemotherapeutic drugs and x-ray therapy but died at the age of 69 of disseminated disease and terminal pulmonary emboli. She had no auditory or vestibular symptoms. Histological studies of the temporal bones show tumor tissue replacing marrow of the petrous apices and in some of the spaces in the mastoids. There are also several discrete osteolytic lesions in the bony labyrinths. The neoplastic tissue consists of sheets of compact cells with no discernible intercellular material. The cells are small and have round, stippled nuclei which substantially fill the cells and resemble plasma cells.

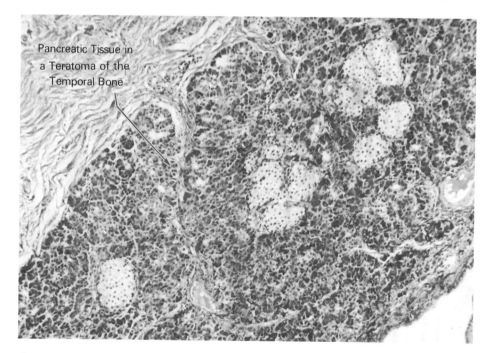

Posterior Semicircular Canal

Multiple Myeloma

Fig. 11.61: Teratoma of the temporal bone. Pancreatic tissue with island of Langerhans appearing in a large teratoma of the temporal bone, which was removed surgically from a 22-year-old female.

Pancreatic Tissue in a Teratoma of the Temporal Bone

the tissues normally reside. The most common sites for teratoma formation in order of frequency are the ovaries, testes, retroperitoneal region, anterior mediastinum, presacral and coccygeal regions, and the base of the skull. They usually occur in tissues which developmentally occupy immediately preaxial, median, or nearly median positions. Teratomas involving the temporal bone are relatively rare. Adam and Gilmour (1930) reported a teratoma of the external auditory canal, Carli and André (1958) observed a large teratoma in the mastoid bone, and Navrátil (1965) described one in the middle ear and another in the eustachian tube. In 1966 Schuknecht removed a huge teratoma from the temporal bone of a 22-year-old woman who had exhibited a post-auricular mass since early childhood. Microscopic examination of the surgical specimen revealed a conglomeration of mature tissues derived from all three germ layers. Part of the tumor consisted of brain tissue which was interlaced and surrounded by irregular connective tissue septa. The tumor also contained ciliated respiratory epithelium, cysts lined with low cuboidal epithelium, intestinal mucous membrane, fatty tssue, mucous glands, hyaline cartilage, nerves, blood vessels, and pancreatic parenchyma with numerous Langerhans' islands and ducts (Fig. 11.61) (Reported by Silverstein et al., 1967).

References

Adam, J., and Gilmour, M., 1930: Teratoid tumor of external auditory meatus. J. Laryng. 45:550.

Alexander, G., 1906: Ueber lymphomatose Ohrenkrankungen: Die Erkrankungen des Gehörorgans bei Leukämie, Chlorom, und der verwandten Krankheiten. Z. Hals-Nas.Ohrenheilk. 7:331.

Alexy, Z., 1968: Fall eines Rhabdomyosarkoms im Mittelohr. Mschr. Ohrenheilk. 102:15.

Alford, B., and Guilford, F., 1962: A comprehensive study of tumors of the glomus jugulare. Laryngoscope 72:765.

Anderson, W., 1966: Bones. In Pathology, 5th ed., Vol. II, C. V. Mosby Co., St. Louis, Mo.

Antoni, N., 1920: Über Rückenmarkstumoren und Neurofibrome. J. F. Bergmann. Wiesbaden.

Ash, J., Beck, M., and Wilkes, J., 1964: Tumors of the upper respiratory tract and ear. In Atlas of Tumor Pathology. Armed Forces Institute of Pathology, Washington, D.C.

Batsakis, J., Hardy, G., and Hishiyama, R., 1967: Ceruminous gland tumors. Arch. Otolaryng. 86:66.

Benitez, J., Lopez-Rios, G., and Novoa, V., 1967: Bilateral acoustic neuroma: A human temporal bone report. Arch. Otolaryng. 86:25.

Bradley, W., and Maxwell, J., 1954: Neoplasms of the middle ear and mastoid: Report of fifty-four cases. Laryngoscope 64:533.

Broders, A., 1921: Epithelioma of the ear: A study of 63 cases. Surg. Clin. N. Amer. 1:1401.

Burman, S., 1955: The vagal body tumor. Ann. Surg. 141:488.

Carli, J., and André, J., 1958: Tumeur dysembryoplasique d'ordre tératologique de la région temporo-mastoidienne. Ann. oto-laryng., Paris 75:791.

Conley, J., 1965: Cancer of the middle ear. Ann. Otol. Rhinol. Laryng. 74:555.

Conte, R., and Sagerman, R., 1971: Embryonal rhabdomyosarcoma of the middle ear with long-term survival. New Eng. J. Med. 284:92.

Costellano, F., and Ruggiero, G., 1953: Meningiomas of the posterior fossa. Acta radiol. Suppl. 104:1.

Coventry, M., and Dahlin, D., 1957: Osteogenic sarcoma, a critical analysis of 430 cases. J. Bone Jt. Surg. 39-A:741.

Crabbe, F., 1966: Le Neurinome de l'acoustique vu par l'otologiste. Acta oto-rhinolaryng. belg. 20:33.

Cushing, H., 1917: Tumors of the Nervus Acusticus and the Syndrome of the Cerebellopontile Angle. W. B. Saunders, Philadelphia, Pa.

Cushing, H., 1935: Intracranial Tumors. Charles C. Thomas, Springfield, Ill.

Dahlin, D., 1957: General aspects and analysis of 2,276 cases. In Bone Tumors. Charles C. Thomas, Springfield, Ill.

Dandy, W., 1934: Removal of cerebellopontile (acoustic) tumors through a unilateral approach. Arch. Surg. 29:337.

De Moura, L., 1967: Inner ear pathology in acoustic neurinoma. Arch. Otolaryng. 85:125.

De Moura, L., 1968: Discussion, in Meniere's Disease. Edited by J. Pulec, W. B. Saunders, Philadelphia, Pa., p. 347.

De Moura, L., Hayden, R., and Conner, G., 1969: Further observations on acoustic neurinoma. Trans. Amer. Acad. Ophthal. Otolaryng. 73:60.

Dill, J., 1959: Tumors of the glomus jugularis. A report of nine cases. Ann. Otol. Rhinol. Laryng. 68:248.

Dix, M., and Hallpike, C., 1950: Observations on the pathological mechanism of conductive deafness in certain cases of neuroma of the VIIIth nerve. J. Laryng. 64:658; Proc. Roy. Soc. Med. 43:291.

Donné, A., 1844: Cours de microscopie complémentaire des études médicales, anatomie, microscopique et, physiologie des fluides de l'économie. J. B. Baillière, Paris.

Druss, J., 1945: Aural manifestations of leukemia. Arch. Otolaryng. 42:267.

Dykstra, P., 1964. The pathology of acoustic neuromas. Arch. Otolaryng. 80:605.

Edwards, C., and Paterson, J., 1951: A review of the symptoms and signs of acoustic neurofibromata. Brain 74:144.

Erickson, L., Sorenson, G., and McGavran, M., 1965: A review of 140 acoustic neurinomas (neurilemmoma). Laryngoscope 75:601.

Figi, F., and Hempstead, B., 1943: Malignant tumors of the middle ear and the mastoid process. Arch. Otolaryng. 37:149.

Fraser, J., 1928: Affections of the labyrinth and eighth nerve in leukemia. Ann. Otol. Rhinol. Laryng. 37:361.

Friedmann, I., and Bird, E., 1960: Electron-microscope investigation of experimental rhabdomyosarcoma. J. Path. 97:375.

Friedmann, I., Harrison, D., Tucker, W., and Bird, E., 1965: Electron microscopy of a rhabdomyosarcoma of the ear. J. Clin. Path. 18:63.

Furstenberg, A., 1924: Primary adenocarcinoma of the middle ear and mastoid. Ann. Otol. Rhinol. Laryng. 33:677.

Gardner, W., and Frazier, C., 1930: Hereditary deafness due to bilateral acoustic tumors. A clinical study and field survey of a family of five generations with a history of deafness in thirty-eight members. Ann. Otol. Rhinol. Laryng. 39:974.

Gardner, W., and Turner, O., 1940: Bilateral acoustic neurofibromas; further clinical and pathologic data on hereditary deafness and Recklinghausen's disease. Arch. Neurol. Chicago 44:76.

Gejrot, T., 1964a: Retrograde jugularography in the diagnosis of abnormalities of the superior bulb of the internal jugular vein. Acta oto-laryng. 57:177.

Gejrot, T., 1964b: Jugular syndrome, with special reference to the diagnostic value of retrograde jugularography. Acta oto-laryng. 57:450.

Gejrot, T., 1965: Surgical treatment of glomus jugulare tumours, with special reference to the diagnostic value of retrograde jugularography. Acta oto-laryng. 60:150.

Gejrot, T., and Laurén, T., 1964a: Retrograde venography of the internal jugular veins and transverse sinuses: Technique and roentgen anatomy. Acta oto-laryng. 57:556.

Gejrot, T., and Laurén, T., 1964b: Retrograde jugularography in diagnosis of glomus tumours in the jugular region. Acta oto-laryng. 58:191.

Glasscock, M., III, 1969: Middle fossa approach to the temporal bone: An otologic frontier. Arch. Otolaryng. 90:15.

Gonzalez-Revilla, A., 1947: Neurinomas of the cerebellopontile recess: clinical study of 160 cases including operative mortality and end results. Bull. Johns Hopkins Hosp. 80:254.

Gonzalez-Revilla, A., 1948: Differential diagnosis of tumors at the cerebellopontile recess. Bull. Johns Hopkins Hosp. 83:187.

Greifenstein, A., 1936: Zur Kenntnis der isolierten Facialisneurome. Arch. Ohr.-Nas-KehlkHeilk. 142:50.

Grubb, W., Jr., and Lampe, I., 1965: The role of radiation therapy in the treatment of chemodectomas of the glomus jugulare. Laryngoscope 75:1861.

Guild, S., 1941: A hitherto unrecognized structure, the glomus jugularis, in man. Anat. Rec. 79:28.

Guild, S., 1953: The glomus jugulare, a non-chromaffin paraganglion, in man. Ann. Otol. Rhinol. Laryng. 62:1045.

Hallberg, O., Uihlein, A., and Siekert, R., 1959: Sudden deafness due to cerebellopontine-angle tumor. Arch. Otolaryng. 69:160.

Hallpike, C., and Harrison, M., 1950: Clinical and pathological observations on a case of leukaemia with deafness and vertigo. J. Laryng. 64:427.

Hambley, W., Gorshenin, A., and House, W., 1964: The differential diagnosis of acoustic neuroma. Arch. Otolaryng. 80:708.

Harbert, F., Liu, J. C., and Berry, R., 1969: Metastatic malignant melanoma to both VIIIth nerves. J. Laryng. 83:889.

Hardy, M., and Crowe, S., 1936: Early asymptomatic acoustic tumors: report of six cases. Arch. Surg. 32:292.

Henschen, F., 1915: Zur Histologie und Pathogenese der Kleinhirnbrückenwinkeltumoren. Arch. Psychiat. Nervenkr. 56:20.

Hilding, D., and House, W., 1965: "Acoustic neuroma": Comparison of traumatic and neoplastic. J. Ultrastruct. Res. 12:611.

Hippel, E. von, 1904: Über eine sehr seltene Erkrankung der Netzhaut. Graefes Arch. Ophthal. 59:83.

Hitselberger, W., and Gardner, G., Jr., 1968: Other tumors of the cerebellopontine angle. Arch. Otolaryng. 88:712.

Hitselberger, W., and House, W., 1966: Classification of acoustic neuromas. Arch. Otolaryng. 84:245.

House, W., 1961: Surgical exposure of the internal auditory canal and its contents through the middle, cranial fossa. Laryngoscope 71:1363.

House, W., 1964a: Evolution of transtemporal bone removal of acoustic tumors. Arch. Otolaryng. 80:731.

House, W., 1964b: Differential diagnosis of cerebellopontine angle lesions. Laryngoscope 74:1283.

House, H., and House, W., 1964: Historical review and problem of acoustic neuroma. Arch. Otolaryng. 80:601.

Igarashi, M., Alford, B., Herndon, J., and Saito, R., 1971: Cerebellopontine meningiomas and the temporal bone. Arch. Otolaryng. 94:224.

Jaffe, B., Fox, J., and Batsakis, J., 1971: Rabdomyosarcoma of the middle ear and mastoid. Cancer 27:29.

Johnstone, J., Lennox, B., and Watson, A., 1957: Five cases of hidradenoma of external auditory meatus: so-called ceruminoma. J. Path. Bact. 73:421.

Juby, H., 1957: Tumours of the ceruminous glands—so-called ceruminoma. J. Laryng. 71:832.

Karatay, S., 1949: Rhabdomyosarcoma of the middle ear. Arch. Otolaryng. 50:330.

Kawabata, I., Duvall, A., III, and Paparella, M., 1969: Ultrastructure of the glomus jugulare tumor. Arch Ohr. Nas.-Kehlk-Heilk. 195:97.

Kos, C., 1940: Tumor of the facial nerve within the mastoid bone. Ann. Otol. Rhinol. Laryng. 49:151.

Kretschmann, F., 1886: Ueber Carcinome des Schläfenbeines. Arch. Ohr.Nas.-KehlkHeilk. 24:231.

Lange, W., 1929: Kleine Acusticustumoren. Z. Hals-Nas.-Ohrenheilk. 23:1.

Lattes, R., and Waltner, J., 1949: Nonchromaffin paraganglioma of the middle ear. Cancer 2:447.

LeCompte, P., 1951: Tumors of the carotid body and related structures (chemoreceptor system). In Atlas of Tumor Pathology. Sect. 4. Fascicle 16. Armed Forces Institute of Pathology, Washington, D.C.

Leonard, J., and Talbot, M., 1970: Asymptomatic acoustic neurilemoma. Arch. Otolaryng. 91:117.

Lewis, J., 1960: Cancer of the ear: A report of 150 cases. Laryngoscope 70:551.

Lichtenstein, L., and Jaffe, H., 1947: Multiple myeloma: A survey based on thirty-five cases, eighteen of which came to autopsy. Arch. Path. 44:207.

Lindbom, A., Soderberg, G., and Spjut, H., 1961: Primary chondrosarcoma of bone. Acta radiol. 55:81.

Litton, W., and McCabe, B., 1966: III.

Neural vs. sensory lesion: Vestibular signs. Laryngoscope 76:1113.

Lukens, R., 1936: Adenocarcinoma of the external auditory canal. Ann. Otol. Rhinol. Laryng. 45:567.

Luse, S., 1960: Electron microscopic studies of brain tumors. Neurology 10:881.

Marshall, R., and Horn, R., 1961: Nonchromaffin paraganglioma: A comparative study. Cancer 14:779.

Marx, H., 1926: Die Geschwülste des Ohres. In Handbuch der Speziellin Pathologischen Anatomie und Histologie. Chap. V. Julius Springer, Berlin.

McCabe, B., and Fletcher, M., 1969: Selection of therapy of glomus jugulare tumors. Arch. Otolaryng. 89:156.

Melmon, K., and Rosen, S., 1964: Lindau's disease: Review of literature and study of large kindred. Amer. J. Med. 36:595.

Miller, D., Silverstein, H., and Gacek, R., 1972: Cryosurgical treatment of carcinoma of the ear. Trans. Amer. Acad. Ophthal. Otolaryng. 76:1363.

Montgomery, W., Ojemann, R., and Weiss, A., 1966: Suboccipital-translabyrinthine approach for acoustic neuroma. Arch. Otolaryng. 83:566.

Mulligan, R., 1950: Chemodectoma in the dog. Amer. J. Path. 26:680.

Murray, M., 1942: Comparative data on tissue culture of acoustic neurilemmoma and meningioma. J. Neuropath. Exp. Neurol. 1:123.

Myers, E., Newman, L., Kaseff, L., and Black, F., 1971: Glomus jugulare tumor: A radiographic-histologic correlation. Laryngoscope 81:1838.

Myers, E., Stool, S., and Weltschew, A., 1968: Rhabdomyosarcoma of the middle ear. Ann. Otol. Rhinol. Laryng. 77:949.

Naessen, R., 1965: Sweat gland adenoma of the external auditory canal—ceruminoma. J. Laryng. 79:637.

Nager, F., 1938: Ueber die Knochenopathologie der Labyrinthkapsel. Acta oto-laryng. 26:127.

Nager, G., 1964a: Association of bilateral VIIIth nerve tumors with meningiomas in von Recklinghausen's disease. Laryngoscope 74:1220.

Nager, G., 1964b: Meningiomas Involving the Temporal Bone: Clinical and Pathological Aspects. Charles C. Thomas, Springfield, Ill.

Nager, G., 1969: Acoustic neurinomas: Pathology and differential diagnosis. Arch. Otolaryng. 89:252.

Navrátil, J., 1965: Teratome der Paukenhöhle und der Tuba Eustachii. Acta oto-laryng. 60:360.

New England Journal of Medicine, 1969: Presentation of a case; case records of the Massachusetts General Hospital. New Eng. J. Med. 275:950.

Ojemann, R., Montgomery, W., Weiss, A., 1972: Evaluation and surgical treatment of acoustic neuroma. New Eng. J. Med. 287:895.

Olivecrona, H., 1940: Acoustic tumors. J. Neuropsychiat. 3:141.

Olivecrona, H., 1950: Analysis of results of complete and partial removal of acoustic neuromas. J. Neurol. Neurosurg. Psychiat. 13:271.

Olsen, A., and Horrax, G., 1944: The symptomatology of acoustic tumours with special reference to atypical features. J. Neurosurg. 1:371.

O'Neal, L., and Ackerman, L., 1952: Chondrosarcoma of bone. Cancer 5:551.

O'Neill, P., and Parker, R., 1957: Sweat gland tumours ("ceruminomata") of external auditory meatus. J. Laryng. 71:824.

Panse, R., 1904: Ein Gliom des Akustikus. Arch. Ohr. Nas.-KehlkHeilk. 61:251.

Penfield, W., 1927: Encapsulated tumors of the nervous system; meningeal fibroblastomata, perineural fibroblastomata and neurofibromata of von Recklinghausen. Surg. Gynec. Obstet. 45:178.

Pennybacker, J., and Cairns, H., 1950: Results in 130 cases of acoustic neurinoma. J. Neurol. Neurosurg. Psychiat. 13:272.

Plester, D., 1959: Das Operative Vorgehen bei den Tumoren des Mittleohres. Arch. Ohr. Nas.-KehlkHeilk. 175:517.

Politzer, A., 1883: A Text-book of the Diseases of the Ear and Adjacent Organs. Translated and edited by J. Cassells. H. C. Lea's Son, Philadelphia, Pa., p. 729.

Politzer, A., 1884: Pathologische Veränderungen im Labyrinthe bei Leukämischer Taubheit. Cong. Internat. d'Otol., Compt. Rend. 3:139.

Pool, J., and Pava, A., 1957: The Early Diagnosis and Treatment of Acoustic Nerve Tumors. Charles C. Thomas, Springfield, Ill.

Proctor, B., and Lindsay, J., 1947: Tumors involving the petrous pyramid of the temporal bone. Arch. Otolaryng. 46:180.

Pulec, J., 1969: Facial nerve tumors. Ann. Otol. Rhinol. Laryng. 78:962.

Pulec, J., 1972: Symposium on ear surgery. II. Facial nerve neuroma. Laryngoscope 82:1160.

Pulec, J., and House, W., 1964: Special tests in the early diagnosis of acoustic neuromas. Laryngoscope 74:1183.

Pulec, J., Parkhill, E., and Devine, K., 1963: Adenoid cystic carcinoma (cylindroma) of the external auditory canal. Trans. Amer. Acad. Ophthal. Otolaryng. 67:673.

Quix, F., 1911: Ein Acusticustumor. Arch. Ohr.Nas.-KehlkHeilk. 84:252.

Raimondi, A., Mullan, S., and Evans, J., 1962: Human brain tumors: An electron-microscopic study. J. Neurosurg. 19:731.

Rauch, S., 1969: Terminologische Probleme bei Glomustumoren. Arch. Ohr.Nas.-KehlkHeilk. 195:81.

Robbins, S., 1962: The nervous system. In Textbook of Pathology with Clinical Application. 2nd ed. Chap. 32. W. B. Saunders, Philadelphia, Pa.

Robinson, G., 1931: Malignant tumors of the ear. Laryngoscope 41:467.

Rosenwasser, H., 1945: Carotid body tumor of the middle ear and mastoid. Arch. Otolaryng. 41:64.

Rosenwasser, H., 1968: Glomus jugulare tumors. Arch. Otolaryng. 88:3.

Saito, H., and Baxter, A., 1972: Undiagnosed intratemporal facial nerve neurilemomas. Arch. Otolaryng. 95:415.

Schall, L., 1935: Neoplasms involving the middle ear. Arch. Otolaryng. 22:548.

Schmiegelow, E., 1915: Beitrag zur translabyrinthären Entfernung der Akustikustumoren. Z. Ohrenheilk. 73:1.

Schuknecht, H., 1966: The pathophysiology of angle tumors. In The Vestibular System and Its Diseases. Edited by R. Wolfson. University of Pennsylvania Press, p. 428.

Schuknecht, H., Allam, A., and Murakami, Y., 1968: Pathology of secondary malignant tumors of the temporal bone. Ann. Otol. Rhinol. Otolaryng. 77:5.

Schuknecht, H., Igarashi, M., and Chasin, W., 1965: Inner ear hemorrhage in leukemia: A case report. Laryngoscope 75:662.

Schuknecht, H., and Woellner, R., 1955: An experimental and clinical study of deafness from lesions of the cochlear nerve. J. Laryng. 69:75.

Schuman, R., 1966: Mesenchymal tumors. In Pathology. 5th ed. C. V. Mosby, St. Louis, Mo., Chap. 17.

Schwabach, D., 1897: Über Erkrankungen

des Gehörorgans bei Leukämie. Z. Ohrenheilk. 31:103.

cott, P., and Colledge, L., 1939: Discussion of malignant disease of the ear (excluding the pinna). J. Laryng. 54:576.

hambaugh, G., Jr., Arenberg, I., Barney, P., and Valvassori, G., 1969: Facial neurilemmomas: A study of four diverse cases. Arch. Otolaryng. 90:742.

Silverstein, H., Griffin, W., Jr., and Balogh, K., Jr., 1967: Teratoma of the middle ear and mastoid process: A case with aberrant innervation of the facial musculature. Arch. Otolaryng. 85:243.

Silverstein, H., and Schuknecht, H., 1966: Biochemical studies of inner ear fluid in man: Changes in otosclerosis, Ménière's disease and acoustic neuroma. Arch. Otolaryng. 84:395.

Simpson, I., and Dallachy, R., 1958: A review of tumors of the glomus jugulare with reports of three further cases. J. Laryng. 72:194.

Skinner, H., 1929: Origin of acoustic nerve tumors. Brit. J. Surg. 16:440.

Smith, C., Portelli, F., Hermann, L., and Walike, J., 1971: Facial palsy caused by facial nerve tumor. Laryngoscope 81:1542.

Sorensen, H., 1960: Cancer of the middle ear and mastoid. Acta radiol. 54:460.

Stout, A., 1935: Peripheral manifestations of specific nerve sheath tumor (neurilemoma). Amer. J. Cancer 24:751.

Stout, A., 1949: Tumors of the peripheral nervous system. In Atlas of Tumor Pathology, II. Armed Forces Institute of Pathology, Washington, D.C., p. 6.

Taylor, D., Alford, B., and Greenberg, S., 1965: Metastases of glomus jugulare tumors. Arch. Otolaryng. 82:5.

Towson, C., and Shofstall, W., 1950: Carcinoma of the ear. Arch. Otolaryng. 51:724.

Trail, M., and Chambers, R., 1970: Chemodectomas of the vagal body. Laryngoscope 80:568.

Verocay, J., 1910: Zur Kenntnis der "Neurofibrome". Beitr. path. Anat. 48:1.

Vidal, J-B., 1856: De la leucocythémie splénique, ou de l'hypertrophie de la rate avec altération du sang consistant dans une augmentation considérable du nombre des globules blancs. Gaz. Hebd. Méd. Paris, vol. 3.

Walshe, F., 1931: Intracranial tumours: a critical review. Quart. J. Med. 24:587.

Warren, S., and Gates, O., 1941: Carcinoma of the ceruminous gland. Amer. J. Path. 17:821.

Watzka, M. von, 1943: Die Paraganglien. Handbuch Mikr. Anat. des Menschen 4:262.

Wronski, J., Bryc, S., Kaminski, J., and Chibowski, D., 1964: Chondrosarcoma of cervical spine causing compression of the cord. J. Neurosurg. 21:419.

Yates, E., 1936: Primary carcinoma of the middle ear. Kentucky Med. J. 34:501.

Young, D., Eldridge, R., and Gardner, W., 1970: Bilateral acoustic neuroma in a large kindred. J. Amer. Med. Assn. 214:347.

Young, J., 1942: Functional repair of nervous tissue. Physiol. Rev. 22:318.

Zechner, G., and Altmann, F., 1969: The temporal bone in leukemia: Histological studies. Ann. Otol. Rhinol. Laryng. 78:375.

Zülch, K., 1957: Brain Tumors: Their Biology and Pathology. J. Springer, New York.

12 Disorders of Unknown or Multiple Causes

A. MÉNIÈRE'S DISEASE

Prosper Ménière must be credited with first recognizing this vertiginous syndrome as a separate entity. His original papers describing this disorder, four in number, appeared in Volume XVI of the *Gazette Médicale de Paris* (1861a, 1861b, 1861c, 1861d) and have been translated into German by Blumenbach (1955), into English by Atkinson (1961), and into Spanish by Velasco (1968). In 1842 Ménière performed a postmortem study on the temporal bones of a young girl who had a sudden and severe attack of vertigo and deafness and died five days later. He reported finding a "reddish plastic lymph" in the semicircular canals. It seems improbable, however, that this individual suffered from the same disorder which he described so well nineteen years later

In 1938, Hallpike and Cairns first observed labyrinthine hydrops in the temporal bones of two patients with Ménière's disease who came to autopsy This pathological finding has been confirmed in numerous subsequent reports (Hallpike and Wright, 1940; Lindsay, 1942; Altmann and Fowler, 1943; Schuknecht et al., 1962a). Altmann and Kornfeld in 1965 reviewed the histological findings in the twenty-nine temporal bone reports of Ménière's disease which had appeared in the literature and noted a remarkably uniform type of pathological change characterized by distention of the endolymphatic system with minimal pathological change in the auditory and vestibular sensory epithelium.

1. CLINICAL MANIFESTATIONS

Ménière's disease is characterized by vertiginous episodes, which usually are severe, prolonged, and associated with nausea and vomiting and a sensorineural hearing loss which may be unilateral or bilateral (Williams, 1952; Alford, 1972). The vestibular and auditory symptoms may begin simultaneously, or one may precede the other by days or years. The frequency of attacks is highly variable and long remissions may occur. In a follow-up study

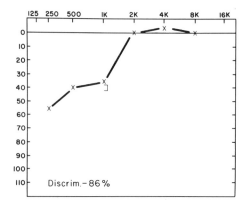

Fig. 12.1: At the age of 28 this patient first experienced episodic vertiginous episodes which recurred at irregular intervals. Repeated audiometric studies were normal until fourteen months later when he suddenly noticed hearing loss, tinnitus, and a feeling of pressure in his left ear. Audiometric studies showed a hearing loss limited to frequencies below 2,000 Hz.

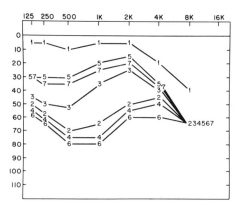

Fig. 12.2: The pure tone audiometric thresholds of this patient with Ménière's disease were determined on seven occasions over a period of four years and showed remarkable fluctuations.

Fig. 12.3: This patient first noted hearing loss in the right ear at the age of 32 and first experienced severe vertiginous episodes with nausea and vomiting at the age of 59. She died at age 65. This photomicrograph shows severe cochlear hydrops in the right ear.

of a large number of patients, Cody (1971) found that 16 percent eventually developed the disease in both ears.

The vertiginous episodes may be preceded by a sensation of fullness or pressure in the ear, increased hearing loss, increased tinnitus, or an alteration in the quality of these symptoms. The onset is frequently sudden, reaching maximum intensity within a few minutes, usually enduring for an hour or more and either subsiding completely or continuing as a sensation of unsteadiness for some hours or days. The attacks are not precipitated by positional changes. Usually, but not always, nystagmus is directed toward the side opposite the involved ear. Vestibular tests frequently show a decreased caloric response in the involved ear. The severity, duration, and frequency of attacks vary greatly in different patients and in the same patient.

The hearing loss is of the sensorineural type and characterized by loudness recruitment, decreased speech discrimination scores, acoustic distortion, and loudness intolerance. Frequently in the early stages of the disease the hearing loss is greater for low frequencies (Fig. 12.1), whereas later the audiometric pattern is flat. Characteristically the hearing fluctuates, particularly in the early stages of the disease, and more for the low frequencies (Fig. 12.2). Decreased hearing may occur immediately preceding or during the vertiginous episodes and for a variable time thereafter. Although it is rare, a total loss of hearing may occur in ears with Ménière's disease. Atypical forms of Ménière's disease are (1) Lermoyez's syndrome in which fluctuation of hearing occurs in reverse relationship to the vertiginous episode; that is, hearing is improved during and immediately after the attack (Lermoyez, 1919); (2) otolithic catastrophe, in which patients experience abrupt falling attacks of fleeting duration (Tumarkin, 1936); (3) cochlear Ménière's disease in which only the characteristic auditory symptoms are present without vertiginous episodes; and (4) vestibular Ménière's disease in which the characteristic vestibular symptoms are present without signs of hearing loss.

2. PATHOLOGY

The principal histological finding is an increase in the volume of endolymph resulting in enormous distention of the endolymphatic system. The distortion of the membranous labyrinth may be accompanied by herniations and ruptures. Sometimes after rupture the membranous labyrinth remains collapsed. The earliest changes are displacement of Reissner's membrane into the scala vestibuli (Fig. 12.3) and dilatation of the saccule (Fig. 12.4). As dilatation progresses, these structures may come to lie against the bony walls; thus, the cochlear duct may occupy the entire scala vestibuli with Reissner's mem-

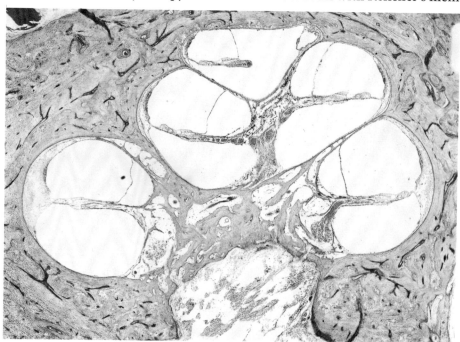

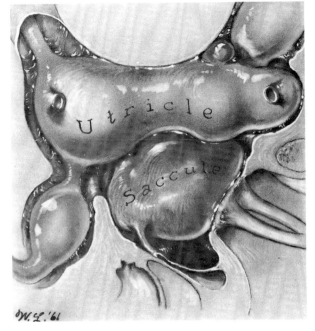

Fig. 12.4: Drawing showing dilatation of the saccule in the right ear of a patient who began having severe vertiginous episodes with nausea and vomiting and progressive right-sided hearing loss at the age of 49. The drawing was made after a three-dimensional model had been developed from serial sections of the ear. The patient died at age 52.

Fig. 12.6: For history see legend, Fig. 12.5. There is severe endolymphatic hydrops. The saccule shows enormous dilatation and herniation into the nonampullated end of the lateral semicircular canal.

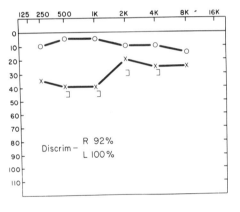

Fig. 12.5: At the age of 52 this woman first experienced severe vertiginous episodes associated with hearing loss and tinnitus in the left ear. Audiometric studies at the age of 56 showed a left sensorineural hearing loss, complete loudness recruitment, and reduced vestibular response to caloric testing. Death occurred at age 59. See Fig. 12.6.

brane abutting the wall of the scala vestibuli while the saccular wall balloons out to make contact with the footplate of the stapes. Sometimes the saccule herniates into the non-ampullated ends of the semicircular canals (Figs. 12.5, 12.6). Reissner's membrane may stretch enormously. At the apex it may herniate through the helicotrema and extend into the scala tympani as far as the second turn, while at its basal end it may balloon into the vestibule and even into the non-ampullated ends of the semicircular canals (Figs. 12.7, 12.8). Usually the dilatation of the utricle and semicircular canals is less severe. Frequently the utricle is displaced posterosuperiorly by the enlarging saccule (Figs. 12.9, 12.10).

Breaks in continuity of the membranous walls are frequent and may involve Reissner's membrane, the saccular wall, and the walls of the utricle and ampullae (Figs. 12.11 to 12.16). Some of these breaks appear to consist of a rupture of the inner cell layer of the membranous labyrinth with an outward bulging of the outer layer, and have been referred to by Altmann and Kornfeld (1965) as "outpouchings."

Ruptures are sometimes followed by collapse of the membranous labyrinth (Figs. 12.17 to 12.20).

Lindsay et al. (1967) found atrophy of the organ of Corti and cochlear neurons in the apical region of the cochlea in two of thirteen ears with Ménière's

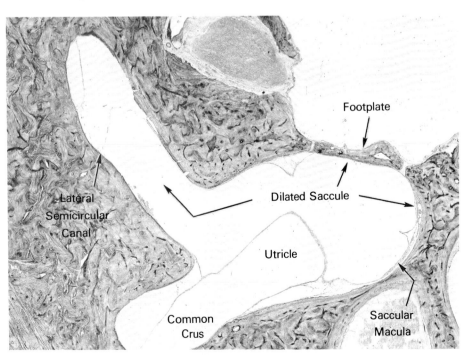

disease. In 1972 Kohut and Lindsay described a similar case. Atrophy of the cochlear neurons of the apical turn is present in three of twenty ears with Ménière's disease in the collection at the Massachusetts Eye and Ear Infirmary (Fig. 12.21). The rarity of atrophic change in the sensory and neural structures has been observed by Schuknecht et al. (1962a) and Altmann and Zechner (1968) (Fig. 12.22).

Several investigators have used the electron microscope to study parts of the membranous labyrinth removed at the time of labyrinthectomy. In several studies the utricular sensory epithelium showed absence of cilia, vesiculation or vacuolization of the cytoplasm, and osmophilic inclusion bodies (Pietrantoni and Iurato, 1960; Litton and Lawrence, 1961; Ireland and Farkashidy, 1963; Friedmann et al., 1963). However, another study (Hilding and House, 1964) showed all of these changes to exist also in the utricles of patients with vestibular schwannomas. Kimura and Schuknecht (1970) examined the stria vascularis in surgical specimens and found atrophic changes which they interpreted to be caused by aging rather than Ménière's disease.

3. PATHOPHYSIOLOGY

a. Elevation of auditory thresholds

The elevation of auditory thresholds cannot be adequately explained on the basis of morphological changes in the structures of the cochlear duct as seen by light microscopy. It is entirely possible, of course, that minor (but important) alterations are present, but undetectable because of postmortem autolysis, preparation artifact, or inadequate resolving power of light microscope techniques. The characteristic flat audiometric pattern suggests that there may be an alteration in the quality of endolymph throughout the cochlear duct. The nature of this change, if it is present, has not been elucidated, as the values for sodium, potassium, and total proteins in the endolymph and perilymph have been found to be normal in Ménière's disease (Silverstein and Schuknecht, 1966).

b. Low-frequency hearing loss

It seems reasonable to associate the low-frequency hearing loss in some way to a functional disorder in the apex of the cochlea. In an experiment utilizing cats it has been demonstrated that apical lesions of the cochlea cause hearing losses which are greater for low frequencies (Schuknecht and Neff, 1952). Degenerative changes restricted to the apical region have been observed in

Fig. 12.7: This man began having attacks of vertigo associated with tinnitus and fluctuating hearing loss in the right ear at the age of 62. The vertiginous episodes recurred over a period of two months after which he had no further attacks. The hearing loss progressed, the last test having been done at the age of 71. Death occurred at age 74. See Fig. 12.8.

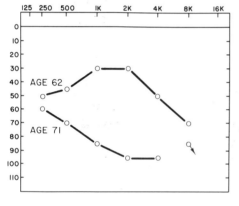

Fig. 12.8: For history see legend, Fig. 12.7. The utricle and saccule are moderately enlarged. The cochlear duct shows an enormous herniation into the vestibule, extending into the nonampullated end of the lateral semicircular canal.

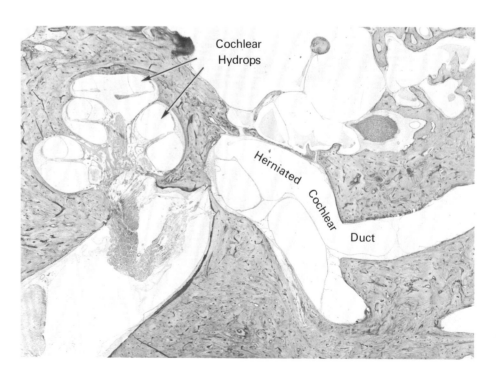

three cases of Ménière's disease (Lindsay and von Schulthess, 1958; Lindsay et al., 1967; Schuknecht, unpublished observation). Most cochleae show no pathological changes in the sensory or neural structures which can be attributed to Ménière's disease. It is of significance that apical lesions in association with endolymphatic hydrops can be produced in animals by destruction of the endolymphatic sac (Kimura and Schuknecht, 1965; Schuknecht et al., 1968).

There are several possible causes for dysfunction of the apical region of the cochlea in Ménière's disease: (1) it is possible that endolymphatic hydrops is associated with a nutritional or metabolic deficiency in the apical region of the cochlea which can lead to atrophic changes in the sensory and neural elements; (2) there may be an alteration in motion mechanics of the cochlear duct (Tonndorf, 1957); and (3) the low-frequency hearing loss may be caused by potassium intoxication of the organ of Corti in the apical region. This theory implies that potassium leaks through Reissner's membrane into the scala vestibuli and reaches the organ of Corti by entering the scala tympani at the apex of the cochlea through the helicotrema. It has been clearly established that endolymph is toxic to the organ of Corti and that toxic fluids can reach the organ only via the scala tympani (see Chapter 3C, The Fluid System).

c. Fluctuations in pure tone thresholds

Fluctuations in pure tone thresholds are common, particularly during the early stages of the disease. Even great threshold losses may be followed by a return to normal within a few days. Temporary losses are probably caused by either chemical alterations in the fluids or by interference with motion mechanics rather than by morphological changes in the sense organs. One possible explanation for the sudden hearing loss is potassium intoxication from leakage of endolymph into the perilymphatic space through ruptures of the membranous labyrinth. This concept derives support from the observation of Tasaki and Fernández (1952) that perfusing the scala tympani with a potassium solution similar to endolymph inhibits the bioelectric activity of the cochlea.

d. Loudness recruitment

Loudness recruitment is a consistent finding in Ménière's disease. Numerous clinical studies have shown that loudness recruitment is associated with hearing losses of sensory origin and is thought to result from abnormal hair

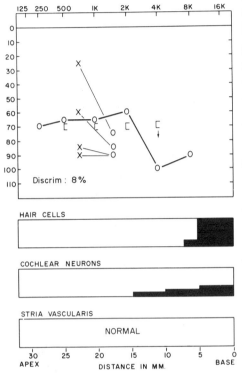

Fig. 12.9: At the age of 51 this woman began having vertiginous episodes and progressive hearing loss in the right ear. From the age of 52 until the time of her death 18 months later she had no attacks of vertigo but felt as if she were tilted to the right and tended to fall to the right. Audiometric studies showed a severe right sensorineural hearing loss with complete loudness recruitment for 1,000 Hz. The 8 percent discrimination score is unusually poor and is not clearly explained by histological studies. Caloric tests showed a greatly decreased response on the right. See Fig. 12.10.

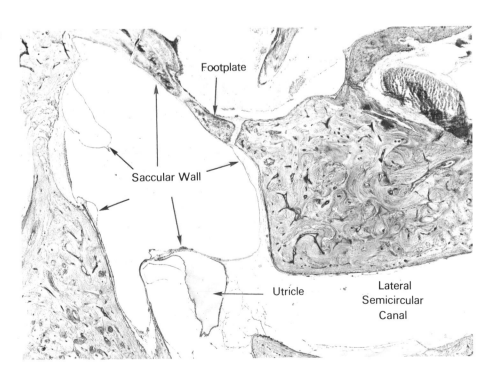

Fig. 12.10: For history see legend, Fig. 12.9. The right ear shows severe endolymphatic hydrops. The enormously dilated saccule occupies most of the space of the vestibule. It has herniated into the sinus of the endolymphatic duct and has displaced the utricle posteriorly.

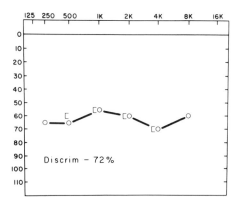

Fig. 12.11: This patient experienced sensori-neural hearing loss in both ears (average loss of about 60 db) associated with episodic vertigo during the last six years of life. The audiogram of the right ear is shown. Death occurred at age 71. See Figs. 12.12 and 12.13.

cell activity. As the hair cell populations are frequently normal in Ménière's disease, hearing loss and recruitment are probably due to an alteration in energy sources, nutrition, metabolism, or biochemistry. For loudness recruitment to exist it appears necessary to have a normal or near normal population of cochlear neurons, a requirement which is met in Ménière's disease (see Chapter 3A5h, Psycho-acoustic manifestations of sensory lesions).

e. Loss of speech discrimination

In Ménière's disease the loss of speech discrimination generally parallels the severity of the hearing loss. It is probably caused by defective stimulus coding by the sense organ because the population of cochlear neurons in these ears is usually normal for age.

f. Episodic vertigo

Episodic vertigo, like fluctuations in hearing, is an expression of sudden alterations in sensory function, presumably due to mechanical, biochemical, nutritional, or metabolic changes of sudden onset. Lawrence and McCabe (1959) and Schuknecht et al. (1962b) have proposed that the spilling of potassium-rich endolymph through ruptures in the distended walls of the membranous labyrinth may cause potassium intoxication of the vestibular nerve fibers. Support for this idea is derived from the animal experiments of Dohlman (1965) and Silverstein (1970) which have shown that perfusion of the perilymphatic space with artificial endolymph produces severe nystagmus. Silverstein has also observed that when this perfusate of artificial endolymph is left in the perilymphatic space, the potassium concentration decreases to normal for perilymph over a period of two to three hours as the nystagmus subsides.

It seems improbable that sudden deformations of the membranous labyrinth, as proposed by Lindsay et al. (1967) and by Altmann and Zechner (1968), are an adequate explanation of the prolonged episodes of vertigo which are so typical of Ménière's disease. On the other hand, it seems reasonable that the fleeting falling attacks, referred to as Tumarkin's otolithic catastrophe, are caused by sudden deformation or displacement of a vestibular sense organ.

4. ETIOLOGY

Numerous proposals have been offered for the etiology of Ménière's disease. Among these are avitaminosis (Selfridge, 1940), sympathetic vaso-motor disturbance (Passe and Seymour, 1948), focal infection (Wright, 1948), acoustic trauma and head blow (Muller, 1950), viral infection (Lempert et al., 1952), allergy (Gundrum, 1953; Derlacki, 1965), endocrine disturbance (God-

Fig. 12.12: For history see legend, Fig. 12.11. This graphic reconstruction shows the location of areas of rupture and atrophy of Reissner's and the tectorial membrane. A photomicrograph made at level A is shown in Fig. 12.13.

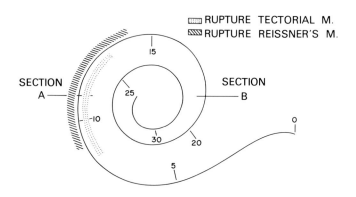

Fig. 12.13: Photomicrograph made at level A shown in Fig. 12.12. In the 9 to 14 mm region of the right cochlea, Reissner's membrane is ruptured and the tectorial membrane is an atrophied encapsulated mass lying on the limbus. Reissner's membrane is collapsed throughout the remainder of the cochlea.

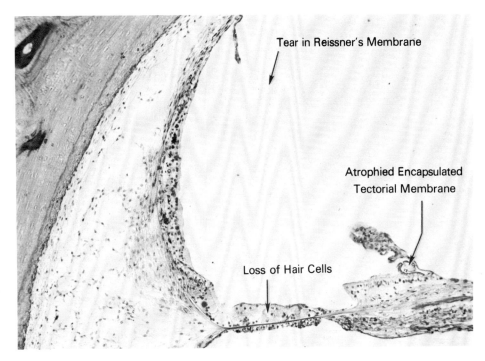

Tear in Reissner's Membrane

Atrophied Encapsulated Tectorial Membrane

Loss of Hair Cells

Fig. 12.14: This patient experienced a slowly progressive bilateral hearing loss for many years. At the age of 73 she began having vertiginous episodes of sudden onset. Audiometric studies showed a bilateral sensorineural hearing loss, much worse on the left. Discrimination score was 28 percent on the right and zero percent on the left. On several occasions she fell at the onset of the vertiginous attacks. Both ears show severe endolymphatic hydrops of the cochlear ducts and vestibular labyrinths. There is a scattered loss of hair cells on the right and 30 to 50 percent loss throughout the cochlea on the left. Both cochleae show patchy atrophy of the striae vasculares in the apical regions and loss of 25 percent of the cochlear neurons to the basal turns. See Figs. 12.15 and 12.25.

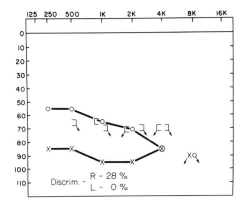

lowski, 1960; Goldman, 1962), psychosomatic disorder (Watson et al., 1967), and others too numerous to mention. A probable hereditary predisposition is indicated by the occasional occurrence of episodic vertigo and hearing loss in families (Brown, 1949; Bernstein, 1965).

There are two findings in the ears of patients with Ménière's disease which seem worthy of mention, although their significance is obscure at this time. First, there is the finding of fibrous proliferation between the distended saccular wall and the footplate of the stapes. This fibrous membrane has been observed both in temporal bone specimens (Figs. 12.23 to 12.25) and during surgical exposure of the oval window (author's observation). Second, there is the occasional appearance of papillary structures within the dilated vestibular end of the cochlear duct and ductus reuniens of some of these ears (Fig. 12.26). The histological appearance is similar to that of the choroid plexus and raises the possibility of secretion of aberrant choroid plexus as a cause for endolymphatic hydrops.

Probably the most significant observation relating to the possible etiology of Ménière's disease has been the experimental production of endolymphatic hydrops in guinea pigs by Naito (1959), and Kimura and Schuknecht

Fig. 12.15: For history see legend, Fig. 12.14. Histological study of the left ear reveals endolymphatic hydrops of both the cochlear duct and vestibular system. This view shows dilatation of the utricle with rupture and herniation of the utricular wall.

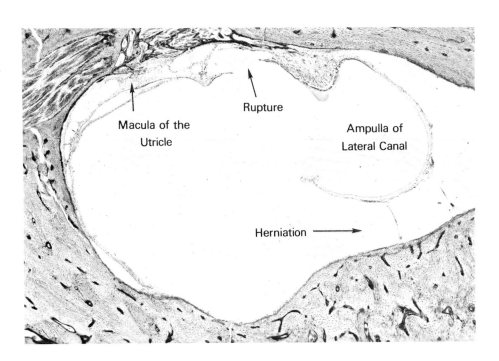

Macula of the Utricle

Rupture

Ampulla of Lateral Canal

Herniation →

Fig. 12.16: Rupture of the ampullary wall of the posterior semicircular canal in a patient with typical Ménière's disease.

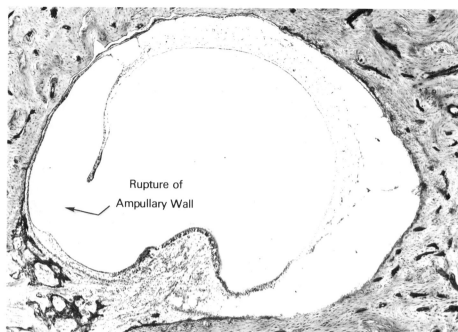

Rupture of
Ampullary Wall

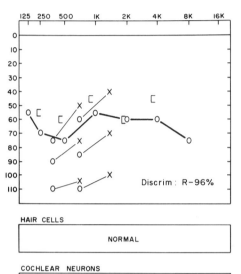

Discrim: R-96%

HAIR CELLS

NORMAL

COCHLEAR NEURONS

STRIA VASCULARIS

30   25   20   15   10   5   0
APEX   DISTANCE IN MM.   BASE

Fig. 12.17: This patient first noted hearing loss in the right ear at the age of 56. This loss was slowly progressive, and seven years later at the age of 63 he experienced the first attack of vertigo associated with nausea and vomiting. During the next eight months he had repeated attacks of severe vertigo and the hearing deteriorated further in the right ear. He had no vertiginous episodes during the final 22 months of life. Audiometric study done five months prior to death revealed a flat audiometric pattern with threshold losses of 60 to 70 db, speech discrimination score of 96 percent, and incomplete loudness recruitment in the involved ear. The hair cell population is normal throughout. There is a 40 to 50 percent loss of cochlear neurons in the basal 20 mm of the cochlea consistent with neural presbycusis. Death occurred at age 66. See also Figs. 12.18 to 12.20.

Fig. 12.18: Same ear as shown in Figs. 12.17 to 12.20. Histological study reveals collapse of the previously distended Reissner's membrane. It is presumed that final rupture and collapse of the membranous labyrinth occurred 22 months before death. In the remaining months he had no further vertiginous episodes.

Fig. 12.19: Same ear as shown in Figs. 12.17 and 12.18. A study of serial sections shows the folded membrane which is in contact with the footplate of the stapes to be a collapsed herniation of the basal end of the cochlear duct. The saccular wall is also collapsed.

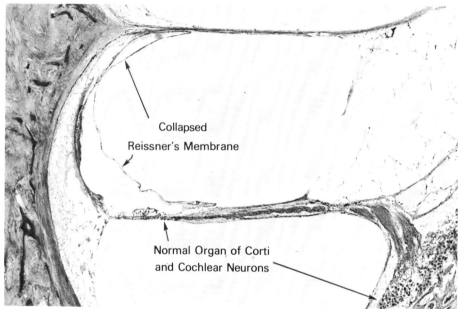

Collapsed
Reissner's Membrane

Normal Organ of Corti
and Cochlear Neurons

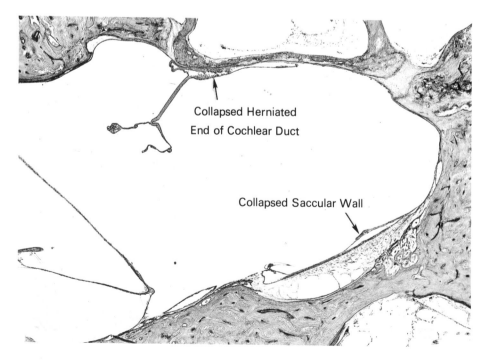

Collapsed Herniated
End of Cochlear Duct

Collapsed Saccular Wall

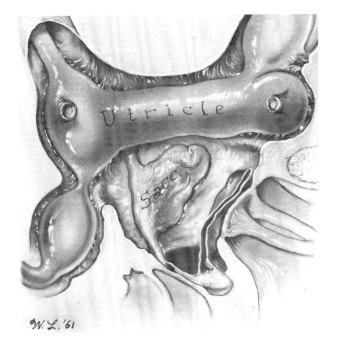

Fig. 12.20: Drawing made from a three-dimensional reconstruction from serial sections of the same ear as shown in Figs. 12.17 to 12.19. There is collapse of both the saccule and the herniated part of the cochlear duct.

Fig. 12.21: This patient had vertiginous episodes and left hearing loss for over 20 years prior to her death at age 86. Histological study of the left ear shows severe endolymphatic hydrops and a loss of cochlear neurons most severe in the apical region. There is a loss of 70 percent of the neurons in the basal end of the cochlea, 40 percent in the remainder of the basal turn and middle turn, and total loss in the apical turn. The right ear without endolymphatic hydrops shows a similar loss of neurons in the basal and middle turns and a normal population in the apical region.

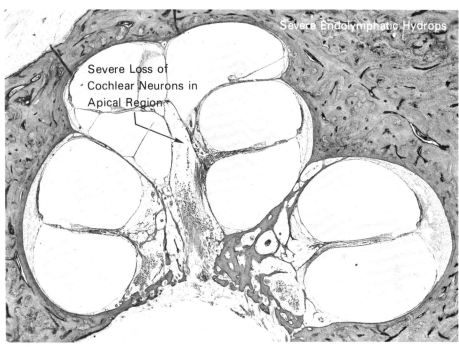

Fig. 12.22: Same ear as shown in Figs. 12.17 to 12.20. The hair cell population throughout the cochlea is normal in spite of a 55 to 80 db sensorineural hearing loss.

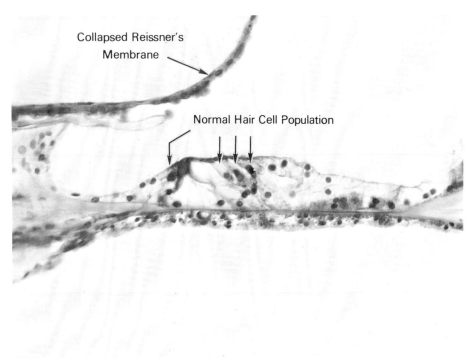

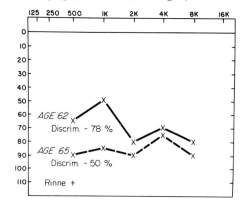

Fig. 12.23: At the age of 62 this man first experienced vertiginous episodes with nausea and vomiting and left hearing loss. The episodic vertigo continued intermittently, the hearing loss progressed and he died at age 67.

(1965), in cats by Schuknecht et al. (1968), and in rabbits by Beal (1968). In these experiments, either blocking the endolymphatic duct or destroying the endolymphatic sac resulted in progressive endolymphatic hydrops. After varying periods of time, degenerative changes were found in the organs of Corti and cochlear neurons, most severe in the extreme apical and basal ends of the cochleae. These findings seem particularly significant in view of the degenerative changes occurring in the sensorineural structures in the apices of the cochleae of some patients with Ménière's disease (Lindsay and von Schulthess, 1958; Lindsay et al., 1967; Schuknecht, unpublished data). Clemis and Valvassori (1968) reported a higher incidence of radiologic nonvisualization of the vestibular aqueduct in Ménière's disease. The vestibular aqueduct is a bony channel through which the endolymphatic duct passes to reach the endolymphatic sac. Yuen and Schuknecht (1972), however, found the vestibular aqueducts of 19 ears exhibiting Ménière's disease to be of similar caliber to ears without Ménière's disease. Considering all the evidence (clinical manifestations, pathological findings, and animal experiments), the most plausible explanation is that Ménière's disease is caused by functional failure of the endolymphatic sac (Arenberg et al., 1970; Gussen, 1971). This hypothesis implies that the loss of resorptive function of the sac results in a slow, progressive accumulation of endolymph with distention of the endolymphatic system, culminating eventually in episodic leakage of endolymph into the perilymphatic system. Thus, the episodes of vertigo and fluctuating hearing could be accounted for by the toxic effect of potassium on the sensory and neural structures which are normally bathed in perilymph.

5. TREATMENT

The management of the acute attack of vertigo consists mainly in the use of sedatives and tranquilizing drugs to control the nausea and vomiting. For the patient with recurring vertiginous episodes, therapy has consisted of regimens involving diets, sedation, diuresis, vitamins, hormones, desensitization, allergic management, vasodilators, and a host of drugs too numerous to mention (Shea and Kitabchi, 1973). Evidence supporting the effectiveness of medical therapy is generally lacking.

In a clinical study Perlman et al. (1953) subjected fifteen patients with active Ménière's disease to measured increases and decreases in sodium serum levels and observed no consistent effects on cochlear or vestibular function,

Fig. 12.24: For history see legend, Fig. 12.23. Histological study reveals severe endolymphatic hydrops. Between the dilated saccular wall and the footplate there is a thin layer of dense fibrous tissue.

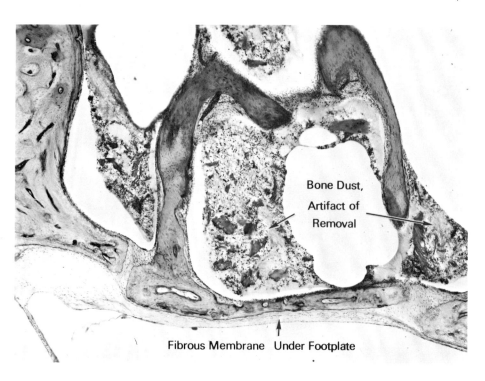

Bone Dust, Artifact of Removal

Fibrous Membrane Under Footplate

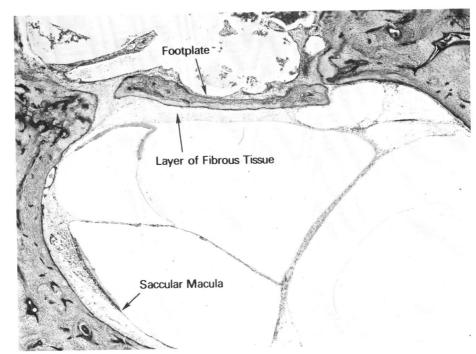

Fig. 12.25: For history see legend, Fig. 12.14. Membranes of the dilated saccule and cochlear duct traverse the vestibule. Between these membranes and the footplate is a dense layer of fibrous tissue.

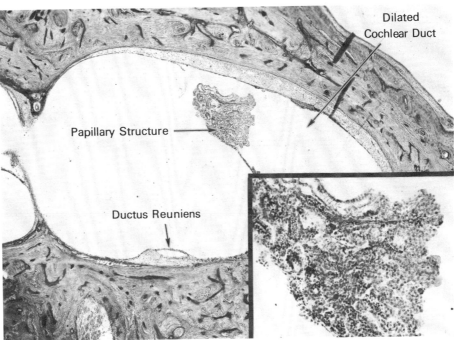

Fig. 12.26: In this ear of a 65-year-old man with typical clinical manifestations and pathological findings of Ménière's disease, there is a papillary structure having a well-developed organoid arrangement in the dilated vestibular end of the cochlear duct. The tissue is histologically similar to choroid plexus.

thus demonstrating the probable lack of therapeutic value of controlled sodium diets in the management of this disease.

Because the disorder is characterized by periods of exacerbation and remission of symptoms, it is difficult to evaluate any treatment. Whether treated or untreated by medical regimens, the vertiginous episodes often continue at irregular intervals for some years. The usual pattern is for the vertiginous attacks to become less severe and for the hearing to stabilize at some level which varies from moderate to severe hearing loss. In some individuals the vertiginous episodes become so frequent and severe as to be socially and occupationally disabling, in which case vestibular ablation may be indicated.

A large number of surgical procedures have been advocated for the patient with disabling unilateral Ménière's disease. A complete description of the surgical procedures which have been advocated, their merits and disadvantages, is not within the scope or purpose of this book. In general, these procedures are designed either to (1) destroy the inner ear completely, (2) selectively ablate vestibular function, or (3) prevent the over-accumulation of endolymph.

Probably the most simple and direct method of destroying the inner ear is transmeatal labyrinthectomy, first described by Lempert (1948) and sub-

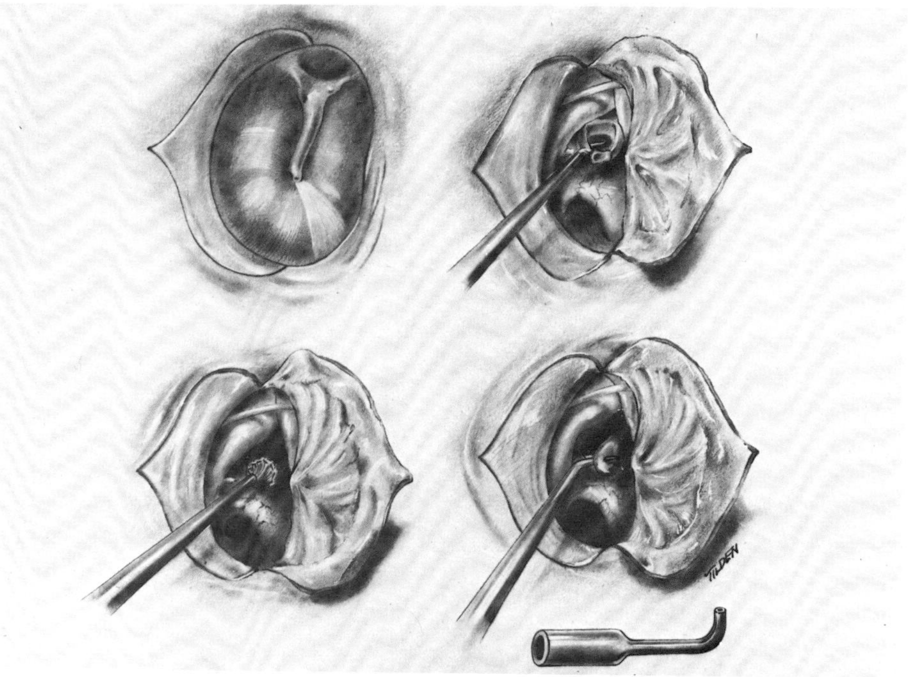

Fig. 12.27: Technique for transmeatal labyrinthectomy. Endaural incisions are made in the skin of the ear canal, and a tympanomeatal flap is elevated to expose the posterior mesotympanum. Fluid may be removed from a small puncture of the footplate to confirm the diagnosis of Ménière's disease (Griffin and Silverstein, 1970). See also Chapter 3C6, Chemistry of the inner ear fluids. The incus and stapes are removed. The oval window is enlarged by removing bone from its inferior margin. The utricular macula is removed, and the ampullated ends of the semicircular canals are probed to disrupt the cristae. The vestibule is filled with Gelfoam or a free graft of adipose tissue from the ear lobe and the tympanomeatal flap is returned to its original position. Rayon cloth strips are placed over the incisions and held in place by a piece of synthetic rubber sponge. This packing is removed one week later.

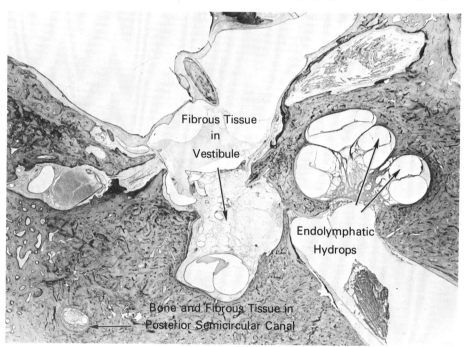

Fig. 12.28: This man experienced a progressive hearing loss in his left ear from the age of 48. Vertiginous episodes began at age 63, and a left labyrinthectomy was performed by the transmeatal approach at the age of 64. He died four months later of unrelated causes. Histological study shows the incus and stapes to be missing. The vestibule and semicircular canals are partly filled with fibrous tissue and bone. The membranous labyrinth is severely degenerated. Cochlear endolymphatic hydrops is present which could have been caused by either pre-existing Ménière's disease or by a response to surgical trauma.

sequently simplified by Schuknecht (1957, 1973), Cawthorne (1957), and Ariagno (1964) (Figs. 12.27, 12.28). Any procedure in which the utricle is removed is almost certain to result in profound loss of all vestibular sensory function and relief of vertiginous episodes. Total ablation of the labyrinth may also be achieved by injection of alcohol into the labyrinth (Wright, 1938, 1942), by electrocoagulation of the labyrinth (Day, 1943, 1952), or by surgical maceration through a fistula in the lateral semicircular canal (Cawthorne, 1943). These procedures are highly successful in alleviating vertiginous episodes and may be utilized for patients with disabling unilateral Ménière's disease who exhibit poor auditory function in the diseased ear.

Selective ablation of vestibular function is most effectively achieved by vestibular nerve section via the posterior cranial fossa (Dandy, 1934; Fluur and Tovi, 1965; Bryan and Bucy, 1973) or via the middle cranial fossa (House, 1961; Fisch, 1973). These procedures are technically demanding and carry some risk of facial nerve injury.

The application of sodium chloride crystals to the round window membrane has been reported to improve the symptomatology (Arslan, 1972); however, the rationale for such therapy is not clear.

The ablation of the vestibular sense organs by the use of ultrasound (Krejci, 1952; Arslan et al., 1963; James et al., 1960; Waltner, 1965; Basek, 1973) and by cryosurgery (Wolfson et al., 1966; House, 1966; Wolfson and Cutt, 1971) have met with some success. A simple procedure which will consistently destroy vestibular function while preserving hearing has not yet been found.

Procedures designed to prevent the over-accumulation of endolymph are the fistulizing operations on the endolymphatic sac (Portmann, G., 1927, 1969; Portmann, M., 1973; House and Hitselberger, 1965; Shambaugh et al., 1969) and the fistulizing operations on the saccule (Fick, 1964; Cody et al., 1967; Cody, 1973). Although some success has been reported with these procedures, there is some question as to whether permanent fistulas can be produced by these methods. Cervicothoracic sympathectomy (Passe and Seymour, 1948) and removal of the stellate ganglion (Golding-Wood, 1960, 1969; Wilmot, 1969) have their advocates but have not gained widespread use.

Experiences with the use of streptomycin sulfate to achieve bilateral ablation of vestibular function for alleviating vertiginous episodes while preserving hearing have been reported by Fowler (1948), Hamberger et al. (1949), Rüedi (1951), Hanson (1951), Schuknecht (1957), Günther (1959), Graybiel et al. (1965), and Singleton and Schuknecht (1968). Relief of vertiginous symptoms is consistently achieved; however, moderately severe ataxia is present for several months following treatment (see Chapter 6A1, Streptomycin).

B. CUPULOLITHIASIS

The term "cupulolithiasis" designates a vestibular disorder which previously has been identified by several names, including postural vertigo, positional vertigo, and positional vertigo of the benign paroxysmal type. Recent pathological studies support the concept that the disorder is caused by an inorganic deposit on the cupula of the posterior semicircular canal which renders this organ sensitive to gravitational force and therefore subject to stimulation with changes in head position. The clinical features of cupulolithiasis are distinctive and serve to differentiate it from positional vertigo caused by lesions of the central nervous system. The diagnosis can be made by inducing the characteristic vestibular manifestations by provocative positional testing.

Bárány (1921) first described the disorder as he observed it in a 27-year-old woman and he wrote as follows:

> The attacks only appeared when she lay on her right side. When she did this, there appeared a strong rotatory nystagmus to the right. The attack lasted about thirty seconds and was accompanied by violent vertigo and nausea. If, immediately after the cessation of the symptoms, the head was again turned to the right no attack occurred and in order to evoke a new attack in this way, the patient had to lie for some time on her back or on her left side.

Bárány and others originally attributed this disorder to lesions in the semicircular canals but, because the dizziness was precipitated by head position and not by head movement, they came to believe that the condition was due to a disorder of the otoliths.

1. SYMPTOMS

The principal complaint of the patient is the occurrence of sudden attacks of vertigo precipitated by certain head positions. Usually the patient volunteers that the attack can be induced by rolling over in bed either to one side or the other but not to both sides. Some state that the attack is provoked by a sudden movement of the head to the right or left, or when extending the neck, as in looking upward, and, more rarely, upon stooping over. Characteristically, there is a severe subjective sensation of disequilibrium which many patients find intensely disagreeable. Those with good motor function rarely fall because the onset, although sudden, is not apoplectiform, so that there is time to grasp for support during the short period of disequilibrium. Aged individuals with a loss of muscle strength and control are more in danger of falling.

Many individuals have mild nausea during and immediately following the attack, and a few experience vomiting.

The sensation of vertigo is usually of short duration (five to ten seconds) which helps to distinguish this condition from other vestibular disorders. Because of the intensity of the vertiginous sensation, affected individuals commonly assign a longer duration to the attack and careful questioning may be required to elicit a reliable history. At the onset of the attack most affected individuals quickly move from the provocative head position and attribute to this the quick termination of the attack; others, however, will relate that if the head is maintained in the provocative position the vertigo will subside in a few seconds.

In many cases the disorder is self-limiting and subsides within a few weeks or months; in others there are remissions and recurrences over time spans of weeks to years and in still others, it is persistent. Some report that the attack is produced only occasionally by the provocative position, a feature which is confirmed by inconsistent responses to the test procedure.

In an attempt to determine a possible etiologic factor, the clinical history should include information relative to recent head injury, ear symptoms (tinnitus, hearing loss, recent or past otorrhea, ear surgery), or a recent severe prolonged vestibular upset.

Although the sex distribution has not been studied, it is Barber's (1964a, 1964b) impression that most patients with the disorder are female.

2. TEST PROCEDURE

After acquiring the history, the diagnosis of cupulolithiasis usually can be promptly confirmed by the positional test procedure (Fig. 12.29).

The patient is seated upon an examining table with the head turned to one side and the gaze fixed on the examiner's forehead. The examiner then grasps the head in his hands and briskly places the patient into the supine head-hanging position. The head should be placed below the level of the table and 30 to 40 degrees to one side. After the position has been assumed, there is a quiescent latent period of one to six seconds (average of three or four seconds). If the vertigo is induced, the patient usually demonstrates a sensation of distress variously manifested by closing the eyes, grasping the examiner, crying out in alarm, and making active efforts to sit up again. If the nystagmus is to be observed, the patient must be instructed, before the test is undertaken, to keep the eyes open. With the eyes in the position of forward gaze the nystagmus is predominantly rotatory. In the right-ear-down position the rotation is to the right (counterclockwise). If the reaction occurs in the left-ear-down position the nystagmus is to the left (clockwise). With the eyes directed toward the uppermost ear the nystagmus is vertical and upward beating. The nystagmus increases in rapid crescendo for three to ten seconds and then rapidly diminishes as the vertigo subsides. The patient is brought back into the sitting position with the head still grasped by the examiner's hands. Almost immediately there is vertigo and nystagmus

Fig. 12.29: This sketch shows the technique for performing the provocative test for cupulolithiasis. When the patient is moved from the sitting to the supine position with the head hanging 30 to 40 degrees and to one side, the labyrinth of the undermost ear is inverted.

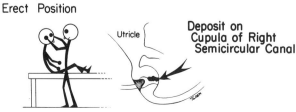

Erect Position

Deposit on
Cupula of Right
Semicircular Canal

Utricle

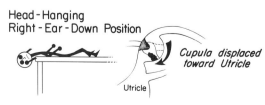

Head-Hanging
Right-Ear-Down Position

Cupula displaced
toward Utricle

Utricle

in reverse direction to that elicited in the previous position, but less severe and for a shorter period of time. Each time the patient is placed into the provocative supine position the reaction is less severe, and often it cannot be elicited more than two or three times. A rest period is required before the phenomenon can be produced again. In the complete test procedure the patient is placed in sequence into both right-ear-down and left-ear-down head-hanging positions.

3. ETIOLOGIC FACTORS

a. Spontaneous degenerative change, vestibular labyrinth

Most affected individuals have no history of antecedent head injury, ear disorder, neurological disease, or ear surgery. They are usually in the fifth, sixth, or seventh decades of life and demonstrate no unusual degenerative changes of aging. Possibly in these cases the disorder is caused by a spontaneous degenerative change in the vestibular labyrinth, consisting specifically of the formation of sediment of high specific gravity (possibly end products of otoconial degeneration) in the endolymph of the pars superior (utricle and canals). The symptoms often subside spontaneously after a few weeks or months, but may recur, and may persist indefinitely. Most patients learn to live with the disorder but consider it an annoyance and wish to be free of it. A few experience disability of sufficient magnitude to require a limitation of social and occupational activities. In aged individuals cupulolithiasis presents as a form of falling disease and may constitute a threat to limb and life.

b. Labyrinthine concussion

Positional vertigo probably is the most common type of vestibular disorder following head injury (Dix and Hallpike, 1952; Cawthorne, 1954; Gordon, 1954; Preber and Silfverskiöld, 1957; Cope and Ryan, 1959; Barber, 1964a, 1964b; Schuknecht, 1969a). Barber (1964b) found this type of positional vertigo in 47 percent of patients with longitudinal fracture of the temporal bone and in 20.8 percent of patients with head injuries of comparable severity but without skull fracture. Characteristically the vertigo occurs when the injured ear is placed in the undermost position during the provocative test procedure (author's observation).

A possible mechanism for the development of positional vertigo following head injury is disruption of the utricular otolithic membrane and release of otoconia into the endolymph of the pars superior.

Postmortem studies of the temporal bone in patients with head injuries thus far have failed to reveal dislodged otoconia, probably because they are absorbed by the decalcification process during histological preparation. Vyslonzil (1963), utilizing a dissection procedure without prior decalcification, found otoconia in the posterior semicircular canals of patients receiving ototoxic doses of streptomycin. Presumably, the reason these patients did not demonstrate positional vertigo was that the function of the posterior canal crista had been abolished by the drug.

c. Otitis media

Dix and Hallpike (1952) were the first to observe that many individuals with the cupulolithiasis syndrome have evidence of previous or current ear infections. In a study of 100 affected individuals evidence of otitis media was found in 26, of which 11 were bilateral and 15 were unilateral. All of the 15 individuals with cupulolithiasis who also showed unilateral evidence of otitis media exhibited nystagmus when the diseased ear was placed undermost during the test procedure.

d. Ear surgery

The cupulolithiasis syndrome is a rare complication of stapes surgery and usually can be attributed to traumatic manipulations within the vestibule. The probable cause in these cases is rupture of the utricular otolithic membrane followed by release of otoconia. Usually the symptom subsides within a few weeks but may persist for months or years. Cupulolithiasis may occur occasionally after other types of temporal bone surgery (fenestration, mastoidectomy, tympanoplasty).

e. Occlusion of the anterior vestibular artery

Lindsay and Hemenway in 1956 described a symptom complex occurring in the latter decades of life which they believed was caused by occlusion of a vessel supplying the vestibular labyrinth. The first manifestation of the disorder was the sudden onset of severe vertigo without deafness or signs of central nervous system disease, followed by gradual recovery over a period of weeks. A second manifestation of the syndrome was the development of positional vertigo, commencing after the original attack had subsided, and persisting for weeks or years. The pathological findings in the temporal bones from a patient with this syndrome were consistent with occlusion of the anterior vestibular artery (Fig. 12.30). This artery supplies the utricular macula and the cristae of the lateral and superior semicircular canals. It seems possible that degeneration of the utricle and its otolithic membrane following loss of blood supply results in release of otoconia which settle upon the cupula of the posterior semicircular canal.

Fig. 12.30: At the age of 65 this patient experienced the sudden onset of severe vertigo associated with vomiting which gradually subsided over a period of one month. Subsequently, she had vertiginous episodes whenever she assumed the supine position with the head turned to the right. The vertigo was readily demonstrated by positional testing. Caloric response was absent in the right ear. The positional vertigo continued until her death 13 years later. Histological study shows degeneration of the superior division of the vestibular nerve and the sense organs supplied by it (utricular macula, superior and lateral canal cristae) in the right ear only. (Courtesy of Lindsay)

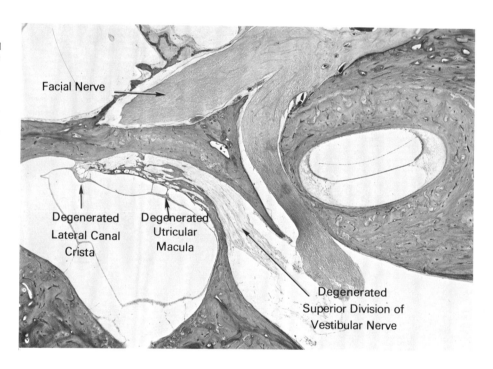

4. PATHOLOGY

Dix and Hallpike (1952), Lindsay and Hemenway (1956), and Cawthorne and Hallpike (1957) reported the pathological findings in the temporal bones of patients with the typical cupulolithiasis syndrome. All three cases showed degeneration of the superior division of the vestibular nerve, the utricular macula, and the cristae of the superior and lateral semicircular canals. In each ear the crista and nerve to the posterior canal appeared intact; however, postmortem autolysis and artifact precluded assessment of their cupulae. It seems probable that these three cases represent cupulolithiasis caused by occlusion of the anterior vestibular artery.

Schuknecht (1969b) reported the findings in two patients with cupulolithiasis presumed to be caused by spontaneous degenerative change in the vestibular labyrinth. Both were female and demonstrated all parameters of the classical syndrome which could be provoked in the supine left-ear-down

Fig. 12.31: At the age of 69, the patient first experienced paroxysmal attacks of vertigo precipitated by stooping over, lying down, and in particular, when rolling onto the left side. On two occasions she fell to the floor at the onset of an attack. The episodes were of short duration, could be precipitated at will, and were not associated with auditory symptoms. Caloric tests were normal (5cc of water at 80° F gave 90 second responses bilaterally). Tests for positional vertigo provoked a severe vertiginous episode of short duration associated with clockwise rotatory nystagmus when she was placed in the supine left-ear-down position. The symptoms continued unchanged and were noted in her medical record on several occasions, the last mention being made when she was 74 years of age. She died at the age of 77. Histological study shows a basophilic staining homogeneous deposit, measuring 300 microns in its greatest dimension, attached to the posterior surface of the cupula of the left posterior semicircular canal. All other vestibular sense organs and the vestibular nerves appear normal.

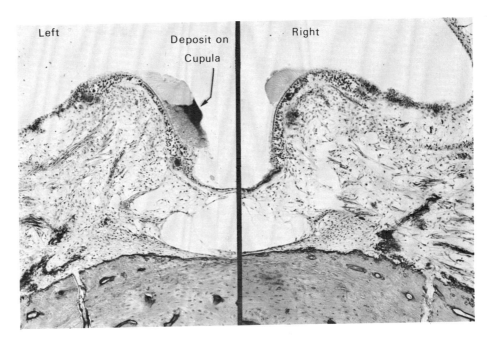

Fig. 12.32: At the age of 64 the patient began having attacks of vertigo precipitated by changes in head position. The duration of each attack was but a few seconds and not associated with auditory symptoms or loss of consciousness. On one occasion she fell to the floor striking the occiput but did not lose consciousness. The attacks were most severe when arising from bed, and she had to sit on the edge of her bed for some seconds before she could rise. Caloric tests were interpreted to be normal. Tests for positional vertigo with eyes in central position provoked clockwise rotatory nystagmus and subjective sensation of vertigo in the supine left-ear-down position. The nystagmus had a latency of 6 seconds and a duration of 7 seconds. With eyes closed and recorded by electronystagmography the latency was 13 seconds and the duration 33 seconds. Upon assuming the upright position there was counterclockwise rotatory nystagmus and subjective vertigo. The nystagmus had a latency of 7 seconds and a duration of 4 seconds. No reaction occurred in the supine right-ear-down position. The vertiginous symtoms continued unchanged until the time of her death at age 68. Attached to the cupula of the left posterior semicircular canal is a granular, basophilic staining mass measuring 350 microns in its greatest dimension. All other vestibular sense organs and the vestibular nerves appear normal. See Fig. 12.33.

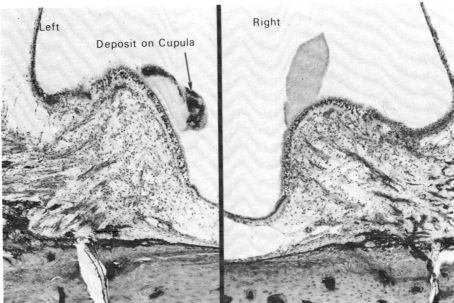

position. Histological studies of both ears revealed basophilic deposits on the cupulae of the posterior canals of the left ears (Figs. 12.31, 12.32) and a layer of granular material in the most inferior part of the posterior canal of one (Fig. 12.33). The cupulae of the other canals as well as those of the opposite ears appeared normal. Schuknecht and Ruby (1973) recently reported the findings in a third case (Fig. 12.34).

The origin of the deposit is not obvious on histological study. It is doubtful that the material was generated from the cupular substance as the cupulae appear identical to the cupulae of the posterior canals of the opposite ears which did not have this deposit. The utricular otolithic membranes appeared normal; however, the integrity of the otoliths could not be evaluated because they had been resorbed by the decalcification process to which they were subjected during histological preparation.

It is possible that the cupular deposits represent calcium carbonate derived from otoconia, perhaps altered to some extent, and embedded in a matrix stained by hematoxylin. Sometimes animal specimens prepared by intravital fixation show the otoconial layer of the otolithic membrane. It is also possible that the deposits represent products of degeneration from other sources.

Schuknecht and Ruby (1973) examined 391 temporal bones from 245 individuals to determine the incidence of cupular deposits and found small deposits in 125, medium deposits in 20, and large deposits in 4. No deposits

Fig. 12.33: Same patient as Fig. 12.32 showing a granular deposit in the most dependent part of the posterior semicircular canal of the left ear.

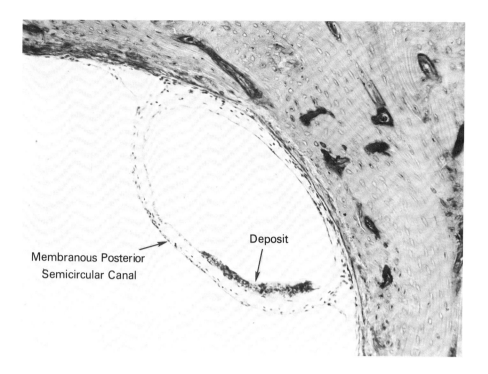

Membranous Posterior Semicircular Canal

Deposit

Fig. 12.34: At the age of 87 this patient fell to the floor and broke his right femur. A daughter relates that although the patient had not complained of vertiginous episodes, the fall in which he broke his femur seemed to be due to a "sudden loss of balance." On this occasion, while in his daughter's home, he arose from a chair, turned to the right to pass through a door into the bedroom and although several individuals, including his daughter, were at arm's length from him, he suddenly fell to the floor as if he had been struck. He did not appear to stumble. He was hospitalized for treatment of the fracture and died 14 days later of staphylococcus pneumonia. Histological study shows a dense basophilic deposit on the cupula of the right posterior semicircular canal. All other vestibular sense organs and the vestibular nerves appear normal.

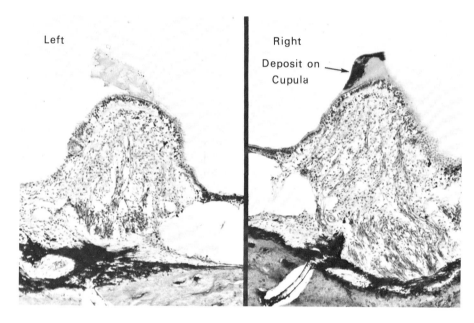

Left

Right

Deposit on Cupula

Fig. 12.35: Experimental section of the anterior vestibular artery and accompanying superior vestibular nerve in the cat resulted in degeneration of the utricular macula and cristae of the superior and lateral semicircular canals. Three weeks following injury the otolithic membrane is undergoing lysis and otoconia are being released into the endolymphatic fluid. The ampullary walls of all three canals and the wall of the utricle are partly collapsed. This may be the result of atrophy of the dark cells in these structures. The dark cells are believed to have a secretory function (Kimura, 1969).

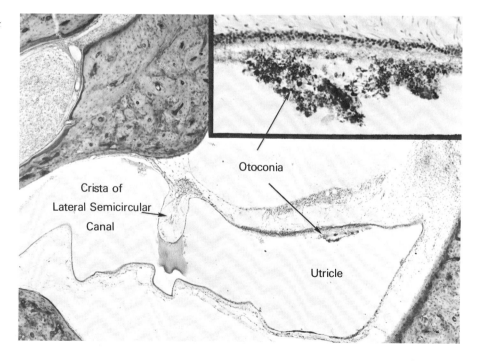

Crista of Lateral Semicircular Canal

Otoconia

Utricle

were found which exceeded in size the deposits found in the cupulolithiasis ears. Most of the deposits appear as a finely granular amorphous substance staining light blue with hematoxylin. They show no evidence of a fibrillar structure, and the granularity is coarser than that of protein precipitate. Some contain round or ovoid forms which may represent nuclear remains of degenerating cells. The presence of deposits bears no relationship to the state of preservation of the temporal bone, the time interval between death and fixation, or the condition of utricular otolithic membrane. Furthermore, the deposits were found as often in temporal bones judged to be normal as in those exhibiting pathological changes.

Experimental evidence compatible with the concept of cupulolithiasis derives from several sources. Schuknecht (1962), working with cats, demonstrated degeneration of the otolithic membrane and loosening of the otoconia following section of the anterior vestibular artery (Fig. 12.35). In another experiment (Schuknecht, 1969b) it was shown that stimulation of the isolated posterior semicircular canal resulted in purely rotatory nystagmus. Harbert (1970) confirmed the observation of Bárány (1921) that with the eyes directed toward the uppermost ear in the provocative test position, the nystagmus becomes purely vertical. Harbert deduced that this effect could only result from the stimulus of the posterior canal on the ipsilateral superior oblique and contralateral inferior rectus muscles. He further postulated that the direction of flow is utriculofugal in the canal being tested.

It was first shown by Wittmaack (1909) and later by Hasegawa (1931) and Kleyn and Versteegh (1933) that intense linear acceleration by centrifugation results in removal of the otoconia and the gelatinous layer of the maculae.

Parker et al. (1968) demonstrated in an experiment on guinea pigs that moderate loss of otoconia from the maculae may be observed following exposure to 12–25 g for 195–330 seconds. There was moderate to severe displacement of otoconia from acceleration exposures of approximately 50 g for 1 minute. Accelerations of 100 g for 30 seconds and 100 g for 15–20 seconds produced severe loss of otoconia from all maculae. They also demonstrated slight to moderate displacements of otoconia following impact decelerations of 240–314 g. They stated that the results of their experiments "support the hypothesis that 'benign paroxysmal positional nystagmus' results from displacement of otoconia into the canal ampullae."

5. PATHOPHYSIOLOGICAL MECHANISM

The concept of cupulolithiasis provides a reasonable explanation for most of the clinical features of positional vertigo of the benign paroxysmal type. It assumes that substances having a specific gravity greater than endolymph and thus subject to movement with changes in the direction of gravitational force come into contact with the cupula of the posterior semicircular canal (Fig. 12.36). It is hypothesized that these particles move about freely in the endolymph or become attached to the cupula.

With the head in the erect position the posterior canal ampulla is located in the most dependent part of the labyrinth, whereas in the provocative test position (supine, head-hanging, ear-down) the posterior canal assumes a superior position. The change in position from erect to the supine, head-hanging, ear-down position would therefore cause a severe utriculofugal displacement of the cupula of the posterior canal, coincident with the action of gravitational force on the cupular deposit.

The delay of onset, which usually is several seconds, may be caused by the period of time required to get the mass in motion. The intense vertiginous sensation may be due to the great magnitude of the cupular displacement, and the limited duration of the vertiginous attack may be the result of the return of the cupula to a normal position after the particles have left it. Fatigability may be caused by dispersement of particles in the endolymph of the pars superior occurring during repeated head positionings and the recur-

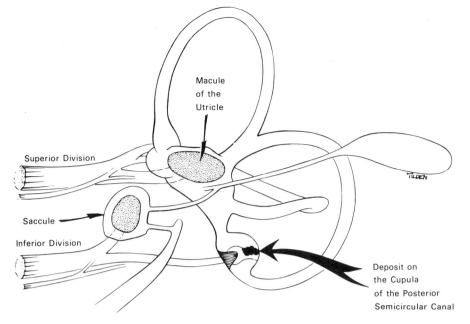

Fig. 12.36: Sketch showing the anatomical relationships of the structures of the vestibular labyrinth. When the head is in the erect position, the ampullary region of the posterior semicircular canal is the most dependent part of the pars superior (utricle and canals) and serves as a "dumping ground" for debris generated in this region.

Macule of the Utricle

Superior Division

Saccule

Inferior Division

Deposit on the Cupula of the Posterior Semicircular Canal

rence after rest may be due to the time required for the sediment to settle again into the posterior canal ampulla so that they can act "en masse" when the pars superior is again inverted.

In an electron microscopic study of the morphologic and physical properties of otoconia, Lim (1973) has shown that when separated from the gelatinous layer of the otolithic membrane the otoconia may dissolve (Fig. 12.37). This might explain the tendency for cupulolithiasis to be self-limiting in most individuals.

The most rational and simplest management of the disorder is avoidance of the provocative position, and most patients accomplish this with little restriction of normal everyday motor activity. The extent to which motor activity must be restricted is determined by the characteristics of the attack, such as suddenness of onset, severity of dysequilibrium, associated nausea and vomiting, and frequency of occurrence. Climbing, swimming, skiing, and other athletic activities may be contraindicated. The operation of mechanical equipment, such as driving an automobile or tending industrial machinery, may have to be curtailed. The extent of occupational handicap will be determined by the need for motor activity, in particular the requirements for head movement. Most individuals will adjust to the disorder with a set of self-imposed restrictions.

In rare cases the disability may be sufficiently severe to justify consideration of some form of ablation of the vestibular labyrinth. Case histories demonstrating that labyrinth ablation is successful in the management of cupulolithiasis have been reported by Citron and Hallpike (1956, 1962) and by Schuknecht (1962). These patients exhibited severe sensorineural hearing loss in the involved ear so that total inner ear ablation constituted rational therapy. Gacek (1974) has shown that section of the nerve to the posterior

Fig. 12.37: Dissolving otoconia of the squirrel monkey. The specimen was fixed in osmic acid and stored in 70 percent alcohol for one week. When otoconia are slightly decalcified they appear to collapse without signs of chemical etching. Otoconia which become separated from the gelatinous layer of the otolithic membrane exhibit similar changes even in the absence of decalcifying agents. (Courtesy of Lim)

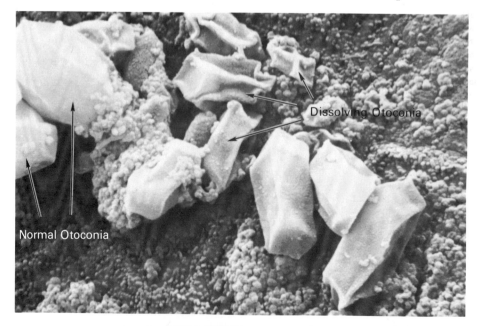

Dissolving Otoconia

Normal Otoconia

canal by an approach through the external auditory canal eliminates the syndrome.

C. SUDDEN DEAFNESS

The numerous and various known etiologies of sudden deafness have been described in some detail in this book. Among the causes for sudden deafness are suppurative labyrinthitis (Chapter 5A10b), viral labyrinthitis (Chapter 5C2), ototoxic drugs (Chapter 6), temporal bone fracture, concussion, noise, surgery, otitic barotrauma, and rupture of the labyrinthine windows (Chapter 7), inner ear hemorrhage (Chapter 8A2), vascular occlusion (Chapter 8B1), multiple sclerosis, carcinomatous encephalomyelitis, and glioma of the pons (Chapter 9), metastatic neoplasms and leukemia (Chapter 11), and Ménière's disease (Chapter 12A).

There are also many cases of sudden deafness in which the etiology is not so obvious. The two most popular concepts to explain these cases are viral labyrinthitis and vascular occlusion. The advocates of these theories necessarily base their judgments on clinical observations because supporting pathological material is lacking.

The deafness may have its onset at any time of the day or night and the patient may be aware of the exact time of onset. Frequently it is first noticed on awakening in the morning, and it may be tinnitus which first alerts the patient to the presence of an otological problem. Characteristically, these individuals are in good health and may be of any age. There is no sex predominance. Although most of these patients have no vestibular symptoms, some have a feeling of unsteadiness which may have its onset immediately or some hours after deafness is first noticed, and a few experience vertigo for some hours or days.

The hearing loss in sudden deafness is usually unilateral, and may vary from a mild loss for a restricted frequency range to profound deafness. Although the natural history of sudden deafness has not been elucidated, it appears that at least some recovery occurs in about 25 to 50 percent of affected individuals.

In 1962, Schuknecht et al. (1962b) described the pathological findings in the ears of four individuals who experienced sudden deafness of unknown cause. The interpretation evolved at that time was that the cochlear changes were similar to those known to occur in human labyrinthitis of known viral etiology such as mumps, rubella, and morbilli, and dissimilar to those occurring in animals following experimental obstruction of the arteries or veins of the inner ear. Since that report, four additional specimens have become available for study (Schuknecht et al., 1973).

The total number of eight ears are from six individuals with unilateral sudden deafness and one individual with bilateral sequential sudden deafness. Four of the seven individuals were male and three were female. Their ages at the time of onset of sudden deafness ranged from 39 to 68 (average 55) years.

The distribution between right and left sides was equal. The time span from deafness to death varied from nine days to thirty-three years. The hearing losses were profound in four ears, severe in three ears, and moderate in one ear. Vertigo as an associated symptom was severe in one case, mild in two cases, absent in four cases, and the history regarding vertigo was noncontributory in one case. Six individuals noted the onset of tinnitus in association with the sudden hearing loss and in two cases the histories regarding tinnitus were noncontributory.

The most spectacular and consistent pathological change in these eight ears is atrophy of the organ of Corti. In four cochleae these changes are limited to the basal turns, with two showing shrinkage of the organ of Corti without loss of hair cells. The other four cochleae exhibit severe atrophy of the organ of Corti in all three turns, with three showing changes of decreasing severity from basal to apical end (see case histories and photomicrographs, Figs. 12.38 to 12.51).

Fig. 12.38: Audiogram and cochlear chart of the right ear of a woman who at the age of 39 years experienced sudden right hearing loss while suffering from a "head-cold." D-A means time interval between death and autopsy and T-A the time lapse between the test of hearing and autopsy. See also Figs. 12.39 and 12.40.

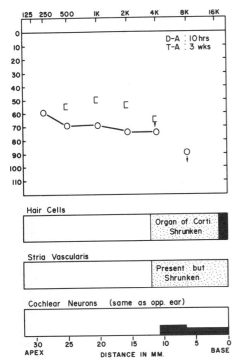

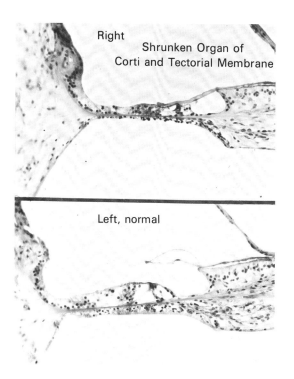

Fig. 12.39: Same case as Figs. 12.38 and 12.40. Photomicrographs of the organs of Corti in the 9 mm regions of the right ear above and the normal left ear below. The organ of Corti and tectorial membrane of the right ear are shrunken. To accomplish rapid fixation, both middle ears were injected with 10 percent formalin thirty minutes after death.

Right Shrunken Organ of Corti and Tectorial Membrane

Left, normal

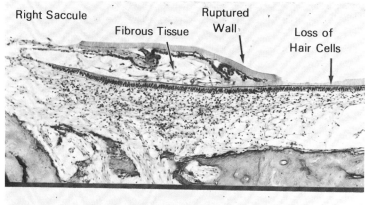

Fig. 12.40: Same case as Figs. 12.38 and 12.39. Photomicrographs of the saccules of the right ear above and normal left ear below. In the right ear the wall of the saccule is ruptured and collapsed. Most of the hair cells of the macula are missing. There is a network of fibrous tissue between the macula and the saccular wall.

Right Saccule   Fibrous Tissue   Ruptured Wall   Loss of Hair Cells

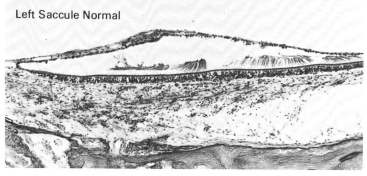

Left Saccule Normal

Fig. 12.41: Audiogram and cochlear chart of the left ear of a woman who at the age of 43 years experienced sudden left deafness during an episode of acute pharyngitis. See Fig. 12.42.

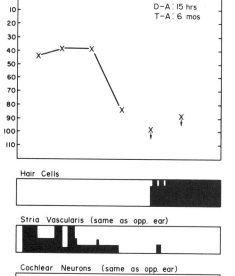

The tectorial membrane is atrophied throughout the cochlear duct in three ears. In one it is shrunken and in two it is atrophied, displaced into the inner sulcus or onto the limbus, and encapsulated. The stria vascularis shows atrophic changes greater than those of the opposite ear in five cases, being shrunken throughout in one, severely atrophied in three, and partially atrophied in one. The six ears from individuals with unilateral sudden deafness show the cochlear neuronal population of the involved ear in each case to be the same as the opposite ear. The neuronal deficits, which are mild in four ears and severe in two ears, logically evolve as degenerative changes of aging which are unrelated to the sudden deafness.

In all specimens it is possible to visualize the external and internal radiating arterioles, capillaries of the spiral ligament, capillaries of the stria vascularis (except in areas where the latter is atrophied) and limbus, as well as the vessels of the tympanic lip and basilar membrane. Among the venous channels, which can be clearly identified in all ears, are the collecting venules of the scala tympani, the anterior and posterior spiral veins, and the vein at the cochlear aqueduct.

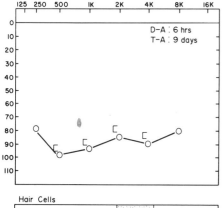

Atrophied Organ of Corti

Fig. 12.42: Same case as Fig. 12.41. The cochlear duct in the 9 mm region of the left ear. The organ of Corti has been reduced to a small mound of undifferentiated cells. The shrinkage of the tectorial membrane is the same as the opposite ear and therefore represents preparation artifact. The stria vascularis is normal in this region.

Fig. 12.43: Audiogram and cochlear chart of the right ear of a man who at the age of 58 years awakened at 4 A.M. to notice hearing loss and tinnitus in his right ear. He stated that he had had a "head-cold" for three days prior to onset of deafness. He died of femoral and splenic artery thrombosis nine days later. See Figs. 12.44 and 12.45.

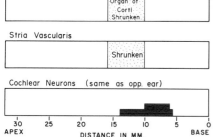

In some of the specimens the arteries and veins contain blood cells and in others they do not. In no case is there obliteration or atrophy of vascular channels except for loss of the capillary network in association with atrophy of the stria vascularis.

Lindsay and Zuidema (1950) studied the clinical features of sixteen cases of sudden deafness and found that four were associated with systemic disease and twelve were unexplainable. They concluded that the high incidence of the disorder in healthy adults under the age of 30 argues against a vascular etiology.

Although it has been established that vascular lesions can produce sudden deafness, these cases occur in association with known systemic vascular disease. For example, massive inner ear hemorrhage has been identified as a cause for sudden deafness in leukemia (Schuknecht et al., 1965). Sudden deafness may also occur in Buerger's disease (thrombo-angiitis obliterans) (Kirikae et al., 1962), macroglobulinemia (Ruben et al., 1969), and disorders characterized by hyperviscosity of the blood serum (Solomon and Fahey, 1963; Wilkinson et al., 1966).

Vascular disease was present in only one of the seven patients in the report by Schuknecht et al. (1973). This individual died of femoral and splenic thrombosis nine days following the sudden deafness. It should be noted, however, that he also complained of a "head cold" at the time of onset of deafness.

Following temporary obstruction of the labyrinthine artery (Perlman et al.,

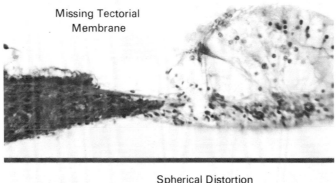

Missing Tectorial Membrane

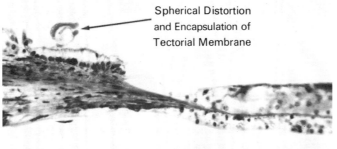

Spherical Distortion and Encapsulation of Tectorial Membrane

Fig. 12.44: Same case as Figs. 12.43 and 12.45. Photomicrographs of the organ of Corti of the right ear. The upper view from the 20 mm region shows all cytological elements to be present but severely swollen, which would be consistent with postmortem autolysis. The tectorial membrane is missing. The lower view from the 12 mm region shows shrinking of the organ of Corti with all cytological elements present. The tectorial membrane is distorted into a sphere, displaced onto the limbus, and partly encapsulated in a dark-staining substance.

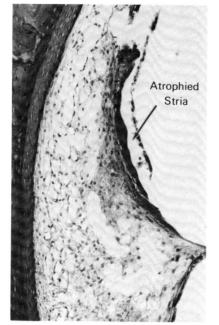
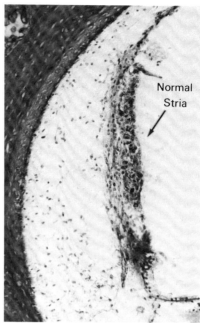

Atrophied Stria

Normal Stria

Fig. 12.45: Same case as Figs. 12.43 and 12.44. Views of the stria vascularis of the right ear. In the 20 mm region (right view) the swollen tissue is consistent with postmortem autolysis. In the 12 mm region (left view) the stria appears as a deeply basophilically staining ribbon with no clearly identifiable cytological structure. The appearance of the spiral ligament in both views is judged to be normal for age.

Fig. 12.46: Audiogram and cochlear chart of the left ear of a man who at the age of 63 years experienced a sudden hearing loss in his left ear associated with severe vertigo, nausea, and vomiting. There was no history of an associated illness. See Figs. 12.47 and 12.48.

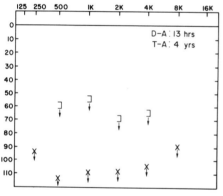

Hair Cells

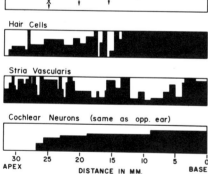

Stria Vascularis

Cochlear Neurons (same as opp. ear)

1959) there are several pathological changes which are distinctly different from those of the sudden deafness ears. The animal ears show (1) a greater loss of cochlear neurons, (2) greater atrophy of the spiral ligament, (3) variable spatial pattern of hair cell loss in the organ of Corti, and (4) little effect on the tectorial membrane.

Permanent obstruction of the labyrinthine arteries of animal ears (Kimura and Perlman, 1958) produced diffuse degeneration of the membranous labyrinth. An orderly sequence of pathological changes occurred beginning in one-half hour with hair cell changes, followed in a few hours by degeneration of the supporting structures, and finally in six months by fibrous tissue invasion and ossification of the inner ear spaces. None of the human cases of sudden deafness reported by Schuknecht et al. (1973) showed fibrous or bony proliferation in the inner ear.

Obstruction of the vein at the cochlear aqueduct and its collaterals (Kimura and Perlman, 1956) resulted in engorgement of the vascular system and scattered hemorrhages followed by progressive loss of external hair cells, severe atrophy of the stria vascularis, and mild atrophy of the spiral ligament, but no changes in the tectorial membrane. The late pathological changes following venous obstruction, while bearing some resemblance to the human ears with sudden deafness, differ in that the stria vascularis is consistently severely

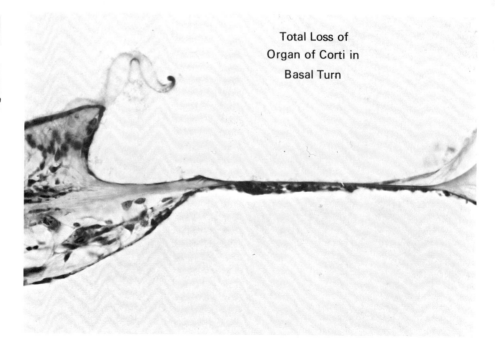

Total Loss of Organ of Corti in Basal Turn

Fig. 12.47: Same case as Figs. 12.46 and 12.48. This view from the 10 mm region of the left ear shows the organ of Corti to be totally missing. The tectorial membrane is normal.

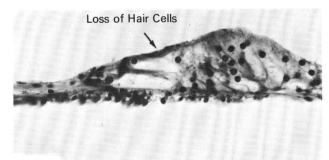
Loss of Hair Cells

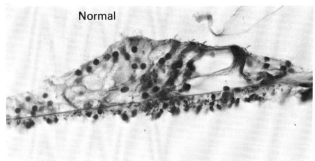
Normal

Fig. 12.48: Case PC. The left view is from the 22 mm area of the left cochlea and shows a partial loss of hair cells. The right view for comparison is from the 22 mm region of the right and shows normal hair cells.

Fig. 12.49: Audiogram and cochlear chart of the left ear of a man who at the age of 68 years experienced a severe loss of hearing in his left ear while hospitalized for "viral pneumonia." See Figs. 12.50 and 12.51.

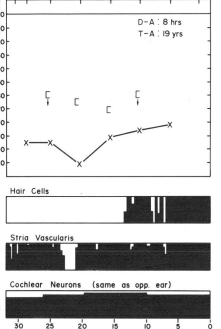

Fig. 12.50: Same case as Figs. 12.49 and 12.51. Cochlear duct in the middle turn of the left cochlea showing the pillar cells and Deiters' cells to be missing, whereas hair cells can be identified. The tectorial membrane is displaced into the inner sulcus, and has undergone spherical distortion and partial cellular encapsulation. About 60 percent of the stria vascularis is degenerated.

atrophied and the tectorial membrane is consistently spared. In the human ears from individuals with sudden deafness, the various venous tributaries, including the two principal veins which drain the labyrinth, (the vein at the cochlear aqueduct and the vein at the vestibular aqueduct) appear patent and normal.

Virus infection has commonly been implicated as an etiological factor for sudden deafness. The labyrinth may become involved in the course of specific viral infections such as measles, mumps, and infectious mononucleosis (Gregg and Shaeffer, 1964). It is also probable that sudden deafness may be caused by viral infection without clinical evidence of systemic involvement; for example, sudden deafness occurring in apparently healthy children or adults may be due to a subclinical mumps infection. During a mumps epidemic a considerable number of healthy contact individuals will show positive serological tests (Wolff, 1953). Van Dishoeck and Bierman (1957) performed serological tests and viral cultures of the blood and stools on sixty-six patients with sudden severe unilateral hearing loss and found that four had mumps and two others probably had mumps. None of their patients had parotitis, and each clearly recalled a previous childhood mumps infection.

A large number of viruses of several morphologically different groups are known to cause illnesses of the upper respiratory tract (Mufson et al., 1966). Although most of these viruses are associated with benign disease, they are capable of extremely virulent attacks upon the central nervous system.

Lindsay (1959) found unilateral sudden deafness, tinnitus, and vertigo in four patients who had acute upper respiratory infections with all experiencing partial recovery of hearing during the subsequent few months. Heller and Lindenberg (1955) reported five cases and Lieberman (1957) four patients who experienced sudden deafness with upper respiratory infections.

Some support for a viral etiology of sudden deafness is found in the high incidence of acute respiratory disease in the clinical histories of the seven cases reported by Schuknecht et al. (1973). At the time of onset of sudden

Spherical Distortion and
Encapsulation of Tectorial Membrane

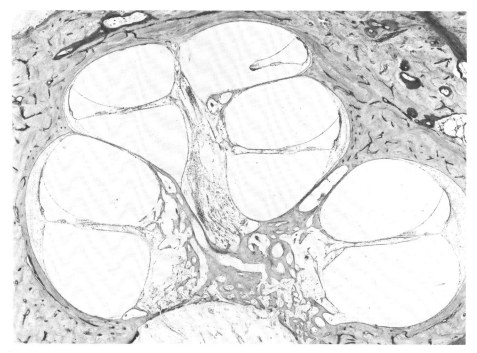

Fig. 12.51: Same case as Figs. 12.49 and 12.50 Mid-modiolar section of the cochlea of the left ear showing severe atrophy of the stria vascularis and severe loss of cochlear neurons in all three turns. The loss of cochlear neurons was of equal severity in the opposite ear.

deafness two reported having "head-colds", one had acute pharyngitis, and two had pneumonia. Furthermore, two of the patients complained of headache suggestive of an associated viral encephalitis.

The similarity of the pathological changes in the ears of these seven individuals with sudden deafness to those occurring in ears with known viral labyrinthitis provides further support for a viral etiology. Lindsay et al. (1960) reported the pathological findings in the ears of a six-year-old child who suffered bilateral profound deafness from mumps at the age of twenty-eight months. They found atrophy of the organ of Corti, stria vascularis, and tectorial membrane. In the basal turns the organ of Corti was missing, whereas in the apical regions supporting elements as well as hair cells were present. The tectorial membrane was severely atrophied in both ears, appearing either shrunken or transformed into a sphere and encapsulated by a single layer of flat cells. There was a slight loss of cochlear neurons in the basal turns. The vestibular sense organs appeared normal.

Lindsay and Hemenway (1954) described the inner ear pathology of an infant who developed measles at the age of three months and died of complications of the disease four months later. Both ears showed atrophy of the organs of Corti which was most severe in the basal turns. The tectorial membranes were degenerated and partially encapsulated. The stria vascularis was atrophied in both ears with the most severe changes occurring in the basal turns. There was a partial loss of cochlear neurons in the basal turn. There was atrophy of the maculae of the utricle and saccule of one ear.

Pathological studies of the inner ears of infants suffering from maternal rubella have consistently demonstrated cochleosaccular degeneration (Nager, 1952; Lindsay et al., 1953; Hemenway et al., 1969). The changes in cases of maternal rubella were found to be similar to those described for measles and mumps, including atrophy of the organ of Corti, stria vascularis, and tectorial membrane. Typically, the saccular wall was collapsed onto a partly degenerated otolithic membrane and sensory epithelium. The utricles and cristae were normal in these cases.

Beal et al. (1967) reported the pathological findings in the temporal bone of a patient who experienced sudden profound unilateral hearing loss while suffering from a "head-cold." They found severe distortion and degeneration of the organ of Corti and stria vascularis with atrophy and encapsulation of the tectorial membrane.

Goodhill et al. (1973) is of the opinion that some cases of sudden deafness of obscure origin are caused by rupture of the labyrinthine windows. Fistulae of the round and oval windows have been observed following head injury without fracture, scuba diving, impact noise, exertion, etc. When sudden deafness occurs in association with a specific stress incident, it would be reasonable to perform surgical exploration in search of a fistula which, if found, could be closed with an autogenous soft tissue graft. It seems doubtful, however, that sudden deafness occurring without a stress incident is caused by an oval or round window fistula.

The total evidence favors viral infection as the most common etiology for sudden deafness. The viruses which appear to be most commonly involved are those which cause upper respiratory disease. Clinical experience has shown that partial or total recovery of hearing occurs in about 25 percent of the cases. The prognosis for recovery is poor for those cases with severe hearing losses, particularly when vertigo is present. Morrison and Booth (1970) advise that therapy be instituted promptly and that measures used be based on an audiometric determination of the location of the lesion. Thus individuals exhibiting a neural loss are given steroid therapy and those with a sensory loss are given vasodilators.

There is considerable controversy as to whether therapy of any type is helpful for sudden deafness of obscure cause. Controlled therapeutic studies are difficult to perform so that statistical evidence showing success of treatment is lacking. In view of the strong probability that most cases of sudden deafness are of viral etiology, it would seem unlikely that the use of vasodilators, anticoagulants, steroids, or antibiotics would be of any value.

D. APICAL LESIONS OF THE COCHLEA

It is now apparent that degenerative changes involving predominantly the apical region of the cochlea may have several different etiologies. In 1967, Bernstein and Schuknecht presented several examples of apical lesions in animals and human subjects and pointed out that they are much less common than lesions of the basal turn of the cochlea.

1. VASCULAR OCCLUSION

The evidence that vascular occlusion may cause degenerative changes in the sensory and neural structures limited to the apical region of the cochlea derives from several animal experiments.

In 1958, Kimura and Perlman obstructed the arterial supply to the cochleae of a large series of guinea pigs. In thirteen animals in which temporary obstruction of the labyrinthine arteries was accomplished, the hair cell loss was limited to the middle and apical turns. In another group of animals in which the labyrinthine arteries were permanently occluded, there were three with hair cell losses greater in the apical turns.

Neff and Kiang (1970) coagulated the anterior inferior cerebellar artery in several cats and found severe loss of cochlear neurons in the middle and apical turns of the cochleae in two of the animals (Fig. 12.52).

Bernstein and Silverstein (1966) ligated the anterior inferior cerebellar artery or its branches in seven cats and found lesions limited to the apical regions of the cochleae in three of them (Fig. 12.53). One showed a small discrete loss of cochlear neurons only at the extreme apex, and two demonstrated loss of external hair cells as well as cochlear neurons in the apical regions.

Alford et al. (1965) and Igarashi et al. (1969) induced microembolization of the cochlear vessels by the injection of styrene divinylbenzene copolymer beads into the vertebral arteries of dogs. Suga et al. (1970) performed a similar experiment utilizing a suspension of barium sulfate. In both of these experiments some of the animals demonstrated degenerative changes located predominantly in the apical regions of the cochleae.

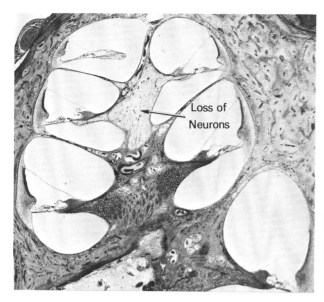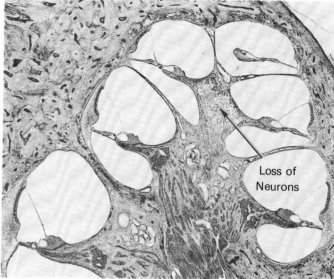

Fig. 12.52: There is severe loss of cochlear neurons in the apical region of the cochlea following occlusion of the anterior inferior cerebellar artery by electrocautery (cat). The organ of Corti and other structures of the cochlear duct appear normal throughout. Postoperative survival time was four months. (Courtesy of Neff and Kiang)

Fig. 12.53: There is severe loss of cochlear neurons and external hair cells in the apical region of the cochlea following ligation of the anterior inferior cerebellar artery with 6–0 silk suture (cat). The postoperative survival time was six weeks. (Courtesy of Bernstein and Silverstein)

2. ENDOLYMPHATIC HYDROPS

Kimura and Schuknecht (1965) demonstrated that endolymphatic hydrops can be produced consistently in both the cochlear and vestibular systems of guinea pigs by obstructing the endolymphatic duct. Kimura (1967) observed degeneration of the hair cells and cochlear neurons in the apical turns in some animals as soon as one month after obstruction of the endolymphatic duct. In several cochleae there was degeneration of the cochlear neurons without reduction of hair cell population in the corresponding area. Some showed degeneration of the stria vascularis limited to the apical region.

Schuknecht et al. (1968) performed a similar experiment in which the endolymphatic sacs of twelve cats were destroyed surgically. After survival times of six months to three years, all were found to have endolymphatic hydrops. Three or four animals with postoperative survival times of 2½ to 3 years demonstrated atrophic changes in the organs of Corti and cochlear neurons, most severe in the apical regions (see Chapter 3C2, Function of the endolymphatic sac).

Beal (1968) ablated the endolymphatic sac of rabbits and found loss of external hair cells and cochlear neurons in the apical regions in several animals with long postoperative survival times.

Lindsay and von Schulthess (1958), Lindsay et al. (1967), and Schuknecht (unpublished data), in studies of the cochleae of patients with Ménière's disease, have found atrophic changes in the organs of Corti and cochlear neurons which were most severe in the apical regions.

Thus, endolymphatic hydrops, whether occurring in Ménière's disease or induced by destruction of the endolymphatic sac, may be associated with atrophy of the sensorineural structures in the apical region. The pathogenesis is not clear at this time.

3. SUPPURATIVE LABYRINTHITIS

Suppurative labyrinthitis uniformly causes severe degeneration of the membranous labyrinth and total loss of auditory and vestibular function. In patients who survive, the labyrinthine spaces often become partially filled with connective tissue and bone, and the modiolus undergoes partial resorption. It is not unusual for these changes to be most severe in the apical regions of the cochleae (see Fig. 12.54).

4. ACQUIRED SYPHILIS

The labyrinthine pathology associated with acquired syphilis has no consistent pattern of auditory and vestibular dysfunction. This is in contradistinction to congenital syphilis in which there is a well-recognized clinical syndrome and pathological findings (see Chapter 5E, Syphilitic Infection). Progressive hearing loss caused by degeneration of cochlear neurons of the apical region of the cochlea has been observed in one case (Fig. 12.55). Possibly the lesion is caused by obliterative endarteritis, which is common to all syphilitic lesions, and may have a common pathogenesis with the apical lesions which result from experimental occlusion of the labyrinthine vessels.

5. POSTOPERATIVE APICAL LESIONS

Several animal experiments have shown that surgical procedures which include fistulization of the oval window can cause degenerative changes of the cochlear neurons and organ of Corti of the apical region of the cochlea.

Igarashi (1967) placed degenerated homografts of fatty connective tissue in the oval windows of cats following stapedectomy. One animal sacrificed six weeks after surgery showed a total loss of cochlear neurons in the apical region of the cochlea (Fig. 12.56). Hayden and McGee (1965) performed an experiment on cats in which crushed subcutaneous fatty connective tissue was

Fig. 12.54: Mid-modiolar section of the cochlea of a 46-year-old woman who was profoundly deaf following meningitis at the age of 3. There is severe atrophy of the auditory and vestibular sense organs. About 50 percent of the cochlear neurons remain in the basal turn of the cochlea. The apical region of the cochlea is obliterated by fibrous tissue and bone. (Courtesy of Rüedi)

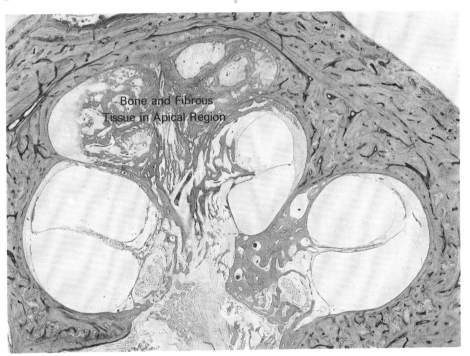

Fig. 12.55: This patient, who died at the age of 58 of aortic aneurysm, was known to have had syphilis for over 30 years. He had a left hearing loss for many years. Histological studies show severe loss of cochlear neurons, most severe in the apical region. The organ of Corti and other structures of the cochlear duct, as well as the vestibular sense organs, appear normal. It is possible that the loss of cochlear neurons is due to syphilitic endarteritis and obliteration of branches of the labyrinthine artery.

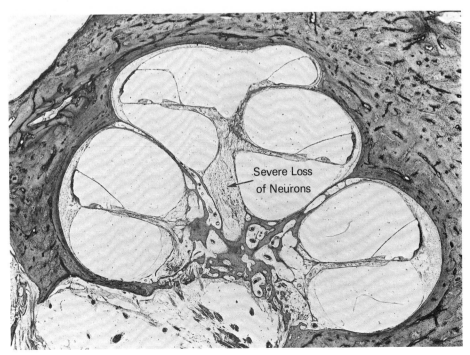

Fig. 12.56: A severe loss of cochlear neurons occurred in the apical region of the cochlea following stapedectomy and introduction of a nonviable homograft of fatty connective tissue into the oval window (cat). Postoperative survival time was six weeks. The organ of Corti and other structures of the cochlear duct appear normal. (Courtesy of Igarashi)

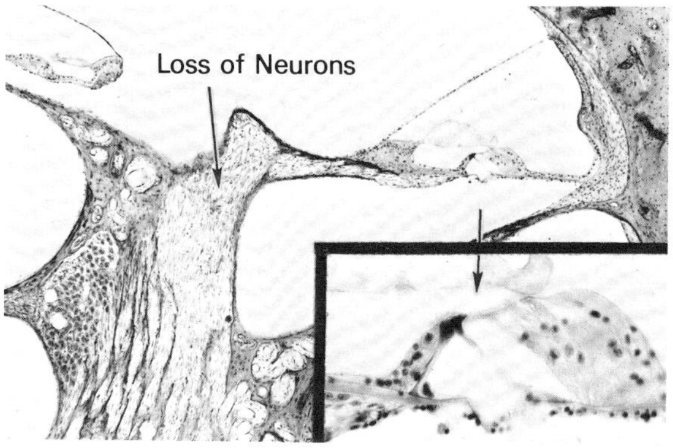

Fig. 12.57: A severe loss of cochlear neurons and a partial loss of external hair cells in the apical region of the cochlea following stapedectomy and the introduction of a viable graft of adipose tissue into the oval window (cat). Postoperative survival time was four months. (Courtesy of Benitez)

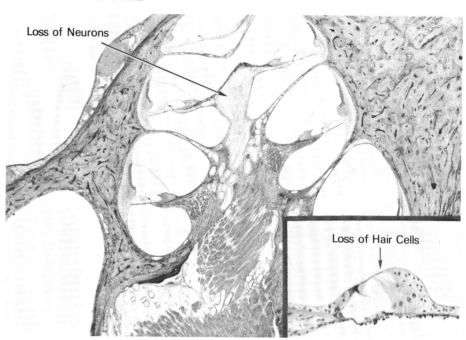

used to seal the oval windows following stapedectomies. An animal with a two-month postoperative survival time showed a diffuse loss of hair cells and a loss of cochlear neurons limited to the apical region. In an experiment on cats, Benitez (1967) subluxated footplates into the vestibules and followed with viable connective tissue homografts in the oval windows. One of these animals, after a survival time of four months, showed a severe loss of cochlear neurons and external hair cells in the apical region (Fig. 12.57).

Sensorineural hearing loss is a recognized complication of stapedectomy in human patients. Frequently the loss is characterized by a particularly severe loss of speech discrimination, suggesting a loss of cochlear neurons. Otte (1968) has found, furthermore, that the neurons located in the middle and apical turns are more important for speech discrimination than those located in the basal turn. The determination of any similarity in the pathology of these human ears to that of the animal ears will have to await the availability of human postmortem specimens.

The mechanism by which oval window surgery causes apical lesions is wholly unknown. Speculation evolves two possible explanations. First, surgical trauma may cause a temporary ischemia, possibly by blood sludging. To support this hypothesis is the experimental evidence that the apical region is exceptionally vulnerable to deprivation of blood supply. A second hypothesis is that apical lesions are caused by toxic products of tissue degeneration or injury generated in the oval window area. Toxic material in the vestibule could reach the apex through the scala vestibuli and, after passing through the helicotrema, could reach the organ of Corti and cochlear neurons through the perilymph channels of the osseous spiral lamina. These perilymph channels have been described by Schuknecht (1959, 1960) and Schuknecht and Seifi (1963), and confirmed by Masuda et al. (1971) (see Chapter 3C4, The perilymph channels).

6. CAUSES UNKNOWN

In 1935 Guild described five human temporal bones showing partial atrophy of the cochlear neurons in the middle and apical turns of the cochleae, all of unknown etiology.

Lurie (1967, personal communication) found a severe loss of cochlear neurons in the apical region of the cochlea of a waltzing mouse, also of unknown cause (Fig. 12.58). Hayden and McGee (1965) described bilateral symmetrical apical lesions involving the modioli and sensorineural structures in a cat. Mature lamellar bone was present in the nerve channels and Rosenthal's canals in the apical 7 mm of the cochleae associated with severe atrophy of the organs of Corti, cochlear neurons, and striae vasculares. At the extreme apex the scalae were partially obliterated by fibrous tissue (Fig. 12.59).

E. COLLAGEN DISEASES

Among the disorders which have been termed collagen diseases are rheumatoid arthritis, acute disseminated lupus erythematosis, generalized scleroderma, dermatomyositis, periarteritis nodosa, temporal arteritis, rheumatic

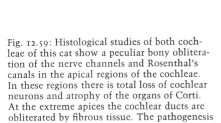

Fig. 12.58: There is a localized area of loss of cochlear neurons in the extreme apical region of the cochlea of this waltzing mouse. (Courtesy of Lurie)

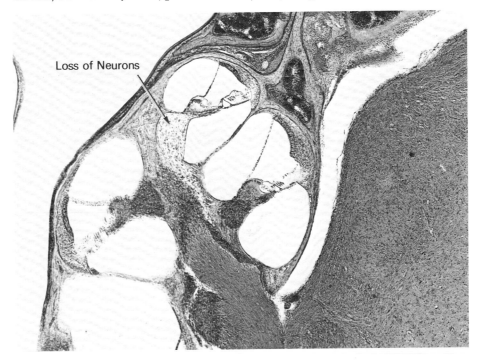

Fig. 12.59: Histological studies of both cochleae of this cat show a peculiar bony obliteration of the nerve channels and Rosenthal's canals in the apical regions of the cochleae. In these regions there is total loss of cochlear neurons and atrophy of the organs of Corti. At the extreme apices the cochlear ducts are obliterated by fibrous tissue. The pathogenesis is unknown. (Courtesy of Hayden and McGee)

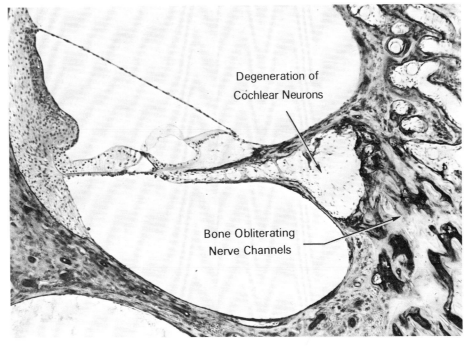

fever, and Wegener's granulomatosis. The basic lesion is a systemic degenerative and prolific alteration of the extracellular portions of the connective tissue. The precise pathogenesis is not known. The most popular concept assumes the presence of an allergic hypersensitivity, probably of the auto-immune variety.

Fudenberg (1968) has shown that auto-immune disease can be a manifestation of immunologic deficiencies rather than immunologic hyperactivity and suggests that an individual may have a genetically determined inability to respond immunologically to a particular antigen.

1. WEGENER'S GRANULOMATOSIS

Wegener (1936, 1939) first described a disorder characterized by destructive granulomatous rhinitis associated with prominent pulmonary symptoms, glomerulonephritis, and generalized angiitis. Wegener, as well as others (Plummer et al., 1957; Milner, 1955; Brown and Woolner, 1960), considers the disease to be a variant of periarteritis nodosa.

The first symptom of Wegener's granulomatosis usually is an acute infection of the upper respiratory tract. This may be followed by bloody nasal discharge and symptoms of acute sinusitis or otitis media. Swelling over the maxilla, ocular proptosis, sagging of the nasal bridge, and palatal ulcerations often occur. The involvement of the nose and sinuses may persist as a low-grade chronic inflammatory and infectious process. The most common otologic manifestation is conductive hearing loss caused by blockage of the eustachian tube resulting in seromucinous otitis media. The nasal septum or turbinates may appear granular with the development of bloody crusts. Occasionally the larynx is involved in a similar process. The patients are usually febrile, lose weight, become anemic, and exhibit leukocytosis and an elevated sedimentation rate. Within a few months there is evidence of arthritis, peripheral neuritis, pulmonary infiltrates, and renal involvement. The average duration of the untreated disease is about six months, and death is usually caused by renal failure.

Godman and Churg (1954) have characterized the pathological lesions of Wegener's granulomatosis as follows:

(1) A necrotizing granulomatous process involving the upper and lower part of the respiratory tract, or both.
(2) Generalized focal necrosing vasculitis involving both arteries and veins, almost always in the lungs and more or less widely disseminated in other sites.
(3) Glomerulitis characterized by necrosis of loops and lobes of the capillary tuft, adhesions, and development of a granulomatous lesion.

Blatt et al. (1959) reviewed reports of 124 cases of Wegener's granulomatosis and found that of eighteen who exhibited ear disease, otitis media and hearing impairment were initial signs of the disease in six. The clinical histories and pathological findings of two patients who developed seromucinous otitis media in association with this disease appear in Figs. 12.60 to 12.63. Blatt and Lawrence (1961) studied the ear of a patient who experienced profound, unilateral sensorineural hearing loss in association with Wegener's granulomatosis. They found that granulomatous tissue extended from the middle ear into the inner ear through the round window niche resulting in destruction of the membranous labyrinth. Cody (1971) also reported a severe bilateral sensorineural hearing impairment in a 69-year-old man with Wegener's granulomatosis. Therapy with prednisone resulted in a dramatic improvement in hearing.

Acute hemorrhage is a common occurrence in association with Wegener's granulomatosis (Castleman, 1969; Shuman, 1970) and can occur into the inner ear (see Chapter 8A2, Hemorrhage into the inner ear).

Malignant granuloma (lethal midline granuloma, granuloma gangraenescens) is presumed by some authors to be a separate clinical entity where the

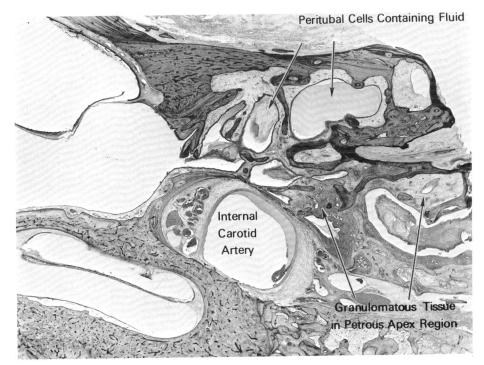

Fig. 12.60: Wegener's granulomatosis. At the age of 29, the patient developed a necrotic lesion of the palate and nasal passages. Her hearing was good and ear drums appeared normal. She received radiotherapy; however, the disease progressed and one year later she complained of left-sided hearing loss. Fluid was removed from the left middle ear by a paracentesis which resulted in temporary subjective improvement in hearing. She died two years later. A granulomatous tumor mass has partly destroyed the peritubal and apical areas of the petrous bone and obstructed the eustachian tube. See Fig. 12.61.

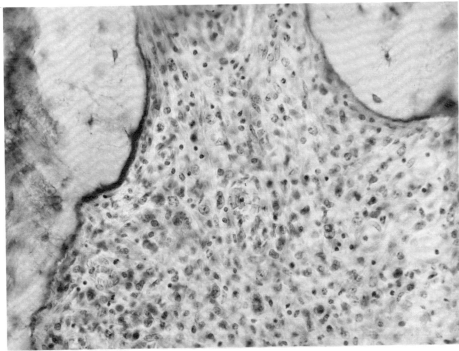

Fig. 12.61: Wegener's granulomatosis. For clinical history see legend, Fig. 12.60. High-power view of the tissue of the petrous apex area showing nonspecific granulation tissue containing large and small round cells, polymorphonuclear leukocytes, and occasional multinucleated giant cells. No mitotic figures are seen.

Fig. 12.62: Wegener's granulomatosis. At the age of 35, this male developed bilateral acute otitis media and was treated with penicillin and myringotomy, which temporarily relieved his symptoms. He also noted sneezing, nonproductive cough, and fever of undetermined etiology. At the age of 36 he exhibited multiple arthralgias, nasal hemorrhages, and bilateral conductive hearing loss. Examination showed fluid-filled middle ears and obstructed eustachian tubes. Pressure-equalizing tubes were introduced through both tympanic membranes. The left tube was successful in maintaining aeration of the middle ear. See Fig. 12.63.

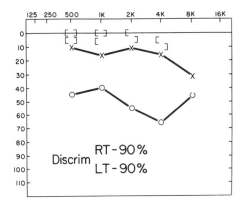

lesion remains confined to the upper respiratory tract (Stewart, 1933; Spear and Walker, 1956). It can often be controlled by local radiotherapy, corticosteroids, and immunosuppressive cytotoxic drugs.

Duvall et al. (1969) presented the case histories of two patients who developed necrotizing granulomatous lesions of the palate and nose during immunosuppressive therapy following kidney transplantation. The symptoms and histological findings were identical to that of Wegener's granulomatosis.

The prognosis of Wegener's granulomatosis remains poor, although treatment with a combination of steroids (e.g., prednisone) and cytotoxic drugs (e.g., azathioprine) has lengthened survival times to as long as fifty months (Froud and Henderson, 1971).

2. PERIARTERITIS NODOSA

Hearing loss associated with periarteritis has been reported by Atkins and Eisman (1959), Brown and Woolner (1960), Herberts et al. (1957), and Toma (1968). The hearing losses were all of the combined sensorineural and conductive type. Peitersen and Carlsen (1966) reported two cases of periarteritis

Fig. 12.63: Wegener's granulomatosis. For clinical history see legend, Fig. 12.62. The left middle ear and mastoid are aerated by a pressure-equalizing tube in the tympanic membrane. The lining membrane of the middle ear is thickened by a granulomatous tissue which has obliterated the eustachian tube. [This case was reported in the New England Journal of Medicine, Weekly Clinicopathological Exercises, 280:828–834, April 10, 1969.]

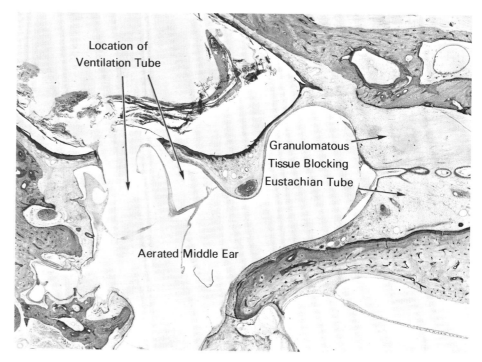

nodosa in which hearing impairment was an initial sign. Both patients experienced combined sensorineural and conductive hearing losses which were improved with prednisone therapy.

3. TEMPORAL ARTERITIS

Cody (1971) reported the findings in a 66-year-old woman with temporal arteritis in whom the first symptoms were rapidly progressive hearing loss and tinnitus. She experienced the typical symptoms of bitemporal headaches, scalp tenderness, fever, and weight loss and on one occasion experienced a severe prolonged attack of vertigo with nausea and vomiting. Ice water caloric tests elicited no response in the left ear. Treatment with cortisone acetate resulted in bilateral hearing improvement and recovery of caloric response in the left ear.

4. COGAN'S DISEASE

Nonsyphilitic interstitial keratitis with vestibulo-auditory symptoms was first recognized as a clinical entity by Cogan in 1945. The syndrome usually occurs in young adults and is of sudden onset, initiated by either ocular or auditory manifestations. The symptoms of both may occur almost simultaneously, or the onset of one may be delayed for several months. Norton and Cogan (1959) studied 13 cases of the syndrome some years after their onset and did not find a common cause.

The vestibulo-auditory symptoms usually are characterized by the sudden onset of vertigo, tinnitus, nausea, and vomiting, associated with the rapid development of deafness. The deafness often is bilateral but, in some cases, is unilateral in the beginning, to be followed by involvement of the second ear after some weeks or months. The hearing loss is of the sensorineural type, may be partial or complete, and usually is severe enough to constitute a handicap. Caloric tests reveal diminution or loss of vestibular function.

The ocular findings are less dramatic and may consist of lacrimation, a sensation of a foreign body in the eye, blurring of vision, and blepharospasm. The symptoms may fluctuate in intensity. Impairment of vision is not severe. There is a granular type of corneal infiltrate, patchy in distribution, situated predominantly in the posterior half of the cornea. Late in the disease the cornea may become vascularized.

The serologic findings are negative, as is the neurologic examination except for the oculo-auditory findings. The family history is noncontributory. There may be mild leukocytosis and eosinophilia.

Whereas the etiology is not definitely known, several cases have resembled periarteritis nodosa. Three patients with the syndrome have had autopsy studies. One of these showed necrotizing angiitis of the dura, brain, gastrointestinal tracts, spleen, and kidneys (Fisher and Hellstrom, 1961), another showed healed endocarditis and disease of the aortic cusps with acute periarteritis of a coronary artery (Eisenstein and Taubenhaus, 1958), and the third showed arteritis of the extremities and viscera resembling polyarteritis nodosa (Crawford, 1957). Cogan and Dickersin (1964) found acute aortitis involving all three layers with acute and chronic inflammation in a patient with typical ocular and vestibulo-auditory symptoms. Thus, it may be that the eye and ear involvement is a part of the syndrome of necrotizing angiitis (periarteritis nodosa). Cody and Williams (1960) reviewed the literature and reported four additional cases. They, too, believe that the disorder is a local manifestation of periarteritis nodosa. Wolff et al. (1965) have recently reported the pathological findings in the temporal bone of a patient said to have Cogan's disease. The pathological findings of significance were endolymphatic hydrops, degeneration of the organ of Corti and cochlear neurons most severe in the basal turn, and bone in the scala tympani of the basal turn and posterior semicircular canal.

The onset of the syndrome should be regarded as a medical emergency and treated with large doses of steroids (Smith, 1970).

5. RELAPSING POLYCHONDRITIS

In 1923 Jaksch-Wartenhorst first described this disease entity which is characterized by an inflammatory reaction in multiple cartilages. Pearson et al. (1960) subsequently named the disorder "relapsing polychrondritis." Initial symptoms may consist of hyperemic and edematous auricles, joint pains, tender and swollen nasal septum, conjunctivitis, iritis, dyspnea, cough, fever, malaise, fatigue, vertigo, and hearing loss. In 88 percent of published cases the auricles are the first areas to be involved (Ödkvist, 1970).

Several reports in the literature indicate that hearing loss may be purely conductive, purely sensorineural, or combined (Daly, 1966; Dolan et al., 1966; Rabuzzi, 1970). The conductive hearing loss is presumed to be the result of serous otitis media secondary to involvement of the cartilage of the eustachian tubes.

In a study of 40 cases, Cody and Sones (1971) found the mean age to be 45 years (range 20–57), and the mean duration of the disease prior to the onset of auditory and vestibular symptoms to be 2⅓ years. Of eight patients with sensorineural hearing impairment, the loss was bilateral in five and unilateral in three. In four the hearing impairment occurred suddenly, reaching a maximum within 24 hours; in two the impairment was progressive, reaching a maximum within two to three weeks; and in two, the impairment was slowly progressive, reaching a maximum in nine to 24 months. Audiometric evaluations indicate that the hearing losses are of cochlear origin and are presumed to be caused by impairment of blood supply associated with the vasculitis characteristic of this disease. Cody and Sones (1971) found that eight of their patients with hearing impairment had vestibular symptoms, and abnormal caloric responses were elicited in all of these patients. The abnormal responses were unilateral in five and bilateral in three. In seven ears there was no response to 30 ml of ice water.

The administration of corticosteroids is the only effective means of suppressing the inflammatory lesions in relapsing polychondritis. The administration of prednisone to individuals with early mild sensorineural hearing loss can result in recovery of hearing. Cody and Sones (1971) noted that the hearing loss recurred in several of their patients when the maintenance doses of prednisone were reduced.

The etiology of relapsing polychondritis is not known; however, the histological appearance of the cartilaginous structures is quite characteristic. The chondrocytes lose their cytoplasm until only nuclear remnants are found in involved areas. Fibrous tissue grows inward from the edge of the cartilaginous plate to replace the destroyed and fragmented areas of cartilage. At the interface of cartilage and connective tissue an inflammatory infiltration of plasma cells and lymphocytes is seen during periods of acute inflammation (Kaye and Sones, 1964). The condition may be an auto-immune reaction. The resemblance to rheumatoid arthritis and the success of corticosteroid therapy supports this contention.

F. VOGT-KOYANAGI-HARADA SYNDROME

In 1906 Vogt reported a case of nontraumatic, bilateral uveitis associated with poliosis (white eyelashes). Koyanagi (1929) reported six cases in detail and included in the syndrome vitiligo and deafness. It came to be known as Vogt-Koyanagi syndrome and included nontraumatic bilateral uveitis associated with some or all of the following symptoms: alopecia, poliosis, deafness, and vitiligo.

Ordinarily, three stages of the disease may be recognized: the meningeal, the ophthalmic, and the convalescent stages. The meningeal stage is present in at least 50 percent of the patients. There is elevated cerebrospinal fluid pressure and spinal fluid lymphocytic pleocytosis. The patient may have severe headache, dizziness, deep orbital pain, lethargy, and malaise. This stage may last from two to four weeks.

The ophthalmic stage often is ushered in by a mild or fulminating uveitis. Retinal detachment is common. Deafness and tinnitus may ensue during this second stage, and appears to occur in about one-half of the cases.

From several weeks to months after onset of the uveitis, the third stage ensues. This consists of poliosis (80 to 90 percent), vitiligo (50 to 60 percent), and alopecia areata (30 to 50 percent). The uveitis usually subsides during the third stage of the disorder. Complications may be a residual detached retina and glaucoma.

Peters (1912) suggested that the disorder might be due to sensitization to uveal pigment. Thus, other pigmented areas might also be involved, such as the cochlea (stria vascularis), the skin, and the meninges. Other investigators have suggested a viral etiology; however, attempts to isolate a virus in patients with the disease have been unsuccessful.

In 1926 Harada described a disease which was characterized by bilateral ocular involvement with massive subretinal fluid leading to detachment but without uveal involvement. The patients showed pleocytosis of the spinal fluid and retinal detachment. Harada's syndrome now is generally considered to be a variant of Vogt-Koyanagi syndrome (Hodgkinson, 1961).

In Vogt-Koyanagi syndrome a sensorineural hearing loss may occur at or near the time the blindness occurs. Varying degrees of bilateral loss, usually associated with tinnitus and vertigo, have been noted. Usually the tinnitus and vertigo subside in one to three weeks and the hearing returns to normal. Audiometric documentation of a case was acquired by Maxwell (1963). The fact that the hearing loss may be unilateral and may not always recover has been pointed out by von Dietzel (1960). His patient had mild hearing loss in the left ear and developed a severe hearing loss in the right ear which was still present two years following the onset of the disease.

References

Alford, B., 1972: Ménière's disease: criteria for diagnosis and evaluation of therapy for reporting. Report of Subcommittee on Equilibrium and its Measurement. Trans. Amer. Acad. Ophthal. Otolaryng. 76:1462.

Alford, B., Shaver, E., Rosenberg, J., and Guilford, F., 1965: Physiologic and histopathologic effects of microembolism of the internal auditory artery. Ann. Otol. Rhinol. Laryng. 74:728.

Altmann, F., and Fowler, E., Jr., 1943: Histological findings in Ménière's symptom complex. Ann. Otol. Rhinol. Laryng. 52:52.

Altmann, F., and Kornfeld, M., 1965: Histological studies of Ménière's disease. Ann. Otol. Rhinol. Laryng. 74:915.

Altmann, F., and Zechner, G., 1968: The pathology and pathogenesis of endolymphatic hydrops. New investigations. Arch. klin. exper. Ohr.-Nas.-Kehlkheilk. 192:1.

Arenberg, I., Marovitz, W., and Shambaugh, G., Jr., 1970: The role of the endolymphatic sac in the pathogenesis of endolymphatic hydrops in man. Acta oto-laryng. Suppl. 275.

Ariagno, R., 1964: Transtympanic labyrinthectomy. Arch. Otolaryng. 80:282.

Arslan, M., 1972: Symposium on Ménière's disease: IV. Treatment of Ménière's disease by apposition of sodium chloride crystals on the round window. Laryngoscope 82:1736.

Arslan, M., Sala, O., and Molinari, G., 1963: The ultrasonic irradiation of the posterior labyrinth in Ménière's disease. Acta oto-laryng. 56:154.

Atkins, J., and Eisman, S., 1959: Wegener's granulomatosis. Ann. Otol. Rhinol. Laryng. 68:524.

Atkinson, M., 1961: Ménière's original papers: Reprinted with an English translation together with commentaries and biographical sketch. Acta oto-laryng. Suppl. 162.

Bárány, R., 1921: Diagnose von Krankheitserscheinungen im Bereiche des Otolithenapparates. Acta oto-laryng. 2:434.

Barber, H., 1964a: Positional nystagmus, especially after head injury. Laryngoscope 74:891.

Barber, H., 1964b: Positional nystagmus: testing and interpretation. Ann. Otol. Rhinol. Laryng. 73:838.

Basek, M., 1973: Ultrasound for Ménière's disease. Arch. Otolaryng. 97:133.

Beal, D., 1968: Effect of endolymphatic sac ablation in the rabbit and cat. Acta oto-laryng. 66:333.

Beal, D., Hemenway, W., and Lindsay, J., 1967: Inner ear pathology of sudden deafness: Histopathology of acquired deafness in the adult coincident with viral infection. Arch. Otolaryng. 85:591.

Benitez, J., 1967: Personal communication.

Bernstein, J., 1965: Occurrence of episodic vertigo and hearing loss in families. Ann. Otol. Rhinol. Laryng. 74:1011.

Bernstein, J., and Schuknecht, H., 1967: Lesions of the apical region of the cochlea. J. Laryng. 81:1.

Bernstein, J., and Silverstein, H., 1966: Anterior cerebellar and labyrinthine arteries: A study in the cat. Arch. Otolaryng. 83:422.

Blatt, I., and Lawrence, M., 1961: Otologic manifestations of fatal granulomatosis of respiratory tract: Lethal midline granuloma—Wegener's granulomatosis. Arch. Otolaryng. 73:639.

Blatt, I., Seltzer, H., Rubin, P., Furstenberg, A., Maxwell, J., and Schull, W., 1959: Fatal granulomatosis of the respiratory tract (lethal midline granuloma—Wegener's granulomatosis). Arch. Otolaryng. 70:707.

Blumenbach, L., 1955: Ménière's Originalarbeiten. Musterschmidt Verlag, Göttingen.

Brown, H., and Woolner, L., 1960: Findings referable to the upper part of the respiratory tract in Wegener's granulomatosis. Ann. Otol. Rhinol. Laryng. 69:810.

Brown, M., 1949: The factor of heredity in labyrinthine deafness and paroxysmal vertigo (Ménière's syndrome). Ann. Otol. Rhinol. Laryng. 58:665.

Bryan, V., and Bucy, P., 1973: Vestibular nerve section for Ménière's disease. Arch. Otolaryng. 97:115.

Castleman, B., 1969: "Draining ears and renal failure in a 36-year-old man." Case report, Case 15—1969—Case Records of the Massachusetts General Hospital Weekly CPC Exercises. B. Castleman, Editor, B. McNeely, Assistant Editor, New Eng. J. Med. 280:828.

Cawthorne, T., 1943: The treatment of Ménière's disease. J. Laryng. 58:563.

Cawthorne, T., 1954: Positional nystagmus. Ann. Otol. Rhinol. Laryng. 63:481.

Cawthorne, T., 1957: Membranous labyrinthectomy via the oval window for Ménière's disease. J. Laryng. 71:524.

Cawthorne, T., and Hallpike, C., 1957: A study of the clinical features and pathological changes within the temporal bones, brain stem and cerebellum of an early case of positional nystagmus of the so-called benign paroxysmal type. Acta oto-laryng. 48:89.

Citron, L., and Hallpike, C., 1956: Observations upon the mechanism of positional nystagmus of the so-called "benign paroxysmal type." J. Laryng. 70:253.

Citron, L., and Hallpike, C., 1962: A case of positional nystagmus of the so-called benign paroxysmal type and the effects of treatment by intracranial division of the VIIIth nerve. J. Laryng. 76:28.

Clemis, J., and Valvassori, G., 1968: Recent radiographic and clinical observations on the vestibular aqueduct—a preliminary report. Otolaryng. Clin. N. Amer., October, p. 339.

Cody, D., 1971: Rehabilitation for sensorineural hearing loss, I. Clin. Otol.—An Int. Symp., Edited by M. Paparella, A. Hohmann, and J. Huff., C. V. Mosby Co. St. Louis, Mo.

Cody, D., 1973: The tack operation. Arch. Otolaryng. 97:109.

Cody, D., Simonton, K., and Hallberg, O., 1967: Automatic repetitive decompression of the saccule in endolymphatic hydrops (Tack operation): Preliminary report. Laryngoscope 77:1480.

Cody, D., and Sones, D., 1971: Relapsing polychondritis: Audiovestibular manifestations. Laryngoscope 81:1208.

Cody, D., and Williams, N., 1960: Cogan's syndrome. Laryngoscope 70:447.

Cogan, D., 1945: Syndrome of nonsyphilitic interstitial keratitis and vestibuloauditory symptoms. Arch. Ophthal. 33:144.

Cogan, D., and Dickersin, G., 1964: Nonsyphilitic interstitial keratitis with vestibuloauditory symptoms. Arch. Ophthal. 71:172.

Cope, S., and Ryan, G., 1959: Cervical and otolith vertigo. J. Laryng. 73:113.

Crawford, W., 1957: Cogan's syndrome associated with polyarteritis nodosa: A report of 3 cases. Penn. Med. J. 60:835.

Daly, J., 1966: Relapsing polychondritis of the larynx and trachea. Arch. Otolaryng. 84:570.

Dandy, W., 1934: Effects on hearing after subtotal section of the cochlear branch of the auditory nerve. Bull. Johns Hopkins Hosp. 55:240.

Day, K., 1943: Labyrinth surgery for Ménière's disease. Laryngoscope 53:617.

Day, K., 1952: Surgical treatment of hydrops of the labyrinth. (a) Surgical destruction of the labyrinth for Ménière's disease. Laryngoscope 62:547.

Derlacki, E., 1965: Medical management of endolymphatic hydrops. Laryngoscope 75:1518.

Dietzel, K. von, 1960: On the causal genesis of the Vogt-Koyanagi syndrome (nontraumatic uveitis and deafness). H.N.O. 8:214.

Dishoeck, H. van, and Bierman, Th., 1957: Sudden perceptive deafness and viral infection (report of the first one hundred patients). Ann. Otol. Rhinol. Laryng. 66:963.

Dix, M., and Hallpike, C., 1952: The pathology, symptomatology and diagnosis of certain disorders of the vestibular system. Ann. Otol. Rhinol. Laryng. 61:987.

Dohlman, G., 1965: The mechanism of secretion and absorption of endolymph in the vestibular apparatus. Acta oto-laryng. 59:275.

Dolan, D., Lemmon, G., Jr., and Teitelbaum, S., 1966: Relapsing polychondritis: Analytical literature review and studies on pathogenesis. Amer. J. Med. 41:285.

Duvall, A., III, Nelms, C., and Williams, H., 1969: Necrotizing granuloma of the midline tissues following renal transplantation. Trans. Amer. Acad. Ophthal. Otolaryng. 73:1187.

Eisenstein, B., and Taubenhaus, M., 1958: Nonsyphilitic interstitial keratitis and bilateral deafness (Cogan's syndrome) associated with cardiovascular disease. New Eng. J. Med. 258:1074.

Fick, I., 1964: Decompression of the labyrinth: A new surgical procedure for Ménière's disease. Arch. Otolaryng. 79:447.

Fisch, U., 1973: Excision of Scarpa's ganglion. Arch. Otolaryng. 97:147.

Fisher, E., and Hellstrom, H., 1961: Cogan's syndrome and systemic vascular disease: Analysis of pathologic features with reference to its relationship to thromboangiitis obliterans (Buerger). Arch. Path. 72:572.

Fluur, E., and Tovi, D., 1965: Microscopic intracranial section of the vestibular nerve in Ménière's disease. Acta oto-laryng. 59:604.

Fowler, E., Jr., 1948: Streptomycin treatment of vertigo. Trans. Amer. Acad. Ophthal. Otolaryng. 52:293.

Friedmann, I., Cawthorne, T., McLay, K., and Bird, E., 1963: Electron microscopic observations on the human membranous labyrinth with particular reference to Ménière's disease. J. Ultrastruct. Res. 9:123.

Froud, P., and Henderson, A., 1971: The treatment of Wegener's granulomatosis with immunosuppressive-cytotoxic drugs. J. Laryng. 85:703.

Fudenberg, H., 1968: Are autoimmune diseases immunologic deficiency states? Hosp. Practice 3:43.

Gacek, R., 1974: Transection of the posterior ampullary nerve for relief of benign paroxysmal positional vertigo. Ann. Otol. Rhinol. Laryng. in press.

Godlowski, Z., 1960: Endocrine management of selected cases of allergy based on enzymatic mechanism of sensitization. Arch. Otolaryng. 71:513.

Godman, C., and Churg, J., 1954: Wegener's granulomatosis. Arch. Path. 58:533.

Golding-Wood, P., 1960: Observations on sympathectomy in the treatment of Ménière's disease. J. Laryng. 74:951.

Golding-Wood, P., 1969: The role of sympathectomy in the treatment of Ménière's disease. J. Laryng. 83:741.

Goldman, H., 1962: Hypoadrenocorticism and endocrinologic treatment of Ménière's disease. N.Y. J. Med. 62:377.

Goodhill, V., Harris, I., Brockman, S., Hantz, O., 1973: Sudden deafness and labyrinthine window ruptures: audio-vestibular observations. Ann. Otol. Rhinol. Laryng. 82:2.

Gordon, N., 1954: Post traumatic vertigo, with special reference to positional nystagmus. Lancet 1:1216.

Graybiel, A., Schuknecht, H., Fregly, A., Miller, E., and McLeod, E., 1965: Practical and theoretical implications based on long-term follow-up of Ménière's patients treated with streptomycin sulfate. Joint report, U.S. Naval Aerospace Medical Institute and National Aeronautics and Space Administration, October 25.

Gregg, J., and Shaeffer, J., 1964: Unilateral inner ear deafness complicating infectious mononucleosis. S. Dak. J. Med. Pharm. 17:22.

Griffin, W., Jr., and Silverstein, H., 1970: Inner ear fluids in certain human otologic disorders. Chap. 23 in Biochemical Mechanisms in Hearing and Deafness—Res. Otol. Int. Symp. Edited by M. Paparella. C. C. Thomas, Springfield, Ill., p. 318.

Guild, S., 1935: II. Discussion from the point of view of studies on human temporal bones. Symposium: Is there localization in the cochlea for low tones? Ann. Otol. Rhinol. Laryng. 44:738.

Gundrum, L., 1953: Etiologic analysis of one hundred cases of Ménière's symptom-complex. Arch. Otolaryng. 57:123.

Günther, H., 1959: Erfahrungen bei der Streptomycinbehandlung der Ménièreschen Krankheit. Z. Laryng. Rhinol. Otol. 38:319.

Gussen, R., 1971: Ménière's disease: New temporal bone findings in two cases. Laryngoscope 81:1695.

Hallpike, C., and Cairns, H., 1938: Observations on the pathology of Ménière's syndrome. J. Laryng. 53:625.

Hallpike, C., and Wright, A., 1940: On the histological changes in the temporal bones of a case of Ménière's disease. J. Laryng. 55:59.

Hamberger, C., Hydén, H., and Koch, H., 1949: Streptomycin bei der Ménièreschen Krankheit. Arch. Ohr.-Nas.-KehlkHeilk. 155:667.

Hanson, H., 1951: The treatment of endolymphatic hydrops (Ménière's disease) with streptomycin. Ann. Otol. Rhinol. Laryng. 60:676.

Harada, Y., 1926: Beitrage zur klinischen Kenntniss von nichteitriger Choroiditis. Nipp. Gank. Zass. 30:356.

Harbert, F., 1970: Benign paroxysmal positional nystagmus. Arch. Ophthal. 84:298.

Hasegawa, T., 1931: Die Veränderung der Labyrintharen Reflexe bei zentrifugierten Meerschweinchen. Pflügers Arch. ges. Physiol. 229:205.

Hayden, R., and McGee, T., 1965: Traumatized oval window fat grafts. Arch. Otolaryng. 81:243.

Heller, M., and Lindenberg, P., 1955: Sudden perceptive deafness: report of five cases. Ann. Otol. Rhinol. Laryng. 64:931.

Hemenway, W., Sando, I., and McChesney, D., 1969: Temporal bone pathology following maternal rubella. Arch. klin. exper. Ohr.-Nas.-KehlkHeilk. 193:287.

Herberts, G., Hillerdal, O., and Ranström, S., 1957: Rhinitis, sinusitis and otitis as initial symptoms in periarteritis nodosa (Wegener's granulomatosis). Acta oto-laryng. 48:205.

Hilding, D., and House, W., 1964: An evaluation of the ultrastructural findings in the utricle in Ménière's disease. Laryngoscope 74:1135.

Hodgkinson, C., 1961: Vogt-Koyanagi-Harada syndrome. Henry Ford Hosp. Med. Bull. 9:539.

House, W., 1961: Surgical exposure of the internal auditory canal and its contents through the middle cranial fossa. Laryngoscope 71:1363.

House, W., 1966: Cryosurgical treatment of Ménière's disease. Arch. Otolaryng. 84:616.

House, W., and Hitselberger, W., 1965: Endolymphatic subarachnoid shunt for Ménière's disease. Arch. Otolaryng. 82:144.

Igarashi, M., 1967: Personal communication.

Igarashi, M., Alford, B., Konishi, S., Shaver, E., and Guilford, F., 1969: Functional and histopathological correlations after microembolism of the peripheral labyrinthine artery in the dog. Laryngoscope 79:603.

Ireland, P., and Farkashidy, J., 1963: Electron microscopic studies of Ménière's disease: Twelve fresh specimens taken at operation. Trans. Amer. Acad. Ophthal. Otolaryng. 67:28.

Jaksch-Wartenhorst, R., 1923: Polychondropathia. Arch. inn Med. (Vienna) 6:93.

James, J., Dalton, G., Bullen, M., Freundlich, H., and Hopkins, J., 1960: The ultrasonic treatment of Ménière's disease. J. Laryng. 74:730.

Kaye, R., and Sones, D., 1964: Relapsing polychondritis: Clinical and pathologic features in 14 cases. Ann. Intern. Med. 60:653.

Kimura, R., 1967: Experimental blockage of the endolymphatic duct and sac and its effect on the inner ear of the guinea pig. Ann. Otol. Rhinol. Laryng. 76:664.

Kimura, R., 1969: Distribution, structure and function of dark cells in the vestibular labyrinth. Ann. Otol. Rhinol. Laryng. 78:542.

Kimura, R., and Perlman, H., 1956: Extensive venous obstruction of the labyrinth. A. Cochlear changes. Ann. Otol. Rhinol. Laryng. 65:332.

Kimura, R., and Perlman, H., 1958: Arterial obstruction of the labyrinth. Part I. Cochlear changes. Ann. Otol. Rhinol. Laryng. 67:5.

Kimura, R., and Schuknecht, H., 1965: Membranous hydrops in the inner ear of the guinea pig after obliteration of the endolymphatic sac. Pract. oto-rhino-laryng. 27:343.

Kimura, R., and Schuknecht, H., 1970: The ultrastructure of the human stria vascularis. Part I. Acta oto-laryng. 69:415, Part II. Acta oto-laryng. 70:301.

Kirikae, I., Nomura, Y., Shitara, T., and Kobayashi, T., 1962: Sudden deafness due to Buerger's disease. Arch. Otolaryng. 75:502.

Kleyn, A. de, and Versteegh, C., 1933: Labyrinthreflexe nach Abschleuderung der Otolithenmembranen bei Meerschweinchen. Pflügers Arch ges. Physiol. 232:454.

Kohut, R., and Lindsay, J., 1972: Pathologic changes in idiopathic labyrinthine hydrops, correlations with previous findings. Acta oto-laryng. 73:402.

Koyanagi, Y., 1929: Dysakusis, Alopecia und Poliosis bei schwerer Uveitis nicht traumatischen Ursprungs. Klin. Mbl. Augenheilk. 82:194.

Krejci, F., 1952: Experimentelle Grundlagen einer extralabyrinthären chirurgischen Behandlungsmethode der Ménièreschen Erkrankung. Pract. oto-rhino-laryng. 14:18.

Lawrence, M., and McCabe, B., 1959: Inner ear mechanics and deafness. Special considerations of Ménière's syndrome. J. Amer. Med. Assn. 171:1927.

Lempert, J., 1948: Lempert decompression operation for hydrops of the endolymphatic labyrinth in Ménière's disease. Arch. Otolaryng. 47:551.

Lempert, J., Wolff, D., Rambo, J., Wever, E., and Lawrence, M., 1952: New theory for the correlation of the pathology and the symptomatology of Ménière's disease. Ann. Otol. Rhinol. Laryng. 61:717.

Lermoyez, M., 1919: Le Vertige qui fait entendre (angiospasme labyrinthique). Presse Méd. 27:1.

Lieberman, A., 1957: Unilateral deafness.

Laryngoscope 67:1237.

Lim, D., 1973: Formation and fate of the otoconia. Scanning and transmission electron microscopy. Ann. Otol. Rhinol. Laryng. 82:23.

Lindsay, J., 1942: Labyrinthine dropsy and Ménière's disease. Arch. Otolaryng. 37:853.

Lindsay, J., 1959: Sudden deafness due to virus infection. Arch. Otolaryng. 69:13.

Lindsay, J., Caruthers, D., Hemenway, W., and Harrison, S., 1953: Inner ear pathology following maternal rubella. Ann. Otol. Rhinol. Laryng. 62:1201.

Lindsay, J., Davey, P., and Ward, P., 1960: Inner ear pathology in deafness due to mumps. Ann. Otol. Rhinol. Laryng. 69:918.

Lindsay, J., and Hemenway, W., 1954: Inner ear pathology due to measles. Ann. Otol. Rhinol. Laryng. 63:754.

Lindsay, J., and Hemenway, W., 1956: Postural vertigo due to unilateral sudden partial loss of vestibular function. Ann. Otol. Rhinol. Laryng. 65:692.

Lindsay, J., Kohut, R., and Sciarra, P., 1967: Ménière's disease: pathology and manifestations. Ann. Otol. Rhinol. Laryng. 76:1.

Lindsay, J., and Schulthess, G. von, 1958: An unusual case of labyrinthine hydrops. Acta oto-laryng. 49:315.

Lindsay, J., and Zuidema, J., 1950: Inner ear deafness of sudden onset. Laryngoscope 60:238.

Litton, W., and Lawrence, M., 1961: Electron microscopy in Ménière's disease. Arch. Otolaryng. 74:32.

Lurie, M., 1967: Personal communication.

Masuda, Y., Sando, I., and Hemenway, W., 1971: Perilymphatic communication routes in guinea pig cochlea. Arch. Otolaryng. 94:240.

Maxwell, O., 1963: Hearing loss in uveitis. Arch. Otolaryng. 78:138.

Ménière, P., 1842: De l'exploration de l'appareil auditif ou recherches sur les moyens progres à conduire au diagnostic des maladies de l'oreille. Gaz. méd. Paris 10:114.

Ménière, P., 1861a: Congestions cérébrales apoplectiformes. Gaz. méd. Paris 16:55.

Ménière, P., 1861b: Maladies de l'oreille interne offrant les symptômes de la congestion cérébrale apoplectiforme. Gaz. méd. Paris 16:88.

Ménière, P., 1861c: Nouveaux documents relatifs aux lesions de l'oreille interne caractérisées par des symptômes de congestion cérébrale apoplectiforme. Gaz. méd. Paris 16:239.

Ménière, P., 1861d: Auricular pathology, Mémoire sur des lésions de l'oreille interne donnant lieu à des symptômes de congestion cérébrale apoplectiforme. Gaz. méd. Paris 16:597. Translated by M. Atkinson, Acta oto-laryng. Suppl. 162.

Milner, P., 1955: Nasal granuloma and periarteritis nodosa: report of a case. Brit. Med. J. 2:1597.

Morrison, A., and Booth, J., 1970: Sudden deafness: an otological emergency. Brit. J. Hosp. Med. 4:287.

Mufson, M., Webb, P., Kennedy, H., Gill, V., and Chanock, R., 1966: Etiology of upper respiratory tract illnesses among civilian adults. J. Amer. Med. Assn. 195:91.

Muller, A., 1950: Traumatisime acoustique et maladie de Ménière. Pract. oto-rhino-laryng. 12:338.

Nager, F., 1952: Histologische Ohruntersuchungen bei Kindern nach mütterlicher Rubella. Pract. oto-rhino-laryng. 14:337.

Naito, T., 1959: Clinical and pathological studies of Ménière's disease. Sixtieth Annual Meeting of the Oto-Rhino-Laryng. Soc. of Japan, Tokyo, (March).

Neff, W., and Kiang, N., 1970: Personal communication.

Norton, E., and Cogan, D., 1959: Syndrome of nonsyphilitic interstitial keratitis and vestibuloauditory symptoms. Arch. Ophthal. 61:695.

Ödkvist, L., 1970: Relapsing polychondritis. Acta oto-laryng. 70:448.

Otte, J., 1968: Estudio del ganglio espiral y su relación con la discriminación. Rev. Otorinolaring. 28:89.

Parker, D., Covell, W., and Gierke, H. von, 1968: Exploration of vestibular damage in guinea pigs following mechanical stimulation. Acta oto-larying. Suppl. 239.

Passe, E., and Seymour, J., 1948: Ménière's syndrome; successful treatment by surgery on the sympathetic. Brit. med. J. 2:812.

Pearson, C., Kline, H., and Newcomer, V., 1960: Relapsing polychondritis. New Eng. J. Med. 263:51.

Peitersen, E., and Carlsen, B., 1966: Hearing impairment as the initial sign of polyarteritis nodosa. Acta oto-laryng. 61:189.

Perlman, H., Goldinger, J., and Cales, J., 1953: Electrolyte studies in Ménière's disease. Laryngoscope 63:640.

Perlman, H., Kimura, R., and Fernández, C., 1959: Experiments on temporary obstruction of the internal auditory artery. Laryngoscope 69:591.

Peters, A., 1912: Sympathische Ophthalmie und Gehörstörungen. Klin. Mbl. Augenheilk. 50:433.

Pietrantoni, L., and Iurato, S., 1960: Some initial electron-microscope investigations of a case of Ménière's syndrome. Acta oto-laryng. 52:15.

Plummer, N., Angel, J., Shaw, D., and Hinson, K., 1957: Respiratory granulomatosis with polyarteritis nodosa (Wegener's syndrome). Thorax 12:57.

Portmann, G., 1927: Vertigo: surgical treatment by opening saccus endolymphaticus. Arch. Otolaryng. 6:309.

Portmann, G., 1969: Surgical treatment of vertigo by opening of the saccus endolymphaticus. Arch. Otolaryng. 89:809.

Portmann, M., 1973: Decompression and drainage of the endolymphatic sac. Arch. Otolaryng. 97:125.

Preber, L., and Silfverskiöld, B., 1957: Paroxysmal positional vertigo following head injury: Studied by electronystagmography and skin resistance measurements. Acta oto-laryng. 48:255.

Rabuzzi, D., 1970: Relapsing polychondritis. Arch. Otolaryng. 91:188.

Ruben, R., Distenfeld, A., Berg, P., and Carr, R., 1969: Sudden sequential deafness as the presenting symptom of macroglobulinemia. J. Amer. Med. Assn. 209:1364.

Rüedi, L., 1951: Therapeutic and toxic effects of streptomycin in otology. Laryngoscope 61:613.

Schuknecht, H., 1957: Ablation therapy in the management of Ménière's disease. Acta oto-laryng. Suppl. 132.

Schuknecht, H., 1959: Discussion. Trans. Amer. Otol. Soc. 47:112.

Schuknecht, H., 1960: Discussion of peripheral auditory mechanisms. In Neural Mechanisms of the Auditory and Vestibular Systems, Edited by G. Rasmussen and W. Windle, C. C. Thomas, Springfield, Ill., pp. 94–95.

Schuknecht, H.: Unpublished data.

Schuknecht, H., 1962: Positional vertigo: clinical and experimental observations.

Trans. Amer. Acad. Ophthal. Otolaryng. 66:319.

Schuknecht, H., 1969a: Mechanism of inner ear injury from blows to the head. Ann. Otol. Rhinol. Laryng. 78:253.

Schuknecht, H., 1969b: Cupulolithiasis. Arch. Otolaryng. 90:765.

Schuknecht, H., 1973: Destructive labyrinthine surgery. Arch. Otolaryng. 97:150.

Schuknecht, H., Benitez, J., and Beekhuis, J., 1962a: Further observations on the pathology of Ménière's disease. Ann. Otol. Rhinol. Laryng. 71:1039.

Schuknecht, H., Benitez, J., Beekhuis, J., Igarashi, M., Singleton, G., and Ruedi, L., 1962b: The pathology of sudden deafness. Laryngoscope 72:1142.

Schuknecht, H., Igarashi, M., and Chasin, W., 1965: Inner ear hemorrhage in leukemia. Laryngoscope 75:662.

Schuknecht, H., Kimura, R., and Naufal, P., 1973: The pathology of sudden deafness. Acta oto-laryng 76:75.

Schuknecht, H., and Neff, W., 1952: Hearing losses after apical lesions in the cochlea. Acta oto-laryng. 42:263.

Schuknecht, H., Northrop, C., and Igarashi, M., 1968: Cochlear pathology after destruction of the endolymphatic sac in the cat. Acta oto-laryng. 65:479.

Schuknecht, H., and Ruby, R., 1973: Cupulolithiasis. Adv. Oto-Rhino-Laryng. (Karger) 20:434.

Schuknecht, H., and Seifi, A. el, 1963: Experimental observations on the fluid physiology of the inner ear. Ann. Otol. Rhinol. Laryng. 72:687.

Selfridge, G., 1940: A survey of the relation between nutrition and the ear. Ann. Otol. Rhinol. Laryng. 49:674.

Shambaugh, G., Jr., Clemis, J., and Arenberg, I., 1969: Endolymphatic duct and sac in Ménière's disease. Arch. Otolaryng. 89:816.

Shea, J., and Kitabchi, A., 1973: Management of fluctuant hearing loss. Arch. Otolaryng. 97:118.

Shuman, H., 1970: Hemorrhage in Wegener's granulomatosis. Correspondence to the Editor re case report by B. Castleman. New Eng. J. Med. 282:513.

Silverstein, H., 1970: The effects of perfusing the perilymphatic space with artificial endolymph. Ann. Otol. Rhinol. Laryng. 79:754.

Silverstein, H., and Schuknecht, H., 1966: Biochemical studies of inner ear fluid in man: Changes in otosclerosis, Ménière's disease, and acoustic neuroma. Arch. Otolaryng. 84:395.

Singleton, E., and Schuknecht, H., 1968: Streptomycin sulfate in the management of Ménière's disease. Otolaryng. Clin. N. Amer., October, p. 531.

Smith, J., 1970: Cogan's syndrome. Laryngoscope 80:121.

Solomon, A., and Fahey, J., 1963: Plasmapheresis therapy in macroglobulinemia Ann. Intern. Med. 58:789.

Spear, G., and Walker, W., Jr., 1956: Lethal midline granuloma (Granuloma Gangraenescens) at autopsy: Report of a case and review of literature. Bull. Johns Hopkins Hosp. 99:313.

Stewart, J., 1933: Progressive lethal granulomatous ulceration of the nose. J. Laryng. 48:657.

Suga, F., Preston, J., and Snow, J., 1970: Experimental microembolization of cochlear vessels. Arch. Otolaryng. 92:213.

Tasaki, I., and Fernández, C., 1952: Modification of cochlear microphonics and action potentials by KCl solution and by direct currents. J. Neurophysiol. 15:497.

Toma, G., 1968: Lethal midline granuloma and Wegener's granulomatosis. J. Laryng. 82:129.

Tonndorf, J., 1957: The mechanism of hearing loss in early cases of endolymphatic hydrops. Ann. Otol. Rhinol. Laryng. 66:766.

Tumarkin, I., 1936: Otolithic catastrophe; a new syndrome. Brit. Med. J. 2:175.

Velasco, R., 1968: Patologia auricular. (Translated from the original by P. Ménière. Gaz. méd. Paris. 16:597, 1861.) Rev. Otorinolaring. 28:82.

Vogt, A., 1906: Frühzeitiges Ergrauen der Zilien und Bemerkungen über den sogenannten plötzlichen Eintritt dieser Veränderung. Mbl. Augenheilk. 45:228.

Vyslonzil, E., 1963: Über eine umschriebene Ansammlung von Otokonien im hinteren häutigen Bogengang. Mschr. Ohrenheilk. 97:63.

Waltner, J., 1965: Ultrasonic surgery in Ménière's disease. Ann. Otol. Rhinol. Laryng. 74:174.

Watson, C., Barnes, C., Donaldson, J., and Klett, W., 1967: Psychosomatic aspects of Ménière's disease. Arch. Otolaryng. 86:543.

Wegener, F., 1936: Über generalisierten, septischen Gefässerkrankungen. Verh. dtsch. Ges. Path. 29:202.

Wegener, F., 1939: Über eine eigenartige rhinogene Granulomatose mit besonderer Beteiligung des Arteriensystems und der Nieren. Beitr. path. Anat. 102:36.

Wilkinson, P., Davidson, W., Sommaripa, A., 1966: Turnover of 131 I-labeled autologous macroglobulinemia in Waldenstrom's macroglobulinemia. Ann. Intern. Med. 65:308.

Williams, H., 1952: Ménière's Disease. C. C. Thomas, Springfield, Ill.

Wilmot, T., 1969: Sympathectomy for Ménière's disease—a long-term review. J. Laryng. 83:323.

Wittmaack, K., 1909: Über die Veränderungen im Innen-Ohr nach Rotationen. Verh. dtsch. Ges. Otol. 18:150.

Wolff, H., 1953: Early diagnosis of mumps.

Acta Leidensia Sch. med. trop. 23:130.

Wolff, D., Bernhard, W., Tsutsumi, S., Ross, I., and Nussbaum, H., 1965: The pathology of Cogan's syndrome causing profound deafness. Ann. Otol. Rhinol. Laryng. 74:507.

Wolfson, R., and Cutt, R., 1971: Long-term results with cryosurgery for Ménière's disease. Arch. Otolaryng. 93:483.

Wolfson, R., Cutt, R., Ishiyama, E., and Myers, D., 1966: Cryosurgery of the labyrinth—preliminary report of a new surgical procedure. Laryngoscope 76:733.

Wright, A., 1938: Labyrinthine giddiness: Its nature and treatment. Brit. Med. J. 1:668.

Wright, A., 1942: Ménière's disease: alcohol injection of the labyrinth. J. Laryng. 57:120.

Wright, A., 1948: Ménière's disease. Proc. Roy. Soc. Med. 41:801.

Yuen, S., and Schuknecht, H., 1972: Vestibular aqueduct and endolymphatic duct in Ménière's disease. Arch. Otolaryng. 96:553.

Acknowledgments

In a book of this kind, in which the accumulated experience and observations of the author (and his clinical and research associates) have been compiled into a single volume, it is obvious that numerous illustrations will have been previously published in a number of journals and books.

The author is grateful to these publishers for permission to use illustrations which have appeared previously as indicated below:

Academic Press, Incorporated:

Foundations of Modern Auditory Theory, Volume I, 1970
Figures 1, 3, 4, 5, 7 and 10

Contributions to Sensory Physiology, Volume 4, 1970
Figures 1, 2, 3, 4, 5, 6, 7, 9, 10, 11, 12, 13, 14 and 16

Acta Otolaryngologica:

Supplement 132, 1957—Figure 14
54:336–348, 1962—Figures 8 and 9A
59:154–167, 1965—Figures 1A, 2A, 2B, 2C, 4, 6A and 7A
65:479–487, 1968—Figures 4 and 5
65:586–598, 1968—Figures 1 and 3
76:75–97, 1973—Figures 1, 2, 3, 5, 6, 13, 14, 15, 16, 17, 18, 20, 21 and 22
77:1–12, 1974—Figures 1, 6 and 8

Annals of Otology, Rhinology and Laryngology:

63:727–754, 1954—Figures 2B, 7A, 9B and 10B
71:1039–1054, 1962—Figures 3B, 6A, 6B and 7
72:687–723, 1963—Figures 1, 3B, 13B, 14 and 15
74:289–303, 1965—Figures 6 and 8A
75:423–436, 1966—Figures 1, 2, 5 and 6
76:1008–1018, 1967—Figure 4
77:5–23, 1968—Figures 5 and 6
77:37–43, 1968—Figures 2, 6 and 8
78:253–262, 1969—Figures 2 and 3
80:397–399, 1971—Figures 1 and 2
80:415–418, 1971—Figure 1

Archives of Otolaryngology:

57:129–142, 1953—Figures 1A, 2A, 6B and 8B
58:377–397, 1953—Figure 11
63:513–528, 1956—Figures 4 and 6
69:549–559, 1959—Figures 1A and 4B
71:562–572, 1960—Figures 2A, 5 and 7
75:192–197, 1962—Figures 1, 2 and 3B

76:126–130, 1962—Figures 4A and 5
79:437–446, 1964—Figure 3
80:369–382, 1964—Figures 1, 5A, 6, 8A, 9A and 10B
83:18–27, 1966—Figures 3, 6, 8, 9 and 10
83:439–445, 1966—Figures 1, 4, 5 and 6
86:497–502, 1967—Figures 1, 2 and 5
87:27–41, 1968—Figures 1, 2, 4, 8 and 9
87:129–137, 1968—Figures 1, 2, 3, 4, 6, 7 and 8
90:765–778, 1971—Figures 2, 3, 4, 5, 6 and 7
96:16–21, 1972—Figures 3 and 9
96:468–474, 1972—Figures 2 and 4
97:150–151, 1973—Figures 2 and 4

Archives of Oto-Rhino-Laryngology:

195:207–225, 1970—Figures 4, 7, 11, 13 and 14

Clinical Pediatrics:

3/12:718–727, 1964—Figure 5

Journal of Otolaryngology, Japan:

69:1825–1833, 1966—Figures 3, 8 and 9

Charles C. Thomas, Publishers:

Neural Mechanisms of Auditory and Vestibular Systems, Rasmussen and Windle
page 79 —Figure 64
page 84—Figure 70
page 85—Figure 72

Henry Ford Hospital Bulletin:

7:202–210, 1959—Figures 3 and 6A

Journal of Laryngology and Otology:

69:75–97, 1955—Figure 3
78:115–123, 1964—Figures 1, 2, 4 and 5
80:1–10, 1966—Figures 1, 2A, 3B, 4C, 6 and 7
81:1–26, 1967—Figures 1, 6, 7, 8, 15, 25 and 30
82:321–329, 1968—Figures 1, 2, 7 and 8

The Laryngoscope:

66:859–870, 1956—Figures 2 and 7
68:429–439, 1958—Figure 5
69:614–643, 1959—Figure 13A
72:1–9, 1962—Figures 4A and 7A
72:1142–1157, 1962—Figures 5, 6, 8 and 9
73:651–665, 1963—Figures 1B, 4, 7 and 9A
75:662–668, 1965—Figure 1
76:1416–1428, 1966—Figures 2, 3, 4 and 6

88:1813–1832, 1968—Figures 2, 4, 6, 7, 12 and 14

Little Brown and Company, Incorporated:

Otosclerosis, Edited by H. F. Schuknecht, 1962
Page 101—Figure 3A and B
Page 102—Figure 4
Page 103—Figure 5
Page 342—Figure 4
Page 343—Figure 5B
Page 344—Figure 9A

Sensorineural Hearing Processes and Disorders, Edited by B. Graham, 1967

Figures 1, 2, 3 and 5

Stapedectomy, H. F. Schuknecht, 1971

Figures 2, 5, 6, 7, 11, 12, 15, 18, 21, 23, 24, 25, 28, 32, 33, 34, 38, 45 and 49

New England Journal of Medicine:

280:1154–1160, 1969—Figures 1 and 2

Advances in Oto-Rhino-Laryngology:

20:434–443, 1973—Figures 1, 2, 3, 4 and 5

Southern Medical Journal:

57:1161–1167, 1964—Figures 2, 5B and 6B

Transactions of the American Academy of Ophthalmology and Otolaryngology:

57:366–382, 1953—Figures 2, 3 and 6B
62:601–606, 1958—Figures 2 and 4
63:684–692, 1959—Figures 2, 3 and 6
66:319–332, 1962—Figures 1B and 5
68:222–242, 1964—Figures 1A, 3A, 4B, 9B, 10, 11A and 12
77:257–266, 1973—Figures 1, 2 and 3

W. B. Saunders Publishing Company:

Otolaryngologic Clinics of North America, October 1968
pages 331–337   Figures 3, 7, 8 and 9
pages 433–440   Figures 2, 5 and 7

Diseases of the Nose, Throat and Ear (Second Edition)

page 386   Figures 49A, B and C
page 391   Figures 53A and B
page 397   Figure 57

Index